DRUG DISCOVERY AND DEVELOPMENT – PRESENT AND FUTURE

Edited by **Izet M. Kapetanovic**

INTECHOPEN.COM

Drug Discovery and Development – Present and Future
Edited by Izet M. Kapetanovic

CBS, Edition 2016

Published by InTech

Janeza Trdine 9, 51000 Rijeka, Croatia

Publishing Process Manager Ivana Zec

Technical Editor Teodora Smiljanic

Cover Designer InTech Design Team

Image Copyright Olga Miltsova, 2011. Used under license from Shutterstock.com

Additional hard copies can be obtained from orders@intechopen.com

Drug Discovery and Development – Present and Future, Edited by Izet M. Kapetanovic
p. cm.
978-953-307-615-7

INTECH

open science | open minds

Contents

Preface

Drug discovery and development process aims to make available medications that are safe and effective in improving the length and quality of life and relieving pain and suffering. However, the process is very complex, time consuming, and resource intensive, requiring multi-disciplinary expertise and innovative approaches. Recent estimates suggest that it takes up to 13.5 years and 1.8 billion U.S. dollars to bring a new drug to the market. There is a growing urgency to identify and develop more effective, efficient, and expedient ways to bring safe and effective products to the market. The drug discovery and developmental process relies on utilizing relevant and robust tools, methods, and models that are predictive of clinical effects in terms of diagnosis, prevention, therapy, and prognosis. There is a growing emphasis on translational research, a bidirectional bench to the bedside approach. The all-important predictivity depends on having robust, relevant, validated and qualified biomarkers for physiological and pathological effects of interest.

The first section, Introduction, presents an overview of the principles, approaches, processes, and status of drug discovery today with an eye towards the future.

The second section, Current Status and Future Directions, presents a broad picture of the current, emerging, and evolving state of the drug discovery and development. It discusses topics such as chemical genetics, combination of ancient traditional, conventional and evolving systems, biology approaches, role of evolutionary biology, personalized medicine, and interaction. Other topics, such as collaboration between academia, government, and a private sector, and a practical overview of drug development from a big pharma perspective are also explored.

Section 3, Models, deals with the existing and emerging models for evaluating efficacy and safety. While model systems provide useful information and approximation to human pathophysiology and pharmacology, it is important to keep in mind that these are only models. They may only be applicable to addressing specific questions, and care must be exercised in their extrapolations.

As discussed in Section 4, Tools, Methods and Biomarkers, having and utilizing the right tools is critical during the drug discovery and development process. Biomarkers represent physiological, biochemical, or pathophysiological parameters or sentinels which are intended to detect or monitor diseases, or the health status of an organism. The aim is to decrease probability of failure, decrease drug development time, and improve resource utilization. Also, biomarkers can provide information that is not readily available otherwise, such as that due to a lack of acceptably invasive procedures or unrealistic time frames. Biomarkers can be used as indices of efficacy, toxicity and for selection of appropriate patient populations. However, there are many caveats and few validated biomarkers. Some of the issues include inter-laboratory variation, lack of adequate sensitivity, specificity and predictability, or adequate knowledge if the biomarkers are within a causative or only a correlative pathway.

The final section 5, Drug Delivery, discusses development of appropriate formulations for drug delivery to achieve reasonable bioavailability, access to a target site, desirable pharmacokinetic profile, and a practical dosing regimen. Many drug candidates due to their physicochemical properties suffer from a poor solubility and/or poor permeability. Consequently, the Biopharmaceutics Classification System (BCS) was developed to predict intestinal drug absorption, identify strategies, and improve the efficiency of drug development. Perhaps the most rapidly growing area in drug delivery involves nanotechnology and use of nanoparticles. Nanoparticles range in size between 1 and 100 nm. and have shown usefulness in enhancing bioavailability, providing sustained drug release, and enabling targeted delivery to specific sites in the body. These effects can help improve efficacy and decrease toxicity of drugs. Furthermore, specific forms of nanoparticles, in addition to serving as drug delivery vehicles, can also serve as imaging agents, biosensors, and diagnostic agents. Another new approach involves the use of mesenchymal stem cells for targeted delivery of drugs and nanoparticles to tumors and sites of inflammation.

It is our hope that the readers find the book informative and that it stimulates new and innovative ideas to apply to drug discovery and development of the future.

Izet M. Kapetanovic
Division of Cancer Prevention, National Cancer Institute, Bethesda,
USA

Introductory Chapter

Overview of Current Drug Discovery and Development with an Eye Towards the Future

Izet M. Kapetanovic
Division of Cancer Prevention, National Cancer Institute, Bethesda, MD USA

1. Introduction

Drug discovery and development process aims to make available new pharmacological interventions to prevent, treat, mitigate, or cure disease in a safe and effective manner. It is a slow, complex, multi disciplinary and costly process. Drug development starts with a target identification and validation, followed by drug candidates (hits) discovery, and lead drug (compound with favorable pharmaceutical, safety, efficacy, and pharmacokinetic profile) selection and optimization. Preclinical (non clinical) efficacy, pharmacology, toxicology, and mechanistic studies may include *in silico* (computational) methods, use of *in vitro* animal or human tissues (including cells and subcellular fractions), and *in vivo* animals. The studies rely on models that are thought to be predictive of the subsequent preclinical or clinical effects. Guidances (government-regulated standards of normal expectations) for different steps are readily available from the regulatory agencies (http://www.fda.gov/drugs/guidancecomplianceregulatoryinformation/guidances/default.htm). The required toxic ology studies must be performed according to the Good Laboratory Practice (GLP) guidelines. Medicinal chemistry and pharmaceutics also play a crucial role from the beginning of the drug discovery and development process, involving chemical synthesis (including compliance with current Good Manufacturing Practice, cGMP), characterization, purification, chemical alteration, stability determination, and formulation of the drug candidate. The first-in-human (FIH) doses are based on the No-Observed-Adverse-Event-Level (NOAEL) values obtained in the relevant and more sensitive toxicology specie (rodent and non-rodent, commonly rat and dog), interspecies dose extrapolation, and a selection of an appropriate safety factor. Subsequent to preclinical evaluation, an Investigational New Drug (IND) application is submitted to the regulatory agency (e.g. United States Food and Drug Administration, FDA or European Medicine Agency, EMEA) summarizing all preclinical data (chemical, pharmaceutical, efficacy, toxicology and other) along with a rationale for the proposed clinical study and a clinical study protocol. Clinical drug development can commence after review of the IND by the regulatory agency and a clinical study approval by a local Institutional Review Board (IRB, a committee of scientists and non-scientists overseeing the clinical research). Phase 1 studies commonly use human volunteers to determine human safety and pharmacokinetics. Frequently, these studies also include biomarkers of efficacy as secondary endpoints. Drugs with acceptable safety profiles then enter Phase 2 for efficacy evaluations. These include the proof-of-principle studies to demonstrate effects on disease-relevant biomarkers and the proof-of-concept studies to demonstrate direct effects on the target disease in a small patient sampling. Controlled trials are commonly designed to compare effects of the new drug to a placebo or to a standard of care treatment (for ethical reasons). Drugs showing promising efficacy continue to Phase 3, much larger trials examining efficacy as well as safety. Drugs emerging from these trials with appropriate evidence of safety and efficacy are submitted for marketing approval via a New Drug Application (NDA). Following a review and approval by the regulatory agency, the drug can then be marketed and enters Phase 4 or post-marketing monitoring.

Recent estimates suggest that it takes up to 13.5 years and 1.8 billion U.S. dollars to bring a new drug to the market [17]. There are rising concerns over the diminished productivity (number of new medical entities approved) in face of the escalating cost (R&D spending). In view of this, there is a growing effort and urgency to find new approaches aiming to decrease attrition and increase success in drug development [8, 10, 11, 17]. This is at times when number of drug blockbusters is coming off patent, large personnel layoffs and pharmaceutical consolidation (buying and merging in an effort to shore up pharmaceutical company pipelines). There are strong beliefs that pharmaceutical industry needs to find means of improving efficiency and effectiveness in order to sustain itself. Two independent studies, one by the FDA and the other by the European Federation of Pharmaceutical Industries and Associations (EFPIA), examined the causes behind the decreasing productivity. Based on these studies, improvements in predictivity of safety and efficacy were deemed to have the greatest potential for reversing the trend of diminished productivity and success [10]. This led to formation of public-private initiatives aiming to accelerate the development of better and safer medicines, the Innovative Medicines Initiative, IMI (http://imi.europa.eu) and the Critical Path Institute, C-PATH (http://www.c-path.org/). In 2004, FDA launched the Critical Path Initiative (CPI) as described in its white paper *Innovation/Stagnation: Challenge and Opportunity on the Critical Path to New Medical Products* (http://www.fda.gov/ScienceResearch/SpecialTopics/CriticalPathInitiative/CriticalPathOpportunitiesReports/ucm077262.htm):

"Sounding the alarm on the increasing difficulty and unpredictability of medical product development, the report concluded that collective action was needed to modernize scientific and technical tools as well as harness information technology to evaluate and predict the safety, effectiveness, and manufacturability of medical products. The report called for a national effort to identify specific activities all along the critical path of medical product development and use, which, if undertaken, would help transform the critical path sciences."

This was echoed in subsequent C-PATH reports (http://www.fda.gov/downloads/ScienceResearch/SpecialTopics/CriticalPathInitiative/UCM186110.pdf;http://www.fda.gov/ScienceResearch/SpecialTopics/CriticalPathInitiative/ucm076689.htm). Dr. Raymond Woosley, the president and CEO of the C-PATH is quoted on the C-PATH's website that it presently takes 15 years for drug development and 95% of drug candidate fail along the way. The very ambitious goal cited by the Institute is to shorten the time to 3 years and improve the success to 95%.

Major reasons cited for drug attrition are lack of efficacy, presence of toxicity, and commercial concerns [12]. It was reported that only 5% of the compounds entering the first-in-human studies in oncology achieve successful registration [12]. Majority of failures occurred in Phase 3 and were attributed to the lack of efficacy proof of concept, lack of objective and robust biomarkers, inadequate predictivity and poor translation of scientific discoveries and preclinical information to clinical settings. Innovation was commonly viewed as one of the most needed approaches to reversing the situation [8, 11, 17, 24]. A recent Science editorial by the current FDA commissioner [6] echoed these viewpoints. Commonly cited areas for potential and fruitful innovations include the development process itself, identification, validation and qualification of relevant biomarkers, predictive modeling, clinical trial subject selection, clinical trial design, and collaborative efforts involving pharmaceutical companies, academia, government, and public.

"Fail fast, fail cheap" is a common mantra in the pharmaceutical industry. This is intended to minimize losses of time, resources, and expenses. There are number of go/no-go decision gates along the common drug development path. Earlier an appropriate no-go decision is made, lesser the possibility for waste. Drug developers strive to identify the most effective and efficient means of bringing safe and effective products to the market. Success along the development path hinges on using appropriate and robust models and biomarkers, which are relevant and predictive of a disease process of interest. One frequently proposed solution is to move the clinical proof-of-concept phase to an earlier point on the drug development timeline and in a bidirectional manner with the preclinical development [17]. It's expected that this would result in a lesser number of drug candidates entering later clinical testing phases but with increasing probability of their success.

In an effort to decrease the development time and improve drug development efficiency, the regulatory agencies have recently introduced the Exploratory Phase (also known as Phase 0) option(http://www.fda.gov/downloads/Drugs/GuidanceComplianceRegulatoryInformation/Guidances/ucm078933.pdf). The regu latory requirements for Exploratory Phase are lesser than those for Phase 1 but the doses and scope of the former are also more limited. The Exploratory Phase has no therapeutic or diagnostic intent. Its purpose is to obtain pharmacokinetic and/or pharmacodynamic data and thereby provide an opportunity to obtain the necessary information for an early decision whether to continue the development or to select the optimum candidate or formulation for development [22].

One of the major initiatives in an effort to improve the efficiency and success in drug development deals with identification and validation of robust and predictive biomarkers. Biomarkers play a pivotal role throughout the drug discovery and development process, from the beginning through post-marketing. Biomarker Consortium, composed of the National Institutes of Health, the FDA, the Center for Medicare and Medicaid Services, Pharmaceutical Research and Manufacturers of America (PhRMA), Biotechnology Industry Association (BIO), pharmaceutical companies, academia, and patient groups, was formed in the United States to accelerate development in this area. Present and future perspectives by FDA on molecular biomarkers have been summarized in a recent publication [7]. The Predictive Safety Testing Consortium, PSTC (http://www.c-path.org/pstc.cfm) represents an example of one successful collaborative effort stemming from some of these initiatives. In collaboration with the regulatory agencies (FDA and EMEA), the PSTC worked on defining methodologies and validations for new safety biomarkers and presented an initial path and outline for regulatory qualification of biomarkers [5, 21]). In addition through the efforts of the Nephrotoxicity Working Group, seven renal biomarkers have been qualified for limited use in nonclinical and clinical drug development as a measure of drug safety. These efforts were highlighted in a special issue of Nature Biotechnology (http://www.nature.com/nbt/journal/v28/n5/index.html).

Advances in hardware and software computational power and sophistication are fueling the rapidly growing reliance on computers and computational modeling in an attempt to improve the efficiency and effectiveness in the drug discovery and development process [9]. It's not uncommon to hear statements at drug development conferences that computational modeling will play the major role in drug design and development in not too distant future, similar to its role presently in the automotive and airplane industries. Computational modeling addresses the key critical element in all aspects of the drug discovery and development process, the prediction [13]. This *in silico* approach is thought to obviate some disadvantages of the more traditional approaches (need for large amounts of test agent for *in vivo* testing, poor predictability of *in vivo* animal and *in vitro* models for human toxicity and efficacy, lack of reliable high-throughput *in vitro* assays and a lack of animal models for some common adverse events seen in humans, e.g. headache, nausea, dizziness) [16]. There are also increasing legal requirements, especially in Europe, for use of alternative, non-animal models in the regulatory safety assessment of chemicals and urging development, independent assessment and application of computational methods. [15]. As stated in the *Science* editorial: "The FDA is also working to eventually replace animal testing with a combination of *in silico* and *in vitro* approaches" [6]. In 2007, the National Academy of Sciences also proposed a shift away from the current animal toxicology testing to use of emerging technologies i.e., *in vitro* assays using human cells, non-mammalian model organisms, high throughput testing, imaging technologies, omics technologies, systems biology, and computational modeling. Some of the advantages and disadvantages of these approaches were recently discussed by van Vliet [23]. In order to address the great complexity of the biological systems, extensive computational power is required and there are several major virtual screening efforts utilizing grid or distributed computing (e.g. http://www.worldcommunitygrid.org/research/hdc/overview.do). *PriceWaterhouse Coopers Pharma 2005: An Industrial Revolution in R&D* report emphasized the growth and value of *in silico* approaches and projected that *in silico* methods will become dominant from drug discovery through marketing (http://www.pwc.com/en_GX/gx/pharma-lifesciences/pdf/industrial_revolution.pdf). Furthermore, the report suggested that we are in a transitional period where the roles of primary (laboratory and clinical studies) and secondary (computational) science are in process of reversal. In a more recent report, *PriceWaterhouseCoopers Pharma 2020: Virtual R&D,* it was stated that pharmaceutical innovation and productivity could be improved significantly via enhanced and more complete molecular understanding of the human body and a more complete knowledge of human disease pathophysiology, thereby enabling development of more predictive computational models (http://www.pwc.be/en/pharma/pdf/Pharma-2020-virtual-rd-PwC-09.pdf). This was envisioned as a path towards predictive biosimulation in form of a "virtual man" and a "virtual patient" in some not too distant future with some of the effort along these lines already in progress.

The rapid growth in scientific knowledge and computational capabilities is also providing means for integrating and analyzing disparate chemical, biochemical, physiological, pathological, and clinical data in a parallel as opposed to a sequential fashion. Systems biology applies principles and mathematical tools of electrical engineering and networks to dynamic modeling and simulation of complex biological systems in a holistic manner. This is facilitating a change in drug discovery and development paradigm away from the reductionist approach. It's becoming more recognized that a commonly utilized reductionist approach may not be well suited for complex human disease processes and that the old magic bullet paradigm needs to be replaced by a magic shotgun for many of the diseases

[19]. Human physiology and pathology are very complex involving multi-factorial and heterogenous processes with dynamic, redundant and interactive networks and signaling pathways [1-4, 14, 18, 20]. In fact, the term "Network Medicine" and what it entails is growing in recognition [2]. Furthermore, one size doesn't fit all and the targets may also change as the disease progresses. In many cases, it's more relevant to understand the system and how to apply and interpret its perturbations in order to achieve desired efficacy and safety as opposed to concentrating on a single target. In fact, a partial modification of several targets may be more effective and safer than a complete modification of a single target.

Based on the above overview, it is clear that changes and innovations in drug discovery and development are needed and that there are ongoing efforts in this area on several fronts. Ultimately, the success hinges on improving the predictivity of efficacy and toxicity, which in turn depends on innovations and having reliable and robust biomarkers and using appropriate tools and methodologies.

2. References

[1] Azmi AS, Wang Z, Philip PA, Mohammad RM, Sarkar FH (2010) Proof of Concept: Network and Systems Biology Approaches Aid in the Discovery of Potent Anticancer Drug Combinations. Molecular Cancer Therapeutics 9: 3137-3144

[2] Barabási AL, Gulbahce N, Loscalzo J (2011) Network medicine: A network-based approach to human disease. Nature Reviews Genetics 12: 56-68

[3] Boran ADW, Iyengar R (2010) Systems pharmacology. Mount Sinai Journal of Medicine 77: 333-344

[4] Csermely P, Agoston V, Pongor S (2005) The efficiency of multi-target drugs: the network approach might help drug design. Trends Pharmacol Sci 26: 178-82

[5] Dieterle F, Sistare F, Goodsaid F, Papaluca M, Ozer JS, Webb CP, Baer W, Senagore A, Schipper MJ, Vonderscher J, Sultana S, Gerhold DL, Phillips JA, Maurer G, Carl K, Laurie D, Harpur E, Sonee M, Ennulat D, Holder D, Andrews-Cleavenger D, Gu YZ, Thompson KL, Goering PL, Vidal JM, Abadie E, Maciulaitis R, Jacobson-Kram D, Defelice AF, Hausner EA, Blank M, Thompson A, Harlow P, Throckmorton D, Xiao S, Xu N, Taylor W, Vamvakas S, Flamion B, Lima BS, Kasper P, Pasanen M, Prasad K, Troth S, Bounous D, Robinson-Gravatt D, Betton G, Davis MA, Akunda J, McDuffie JE, Suter L, Obert L, Guffroy M, Pinches M, Jayadev S, Blomme EA, Beushausen SA, Barlow VG, Collins N, Waring J, Honor D, Snook S, Lee J, Rossi P, Walker E, Mattes W (2010) Renal biomarker qualification submission: a dialog between the FDA-EMEA and Predictive Safety Testing Consortium. Nat Biotechnol 28: 455-62

[6] Hamburg MA (2011) Advancing regulatory science. Science 331: 987

[7] Hong H, Goodsaid F, Shi L, Tong W (2010) Molecular biomarkers: a US FDA effort. Biomark Med 4: 215-25

[8] Kaitin KI (2008) Obstacles and Opportunities in New Drug Development. Clin Pharmacol Ther 83: 210-212

[9] Kapetanovic IM (2008) Computer-aided drug discovery and development (CADDD): in silico-chemico-biological approach. Chem Biol Interact 171: 165-76

[10] Koening J (2011) Does process excellence handcuff drug development? Drug Discov Today 16: 377-381

[11] Kola I (2008) The State of Innovation in Drug Development. Clin Pharmacol Ther 83: 227-230

[12] Kola I, Landis J (2004) Can the pharmaceutical industry reduce attrition rates? Nat Rev Drug Discov 3: 711-5

[13] Kumar N, Hendriks BS, Janes KA, de Graaf D, Lauffenburger DA (2006) Applying computational modeling to drug discovery and development. Drug Discovery Today 11: 806-811

[14] Lowe JA, Jones P, Wilson DM (2010) Network biology as a new approach to drug discovery. Current Opinion in Drug Discovery and Development 13: 524-526

[15] Mostrag-Szlichtyng A, ZaldÃ-var Comenges J-M, Worth AP (2010) Computational toxicology at the European Commission's Joint Research Centre. Expert Opinion on Drug Metabolism & Toxicology 6: 785-792

[16] Muster W, Breidenbach A, Fischer H, Kirchner S, Muller L, Pahler A (2008) Computational toxicology in drug development. Drug Discov Today 13: 303-10

[17] Paul SM, Mytelka DS, Dunwiddie CT, Persinger CC, Munos BH, Lindborg SR, Schacht AL (2010) How to improve R&D productivity: the pharmaceutical industry's grand challenge. Nat Rev Drug Discov 9: 203-214

[18] Rosenfeld S, Kapetanovic I (2008) Systems biology and cancer prevention: all options on the table. Gene Regul Syst Bio 2: 307-19

[19] Roth BL, Sheffler DJ, Kroeze WK (2004) Magic shotguns versus magic bullets: selectively non-selective drugs for mood disorders and schizophrenia. Nat Rev Drug Discov 3: 353-9

[20] Roukos DH (2011) Networks medicine: From reductionism to evidence of complex dynamic biomolecular interactions. Pharmacogenomics 12: 695-698

[21] Sistare FD, Dieterle F, Troth S, Holder DJ, Gerhold D, Andrews-Cleavenger D, Baer W, Betton G, Bounous D, Carl K, Collins N, Goering P, Goodsaid F, Gu YZ, Guilpin V, Harpur E, Hassan A, Jacobson-Kram D, Kasper P, Laurie D, Lima BS, Maciulaitis R, Mattes W, Maurer G, Obert LA, Ozer J, Papaluca-Amati M, Phillips JA, Pinches M, Schipper MJ, Thompson KL, Vamvakas S, Vidal JM, Vonderscher J, Walker E, Webb C, Yu Y (2010) Towards consensus practices to qualify safety biomarkers for use in early drug development. Nat Biotechnol 28: 446-54

[22] Sugiyama Y, Yamashita S (2011) Impact of microdosing clinical study -- Why necessary and how useful? Advanced Drug Delivery Reviews 63: 494-502

[23] van Vliet E (2011) Current Standing and Future Prospects for the Technologies Proposed to Transform Toxicity Testing in the 21(st) Century. Altex-Alternatives to Animal Experimentation 28: 17-44

[24] Wagner JA (2008) Back to the future: driving innovation in drug development. Clin Pharmacol Ther 83: 199-202

Part 1

Current Status and Future Directions

1

Drug Discovery and Ayurveda: Win-Win Relationship Between Contemporary and Ancient Sciences

Bhushan Patwardhan[1] and Kapil Khambholja[2]
[1]*Symbiosis International University, Pune,*
[2]*Novartis Healthcare Pvt. Limited, Hyderabad,*
India

1. Introduction

The present medicinal system is dominated by the Allopathy or western medicine which is prominently taught and practiced in most of the countries world wide. This system is still evolving and during last few decades focus was based on chemical origin of most of the medicines. Thus majority of drugs in current practice are from synthetic origin. Even so, a large number of these synthetic molecules are based directly or indirectly on natural products or phytoconstituents (Gupta *et al.* 2005; Harvey 2008) . The interesting question is - what type of medicines were people using for thousands of decades? Another interesting futuristic question is - What type of medicine / therapy would emerge and sustain in future? Answers to such questions can be obtained by doing a systemic review of existing scientific literature and also by making a forecast based on emerging technologies based on genetic sciences. Another important arena of brainstorming is how we link such questions with each other. We need to understand medicines or systems those were existing in use before emergence of current "synthetic era" and visualize the future of medicine and health care in the "technology era". The linkage between "the past" and "the future" of medicine is much more important and can give us "new directions" for better understanding health, disease and possible solutions.

Ayurveda, one of the oldest systems used by mankind for well being(Sharma 1995), originated in ancient India many thousand years ago (about 4500 BC as agreed by most scientists). The origin, development, existence and even practice of Ayurveda has many dimensions and complex theories based on religions, faith and ancient Vedic science (Patwardhan & Mashelkar 2009). Discussion on all these aspects is beyond the scope of this book chapter. Ayurveda, as a system of medicine, is one of the official systems of medicine in India (Mashelkar 2008) and is also widely practiced in many other countries (Mashelkar 2008). Evidence for effectiveness of many ayurvedic drugs and therapies is being generated rapidly from many research institutes and also there are projects under way to decipher unanswered questions related to Ayurveda. In this chapter we have tried to cover different but important aspects which give us a futuristic vision. After giving an overview of basics of Ayurveda, a comprehensive review of current status of research in Ayurveda is attempted. In later part of the chapter a dialogue on the key term "Drug Rediscovery" is being presented for the first time with a scientific perspective. The later part of the chapter also covers futuristic discussion where possibilities of linking Ayurveda with drug discovery process are described. We have tried to lay down conceptual framework for win-win relationship between ancient and contemporary health care sciences backed by strong scientific evidence being generated in recent years. We hope to provide innovative material for use in further development by scientific fraternity for ultimate benefit of health care and humanity.

1.1 Introduction to Ayurveda

There exist a plethora of information on Ayurveda through many books and commentaries published in past few decades. Most of these books are based on the traditional books which are thought to carry the knowledge and know-how of Ayurveda which, in ancient time, was existing in the form of memorised shlokas and manuscripts written in Sanskrit language. In this part of the chapter we have tried to present brief and comprehensive introduction to Ayurveda and its' fundamentals. The information provided is just a drop in the ocean and represents only that which is relevant to understanding the concept of Ayurveda and its further use in drug discovery process.

1.2 What is Ayurveda?

Ayurveda literally means "science of life" in Sanskrit (Ayur: Life; Veda: Science). It is not only a medical system but a way of life. As discussed earlier Ayurveda aims at a holistic management of health and diseases. It is widely practiced in the Indian subcontinent and is also one of the official systems of medicine in India. Its concepts and approaches are considered to have been perfected between 2500-500 BC.

Charak Samhita and *Sushrut Samhita* (100-500 BC) are the two main Ayurvedic classics, wherein more than 700 plants along with their classification, pharmacological and therapeutic properties have been described. Ayurveda during course of ancient times developed as sound scientific system and it is evident as it is divided into eight major disciplines known as *Ashtanga Ayurveda.* It is important to note that these specialisations or super specialisations were in existence and practiced by experts hundreds of years before the emergence of modern Anatomy, physiology and contemporary medicinal system!

1.3 Fundamentals and perspectives

1.3.1 Ashtanga Ayurveda: Specialities of knowledge in Ayurveda

Eight major divisions of Ayurveda have been described and followed for specialized knowledge. These categories are:

1. Kayachikistsa : The closest synonym would be internal medicine,
2. Shalya: General Surgery,
3. Shalakya: Speciality dealing with head and neck disorders,
4. Kaumar-bhritya: obstetrics and pediatrics
5. Rasayana: geriatrics and rejuvenative/reparative medicine
6. Vajikaran: Sexology and reproductive medicine,
7. Agad-Tantra: the body of knowledge on poisons, venoms and toxic substances,
8. Bhuta-Vidya: infectious diseases and mental illness. The fact that such a systemic categorization was established so early speaks of the knowledge and skills being central to the practice of Ayurveda.

Another fundamental concept of Ayurveda is the well defined system for classifying the individuals on basis of their body constitution, physiology and other relevant factors. The concept of "Prakruti" is thought to be at the base of many important steps in Ayurvedic diagnosis and therapy.

Prakriti is a consequence of the relative proportion of three entities (Tri-Doshas), Vata (V), Pitta (P) and Kapha (K), which are not only genetically determined (Shukra Shonita), but also influenced by environment (Mahabhuta Vikara), maternal diet and lifestyle (Matur Ahara Vihara), and age of the transmitting parents (Kala -Garbhashaya).

In an individual, the Tri-Doshas work in conjunction and maintain homeostasis throughout the lifetime starting from fertilization. Distinct properties and functions have been ascribed to each Dosha. For instance, Vata contributes to manifestation of shape, cell division, signaling, movement, excretion of wastes, cognition and also regulates the activities of Kapha and Pitta. Kapha is responsible for anabolism, growth and maintenance of structure, storage and stability. Pitta is primarily responsible for metabolism, thermo-regulation, energy homeostasis, pigmentation, vision, and host surveillance.

1.4 Drugs of Ayurveda

Drugs used in Ayurvdea are mostly herbs (crude or processed), minerals products, metals (in different oxidised forms prepared by specialised manufacturing techniques) and also some times animal products. It is to be noted that in many instances a combination of one or more of above type of drugs are prescribed. As per Ayurveda- drugs alone cannot fulfil the goal of achieving, improving or maintaining the healthy state of the body. The lifestyle, food habits, environment and more importantly the mind plays an important role in Health. Thus the Vaidya (Ayurvedic physician) suggests a complete regime which is composed of a set of ayurvedic drugs (herbs/ herbo-mineral formulations) to be taken in specified manner in combination of food and life style changes are to be followed strictly, to achieve a healthy state of mind and body.

In last few years lots of research has been undertaken on medicinal properties, possible mechanisms and other relevant information on many popular herbs mentioned in traditional texts and used by Vaidyas. These research projects, mainly pre-clinical studies, help to generate evidence behind ayurvedic drugs' clinical use. Many interesting leads are emerging for further drug discovery from Ayurvedic drugs (Patawardhan et al. 2004,). These contributions are sometimes forgotten in the current dominance of the reductionist paradigm. Table 1 enlists some of the Ayurvedic herbs, which have been widely used and subject to pharmacological research. The structural modifications of active principles of these plants have led to a plethora of new "chemical" drugs and still there exist a vast unexplored arena for SAR based studies which may lead to unique molecules with unprecedented safety and efficacy. Since many decades several of these plants are being globally used by thousands of licensed Vaidyas and other practitioners and even as a part of household tradition. Looking into this background it is desirable to understand the Ayurvedic properties of herbs. This approach would assist in evolving innovative combinations, investigate new uses and conduct clinical trials with appropriate targets. As for example, a judicious and standardized combination of Aloe vera gel and Curcuma longa rhizome powder may yield a potent wound and burn healing new product. Similarly, a combination of *Glycyrrhiza glabra* and *Zingiber officinale* would be more useful in acid-peptic disease than the single ingredients. But any such combination must have a rational Ayurvedic basis, rather than herbal concoctions. Understanding the ayurvedic basis of any

combination of herbs and its use in different condition requires knowledge of ayurvedic fundamentals and its correlation with contemporary concepts. Table 1 represent some examples of current evidence for ayurvedic drugs and their untapped potential yet to be established extending their scientific basis from Ayurveda (Vaidya AB 2006).
For further information and detailed knowledge readers are advised to study following subjects / specialisations of Ayurveda.

1.5 Ayurvedic pharmaceuticals

Bhaisajya Kalpana (Ayurvedic Pharmaceutics) forms a branch of Ayurveda, which mainly deals with collection and selection of ayurvedic drugs, purification as well as preparation, preservation, besides mode of administration and dosage specification. The ancient Ayurvedic scholars were very much rational and had a strong scientific background in fundamental principles, which are concerned with drug manufacturing.
Dravyagunavigyana includes identification (pharmacognosy-Namarupa vigyanya), preparation (pharmacy-Kalpa Vigyana) and administration (clinical pharmacology-Yoga Vigyana). The later deals with the effects of drugs on various systems (pharmacodynamics-Gunakarma Vigyana) and their application in different diseases (therapeutic-Pryoga Vigyana)

Ayurvedic Plant	**Impact**	**Untapped potential**
Aloe vera	Cosmetopharmaocolgy/ Burns	Menopause/Andropause
Atropa belladona	Acetyl choline pharmacology	Cigarrete for asthama
Azadirachta indica	Antiinsect/Antifungal	Head and neck cancer
Cassia angustifolia	Laxative/Indigetion	Chronic infections
Curcuma longa	Antiinflammatory/Antidiabetic	Cancer
Commiphora wightii	Antiarthritic/Obesity	Tuberculosis/Anti cancer
Glycyrrhiza glabra	Peptic ulcer/Sore throat	Anti viral/Anti cancer
Psoralea coryllifolia	Leucoderma/Psoriasis	Antimicrobial/Alopecia
Rauwolfia serpentina	Antihypertensive/tranquillizer	Antivenom
Strychnos nux-vomica	Digestive/Nervine tonic	Glycinergic receptors
Tinospora cordifolia	Immuostimulant/Anticancer	Hepatoprotective
Withania somnifera	Sedative/Phytoestrogen	Anticancer
Zingiber officinalis	Indigetion/Nausea	Arthritis

Table 1. Ayurvedic plants and impact on therapy and drug discovery

2. Contemporary drug discovery / development research on Ayurvedic concepts and medicines

As discussed above Ayurvedic concepts differ significantly when it comes to diagnosis, use of drugs or even treatment pedagogy. It is well-known that Ayurveda tries to heal or cure any disease condition from its grass-root level. It means, it does not only remove the symptoms of the condition, but also alleviates the cause or factors behind the disease. In this part of the chapter we would share and discuss few examples of research done on ayurvedic concepts and medicines using contemporary technologies or methodologies.

2.1 Exploring targets - Understanding mechanisms

There are many studies reported where preclinical or even clinical evidence has been generated for understanding targets or even mechanisms for Ayurvedic therapies. Another important aspect of research is to correlate ayurvedic fundamentals behind etiology, disease progression and its possible interventions in terms of contemporary medical/life science.

2.2 Correlating ancient science with contemporary pathophysiology and medicinal system

An article published by Sharma and Chandola, discusses the details of "Prameha" of Ayurveda and its correlation with obesity, metabolic syndrome, and diabetes mellitus (Sharma& Chandola 2011). The authors have given scientific basis of correlation and have described etiology, classification, and pathogenesis of these conditions both in terms of ayurvedic and modern concepts. According to this article there are 20 subtypes of Prameha due to the interaction of the three Doshas and 10 Dushyas (disturbed functioning of the principles that support the various bodily tissues); several of these subtypes have sweet urine, whereas some of them have different coloration of the urine, highlighting the inflammatory conditions involved in the metabolic syndrome. This disease has close ties to Sthaulya (i.e., obesity). With regard to diabetes mellitus, Sahaja Prameha and Jatah Pramehi correlate with type 1 diabetes; Apathyanimittaja Pramehacorrelates with type 2 diabetes. Madhumeha is a subtype of Vataja Prameha (Prameha withVata predominance) that can occur as the terminal stage of type 2 diabetes (in which insulin is required), or as type 1 diabetes beginning in early childhood. The latter is defined as Jatah Pramehi Madhumehino in Charaka Samhita, one of the classical Ayurvedic texts. The authors have concluded that various dietary, lifestyle, and psychologic factors are involved in the etiology of Prameha, particularly in relation to disturbances in fat and carbohydrate metabolism. The ancient Ayurvedic knowledge regarding Prameha can be utilized to expand the current understanding of obesity, metabolic syndrome, and diabetes.

2.3 Discovery through pre-clinical studies for understanding mechanism and targets for Ayurvedic drugs

As discussed earlier there are many papers being published regularly in national and international journals which provide evidence based on pre clinical studies and also some times provide probable mechanism of the ayurvedic drug / formulation under study. Few such examples are quoted here to reiterate the fact that ayurvedic drugs and therapies are having sound scientific background and one of the primary things remaining is to generate evidence so as to understand their utility and mechanism from contemporary science's point of view. In 2009 our team published results for understanding the immunomodulatory effect of "Shatavri" (*Asparagus racemosus*). Shatavri is one of the reputed and widely used rasayana herb of Ayurveda and is responsible for providing rejevunating effect along with other beneficial effects. In this article mixed Th1/Th2 activity of shatavri extracts is proven supporting its immunoadjuvant potential (Gautam *et al.* 2009).

In another mechanistic study Chondroprotective potential of Extracts of Almalki Fruits *(Phyllanthus emblica)* in Osteoarthritis was undertaken to understand mechanism behind the traditional use of Almalki. Chondroprotection was measured in three different assay systems. First, the effects of fruit powder were studied on the activities of the enzymes hyaluronidase and collagenase type 2. Second, an in vitro model of cartilage degradation was set-up with explant cultures of articular knee cartilage from osteoarthritis patients. Cartilage damage was assayed by measuring glycosaminoglycan release from explants treated with/without *P. emblica* fruit powders. Aqueous extracts of both fruit powders significantly inhibited the activities of hyaluronidase and collagenase type 2 in vitro. Third, in the explant model of cartilage matrix damage, extracts of glucosamine sulphate and selected extract exhibited statistically significant, long-term chondroprotective activity in cartilage explants from 50% of the patients tested (Sumantran *et al.* 2008).

2.4 Clinical evidence for medicinal uses of Ayurvedic drugs

Apart from pre-clinical studies many clinical studies of various depths are also being reported recently. Additionally the Government of India supported Department of AYUSH undertakes many clinical research based projects on prioritised ayurvedic medicines and formulations. One of the clinical studies we would like to quote here as reference is for studying efficacy of standardised ayurvedic formulation in arthritis. The multidisciplinary "New Millennium Indian Technology Leadership Initiative" Arthritis Project was supported by Government of India. It included randomised controlled exploratory trial with *Zingiber officinale* and *Tinospora cordifoliaas* as main drugs in the formulations under study. Total 245 eligible patients suffering from symptomatic osteo arthritic knees gave consent for it and were randomized into seven arms (35 patients per arm) of a double blind, parallel efficacy, and multicentre drug trial of sixteen weeks duration. The trial was controlled for placebo and glucosamine sulphate use. No dietary or other restrictions were advised. The groups matched well at baseline. There were no differences between the groups for patient withdrawals (total forty three) or adverse events (AE) which were all mild. In an intention-to-treat primary efficacy analysis, there were no significant differences ($P < .05$) for pain (weight bearing) and WOMAC questionnaire (knee function); a high placebo response was recorded. Based on better pain relief, significant ($P < .05$) least analgesic consumption, and improved knee status, one of the formulations under study "C" formulation was selected for further development. This study gives overview suggesting that how the clinical research on ayurvedic herbs or formulations can generate the evidence and also in understanding their possible mechanism of action (Chopra et al. 2011).

2.5 Clinical evidence for Ayurvedic therapy

As discussed earlier most of the time Ayurvedic physicians undertake different approaches for treatment where multiple drugs or formulations are used at one or different stages therapy. One such popular approach in Ayurveda is "Pachkarma therapy" which is used for variety of conditions where detoxification is required to cope up with stress or unbalanced physiology. Ayurvedic drugs or formulations used in such therapy can lead to a very different approach of drug discovery where multiple drugs are working together on multiple targets to achieve the objective of balancing the body physiology.

One such study is reported by Tripathi et al. (2010). This was a comparative clinical trial on the role of Panchakarma therapy and Unmada Gajankusha Rasa in the cases of major depressive disorder vis-à-vis kaphaja Unmada.

2.6 Safety pharmacology and drug interaction studies as part of drug discovery based on ayurvedic drugs

In contemporary Drug discovery programs safety has prime importance and any molecule must have a favorable risk benefit ratio to be considered and approved as drug. Even though ayurvedic drugs and/or formulations are in use by public and vaidyas since antiquities, most of them have a proven record of safety and tolerability. Any change or deviation in method of preparation or use other then that mentioned in traditional text requires additional studies to evaluate safety. Another safety aspect includes understanding of drug interactions if ayurvedic drugs are to be taken with other form of medicines. These sub parts of drug discovery process can be addressed by undertaking invitro toxicology studies and pharmacokinetic studies to understand drug interactions. In one of the studies we have reported Safety Pharmacology and Drug Interaction aspects of *Cassia auriculata*. In this study routine safety pharmacology with focus on cardiovascular variables and pharmacokinetic herb-drug interaction studies on rats fed with standardized traditional hydro-alcoholic extract and technology-based supercritical extract of Cassia auriculata for 12 weeks were undertaken. These studies indicate that both these extracts are pharmacologically safe and did not show any significant adverse reactions at the tested doses. The traditional hydro-alcoholic extract did not show any significant effect on pharmacokinetics; however, the technology-based supercritical extract caused a significant reduction in absorption of Metformin (Puranik et al. 2011).

These and many other such studies describe the way of incorporation of safety aspect in drug discovery process for Ayurvedic drugs.

3. Concept of "Drug rediscovery"

Contemporary Drug discovery and development (DD) process is becoming longer and expensive. Establishing the right balance between efficacy and safety is the crucial part of DD process. As the chemical entity under study would be completely new and no prior human exposure is reported, there are chances of many unexpected side effects being observed at various stages of development. These require multiple efforts for optimisation of the molecule for its safety and efficacy and many times the molecule under study has to be dropped from study due to high toxicity or side effects.

Most ayurvedic drugs / herbs are in use since times immemorable and experience of thousands of physicians is available to vindicate their safety and efficacy. Thus drug discovery process needs to be modified if benefits from Ayurvedic science are to be tapped. Many scholars have previously reported different approaches for this. "Reverse pharmacology" approach starts with clinical studies and goes upto the mechanistic pre-clinical studies (Patwardhan 2004).

Here we deploy a term "Drug rediscovery" which is more relevant for research involving ayurvedic herbs and drugs. As ayurvedic drugs are already in use as part of medicinal system any further research on these drugs would aid only in understanding their mechanisms and / or help in optimising their doses either alone or in combination. Thus the term "Drug rediscovery" would help differentiate process of discovering a drug from totally new chemical entity from the process of understanding a drug which is not totally new to mankind.

Another extension of Drug rediscovery from ayurvedic drugs can be done for benefit of contemporary science of medicine and that would be "stage 2 drug discovery" based on results of research done during drug rediscovery of ayurvedic drugs and herbs. This stage 2 DD would start only after bio-marker based research which is a part of Drug rediscovery of ayurvedic drugs. This may generate to newer leads with multiple targets and can give new direction to speed up the existing discovery path adopted. This concept is explained in Table 2.

Stage I :

DRUG REDISCOVERY **on Ayurvedic Drugs**

- Proven Ayurvedic drugs to be studied for phytoconstituents
- Activity guided fractionation of Biomarkers
- SAR studies of active constituents
- Mechanistic studies (Preclinical & Clinical)
- **All these leads to optimized therapy based on new evidences to be clubbed with traditional knowledge**

↓

Stage II:

Drug Discovery: Outputs of SAR studies (Stage I) from Ayurvedic Drug rediscovery program

- New LEADS

- Lead optimization and study on new molecule with unique safety and efficacy profile

Outputs of Mechanistic studies of Ayurvedic Drug rediscovery program

- Unique mechanism with multiple targets.
- New target identificaton and validation.
- Systems biology approach potentiating:
  - Single drug / molecule working on multiple targets or even multiple systems.
  - Multi herb-Multi target

Table 2. Unique potential of Ayurvedic Drugs for Drug (Re)discovery

3.1 Accelerated clinical research

The process of rediscovering a drug on basis of its ayurvedic origin involves reverse pharmacology and requires different approaches for undertaking clinical research. One of the approaches can be retrospective study based on hospitals' or clinicians' (vaidya in most of the cases) practice of particular disease or herb. This would be little difficult looking into differences in documentation and record keeping practices in most of the parts of India where Ayurveda is regularly practiced. Another approach for undertaking clinical study can be based on Reverse pharmacology where drug under study can be selected on basis of its clinical use and field experience. We have already discussed one such study earlier in this chapter where randomized, controlled exploratory clinical study on ayurvedic formulation was done for its use in osteoparthritic conditions (Chopra et al. 2011). This study along with standardization of formulation was completed in 23 months and thus the time of generation of evidence is comparatively low as that of contemporary discovery of newer molecules. Even WHO had published guideline mentioning different requirements for clinical research on Traditional medicines (2000). Thus the concepts of "Reverse pharmacology" and "Drug Rediscovery" through Ayurvedic drugs can significantly reduce the time-lag between induction of research project and clinical evidence generation through scientifically designed clinical research.

3.2 AyuGenomis: Role in future of drug discovery

Biotechnology with its specialisations like genomics, proteomics, genetic engineering etc. has made immense advances in deciphering diseases conditions, disease progression, prognosis and even up-to certain level cure for particular conditions. Genomics can play important role both in prevention and treatment of many diseases (Steinberg et al. 2001). The advanced technologies used in genomics and related sciences can help understanding role of genes in diseases and health. The use of these technologies and concepts for generating scientific evidence behind concepts of Ayurveda can open up many interesting avenues.

Structural and functional genetic differences in humans can take the form of single nucleotide polymorphisms (SNP), copy number variations (CNVs), and epigenetic or gene expression modifications. As per current research, in human 99.5 % genetic similarity is found and almost all physiological or anatomical variations amongst person to person are due to 0.5% diversity in single nucleotide polymorphism (SNP) and other variations in nucleotides (Levy *et al.* 2007). These inherited inter-individual variations in DNA sequence contribute to phenotypic variation, influencing an individual's anthropometric characteristics, risk of disease and response to the environment. Characterizing genetic variation may bring improved understanding of differential susceptibility to disease, differential drug response, and the complex interaction of genetic and environmental factors, which go to produce each phenotype.

Ayurveda, the traditional system of Indian medicine, Traditional Chinese medicine and Korean medicine all have well-defined systems of constitutional types used in prescribing medication bearing distinct similarities to contemporary pharmacogenomics. The pharmacognenomics can become useful for understanding genetic basis of concept of "Prakriti". This part of the chapter would discuss about how Pharmacogenomics and Ayurveda can be researched together for unpacking vast possibilities of integrated science.

According to Ayurveda an individual's basic constitution to a large extent determines predisposition and prognosis to diseases as well as therapy and life-style regime. Importance of such individual variations in health and disease is an important basic principle of ayurveda and was underlined by Charaka sometime 4000 years ago as follows:

'Every individual is different from another
and hence should be considered as a different entity.
As many variations are there in the Universe, all are seen in Human being'.

In the Ayurveda system of medicine, predisposition to a disease as well as selection of a preventive and curative regime is primarily based on phenotypic assessment of a person which includes one's body constitution termed "Prakriti". The concept of Prakriti is already discussed in detail earlier in this chapter.

The phenotypic diversity, according to Ayurveda, is a consequence of a continuum of relative proportions of Doshas resulting in seven possible constitutional types namely Vata (V), Pitta(P), Kapha(K), Vata-Pitta, Pitta-Kapha, Vata-Kapha and Vata-Pitta-Kapha. Amongst these, the first three are considered as extremes, exhibiting readily recognizable phenotypes, and are more predisposed to specific diseases.

Better characterization of the human genome has improved the scientific basis for understanding individual variation. The Ayurvedic Prakriti concept should be examined from a genomic perspective. Permutations and combinations of V, P, K attribute characters along with other host factors such as tissue status (Dhatusarata), twenty Gunas, digestive capacity and metabolic power (Agni), psychological nature (Manas Prakriti), habitat (Desha), and season (Kaala), lead to sufficient numbers of variants to define a unique constitution for every individual. Ayurveda thus describes the basis of individual variation(Bhushan 2007).

In the realm of modern predictive medicine, efforts are being directed towards capturing disease phenotypes with greater precision for successful identification of markers for prospective disease conditions.

Ayurveda has been investigated for this purpose, based on the hypothesis that Prakriti types (V, P and K) may offer phenotypic datasets suitable for analysis of underlying genetic variation. As a proof of concept, in the first study done by us, we evaluated 76 subjects both for their Prakriti and HLA DRB1 types, finding significant correlations in support of it (Patwardhan et al. 2005). The study concluded that Ayurveda based phenomes may provide a model to study multigenic traits, possibly offering a new approach to correlating genotypes with phenotypes for human classification.

The three major constitution types described in Ayurveda have unique putative metabolic activities, K being slow, P fast, while V is considered to have variable metabolism. We hypothesized that this might relate to drug metabolism and genetic polymorphism of drug metabolizing enzymes (DME). Inter-individual variability in drug response can be attributed to polymorphism in genes encoding different drug metabolizing enzymes, drug transporters and enzymes involved in DNA biosynthesis and repair. Gene polymorphisms precipitate in different phenotypic subpopulations of drug metabolizer. Poor metabolizers (PM) have high plasma concentration of the drug for longer periods and so retain drugs in the body for longer times. Intermediate metabolizers retain drugs in the body for normal time periods. Extensive metabolizers (EM) retain drugs in the body for the least time, plasma concentrations being high for shorter periods.

In another study we investigated the distribution of drug metabolizing enzymes CYP2C19 and CYP2C9 genotypes in 132 healthy individuals of different Prakriti classes(Ghodke et al. 2009). The results obtained suggest possible association of CYP2C19 gene polymorphism with Prakriti phenotypes.

Overview of few such studies are given in Table No 3 which gives successful lead to new directions for further research.

medicine/intervention	target/enzyme	no. of person	Output	Ref. no
corelation between Human Leucocytes Antigen(HLA) and prakriti type	HLA DRB1 gene	Total 76 person 10 - vata 32 - kapha 34 - pitta prakriti	There is complete absence of HLA DRB1*02 in Vata and HLA DRB1*13 in Kapha	(Bhushan *et al.* 2005)
correlation between CYP2C19 Gene Polymorphism and prakriti type associated with metabolic activity	CYP2C19 (a variant of the enzyme, cytochrome P450)	132 healthy subjects	The extensive metabolizer (EM) genotype was predominant in Pitta Prakriti (91%), Poor metabolizer (31%) in Kapha Prakriti when compared with Vata (12%) and Pitta Prakriti (9%).	(Ghodke *et al.* 2009)
Ayurveda's 'Rasa' correspondence with pharmacological activity	Ibuprofen, oleocanthal (from olive oil)		substances' similarities of 'Rasa' may indicate similar pharmacological activity & assumes a new significance to distinguish all the kinds of molecule	(Joshi *et al.* 2007)
The molecular correlation between the different constitution types	genome wide expression levels, biochemical and hematological parameters, Gene Ontology (GO) and pathway based analysis	Total 96 individuals *Vata*-39 *Pitta*-29 *Kapha*-28	The extreme constitution types revealed differences at gene expression level, biochemical levels. It provide a strong basis for integration of this holistic science with modern genomic approaches for predictive marker discovery and system biology studies.	(Prasher *et al.* 2008)
EGLN1 involvement in high-altitude adaptation revealed through genetic analysis of extreme constitution types defined in Ayurveda	EGLN1 is a key oxygen sensor gene inhibit hypoxia-inducible factor (HIF-1A).	24 different Indian Populations	TT genotype of rs479200 was more frequent in Kapha types and correlated with higher expression of EGLN1, was associated with patients suffering from high-altitude pulmonary edema, whereas it was present at a significantly lower frequency in Pitta and nearly absent in natives of high altitude.	(Aggarwal *et al.* 2010)

Table 3. Advanced studies on Ayurvedic fundamentals

Thus it can be summarised that identification of genetic variations underlying metabolic variability in Prakriti may provide newer approach to Pharmacogenomics. Extensive studies on Prakriti subtypes and genome wide single nucleotide polymorphism (SNP) mapping especially of other important DME polymorphisms like CYP2D6, CYP2C9, CYP3A4, TPMT, etc., would be useful to understand possible Prakriti pharmacogenomics relationship correlating genotype, Prakriti and drug metabolism.

Thus, these studies support that Ayurveda Classification is based on genome differentiation and having correlation with different drug responses and adverse effect. The Ayurvedic classification shows similar principle of pharmacogenomics for selecting "right drug, right dosage and to the right patient". There are many such studies required to prove the scientific basis of many of the un-deciphered complex Ayurvedic principles and fundamentals given in Vedic science of life. It seems that thousands of years before, Ayurvedic experts had known effect of genetic variation on physiology and pharmacology much more in details and current scientific tools fell short of understanding such complex concepts of Ayurveda.

An integration of traditional systems of medicine(Ayurveda, TCM, SCM, Kampo) with pharmacogenomics utilizes the advantage of high throughput DNA sequencing, gene mapping, and bioinformatics to identify the actual genetic basis of 'interindividual' and 'interracial' variation in drug efficacy and metabolism and holds promise for future predictive and personalized medicine.

Combining the strengths of the knowledge base of traditional systems of medicine with the dramatic power of combinatorial sciences and HTS will help in the generation of structure-activity libraries which will converge to form a real discovery engine that can result in newer, safer, cheaper and effective therapies.

The traditional systems of medicine in Asia (Ayurveda, TCM, SCM, Kampo) are considered great living traditions. They are all closely related to each other. For example, all are based on theories of constitution. All identify unique qualities of each individual, and state the necessity of developing personalized medicine in order to obtain optimal response to treatment. This is similar to the science of Pharmacogenomics, which tries to identify individual differences between patients connected to drug metabolism, efficacy and toxicity at the genomic level. Current research in 'Omics' is focusing on the polygenic approach using high throughput technology rather than the single gene approach.

Such research found a genetic basis for the classification of physical constitution in traditional medicine. "These observations are likely to have an impact on phenotype-genotype correlation, drug discovery, pharmacogenomics and personalized medicine." So, "Identifying genetic variations in Asia-based constitution may provide a newer approach to pharmacogenomics and help better understand the scientific classification basis of human population for better therapeutic benefits."

4. Current status: Promises and bottle necks

4.1 Appraisals or evidence for importance of Ayurveda

The evidence is what is required to prove an idea or concept or even a system. There exist plethora of evidence for scientific basis of Ayurveda (Mishra 2003; Patwardhan& Mashelkar 2009; Vaidya AB 2006) and one needs to adopt an unbiased neutral opinion to see the promising way forward for drug discovery with support of Ayurveda. Because ancient sciences are not limited to one religion or geographical area, they should be used for benefit

of health care system in totality. The promising outputs are already available where Ayurveda has given many miracle drugs like Ashwagandha (*Withania somnifera,* Family: Solanaceae), Guggul (*Commiphora wightii,* F: Burseraceae), Shatavari (*Asparagus racemosus,* F: Asparagaceae), Brahmi(*Centella asiatica,* F: Mackinlayaceae), Neem (*Azadirachta indica,* F: Meliaceae), Turmeric (*Curcuma longa,* F: Zingiberaceae), Isabgul (*Plantago ovata,* F: Plantaginaceae) so on and so forth. These drugs can be used both in traditional forms as well as in form of standardized semipurified or purified phytopharmaceuticals. These plants or their parts are regulated differently in different countries. As per Ayurvedic system of medicine they are licensed as drugs and are in Clinical use in India. As these drugs are not fully standardised or as currently there is no globally accepted common regulations for herbals they can be considered as herbal supplement or functional food etc.
The research on preclinical, clinical, Phytochemical, Pharmacokinetics-Pharmacodynemics (PK-PD), safety pharmacology etc. for ayurvedic drugs and formulations are on surge and world needs to have more integrative and planned approach so as to leverage the benefit of this tie-up between ancient and contemporary sciences.

4.2 Possible bottle necks

As many concepts of Ayurveda are more of integrated nature it needs inputs from many branches of science. As for example personalized medicine concept is an integral part of Ayurveda and is based on "Prakriti" of an individual which affects the choice of medicine and the way the particular health condition is treated though Ayurveda. This paradigm is into its infancy in modern science where we are still trying to understand genetic variations and their links with diseases and physiology. One of the possible bottlenecks can be lack of scientific tools which help to understand the detailed concepts of Ayurveda.
Another bottle neck that is already under debate is "marker" based evaluation of herbs. Traditionally ayurvedic herbs are used in crude form (and not as isolated or purified compounds) and many a times in combination with other herbs or preparations and thus science behind chemistry of such complex mixtures is yet to be evolved. Even though Ayurveda has provided many promising leads in terms of isolated molecules it is different part of story where individual phytoconstituents are studied as drugs. Thus we need to differentiate between traditional ayurvedic drugs and modern form of phyto-constituent based drugs (Patwardhan& Mashelkar 2009).

5. Win-win situation for future of health care

To conclude this chapter we would like to elaborate various points where ancient science of Ayurveda and contemporary health care stream can gain from each other for far reaching benefits and newer directions of drug discovery and health.
Table No. 4 discusses benefits that can be gained by Ayurveda and contemporary science.

6. Disclaimer

Dr Kapil M Khambholja is currently affiliated to Novartis Healthcare Pvt. Ltd., India and was earlier affiliated to S K Patel College of Pharmacetuical Education and Research, Ganpat University, India as an Asst. Professor. The views expressed in this chapter are purely of author him self and in no manner reflects views or opinion from affiliating company or organisation.

	Benefits for Ayurveda	Benefits for drug discovery / health care sciences
Benefits in Chemistry domain	- Understanding of chemistry behind success of ayurvedic herbs. - Better understanding of chemical transformation during traditional manufacturing practices	- Availability of new leads based on SAR studies of phytoconstituents. - Herbo-mineral formulations mixed with plants provide unique combination for studying interaction between organic and inorganic constitutents.
Benefits in Process domain	- Ability to provide uniform and consistent products using analytical and standardisation techniques - Traditional manufacturing techniques can be improved using modern unit operation based techniques.	- Traditional ayurvedic manufacturing techniques involve unique type of processes which can form basis of improved unique processes of purification, separation, manufacturing etc.
Benefits in Life science domain	- better understanding of mechanisms of individual herbs using invitro techniques - better understanding of mechanisms of polyherbal formulations using in-vivo animal models - Understanding genetic basis of prakriti and tri-dosha based classification of humans	- Improved understanding of correlation between mind and body linked with quantum physics / chemistry - Newer approaches for maintaing health and /or treating diseased conditions. - Understanding of link between life style, environment and health

Table 4. Win-win situation for Ayurveda, contemporary drug discovery process and health care sciences

7. References

(2000). *General Guidelines for Methodologies on Research and Evaluation of Traditional Medicine.* Geneva: World Health Organisation.

Aggarwal S, Negi S, Jha P, Singh PK, Stobdan T, Pasha MA, Ghosh S, Agrawal A, Prasher B , Mukerji M (2010). EGLN1 involvement in high-altitude adaptation revealed through genetic analysis of extreme constitution types defined in Ayurveda. *Proc Natl Acad Sci U S A.* Vol.107,No., 44, 18961-18966.1091-6490 (Electronic) 0027-8424 (Linking),

Patwardhan B (2007). *Drug discovery and development: traditional medicine and ethnopharmacology.* New Delhi: New India Publishing Agency.

Patwardhan B, Joshi K, Arvind C (2005). Classification of Human Population Based on HLA Gene Polymorphism and the Concept of Prakriti in Ayurveda. *The Journal of Alternative and Complementary Medicine.* Vol.11,No., 2, 349-353,

Bhushan Patwardhan, Ashok Vaidya, Mukund Chorghade (2004). Ayurveda and natural products drug discovery. *Current Science*. Vol.86,No., 6, 789-799,

Chopra A, Saluja M, Tillu G, Venugopalan A, Sarmukaddam S, Raut AK, Bichile L, Narsimulu G, Handa R , Patwardhan B (2011). A Randomized Controlled Exploratory Evaluation of Standardized Ayurvedic Formulations in Symptomatic Osteoarthritis Knees: A Government of India NMITLI Project. *Evidence-based Complementary and Alternative Medicine*. Vol.2011,No.,

Gautam M, Saha S, Bani S, Kaul A, Mishra S, Patil D, Satti NK, Suri KA, Gairola S, Suresh K, Jadhav S, Qazi GN , Patwardhan B (2009). Immunomodulatory activity of Asparagus racemosus on systemic Th1/Th2 immunity: Implications for immunoadjuvant potential. *Journal of Ethnopharmacology*. Vol.121,No., 2, 241-247.0378-8741,

Ghodke Y, Joshi K , Patwardhan B (2009). Traditional Medicine to Modern Pharmacogenomics: Ayurveda Prakriti Type and CYP2C19 Gene Polymorphism Associated with the Metabolic Variability. *Evid Based Complement Alternat Med.*No.1741-4288 (Electronic) 1741-427X (Linking),

Gupta R, Gabrielsen B , Ferguson SM (2005). Nature's medicines: traditional knowledge and intellectual property management. Case studies from the National Institutes of Health (NIH), USA. *Curr Drug Discov Technol*. Vol.2,No., 4, 203-219.1570-1638 (Print) 1570-1638 (Linking),

Harvey AL (2008). Natural products in drug discovery. *Drug Discov Today*. Vol.13,No., 19-20, 894-901.1359-6446 (Print) 1359-6446 (Linking),

Joshi K, Hankey A , Patwardhan B (2007). Traditional Phytochemistry: Identification of Drug by ‘Taste’. *Evidence-based Complementary and Alternative Medicine*. Vol.4,No., 2, 145-148,

Levy S, Sutton G, Ng PC, Feuk L, Halpern AL, Walenz BP, Axelrod N, Huang J, Kirkness EF, Denisov G, Lin Y, MacDonald JR, Pang AWC, Shago M, Stockwell TB, Tsiamouri A, Bafna V, Bansal V, Kravitz SA, Busam DA, Beeson KY, McIntosh TC, Remington KA, Abril JF, Gill J, Borman J, Rogers Y-H, Frazier ME, Scherer SW, Strausberg RL , Venter JC (2007). The Diploid Genome Sequence of an Individual Human. *PLoS Biol*. Vol.5,No., 10, e254,

Mashelkar RA (2008). Second World Ayurveda Congress (Theme: Ayurveda for the Future) - Inaugural address: Part I. *Evidence-based Complementary and Alternative Medicine*. Vol.5,No., 2, 129-131.1741-427X,

Mishra L (2003).*Scientific basis of Ayurvedic Therapies*, CRC Press, 0-8493-1366-X, New Yourk

Patwardhan B , Mashelkar RA (2009). Traditional medicine-inspired approaches to drug discovery: can Ayurveda show the way forward? *Drug Discov Today*. Vol.14,No., 15-16, 804-811.1878-5832 (Electronic)1359-6446 (Linking),

Prasher B, Negi S, Aggarwal S, Mandal AK, Sethi TP, Deshmukh SR, Purohit SG, Sengupta S, Khanna S, Mohammad F, Garg G, Brahmachari SK , Mukerji M (2008). Whole genome expression and biochemical correlates of extreme constitutional types defined in Ayurveda. *J Transl Med*. Vol.6,No., 48.1479-5876 (Electronic) 1479-5876 (Linking),

Puranik AS, Halade G, Kumar S, Mogre R, Apte K, Vaidya ADB , Patwardhan B (2011). Cassia auriculata: Aspects of Safety Pharmacology and Drug Interaction. *Evidence-based Complementary and Alternative Medicine*. Vol.2011,No.,

Sharma H , Chandola HM (2011). Prameha in Ayurveda: Correlation with Obesity, Metabolic Syndrome, and Diabetes Mellitus. Part 1â€"Etiology, Classification, and Pathogenesis. *The Journal of Alternative and Complementary Medicine*. Vol.17,No., 6, 491-496,

Sharma P (1995). *Charak Samhita*. Varanasi, India: Chaukambha Orientallia.

Steinberg KK, Gwinn M , Khoury MJ (2001). The Role of Genomics in Public Health and Disease Prevention. *JAMA: The Journal of the American Medical Association*. Vol.286,No., 13, 1635,

Sumantran VN, Kulkarni A, Chandwaskar R, Harsulkar A, Patwardhan B, Chopra A , Wagh UV (2008). Chondroprotective Potential of Fruit Extracts of Phyllanthus emblica in Osteoarthritis. *Evidence-based Complementary and Alternative Medicine*. Vol.5,No., 3, 329-335,

Tripathi J, Reddy KRC, Gupta S , Dubey S (2010). A comparative clinical trial on the role of *Panchakarma therapy* and *Unmada Gajankusha Rasa* in the cases of major depressive disorder vis-à-vis *kaphaja Unmada. AYU (An international quarterly journal of research in Ayurveda)*. Vol.31,No., 2, 205-209,

Vaidya AB RA (2006). Evidences based Ayurveda Sorting fact from fantasy. In *Ayurveda and its Scientific Aspects - Opportunities for Globalisation*). New Delhi: Department of AYUSH and CSIR, pp. 1-30.

2

Evolutionary Biology and Drug Development

Pierre M. Durand and Theresa L. Coetzer
University of the Witwatersrand and National Health Laboratory Service
South Africa

1. Introduction

Evolution is the unifying framework in biology and scales to all living systems. It is the central organizing concept to explain seemingly disparate biological phenomena; from the very small (individual molecules) to the very large (ecosystems), from the rise and spread of molecular variants to the behavior and body shapes of elephants. In recent times, our appreciation for evolution in medicine has gained momentum. Individuals have championed the cause, dedicated journals have emerged, and new books on the subject are frequently published ("The Evolution and Medicine Review" is an excellent web-based resource providing updated information on the subject, http://evmedreview.com). This union between evolution and medicine has already advanced our understanding of pathological processes (Maccullum, 2007, Nesse & Stearns, 2008).

Drug development and therapeutic strategies are areas in which evolutionary principles may be particularly helpful. The avalanche of bioinformatic methods, genomic data and subsequent emergence of evolutionary genomics in the last few decades means that integrating these fields in drug design is now a possibility. Incorporating evolutionary information is not only helpful *a posteriori* when we may hope to understand why resistance to a particular compound emerged. It is also valuable *a priori*, to design more efficacious drugs, suggest potential resistance profiles and conceptualize novel treatment strategies. Many allopathic treatments, particularly those for chronic non-infectious diseases, relate to the manipulation of cellular functions within one individual's lifespan, for example, developing a drug aimed at a particular cardiac disorder. In these instances, evolutionary biology may explain why a particular disease arose, the evolutionary relationships between genes in the animal model and human or which pathological processes should be targeted. From an evolutionary perspective populations of reproducing individuals are the material on which evolution acts. Adaptive and non-adaptive changes occur over successive generations, and infectious organisms and cancer are therefore the premier examples to illustrate the role of evolution in drug development. In the current age it is almost unthinkable that evolutionary theory, the only scientific framework for studying ultimate causality in biology, doesn't already form the starting point for developing therapeutic interventions affecting evolving populations.

Here we wish to illustrate the role of evolution in allopathic medicine. A brief overview of the typical drug development pipeline is provided, followed by a discussion of relevant evolutionary questions. We discuss in greater detail the molecular evolutionary processes impacting on the emergence of drug resistance and offer suggestions to limit the problem.

Finally, we discuss the rapidly growing areas of evolvability and multilevel selection and how these inform our understanding of therapeutic strategies.

2. Drug discovery strategies

A drug discovery pipeline is a complex, costly and lengthy process involving several discrete stages (Fig. 1). The median time for the development of a new drug is estimated at ~13 years, with a potential cost upwards of ~1 billion US dollars (Paul et al., 2010). The funnel shape of the pipeline reflects the high failure rate between different stages and fewer than 1 in 50 projects deliver a drug to the market (Brown & Superti-Furga, 2003). In the last few years especially the number of new approved drugs has declined sharply despite an increase in research and development spending. Data from a survey of nine large pharmaceutical companies revealed that in 2010 only two new molecular entities from all these companies were approved by the FDA, a very poor return on their expenditure of approximately $60 billion dollars (Bunnage, 2011). Several strategies have recently been proposed to reduce the costs and improve the success rates, including closer cooperation between pharmaceutical companies and academia (Cressey, 2011, Frye et al., 2011); investigation of new uses for approved drugs (Littman, 2011); increased use of translational phenotypic assays (Swinney & Anthony, 2011); and improved target and lead selection (Brown & Superti-Furga, 2003, Bunnage, 2011).

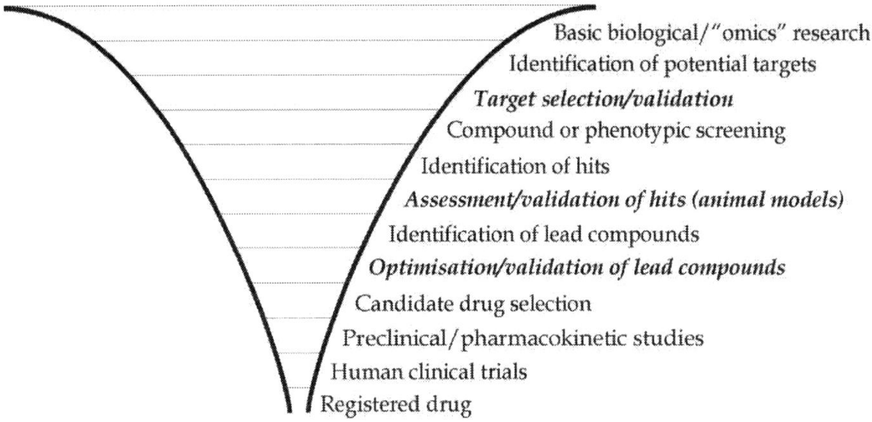

Fig. 1. The drug discovery funnel.

Evolutionary considerations are critical at steps in bold italics.

The availability of whole genome sequences, new discoveries regarding the molecular basis of disease, technological advances in target and lead validation, and high throughput screening strategies, provide exciting opportunities for drug discovery. However, translational research requires improved coordination and integration between different scientific disciplines to ensure a justified transition past key decision points in the drug development pipeline. In this regard, it is critical that evolutionary biologists participate in the process to ensure that fundamental evolutionary principles are taken into account, especially at the validation steps (Fig. 1), to reduce costs and attrition.

3. Evolutionary concepts relevant to drug design

To understand the evolutionary pressures on a potential drug target and the homologous relationships between target genes in the human and the proposed animal model, a few basic concepts should be addressed (Box 1). The reader is referred elsewhere for further discussion of general concepts of molecular evolution (Li, 2006).

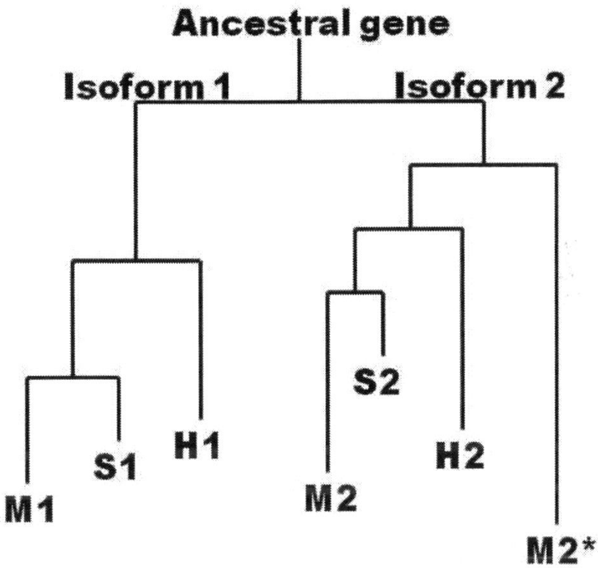

Box 1. Orthology, paralogy and functional shifts. In the hypothetical phylogram an ancestral gene has been duplicated to give paralogous isoforms 1 and 2 in mouse (M), rat (R) and human (H). Speciation events gave rise to orthologues M1, R1 and H1 and orthologues M2, R2 and H2. In the mouse there has been a second duplication event giving rise to M2*. The finding that M2* is isolated on a long branch indicates a functional shift in this gene

3.1 Orthology and paralogy

Homologous genes share a common ancestry and depending on the events in their history are orthologous or paralogous (Box 1). Orthologues arise from speciation events; paralogues arise from gene duplication events and resolving these relationships is best done with phylogenetic reconstructions. A number of methods can be used to re-create phylogeny (Felsenstein, 2004) each with their own strengths and weaknesses, however, it should be borne in mind that phylogenetic reconstructions are not foolproof and may require significant interpretation and re-examination. Processes like concerted evolution, horizontal gene transfer and incongruent evolution cloud the picture (Felsenstein, 2004, Li, 2006). Nevertheless, establishing orthology and paralogy (as best one can) raises major questions and both are important for drug development and assessment of drug targets (Searls, 2003). Orthology informs one about the corresponding gene(s) in the animal model while paralogous relationships are often more important for identifying functional divergence.

3.2 Evolutionary rates

Related to the reconstruction of phylogenetic relationships is the determination of evolutionary rates and patterns. The simplest way of estimating the nature and intensity of the selective pressure is to quantify the ratio of non-synonymous to synonymous nucleotide substitutions in a coding sequence, corrected for opportunity, taking into account various features of sequence evolution such as transition/transversion ratios, base and codon biases, etc (Box 2) (some key references are Goldman & Yang, 1994, Hurst, 2002, Muse & Gaut, 1994, Nei & Gojobori, 1986, Yang, 2006, Yang & Nielsen, 2000). The ratio (*dN/dS* or ω) reflects fitness advantages or disadvantages resulting from changes in the amino acid sequence. A ratio $\omega>1$ indicates positive (diversifying or adaptive) selection; $\omega<1$ is negative (purifying or stabilizing) selection. In positive selection non-synonymous mutations are more prevalent in extant sequences presumably because they confer a fitness advantage. Negative selection indicates a fitness cost to non-synonymous substitutions. Furthermore, the lower the ω value, the stronger the stabilizing pressure as fewer and fewer non-synonymous substitutions are tolerated. If there is no difference between *dN* and *dS* substitution rates ($\omega=1$), the selective pressure is neither stabilizing nor diversifying and evolution is neutral. Examining the evolutionary pressures not only informs one about functional divergence; but guides the researcher in the selection of the target site. Briefly, sites that are fast evolving are typically poor drug targets, while structurally and functionally conserved sites are usually under purifying selection and make more suitable targets.

$$Q_{ij} = \begin{cases} 0 \\ \pi_j \\ \kappa\pi_j \\ \omega\kappa\pi_j \\ \omega\pi_j \\ \omega\kappa\pi_j \end{cases}$$

Box 2. A model for codon evolution (Goldman & Yang, 1994, Muse & Gaut, 1994).
Numerous methods are available to quantify evolutionary rates in nucleotide sequences. An extensively used approach is the maximum likelihood (ML) codon model for evolution. A simplified substitution rate matrix used by the ML method to estimate codon evolution is given (left). The matrix is used to statistically determine evolutionary pressures acting at individual codons: positive, negative or neutral evolution (see text for more discussion and references below). This model determines the probability that codon i mutates to j in a specified time interval and accounts for the transition/transversion rate ratio (κ); the equilibrium frequency of codon j (π_j); and the non-synonymous/synonymous rate ratio (ω). $Q_{ij} = 0$ if i and j differ at more than 1 position.

4. Evolution and target selection

One of the major causes of attrition of a potential drug candidate is poor quality of the target. The critical steps of target selection and validation require greater emphasis and incorporation of additional evolutionary criteria to reduce subsequent failure.

4.1 Has the target undergone functional divergence?

Many genes of therapeutic interest have undergone expansion leading to functional redundancy. Targeting a specific protein isn't helpful if there are other family members that are immune to the drug and at the same time take over the function of the target.

To assess functional shifts, paralogy is a critical consideration. The reason is pleiotropy, which is often associated with paralogous genes. Pleiotropy occurs when a gene product has more than one function and can either precede gene duplications or result from duplication events where the duplicated gene is less constrained and free to evolve multiple functions. The impact of pleiotropy on drug discovery is apparent when one considers that in these situations, one must disentangle the compound's effect on multiple pathways. A good example of gene duplications leading to pleiotropy and functional divergence is that of the caspase family. The ancestral metazoan caspase has undergone numerous gene duplications over time resulting in at least 11 human and 10 murine true caspase genes (Nedelcu, 2009, Uren *et al.*, 2000, Wang & Gu, 2001). In humans, distinct clusters of caspases have been identified (Uren *et al.*, 2000, Wang & Gu, 2001), which may be involved in evolutionarily related but biochemically distinct pathways of inflammation or apoptosis. It also seems likely that some of the caspase family members are implicated in both processes. These proteins are primarily involved in one of the processes but are pleiotropically linked to the other. Disentangling the role of individual caspases in the two pathways would be important for developing drugs targeting either inflammation or apoptosis.

5. Evolution and hit validation

The assessment of hit compounds often requires *in vivo* testing in animal models and an inappropriate choice of model is one of the reasons why an apparently promising lead compound fails during human clinical trials. Understanding the phylogenetic relationships between genes in the two systems is therefore an important initial step.

5.1 What are the evolutionary relationships between genes in the model and target organisms?

The biochemical and pharmacological findings in an experimental model organism cannot be extrapolated to another organism without understanding the evolutionary relationships between the target genes. This is because evolutionary rates and functional divergence between homologous genes in related organisms may vary. It is important; therefore, to establish at the very least the homologous relationships between the gene used in the experimental system and the proposed target gene in the human.

Even a slightly improved understanding of orthologous gene differences between model and target species can have an impact on the progression of a compound with major implications for scientific and financial resources. However, while orthology tells us about the evolutionary relationships between genes in related organisms and *suggests* similar function, this is not guaranteed. A phylogram may reveal that a particular gene in the model organism is orthologous to the gene in the target organism. Despite this orthologous relationship isolation of the gene on its own long branch indicates sequence divergence and a functional shift. This should alert the researcher to be wary of using that particular model as a basis for studying the biochemistry of the protein in the human target. In the example given in Box 1 a duplication event has led to genes M2 and M2* in the mouse. This duplication occurred after the speciation events giving rise to humans and rats and both M2 and M2* are therefore orthologues of R2 and H2. However, the isolation of M2* on its own long branch strongly suggests functional divergence and it should not be used as a model for developing a drug compound targeted at H2.

Molecular evolution of homologous proteins may vary along different lineages, which means that a protein may appear highly stable and conserved in one branch leading to humans, but under a different selective pressure in the experimental model animal. If this is not taken into account inappropriate models may be selected. A good example of this is the finding that leptin is associated with obesity in mice (Chen *et al.*, 1996). The discovery was greeted with tremendous excitement since it implied that rodents could be used as a model organism for studying the pathogenesis of obesity in humans. However, it subsequently emerged that there is evidence for positive selection in leptin in primates (including humans) but not in rodents (Benner *et al.*, 2000). This indicates adaptive evolution and a functional shift in leptin after the divergence of primates from rodents. Using the mouse therefore, as a model for understanding the biochemistry of the protein and its potential use as a drug target in humans is problematic.

6. Harnessing evolution to minimize the emergence of resistance

Drug resistance is an ever present threat that curtails the effective lifespan of a drug and has enormous financial implications for pharmaceutical companies. Resistance can develop very rapidly, for example, resistance to the anti-malaria drugs pyrimethamine and proguanil (Hyde, 2005) developed within a year of introducing the drug to the market. Similarly, chronic myeloid leukaemia (CML) cells have become refractory to treatment with tyrosine kinase inhibitors targeting the bcr-abl oncogenic protein, necessitating the development of second and third generation inhibitors (Kantarjian *et al.*, 2008). It is therefore vital that evolutionary principles are applied to the key decision points in the drug development process relating to the validation of targets, hits and lead compounds to minimize the emergence of resistance.

6.1 What is the possible evolutionary response to drug pressure?

Evolution occurs by non-adaptive and adaptive (Darwinian) means. Non-adaptive evolution includes pleiotropic phenomena and genetic drift, or may appear non-adaptive at one level of selection and adaptive at another. Adaptive evolution occurs by natural selection and is more closely associated with the concept of fitness. For pharmacological interventions against infections and cancer to be effective, they are aimed at killing or at least inhibiting growth of infective organisms or cancer cells. This means they generally act on adaptive traits so that fitness is compromised. Targeting a non-adaptive trait such as the pleiotropic effects of paralogous genes discussed above may have a minimal effect on fitness, limiting the drug's usefulness. Targeting fitness-related traits is important for a drug to be effective, but doing so induces a Darwinian response if there are any survivors following the treatment. Furthermore, the greater the fitness cost resulting from the drug pressure the stronger the evolutionary response (Read *et al.*, 2011), and it is usually a question of *when*, rather than *if*, resistant mutants will emerge.

There is effectively a therapeutic trade-off. From the perspective of treatment efficacy, the trade-off is between maximizing the fitness cost to the target (infectious agent or cancer cell) and minimizing the undesirable evolutionary escape response. Of course, if the fitness cost is absolute and all individuals in the population of infective organisms or cancer cells are killed, there is no trade-off. This is the ideal situation; but often not the case. Unless there is complete cure, there will be a therapeutic trade-off. Optimizing this trade-off is seldom given any consideration and therapy results in a temporary hiatus in the disease. Eventually the most resistant mutants take over and, as indicated, the most aggressive therapies elicit the strongest escape response (Read *et al.*, 2011). In addition, not only does therapy select the most virulent individuals, but the group level dynamic is disrupted, further intensifying the escape response. Studies in mice infected with the malaria parasite *Plasmodium chabaudi* found that more virulent clones are controlled by less virulent ones (Wargo *et al.*, 2007). Treatment that failed to eradicate all clones allowed the more virulent ones to thrive leading to a more serious secondary relapse. Humans living in malaria endemic areas can be infected with over 15 genotypically distinct clones of *P. falciparum* (Juliano *et al.*, 2010). If the mouse model study is extrapolated to humans, then aggressive chemotherapy may actually be harmful in the long-term. Instead, to optimize the therapeutic trade-off, it is suggested that the guiding principle should be to impose no more selection than is absolutely necessary (Read *et al.*, 2011). This holds particular relevance for infections or malignancies where cure is unlikely and therapy is aimed more at disease management, for example, chronic leukaemias and infections like HIV.

An understanding of the evolutionary constraints acting at the molecular level is not only helpful when predicting the intensity of the evolutionary response, but it is also important for identifying the appropriate target sites of a protein.

6.2 Can we identify target sites with minimal risk for resistance?

There are various computational approaches (see Yang, 1997 and later versions) to determine the selective pressures acting on whole genes, specific codons or on lineages in a phylogenetic tree. Whole genes are seldom under positive selection; however, those that are, rapidly escape the fitness cost associated with the drug therapy. Non-synonymous substitutions already confer a fitness advantage in sequences demonstrating positive selection and the added drug pressure rapidly leads to resistance. To obtain a more informative view of a gene's evolutionary rate, it is helpful to examine substitution rates at individual codons in the coding sequence. Maximum likelihood estimates of ω at individual codons will usually reveal variation across the coding sequence. Highly conserved or functionally important amino acids are likely to be under purifying selection, while others in the sequence may be evolving neutrally or be under positive selection. Targeting the positively selected or neutral sites will drive the emergence of resistance mutations and should be avoided, while sites under intense purifying selective pressures are far less likely to produce viable mutations and make suitable targets.

Drug treatments add to the naturally occurring selective pressures and codon sites that code for resistant mutations are frequently evolving more rapidly than others. A good example of this is a study of serially sampled reverse transcriptase coding sequences isolated from a group of HIV-1 subtype C-infected women before and after single-dose nevirapine (Seoighe *et al.*, 2007). Nevirapine is a standard therapy for preventing mother-to-child transmission. A directional selection evolutionary model differentiated codons under positive selection from those subject to purifying selection and the differences in evolutionary rates would reliably have predicted *a priori* the sites of amino acid change leading to nevirapine resistance. This study provided proof of concept that quantifying the evolutionary pressures acting at individual codon sites can predict the likelihood of resistance emerging if the drug-protein binding site is known. Even before this study, others developed iterative approaches for use in development pipelines to guide experimentalists to biologically relevant sites based on sequence conservation. The first approach known as Evolutionary Tracing (ET) (Lichtarge *et al.*, 1996, Lichtarge & Sowa, 2002) and another, Evolutionary Patterning (EP) (Durand *et al.*, 2008), which directly quantifies the evolutionary rate, provide useful examples for further illustration.

6.2.1 Evolutionary tracing

ET generates a trace sequence from multiple sequence alignments of functional classes of a protein family. Clusters of invariant amino acids are identified and incorporated into 3D structures to identify the most suitable target sites in terms of their conservation, functional and structural importance and access. ET is particularly helpful for modeling functional specificity and architecture-defining residues. ET predictions have been verified experimentally. The most complete demonstration that ET anticipates mutational and crystallographic analyses was performed on the regulator of G protein signaling proteins that act to increase G_α GTP hydrolysis rates (Sowa *et al.*, 2000). Based on the ET data specific amino acids were mutated causing profound effects on enzyme activity and led to the prediction of an allosteric binding site (Sowa *et al.*, 2001), which was subsequently confirmed by crystallography (Slep *et al.*, 2001).

6.2.2 Evolutionary patterning

In ET, one of the premises for identifying target sites is that structurally and functionally essential amino acids are conserved in a trace sequence. However, while conservation suggests purifying selection it does not necessarily equate to it. To more accurately quantify the selective pressure acting at a particular amino acid residue, it is important to study the substitution rates at individual codons across a coding sequence. This is the approach adopted by EP, which makes use of a maximum likelihood substitution matrix to estimate the ratio of non-synonymous / synonymous substitutions at individual codons in a coding sequence (Box 2). The Bayes Empirical Bayes posterior probability of the MLE (maximum likelihood estimate) of ω falling into a particular category (for example, positive selection $\omega>1$ or extreme purifying selection $\omega<0.1$) is computed using PAML software (Yang, 2007). The distribution of these probabilities across a potential target protein can be examined and mapped to the predicted 3D structure, guiding the researcher as to which residues to target and which to avoid. It is argued that codons subject to extreme purifying selection are evolutionarily constrained, perhaps because the amino acid is essential for protein structure or function. The data from extant sequences indicate that non-synonymous mutations at these sites are not tolerated and make ideal drug targets if the encoded amino acids are accessible to interactions with lead compounds. In contrast, residues that are subject to positive or neutral selection, or only weakly conserved should be avoided. Non-synonymous mutations at these sites have arisen naturally during the evolutionary history of the protein indicating that amino acid changes do not significantly compromise protein fitness. These sites should not be targeted therapeutically as any mutants that arise are likely to be selected for by the drug pressure. Mapping the amino acids under extreme purifying selection to a structural model is important so that the accessibility and interaction between target sites and lead compounds can be assessed *in silico*. As with ET, this is an iterative process. Docking studies uncover drug-protein interactions and the strength of chemical bonds assessed; interactions with undesirable amino acids are revealed and the lead compound may be modified so that contacts with target sites are optimized. The process can then be repeated as often as necessary to maximize favourable interactions.

The application of EP to a potential drug target, *P. falciparum* glycerol kinase may be used as an illustration (Figures 2 and 3) (Durand *et al.*, 2008). Six separate target sites comprising stretches of contiguous amino acids subject to extreme purifying selection were identified. The targets were mapped to a 3D model generated using the *E. coli* homologue as a template, which revealed that four were accessible to potential lead compounds. These sites were also found to overlap with functional domains and were suggested as therapeutic targets. The EP approach was validated by examining resistance mutations in the *P. falciparum* dihydrofolate reductase-thymidylate synthase protein, which is targeted by the anti-malarial drug pyrimethamine. EP predicted that none of the five known mutations conferring pyrimethamine resistance would have been subject to extreme purifying selection - a factor which would have facilitated the evolution of resistance. This was indeed the case, confirming that the likelihood of an evolutionary escape response was greater if the codon was under more relaxed evolutionary constraints.

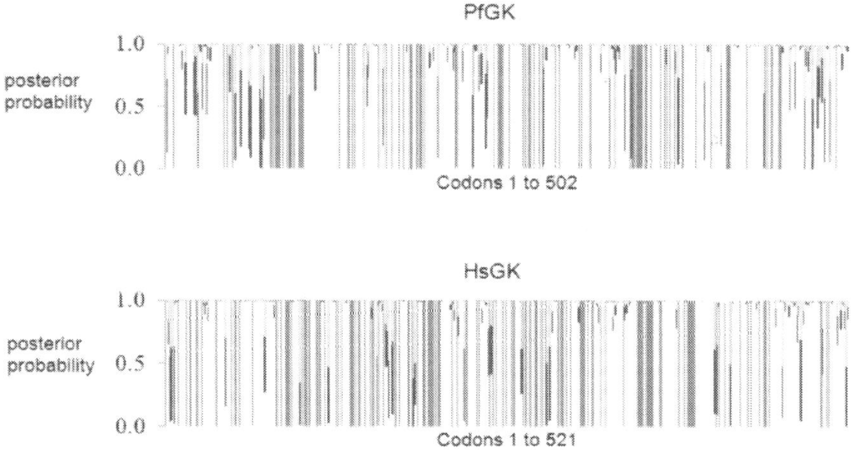

Fig. 2. Posterior probabilities for four categories of ω across GK coding sequences (from Durand *et al.*, 2008). Bayes Empirical Bayes posterior probability estimates for each category of ω across *P. falciparum* (PfGK) and human (HsGK) GK coding sequences are shown. Residues under extreme purifying selection ($\omega \leq 0.1$) are potential drug target sites and were mapped to a 3D model to assess drug accessibility (Fig. 3). Categories for ω are indicated with coloured bars: yellow ($\omega > 1.0$), red ($\omega = 1.0$), white ($0.1 < \omega < 1.0$), and blue ($\omega \leq 0.1$).

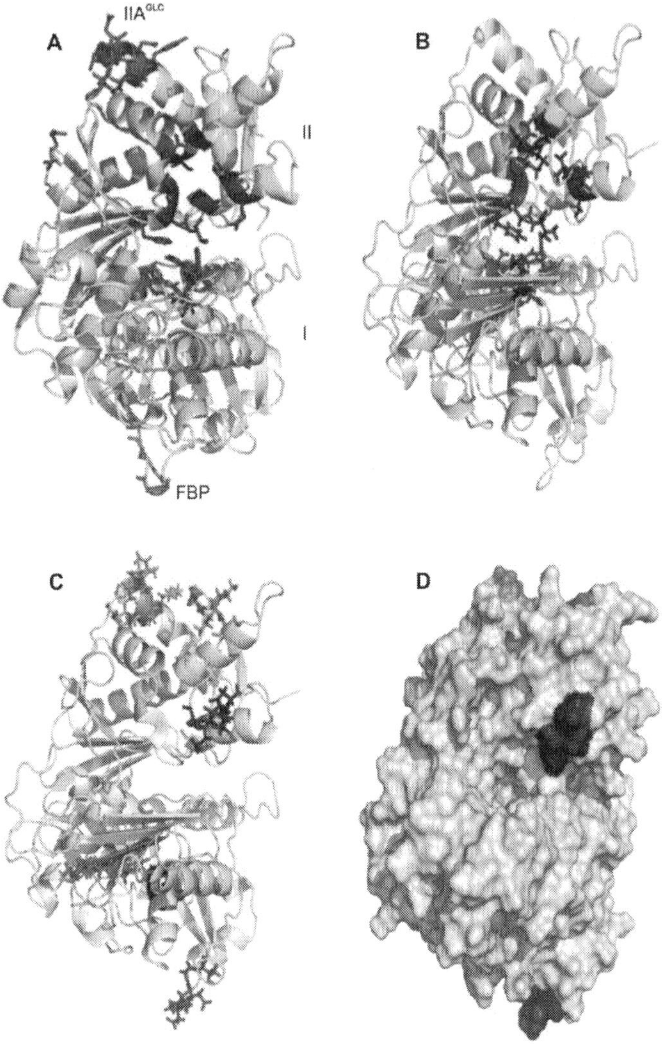

Fig. 3. *E. coli* and *P. falciparum* glycerol kinase 3D models (from Durand *et al.*, 2008). Ribbon models (with functional residues as sticks) of E. coli glycerol kinase (EcGK) (A) and P. falciparum glycerol kinase (PfGK) (B) are displayed. In EcGK, coloured residues are involved in binding to ADP (blue), Mg2+ (yellow), glycerol (red), FBP (fructose-bis-phosphate) (orange) and IIAGLC (purple). Alpha helices and ß sheets in the ATPase site (light green) and subunit interactions (aquamarine) are shown. The PfGK model is based on EcGK. Five regions were identified in Fig. 2 as good target sites and mapped to ribbon (C) and surface (D) models. One of the regions (black) is partly obscured and is in the core of the molecule, indicating the region would not be accessible to drug compounds.

ET and EP provide guidance for selecting the most suitable drug target sites and thus assist in designing more effective drugs, which may limit the emergence of resistance for long periods. However, any drug pressure will still invoke an evolutionary response, so at some point escape mutants are still likely to arise. A truly fundamental shift in the approach to allopathic therapies would involve strategies aimed at having evolution work in our favour rather than against us. Doing so is a major conceptual challenge.

7. Evolvability and multilevel selection: Future avenues for drug research

Basic science research into the fundamental nature of evolution has resulted in what some biologists think is tantamount to a paradigm shift. For a review of these advances see discussions around an "extended theory of evolution" (Danchin *et al.*, 2011). Two areas in which evolutionary thinking has rapidly progressed are the concepts of evolvability and multilevel selection. Both have relevance for future drug development strategies.

7.1 Evolvability

Advances in evolution hold promise for exploiting under-appreciated biological phenomena in drug design. The eloquent statement "Not only has life evolved, but life has evolved to evolve" (Earl & Deem, 2004) implies that the genetically encoded propensity to adapt to environmental pressures (known as evolvability) is a selectable phenotype. The variation in response to changing environments confers heritable variation in fitness. It is argued therefore, that evolvability can be acted on by natural selection leading to populations of organisms that are more or less likely to adapt to environmental pressures. Experimental evolution studies using model organisms like *Escherichia* (Leroi *et al.*, 1994) and *Chlamydomonas* (Bell & Reboud, 1997) date back nearly two decades and seem to support these assertions although whether evolvability itself is always adaptive (as opposed to being non-adaptive) is not always clear (Creavin, 2004). Evolvability also appears to play a role in pathogen virulence. For example, the HIV reverse transcriptase (RT) is notoriously error-prone leading to the evolution of populations of quasispecies that evade host immunity and escape drug pressures (Bebenek *et al.*, 1993). However, as indicated above, whether the error prone nature of HIV RT evolved as an adaptation or whether it is the result of other adaptive or non-adaptive effects is uncertain. Nevertheless, what is clear is that the error rate of HIV RT confers a fitness advantage. Targeting the pathogen's evolvability rather than phenotypic traits that are easily overcome by the propensity to evolve is therefore likely to have a greater impact in the long term. It can be argued that where evolvability forms part of a pathogen's life history strategy, this consideration should be included in drug design efforts. For further discussion on plasticity and evolvability in parasitic infections such as malaria with relevance to chemotherapeutic strategies the reader is referred elsewhere (for example Reece *et al.*, 2009).

7.2 Multilevel selection theory

7.2.1 Multilevel selection, sociobiology and the conceptualization of novel drug strategies

Our understanding of the living world has been transformed by the finding that natural selection acts at multiple levels of biological organization (Box 3). Multilevel selection theory (MLST), which includes group selection and for which there is now a significant body of evidence, describes the living world in terms of hierarchically structured levels where the tenets of selection are applicable to evolutionary units across these levels (Keller, 1999, Lewontin, 1970, Okasha, 2006, Wilson, 1975). Evolutionary transitions gave rise to increasing complexity including groups of genes, which form genomes, which form cells, which form multicellular organisms, which may form social groups and so on (Maynard Smith & Száthmary, 1995). The fact that the units of evolution span levels of biological organization raises the question of whether it may be better to target other levels of organization such as groups rather than individual cancer cells or infectious organisms.

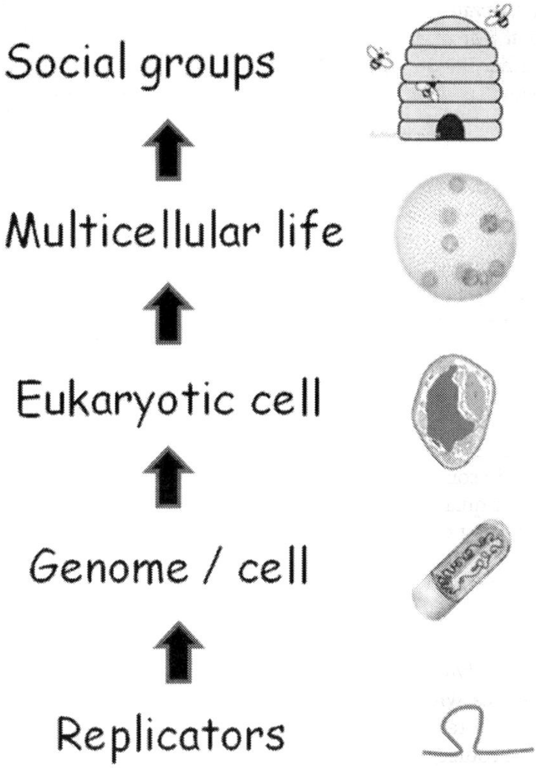

Box 3. The multilevel selection paradigm. The living world is characterized by quantum leaps in organization and complexity. Early replicators cooperated to form genomes and cells, which formed a eukaryotic cell, multicellular life, social groups and so on. Evolution by natural selection acts on any system where there is a group of reproducing individuals, so long as there is heritable variation in fitness. All these levels are therefore subject to natural selection. The related concept of group selection fits into this framework of MLST and describes competition between rather than within groups. While there is ongoing debate regarding the mechanisms, terminology and extent of group selection most researchers accept the fundamentals.

For drug development strategists, there are some key aspects to MLST that must be appreciated. Group level traits and adaptations arise because of selection and dynamics between groups rather than individuals within a group. These traits arise in various ways. They can be aggregates of properties within the group or arise as irreducible 'emergent properties' only existing at the group level (Thompson, 2000). Selection pressures at different levels of organization can vary; a particular trait can be beneficial at one level and harmful at another (see programmed cell death later) or the trait may have differential fitness benefits at two or more levels. Unpacking the relative selection pressures at different levels requires an understanding of Fisher's fundamental theorem of natural selection, which states that "*the rate of increase in fitness of any organism at any time is equal to its genetic variance in fitness at that time*" (Fisher, 1930). Fisher's theorem is applicable at any level of organization, whether it is a population of groups or a population of cells. Drugs targeting more than one level of selection will therefore induce differential responses and the intensity of the evolutionary escape response will depend on fitness variances at the different levels. Targeting the group level, rather than individuals as is the conventional approach has distinct advantages for therapies against infections (Pepper, 2008) and cancer (Pepper *et al.*, 2009). The advantages typically concern the phenomenon of cooperation and the group fitness variance.

The phenomena of cooperation and its more extreme form altruism are commonly found in groups of pathogens or cancer cells. Mechanistically, cooperation can take the form of "public goods" (Wessler *et al.*, 2007), molecules that are produced by individuals but have a group level action. The quantity or quality of molecule produced by one of the individuals is of such a nature that it may have little or no direct benefit for the producer, but in combination with the molecular products from others results in a group level fitness-enhancing trait. For example, in bacterial biofilms quorum-sensing molecules regulate cell division of individuals so that the group responds to challenges as a collective (Wessler *et al.*, 2007). Similarly, in solid tumours angiogenic factors are produced by individual cells but only when sufficient quantities are produced by the group does neo-vascularization occur (Kerbel, 1991). Targeting public goods makes good evolutionary sense.

Consider a situation where individuals (cancer cells or pathogens) secrete molecules that only have a group level benefit. There is initially no benefit for a mutant individual because the concentration of its molecular product is either too low or on its own cannot modify the group phenotype and increase group fitness. More likely, its mutant nature means that its role in the group network is compromised and group fitness is diminished. Unlike conventional therapies which actively select for resistance, there is no immediate fitness benefit to mutants and resistant individuals die along with others in the group or they are selected against. Of course, a larger clone of resistant cells may survive and reproduce, but from the outset and all else being equal, mutants have the same or lower fitness than susceptible cells and generally do not take over the population. This scenario is more than just conceptual. It is supported empirically. One of the most detailed illustrations comes from the 15 year old study of tumour neo-vascularization and drug resistance referred to above (Boehm *et al.*, 1997, Kerbel, 1991).

In solid tumours cancer cells eventually outgrow their nutrient supply. Angiogenesis factors are produced by the tumour leading to neo-vascularization and subsequent survival of the group. Cytotoxic cancer drugs create a powerful selective pressure and in the heterogeneous population of cancer cells resistance rapidly emerges. However, targeting the group level benefit with "anti-angiogenic therapy does not induce drug resistance" (Boehm *et al.*, 1997).

This is because while the angiogenesis blocker is applied, resistant mutants do not produce sufficient angiogenesis factors for neo-vascularization to occur and they die along with others before reaching a critical mass.

Similar strategies have been advocated or used for a number of infectious diseases with some success, including the escalating challenge of methicillin-resistant *S. aureus* (MRSA) (see Pepper, 2008 and references therein). *S. aureus* produces numerous virulence molecules that act at the group level and are required for establishing and maintaining infections. The prototypical public good example in *S aureus* is α-toxin, without which infections in animal models are unsustainable (Bhakdi & Tranum-Jensen, 1991). A literature survey suggests that an appropriate and current opportunity for using MLST in drug development is tuberculosis (TB). TB is one of the major global health challenges and with the emergence of multidrug resistant (MDR) and extreme drug resistant (XDR) strains the need for novel strategies has never been more urgent. Laboratory studies of the resuscitation promoting factors (rpfs) in *Mycobacterium* species indicate that these factors may be prime targets for group level chemotherapy (for a review of rpfs see Kana & Mizrahi, 2010). Knockout experiments suggest rpfs have a negligible role in individual cell fitness; however, at the group level they are important as virulence factors and for the resuscitation of latent infections.

With regards to fitness variance and the rate of evolution, Fisher's theorem bodes well for drug strategies targeting cooperation in groups. The fitness variance of the phenotype decreases as the cooperative behaviour increases and is shared equally within the group (for a detailed discussion see Price, 1972). When fitness variance is zero, the implication is that either all the individuals in the group receive the benefit of the public good or none at all. The evolutionary rate of the group level phenotype is therefore exceedingly slow, as is the likelihood of resistance developing. This is in contrast to the evolutionary rates when the unit of selection is the individual in the group. In these instances fitness variance is usually greater and resistance evolves more rapidly. The fundamental properties of evolutionary rates as they relate to fitness variance coupled with cooperation and group level traits opens a whole new avenue for drug development strategies.

7.2.2 Multilevel selection and the intriguing case of programmed cell death

The phenomenon of programmed cell death (PCD) in unicellular eukaryotes brings together many aspects discussed in this chapter. It provides a useful context for integrating homology, adaptations, evolutionary rates, evolvability and MLST as they relate to infections, cancer and drug development. Our discussion of PCD below is based on a few key papers and requires far more investigation, but as an example it illustrates how evolutionary thinking could lead to a radical shift in drug design.

Programmed cell death (PCD), previously considered a hallmark of multicellularity, has been reported in all major lineages in unicellular eukaryotes and prokaryotes (see Table 1 in Nedelcu *et al.*, 2011). From an evolutionary perspective (with implications for drug design in infections and cancer) the burning question has been: why would an organism actively kill itself? For an individual unicellular organism PCD has no fitness benefit and adaptive evolution cannot explain the phenomenon. Likely explanations are that it is either maladaptive pleiotropy or adaptive in a MLS context (i.e. at a group level). While strong arguments can be made for both scenarios (Nedelcu *et al.*, 2011), laboratory evidence from two model organisms favour the hypothesis that PCD in unicells is adaptive for the group. In *S. cerevisiae* PCD-related aging assists re-growth in a related mutant subpopulation

(Fabrizio *et al.*, 2004, Herker *et al.*, 2004). A direct fitness-related experiment in *C. reinhardtii* demonstrated that molecules released by cells dying by PCD provide fitness benefits to others (Durand *et al.*, 2011). Genomic studies have also revealed that many of the homologues for key protein domains involved in PCD are conserved across a wide range of organisms (for example Nedelcu, 2009), although there has been expansion of many of the gene families, particularly in vertebrates and plants as organism complexity evolved. As discussed in sections 3 and 4, an understanding of the evolutionary rates and relationships between homologues in model and target organisms will be helpful if expanded gene families in the PCD pathway are to be targeted therapeutically.

S. cerevisiae and *C. reinhardtii* are already used as model organisms for a range of diseases including cancer (for example Fang & Umen, 2008). The genomic and empirical data for PCD as an adaptation in these organisms shed new light on PCD in human parasitic infections and cancer and can help explain some puzzling phenomena. With regards to parasitic disease, numerous organisms demonstrate PCD, including apicomplexa, stramenopiles, trichomonads, diplomonads, kinetoplastids and trypanosomatids (see Table 1 in Nedelcu *et al.*, 2011 and references therein). The group effect of PCD in most of these organisms has not been studied; however, in *Leishmania* (a kinetoplastid) infections, PCD as a group level adaptation explains the counterintuitive finding that virulence is associated with PCD (Van Zandbergen *et al.*, 2006). If the infective inoculum contains a proportion of apoptotic (PCD) cells, the population has greater virulence and fitness. Removing the apoptotic forms diminishes disease severity. The interpretation is that apoptotic forms enhance group fitness, which is in keeping with the *C. reinhardtii* findings. Similar experiments have not been performed with cancer cells, but the role of apoptosis is not always clear. Tumour suppressor genes are usually mutated in cancer; however, the apoptosis pathway is malignant cells is frequently activated through the FAS ligand receptor. Curiously, the FAS ligand pathway can also promote tumour growth (Chen *et al.*, 2010). Whether this is due to crosstalk between this pathway and another anti-apoptosis pathway is unclear. However, in light of the *C. reinhardtii* experiments (Durand *et al.*, 2011) and that the essential pathology of cancer is atavism (regression to the ancestral unicellular state) (Davies & Lineweaver), is it possible that apoptosis in some cancers also provides benefits to other cells in the population? In a bizarre twist, can chemotherapy exacerbate a cancer or infection by inducing PCD in some cells, which then provide fitness benefits to others?

8. Concluding remarks

The potential role for evolutionary biology in drug design is vast and can be applied at various stages in the development process. The aim here is to provide the reader with an overview of evolutionary medicine, with specific reference to drug design and the emergence of resistance in infections and cancer. Some key concepts such as phylogenetic relationships and evolutionary rates are introduced to illustrate how evolutionary studies can predict the most suitable drug target sites in a protein and limit resistance. Perhaps the most exciting union between evolution and drug development is the future use of evolvability and multilevel selection, heralding a new era for therapeutic strategies.

9. References

Bebenek, K., Abbotts, J., Wilson, S.H. & Kunkel, T.A. (1993) Error-prone polymerization by HIV-1 reverse transcriptase. Contribution of template-primer misalignment, miscoding, and termination probability to mutational hot spots. *J Biol Chem*, 268, 10324-34.

Bell, G. & Reboud, X. (1997) Experimental evolution in Chlamydomonas II. Genetic variation in strongly contrasted environments. *Heredity*, 78, 498-506.

Benner, S.A., Chamberlin, S.G., Liberles, D.A., Govindarajan, S. & Knecht, L. (2000) Functional inferences from reconstructed evolutionary biology involving rectified databases--an evolutionarily grounded approach to functional genomics. *Res Microbiol*, 151, 97-106.

Bhakdi, S. & Tranum-Jensen, J. (1991) Alpha-toxin of Staphylococcus aureus. *Microbiol Rev*, 55, 733-51.

Boehm, T., Folkman, J., Browder, T. & O'Reilly, M.S. (1997) Antiangiogenic therapy of experimental cancer does not induce acquired drug resistance. *Nature*, 390, 404-7.

Brown, D. & Superti-Furga, G. (2003) Rediscovering the sweet spot in drug discovery. *Drug Discov Today*, 8, 1067-77.

Bunnage, M.E. (2011) Getting pharmaceutical R&D back on target. *Nat Chem Biol*, 7, 335-9.

Chen, H., Charlat, O., Tartaglia, L.A., Woolf, E.A., Weng, X., Ellis, S.J., Lakey, N.D., Culpepper, J., Moore, K.J., Breitbart, R.E., Duyk, G.M., Tepper, R.I. & Morgenstern, J.P. (1996) Evidence that the diabetes gene encodes the leptin receptor: identification of a mutation in the leptin receptor gene in db/db mice. *Cell*, 84, 491-5.

Chen, L., Park, S.M., Tumanov, A.V., Hau, A., Sawada, K., Feig, C., Turner, J.R., Fu, Y.X., Romero, I.L., Lengyel, E. & Peter, M.E. (2010) CD95 promotes tumour growth. *Nature*, 465, 492-6.

Creavin, T. (2004) Evolvability: Implications for drug design. *Drug Discov Today*, 3, 178.

Cressey, D. (2011) Traditional drug-discovery model ripe for reform. *Nature*, 471, 17-8.

Danchin, E., Charmantier, A., Champagne, F.A., Mesoudi, A., Pujol, B. & Blanchet, S. (2011) Beyond DNA: integrating inclusive inheritance into an extended theory of evolution. *Nat Rev Genet*, 12, 475-86.

Davies, P.C. & Lineweaver, C.H. Cancer tumors as Metazoa 1.0: tapping genes of ancient ancestors. *Phys Biol*, 8, 015001.

Durand, P.M., Naidoo, K. & Coetzer, T.L. (2008) Evolutionary patterning: a novel approach to the identification of potential drug target sites in Plasmodium falciparum. *PLoS One*, 3, e3685.

Durand, P.M., Rashidi, A. & Michod, R.E. (2011) How an organism dies affects the fitness of its neighbors. *Am Nat*, 177, 224-32.

Earl, D.J. & Deem, M.W. (2004) Evolvability is a selectable trait. *Proc Natl Acad Sci U S A*, 101, 11531-6.

Fabrizio, P., Battistella, L., Vardavas, R., Gattazzo, C., Liou, L.L., Diaspro, A., Dossen, J.W., Gralla, E.B. & Longo, V.D. (2004) Superoxide is a mediator of an altruistic aging program in Saccharomyces cerevisiae. *J Cell Biol*, 166, 1055-67.

Fang, S.C. & Umen, J.G. (2008) A suppressor screen in chlamydomonas identifies novel components of the retinoblastoma tumor suppressor pathway. *Genetics*, 178, 1295-310.

Felsenstein, J. (2004) *Inferring phylogenies*. Sinauer Ass, ISBN 087893775, Sunderland.

Fisher, R.A. (1930) *The genetical theory of natural selection*. Clarendon Press, Oxford.

Frye, S., Crosby, M., Edwards, T. & Juliano, R. (2011) US academic drug discovery. *Nat Rev Drug Discov*, 10, 409-10.

Goldman, N. & Yang, Z. (1994) A codon-based model of nucleotide substitution for protein-coding DNA sequences. *Mol Biol Evol*, 11, 725-36.

Herker, E., Jungwirth, H., Lehmann, K.A., Maldener, C., Frohlich, K.U., Wissing, S., Buttner, S., Fehr, M., Sigrist, S. & Madeo, F. (2004) Chronological aging leads to apoptosis in yeast. *J Cell Biol*, 164, 501-7.

Hurst, L.D. (2002) The Ka/Ks ratio: diagnosing the form of sequence evolution. *Trends Genet*, 18, 486.

Hyde, J.E. (2005) Drug-resistant malaria. *Trends Parasitol*, 21, 494-8.

Juliano, J.J., Porter, K., Mwapasa, V., Sem, R., Rogers, W.O., Ariey, F., Wongsrichanalai, C., Read, A. & Meshnick, S.R. (2010) Exposing malaria in-host diversity and estimating population diversity by capture-recapture using massively parallel pyrosequencing. *Proc Natl Acad Sci U S A*, 107, 20138-43.

Kana, B.D. & Mizrahi, V. (2010) Resuscitation promoting factors in bacterial population dynamics during TB infection *Drug Discov Today*, 7, e13-e18.

Kantarjian, H., Schiffer, C., Jones, D. & Cortes, J. (2008) Monitoring the response and course of chronic myeloid leukemia in the modern era of BCR-ABL tyrosine kinase inhibitors: practical advice on the use and interpretation of monitoring methods. *Blood*, 111, 1774-80.

Keller, L.K. (1999) *Levels of selection in evolution*. Princeton University Press, Princeton, NJ.

Kerbel, R.S. (1991) Inhibition of tumor angiogenesis as a strategy to circumvent acquired resistance to anti-cancer therapeutic agents. *Bioessays*, 13, 31-6.

Leroi, A.M., Bennett, A.F. & Lenski, R.E. (1994) Temperature acclimation and competitive fitness: an experimental test of the beneficial acclimation assumption. *Proc Natl Acad Sci U S A*, 91, 1917-21.

Lewontin, R.C. (1970) The units of selection. *Annu Rev Ecol Syst*, 1, 1-18.

Li, W.H. (2006) *Molecular evolution*. Sinauer Press, ISBN 0878934804, Sunderland.

Lichtarge, O., Bourne, H.R. & Cohen, F.E. (1996) An evolutionary trace method defines binding surfaces common to protein families. *J Mol Biol*, 257, 342-58.

Lichtarge, O. & Sowa, M.E. (2002) Evolutionary predictions of binding surfaces and interactions. *Curr Opin Struct Biol*, 12, 21-7.

Littman, B.H. (2011) An audience with Francis Collins. *Nature Rev Drug Discov*, 10, 14.

MacCullum, C.J. (2007) Does medicine without evolution make sense? *PLoS Biology*, 5, 679-680.

Maynard Smith, J. & Száthmary, E. (1995) *The major transitions in evolution*. W. H. Freeman, ISBN 019850294X, San Francisco.

Muse, S.V. & Gaut, B.S. (1994) A likelihood approach for comparing synonymous and nonsynonymous nucleotide substitution rates, with application to the chloroplast genome. *Mol Biol Evol*, 11, 715-24.

Nedelcu, A.M. (2009) Comparative genomics of phylogenetically diverse unicellular eukaryotes provide new insights into the genetic basis for the evolution of the programmed cell death machinery. *J Mol Evol*, 68, 256-68.

Nedelcu, A.M., Driscoll, W.W., Durand, P.M., Herron, M.D. & Rashidi, A. (2011) On the paradigm of altruistic suicide in the unicellular world. *Evolution*, 65, 3-20.

Nei, M. & Gojobori, T. (1986) Simple methods for estimating the numbers of synonymous and nonsynonymous nucleotide substitutions. *Mol Biol Evol*, 3, 418-26.

Nesse, R.M. & Stearns, S.C. (2008) The great opportunity: Evolutionary applications to medicine and public health. *Evol Appl*, 1, 28-48.

Okasha, S. (2006) *Evolution and the levels of selection*. Oxford University Press, ISBN 9780199267972, New York.

Paul, S.M., Mytelka, D.S., Dunwiddie, C.T., Persinger, C.C., Munos, B.H., Lindborg, S.R. & Schacht, A.L. (2010) How to improve R&D productivity: the pharmaceutical industry's grand challenge. *Nat Rev Drug Discov*, 9, 203-14.

Pepper, J.W. (2008) Defeating pathogen drug resistance: guidance from evolutionary theory. *Evolution*, 62, 3185-91.

Pepper, J.W., Scott Findlay, C., Kassen, R., Spencer, S.L. & Maley, C.C. (2009) Cancer research meets evolutionary biology. *Evol Appl*, 2, 62-70.

Price, G.R. (1972) Fisher's 'fundamental theorem' made clear. *Ann Hum Genet*, 36, 129-40.

Read, A.F., Day, T. & Huijben, S. (2011) Colloquium Paper: The evolution of drug resistance and the curious orthodoxy of aggressive chemotherapy. *Proc Natl Acad Sci U S A*, 108 Suppl 2, 10871-7.

Reece, S.E., Ramiro, R.S. & Nussey, D.H. (2009) Plastic parasites: sophisticated strategies for survival and reproduction? *Evol Appl*, 2, 11-23.

Searls, D.B. (2003) Pharmacophylogenomics: genes, evolution and drug targets. *Nat Rev Drug Discov*, 2, 613-23.

Seoighe, C., Ketwaroo, F., Pillay, V., Scheffler, K., Wood, N., Duffet, R., Zvelebil, M., Martinson, N., McIntyre, J., Morris, L. & Hide, W. (2007) A model of directional selection applied to the evolution of drug resistance in HIV-1. *Mol Biol Evol*, 24, 1025-31.

Slep, K.C., Kercher, M.A., He, W., Cowan, C.W., Wensel, T.G. & Sigler, P.B. (2001) Structural determinants for regulation of phosphodiesterase by a G protein at 2.0 A. *Nature*, 409, 1071-7.

Sowa, M.E., He, W., Slep, K.C., Kercher, M.A., Lichtarge, O. & Wensel, T.G. (2001) Prediction and confirmation of a site critical for effector regulation of RGS domain activity. *Nat Struct Biol*, 8, 234-7.

Sowa, M.E., He, W., Wensel, T.G. & Lichtarge, O. (2000) A regulator of G protein signaling interaction surface linked to effector specificity. *Proc Natl Acad Sci U S A*, 97, 1483-8.

Swinney, D.C. & Anthony, J. (2011) How were new medicines discovered? *Nat Rev Drug Discov*, 10, 507-19.

Thompson, N.S. (2000) Shifting the natural selection metaphor to the group level. *Behavior and Philosophy*, 28, 83-101.

Uren, A.G., O'Rourke, K., Aravind, L.A., Pisabarro, M.T., Seshagiri, S., Koonin, E.V. & Dixit, V.M. (2000) Identification of paracaspases and metacaspases: two ancient families of caspase-like proteins, one of which plays a key role in MALT lymphoma. *Mol Cell*, 6, 961-7.

van Zandbergen, G., Bollinger, A., Wenzel, A., Kamhawi, S., Voll, R., Klinger, M., Muller, A., Holscher, C., Herrmann, M., Sacks, D., Solbach, W. & Laskay, T. (2006) Leishmania disease development depends on the presence of apoptotic promastigotes in the virulent inoculum. *Proc Natl Acad Sci U S A*, 103, 13837-42.

Wang, Y. & Gu, X. (2001) Functional divergence in the caspase gene family and altered functional constraints: statistical analysis and prediction. *Genetics*, 158, 1311-20.

Wargo, A.R., Huijben, S., de Roode, J.C., Shepherd, J. & Read, A.F. (2007) Competitive release and facilitation of drug-resistant parasites after therapeutic chemotherapy in a rodent malaria model. *Proc Natl Acad Sci U S A*, 104, 19914-9.

Wessler, S.A., Diggle, S.P., Buckling, A., Gardner, A. & Griffin, A.S. (2007) The social lives of microbes. *Annu Rev Ecol Evol Syst*, 38, 53-77.

Wilson, D.S. (1975) A theory of group selection. *Proc Natl Acad Sci U S A*, 72, 143-6.

Yang, Z. (1997) PAML: a program package for phylogenetic analysis by maximum likelihood. *Comput Appl Biosci*, 13, 555-6.

Yang, Z. (2006) *Computational molecular evolution*. Oxford University Press, ISBN-13: 9780198567028 New York.

Yang, Z. (2007) PAML 4: phylogenetic analysis by maximum likelihood. *Mol Biol Evol*, 24, 1586-91.

Yang, Z. & Nielsen, R. (2000) Estimating synonymous and nonsynonymous substitution rates under realistic evolutionary models. *Mol Biol Evol*, 17, 32-43.

3

Novel Oncology Drug Development Strategies in the Era of Personalised Medicine

C.R. Lemech[1,2], R.S. Kristeleit[2] and H.T. Arkenau[1,2]
[1]*Sarah Cannon Research UK, London*
[2]*Cancer Institute, University College London*
UK

1. Introduction

In this era of personalised medicine, the focus of oncology drug development is shifting from classic chemotherapeutic drugs to rationally designed molecularly targeted agents (MTAs). This development has been accelerated by improved understanding of the key features of human tumour biology which have emerged over the last decade. A seminal paper by Hanahan and Weinberg (2000) proposed six vital elements for tumour formation, survival and progression. The six *'Hallmarks of Cancer'* were sustained proliferative signalling, evasion of growth suppressors, resistance to cell death, replicative immortality, angiogenesis and activation of invasion and metastasis. Hanahan and Weinberg updated their findings in 2011 with further evidence describing the complexity of these hallmarks and the addition of further hallmarks, including modification of energy metabolism to fuel cell growth and evasion of immunosurveillance. The tumour micro-environment is also a critical factor in the regulation of tumour growth and progression, with multiple stromal cell types creating a succession of supportive tumour micro-environments enabling invasion of normal tissue and subsequent metastasis.

Recent successes have utilised these advances in understanding to create a strong biologic rationale for drug development, primarily focusing on targets of a single '*Hallmark*'.

However, a number of challenges remain, not only in understanding the complex molecular pathways and networks, their interaction and mechanisms of resistance, but also in the drug development process through early incorporation of biomarkers to create rational drug development strategies. Challenges also lie in defining robust criteria to appropriately select patients for novel therapies. Effective trial design with integration of patient enrichment strategies is paramount to streamline drug development and deliver timely information to guide progress of drugs along the pipeline. The application of new technologies and novel strategies that address these problems will be discussed in detail in this chapter.

2. From hypothesis to proof of concept

Historically, the emphasis for drug development has focused on evidence-based medicine in large trials of unselected patient populations, with the benchmark endpoint for new drugs being overall survival or other intermediate endpoints. This *'one size fits all'* paradigm did not always take into account intra- and interpatient tumour heterogeneity commonly leading to large scale failure rates of multinational phase-III trials.

Incorporating measures of pathway activity and tumour efficacy into early phase trials may help avoid failure in later phases of drug development. Early validation of pharmacodynamic assays to measure target blockade and assess optimal dose range and dosing schedule is essential. Establishing *'proof-of-concept'* can then correlate anti-tumour activity in a selected patient population with validated predictive and intermediate endpoint biomarkers (De Bono & Ashworth., 2010).

For example, in patients with non-small cell lung cancer (NSCLC), correlation of epidermal growth factor receptor (EGFR) mutations with response to the EGFR inhibitors, gefitinib or erlotinib, occurred only after a number of negative trials. Although phase-II data in the second-line setting in patients with NSCLC was encouraging, when taken to a phase-III trial in an unselected group of patients with refractory disease, gefitinib failed to show a benefit in either overall survival or time-to-treatment failure when compared to placebo (Thatcher et al., 2005). In this context, it was only that retrospective analyses could help identify a sub-population benefiting from treatment including being a female, never-smoker and of Asian origin. Similarly, erlotinib demonstrated progression-free and overall survival benefits both in the second-line setting and as maintenance therapy in patients with stable disease after first-line chemotherapy (Cappuzzo et al., 2010; Shepherd et al., 2005). However, the incremental benefits in these unselected patient populations were small, measured in weeks for progression-free survival and 1-2 months for overall survival. Ultimately it was the selection of patients based on EGFR mutation status that demonstrated a marked improvement in response rates and survival in phase-III trials comparing chemotherapy and gefitinib (Fukuoka et al., 2011), as well as chemotherapy and erlotinib in the first-line setting (Rosell et al., 2011).

We have witnessed similar studies in patients with advanced colorectal cancer (ACRC) treated with the monoclonal antibody cetuximab. Initially, treatment with cetuximab was conducted in patients with EGFR over-expression, assessed by immunohistochemistry (IHC) on formalin-fixed paraffin-embedded (FFPE) tumour specimens (Cunningham et al., 2004). It was only later that the importance of Kirsten rat sarcoma-2 virus oncogene (KRAS) mutation was demonstrated; and this, in combination with an increased understanding of the complex EGFR downstream signalling cascade were the first steps in identifying a predictive biomarker for EGFR directed therapies in patients with ACRC. Several studies identified that patients with KRAS mutation did not respond to EGFR directed therapies, whereas patients who had wildtype (wt) KRAS tumours had response rates of over 50% (Lievre et al., 2006; Karapetis et al., 2008). More recently, it has been demonstrated that in fact, not all KRAS mutations are created equal. Although the presence of the majority of KRAS mutations precludes response to the EGFR inhibitors in ACRC, other KRAS mutations, particularly in codon 13, may predict a response similar to that demonstrated in wt KRAS tumours (De Roock et al., 2010).

These are just a few examples that demonstrate how the improved understanding of tumour biology supports a hypothesis-driven approach to the discovery of compounds to potentially generate more selective inhibition of key signalling proteins, pathways and networks. In this context, one of the most challenging tasks is the identification of the right target and more importantly whether this target is 'druggable'. For example, although we know that RAS mutations are an early component of tumorigenesis and are identified in approximately 30% of human cancers, attempts to target RAS have been unsuccessful to date as complex molecular structures constrain binding to the active site or pocket (Gysin et al., 2011). In contrast, selective inhibition of the v-raf murine sarcoma viral oncogene homologue B1 (BRAF) in patients with BRAF V600 mutant melanoma is associated with a dramatic improvement in response rates and survival. The strong biologic rationale of this approach was established through identification of the importance of the mitogen-activated protein kinase (MAPK) pathway in this disease and will be discussed at a later point in this chapter.

3. Biomarker development

Predictive and prognostic biomarkers are increasingly important in tailoring treatment decisions for individual patients. These markers are objectively measured to evaluate pathological processes or pharmacological responses to a therapeutic intervention, and can be any kind of molecule, substance, or genetic marker which is traceable (Atkinson et al., 2001). Predictive biomarkers provide information on response to a treatment, whereas prognostic biomarkers give information about outcome independent of the treatment effect. Historically, biomarkers have often been developed in retrospective analyses and were only in some cases prospectively applied. The retrospective approach was often criticised for being slow and difficult in practice, as well as raising concerns regarding heterogenous sample collection and validity. There are increasing efforts to incorporate new biomarker strategies into the earliest stages of clinical trial design, whether these are mutational analyses, clinical, or imaging measures, so that information can be gathered early and continually revisited during and after trial completion to inform the clinical development process.

As witnessed with a number of targeted agents, such as trastuzumab in human epidermal growth factor receptor-2 (HER2) positive breast cancer, the prospective analysis of HER2 as a predictive biomarker in clinical trials resulted in higher response rates and increased survival in this selected patient population, both in the metastatic and adjuvant setting (Slamon et al., 2001; Romond et al., 2005). This selective approach not only led to better outcomes for this subgroup, but ultimately to shorter and streamlined regulatory approval timelines. The use of trastuzumab in an unselected breast cancer population would undoubtedly have masked its true efficacy and potentially curtailed its development.

Importantly this selective biomarker approach became a good example of what challenges researchers are facing when developing accurate, functional and standardised biomarker assays.

HER2 gene amplification was first observed to be a potential biomarker in breast cancer when its presence in 25% of axillary lymph-node positive breast cancers was correlated with worse prognosis (Slamon et al., 1987). Additional studies confirmed that HER2 protein over-expression was also a poor prognostic marker in breast cancer, correlating with decreased relapse-free and overall survival (Ravdin et al., 1995). The trastuzumab clinical trials were initially designed using HER2 over-expression measured by IHC with a centralised sponsor developed assay, which was particularly important as there was no standardised assay at that time. As the testing of HER2 was expanded from central to local laboratories, with incorporation of fluorescence in-situ hybridisation (FISH) in addition to IHC, there were concerns about the correlation and regulation of such assays.

Although the results of the five adjuvant trastuzumab trials in HER2 positive early stage breast cancer clearly showed a significant clinical benefit in both progression-free and overall survival, the testing algorithms for HER2 were not consistent across these trials. HER2 testing included either IHC supported by FISH testing for intermediate IHC result (IHC2+) or reliance on FISH testing alone to assess gene amplification ratios. Concern was generated at the lack of accuracy and validation of HER2 testing in some instances as several assays were in use, including both validated assays, but also so called "home brew" assays developed in local pathology laboratories. Sub-studies from two of the adjuvant trials demonstrated that approximately 20% of HER2 assays performed at the primary treatment site were incorrect compared to re-evaluation in a high volume, central laboratory (Paik et al., 2002; Roche et al., 2002). Furthermore, the sensitivity of IHC itself was of concern. For example, one study demonstrated that commercially available US Food and Drug Administration (FDA) approved IHC methods were significantly less accurate than FISH at correctly characterising tumours with known HER2 status. Depending on the IHC method and use of HER2 antibody, correlation with FISH positivity ranged between 67-83%, with greater susceptibility to inter-observer variation (Bartlett et al., 2001).

Clearly in the case of IHC testing, several contributing factors may further impact on sensitivity and specificity including initial sample processing, time to and type of fixation, analytic variables of assay validation, equipment calibration, use of standardised laboratory procedures, training of staff, test reagents, use of standardised control materials and use of automated laboratory methods.

Slamon et al. (1989) demonstrated that a proportion of breast cancers known to have gene amplification and over-expression of HER2, in fact lose membrane staining after paraffin embedding and are negative on IHC assessment. Loss of antigenicity resulting in a potential false negative IHC can be affected by poor standardisation of fixative methods.

To overcome this lack of concordance in HER2 testing, which can so markedly impact on patients' prognosis and survival, an American Society of Clinical Oncology (ASCO) panel developed guidelines to improve the accuracy of HER2 testing (Wolff et al., 2007). These recommendations covered over 30 aspects of testing and requirements including the HER2 testing algorithm, optimal FISH and IHC testing and interpretation, tissue handling, internal validation and quality assurance procedures, optimal external proficiency, laboratory accreditation and regulatory requirements, statistical requirements for assay validation and international external quality assessment initiatives. Despite these guidelines, there were concerns that IHC assessment still lacked sufficient sensitivity to be used alone to decide on HER2 status (Carlson., 2008) though this remains the standard initial assessment in most laboratories.

In 2010, the addition of trastuzumab to first-line chemotherapy in HER2 positive advanced gastric cancer demonstrated a survival benefit (Bang et al., 2010). Similar to breast cancer, approximately 20-30% of gastric and gastro-oesophageal junction (GOJ) cancers show HER2 over-expression, but the testing criteria in gastric specimens differs significantly (Albarello et al., 2011). This is related to the increased frequency of heterogeneity of HER2 positivity in gastric cancer compared with breast cancer, as well as variations in membrane staining and the number of stained cells necessary to diagnose a positive case. In addition there is also less stringent correlation between HER2 amplification and protein over-expression with more than 20% of cases carrying HER2 amplification, often of low level, without HER2 expression. Clinically in this group of patients, there is no apparent benefit from adding trastuzumab to chemotherapy (Bang et al., 2010). Similarly, Hofmann et al. (2008a) demonstrated concordance between FISH and IHC of 93%, with 7% of specimens demonstrating FISH positivity with negative or equivocal IHC staining.

melanoma, nor were the pharmacodynamic markers from the early phase trials translated into the design of the phase-III trials. The failure of this drug development programme in melanoma could have been mitigated if phase-II data had been critically reviewed and early *'go or no-go'* decisions had been incorporated in the decision making process for the phase-III trials.

Similarly, the development of bevacizumab as a drug targeting the *'angiogenic switch'* and tumour-associated neo-vasculature met with much anticipation (Hanahan & Folkman, 1996). Bevacizumab is a humanised monoclonal antibody targeting VEGF-A and its binding to VEGFR2. There was early pre-clinical evidence that it not only inhibited the formation of new blood vessels, but also caused regression of existing micro-vessels and stabilised the mature vasculature to improve drug delivery. Significant clinical benefit Has been demonstrated with bevacizumab in combination with chemotherapy in advanced colorectal cancer but despite promising data regarding potential clinical, biochemical and radiological parameters, a predictive biomarker remains elusive (Hurwitz et al., 2004; Jubb & Harris, 2010). Although bevacizumab is now approved in several disease entities, the broad use in many tumour types remains controversial, bearing in mind its associated cost and toxicity. In this context, the lack of proven and validated biomarkers to predict the patient population most likely to benefit is often criticised and in part may have contributed to the withdrawal by the FDA of its approval in metastatic breast cancer.

On the contrary, the development of selective BRAF inhibitors for BRAF V600 mutation positive advanced cutaneous melanoma commenced with a strong biologic rationale and its success was facilitated by the validation of an associated predictive biomarker (Figure 2). Aberrant activation of the MAPK pathway has been demonstrated in over 80% of primary melanomas, due to abnormalities at various levels' along the RAS-RAF-MEK-ERK pathway with subsequent acceleration of cell growth, proliferation and differentiation (Platz et al., 2008). BRAF mutations are among the most studied, occurring in 36-59% of primary melanomas (Houben et al., 2004; Jakob et al., 2011; Long et al., 2011) and 42-66% of metastatic melanomas and have been characterised as oncogenic mutations (Davies et al., 2002; Karasarides et al., 2004). Early phase trials with the selective BRAF inhibitors, vemurafenib (PLX4032) and GSK 2118436, have demonstrated response rates far higher than standard chemotherapy with impressive improvements in survival (Chapman et al., 2011; Flaherty et al., 2010; Kefford et al., 2010; Ribas et al., 2011.). Thus, the identification of *'the right target'*, the BRAF mutation, lent itself to the development of *'the right drug'*, the selective BRAF inhibitors, whose efficacy could be predicted by *'the right biomarker'*, presence of a BRAF mutation.

Activating mutations or translocations of the anaplastic lymphoma kinase gene (ALK) have been identified in several types of cancer, with the EML4-ALK fusion gene evident in 2-7% of all NSCLC. EML4-ALK is an aberrant fusion gene that encodes a cytoplasmic chimeric protein with constitutive kinase activity. It is more prevalent in patients who are never or light smokers and in patients with adenocarcinoma histology. Crizotinib is a selective inhibitor of the ALK and MET tyrosine kinases and has shown unprecedented response rates and clinical benefit in a phase-I trial of heavily pretreated patients with advanced NSCLC harbouring ALK rearrangement (Kwak et al., 2010). The study incorporated molecular analysis of tumour samples with prospective tumour genotyping, including analysis via FISH, IHC and reverse-transcriptase-polymerase-chain-reaction (RT-PCR). FISH positivity for ALK rearrangement strongly correlated with aberrant expression of the ALK protein on IHC and many patients, though not all, also had positive results for EML4-ALK on the RT-PCR assay. The use of prospective tumour genotyping not only potentiated the development of diagnostic approaches for these patients but has also streamlined rapid drug development for crizotinib. Remarkably, there were only three years between target identification, initiation of the phase-I trial and enrolment on the phase-III registration trial and stands in contrast to more than ten years from the initial unsuccessful trials of EGFR inhibitors in non-genotyped unselected patients to the phase–III trials that demonstrated benefit of EGFR inhibitors in EGFR-mutant tumours (Kwak et al., 2010). Again, there is strong supporting evidence for *'the right target'* and *'the right drug'* in this setting, whilst development of *'the right biomarker'* has been incorporated into the phase-I trials to assist in overcoming the many complexities inherent with new assay validation.

1. Development of a strong biologic rationale Mutations along the MAPK pathway present in up to 80% of metastatic melanomas In vitro evidence with vemurafenib (PLX4032) and GSK 2118436 of selective inhibition of BRAF V600E and impaired tumour growth in mouse models
2. Biomarkers for early phase trials Prognostic Biomarker: BRAF aberrations Predictive Biomarker: BRAF V600E aberrations (and V600K with GSK118436) Pharmacodynamic Biomarkers: pMEK and pERK
3. Confirmation of a clinical response Phase 1/2 trials (vemurafenib): RR 50-80%; PFS >7m Phase 1/2 trials (GSK 2118436): RR 60%; PFS 8.3m Phase 3 trial (vemurafenib vs dacarbazine): RR 48% v 5%; PFS 5.3m v 1.6m OS at 6m 84% v 64%
4. Dissecting the Mechanisms of Resistance Longitudinal biopsies pre-treatment, on treatment and on progression On-target effect demonstrated by suppression of pMEK and pERK, and decreased staining of proliferative markers on IHC (cyclin D1 and Ki67) Resistance possible through alternate signalling in MAPK pathway or via bypass pathway signalling **Vemurafenib** Some tumours demonstrate increased pMEK/pERK on progression with reactivation of MAPK pathway Evidence of NRAS and MEK mutations which mediate signalling via the MAPK pathway Evidence of PTEN loss and increase pAkt demonstrates activation of PI3K-AKT-mTOR pathway **GSK 2118436** Abnormal PTEN associated with shorter PFS and loss of inhibition of the PI3K-AKT pathway CDKN2A and KIT deletion associated with shorter PFS

MAPK: mitogen-activated protein kinase; IHC: immunohistochemistry;
BRAF: v-raf murine sarcoma viral oncogene homologue B1;
pMEK: phosphorylated MEK; pERK: phosphorylated ERK; pAKT: phosphorylated AKT; RR: response rate; PFS: progression-free survival, OS: overall survival;
PI3K: phosphatidylinositol 3-kinase; mTOR: mammalian target of rapamycin

Fig. 2. Selective BRAF Inhibitors for BRAF mutant Metastatic Melanoma

In haematological malignancies, the development of the phosphatidylinositol 3-kinase (PI3K) inhibitor, CAL-101, has shown encouraging results in advanced non-hodgkins lymphoma (NHL), mantle cell lymphoma and chronic lymphocytic leukaemia (CLL) (Herman et al., 2010). CAL-101 is a selective inhibitor of the PI3K p110 δ isoform that is primarily expressed on cells of haematopoietic origin and has a key role in B cell maturation and function. Through inhibition of PI3K signalling, CAL-101 can induce apoptosis of primary CLL and acute myelogenous leukaemia (AML) cells and a range of other leukaemia and lymphoma cell lines (Lannutti et al., 2010). In phase-I studies, CAL-101 has demonstrated durable clinical responses in a number of haematological malignancies, including NHL (Flinn et al., 2009). Reduction in phosphorylated AKT (pAKT) as a marker of PI3K activation provides *'proof-of-mechanism'* for this agent and later phase trials are underway in B cell malignancies with markers along the PI3Kδ pathway acting as predictive biomarkers.

These recent *'proof-of-concept'* studies were the first of their kind where molecular profiles were used for selection of *'new in class'* compounds and demonstrate that when patients are appropriately selected, convincing benefit can be realised in the earliest of trials, setting the stage for rapid drug approval. This phase-I experience has convinced investigators that tumour profiling and patient selection will become a routine part of cancer drug development.

5. Challenges in drug development

5.1 Mechanisms of resistance

Despite the advances in parallel drug and biomarker development in early clinical trials, one of the major challenges remaining is the understanding of mechanisms that cause primary and acquired or secondary resistance. Primary resistance is characterised by lack of efficacy of an agent from treatment initiation, whereas acquired resistance develops after an initial response of some degree over a period of time.

As evidenced by all currently approved molecularly targeted agents, initial treatment may yield response rates far higher than standard chemotherapy with impressive disease control, but inevitably resistance and tumour progression develops. Importantly, understanding the mechanisms of resistance can lead to rationally designed drug combinations incorporating targeted agents, antibodies, or cytotoxics. This approach should include continuous analysis of tumour material via biopsies on disease progression or surrogate markers such as circulating tumour cells (CTCs) or circulating free DNA (cfDNA). In this context, cancer treatment could follow strategies as witnessed by the treatment of tuberculosis with quadruple combination regimens or human immunodeficiency virus (HIV) with highly active antiretroviral therapy (HAART). In a similar way, cancer drugs will be used in parallel or sequentially to block different driver pathways and networks simultaneously.

Although there are a number of mechanisms of resistance that are particular to molecularly targeted agents and are intrinsic to the pathway they inhibit, there are other mechanisms that are common to both cytotoxic chemotherapy and molecularly targeted agents falling into three main categories: decreased uptake, such as occurs with water-soluble drugs like the folate antagonists; impaired capacity of cytoxic drugs to induce cell kill via a combination of altered cell cycle checkpoints, increased or altered drug targets, repair of DNA damage and inhibition of apoptosis; or increased drug efflux (Gottesman et al., 2002; Szakacs et al., 2006).

The presence of efflux pumps is one of the best described mechanisms of resistance and is thought to be common to both cytotoxic chemotherapy and the molecularly targeted agents. P-glycoprotein (P-gp), otherwise known as the multidrug transporter, is an energy dependent efflux pump that has been identified as a major mechanism of multidrug resistance (MDR) in cultured cancer cells. It is the product of the MDR1 gene in humans and is one member of a large family of ATP-dependent transporters known as the ATP-binding cassette (ABC family). P-gp is widely expressed in many human cancers including cancers of the gastrointestinal tract, hematopoietic system, genitourinary system and childhood cancers. P-gp can detect and bind a large variety of hydrophobic natural-product drugs as they enter the plasma membrane including chemotherapeutic agents such as doxorubicin, vinblastine and paclitaxel, as well as anti-arrhythmics, antihistamines and the HIV protease inhibitors (Robert., 1999). Increased drug efflux was initially thought to be a significant mechanism of resistance for the tyrosine kinase inhibitor imatinib in patients with CML (Mahon et al., 2003). However, it is not fully understood how much impact this resistance mechanism has on molecularly targeted drugs as a prime source of resistance.

Another relevant mechanism of resistance that has been illustrated in a number of cancers involves the disruption of interacting proteins and receptors on the plasma membrane level impacting on receptor binding and subsequent drug efficacy. For example, EGFR is a membrane-bound receptor whose signalling involves a complex pathway of ligand binding, receptor homo- and heterodimerisation with ERBB2 and other family members, followed by internalisation and recycling of the ligand-bound receptor. Significant EGF-dependent signalling may occur during the process of internalisation and alterations in EGFR trafficking have been linked to cellular responses (Wiley et al., 2003). Analysis of EGFR trafficking in resistant lung cancer cell lines demonstrated increased internalisation of EGFR compared to parental drug-sensitive cells, which interestingly could be overcome by the action of irreversible EGFR inhibitors (Kwak et al., 2005). Similarly in breast cancer, one of the proposed mechanisms of resistance to trastuzumab involves membrane-associated glycoprotein mucin-4 (MUC4) which may block the inhibitory actions of trastuzumab by directly binding with HER2 and preventing interaction between the drug and the molecular target (Nagy et al., 2005).

Primary or secondary mutations and aberrations at the level, up- or downstream of the target are also frequently studied mechanisms of resistance to the molecularly targeted agents. For example, primary resistance to the EGFR targeted agents, gefitinib and erlotinib, has been associated with the presence of a KRAS mutation in 20-30% of NSCLC patients, or via an insertion mutation in exon 20 of EGFR, which represents fewer than 5% of all known mutations in the EGFR gene (Hammerman et al., 2009). Secondary resistance to the EGFR inhibitors after an initial response is mediated by the T790M mutation in 50-59% of patients, characterised by the substitution of methionine for threonine at position 790 (T790M) in EGFR (Pao et al., 2005). In this case, biological understanding of primary and secondary resistance allows for development of rationally designed drugs. Pre-clinical evidence demonstrated that an irreversible inhibitor of EGFR, such as neratinib (HKI-272), could overcome resistance induced by T790M-mutant EGFR and such agents are currently in clinical development (Kobayashi et al., 2005; Kwak et al., 2005).

Recent advances in the treatment of melanoma have further assisted in the understanding of the complexity of resistance mechanisms. For example although secondary BRAF mutations have not been identified as a cause of BRAF inhibitor resistance, mutations elsewhere along the MAPK pathway have been implicated, including secondary NRAS and MEK mutations.

MEK mutations have been demonstrated to cause reactivation of ERK signalling despite BRAF or MEK inhibition both in vitro and in vivo (Corcoran et al., 2011; Emery et al., 2009; Wagle et al., 2011). Similarly NRAS mutations, such as the NRAS Q61K mutation, have been demonstrated in BRAF mutant melanoma cell lines resistant to vemurafenib, and in a nodal biopsy from a patient who progressed after an initial response on treatment (Nazarian et al., 2010). The presence of an NRAS mutation can result in persistently elevated pMEK and pERK levels despite BRAF inhibition and is thought to signal through RAS and subsequently through RAF isoforms other then BRAF (Nazarian et al., 2010).

Signalling via the CRAF isoform is also a significant mechanism of resistance, with increased CRAF activity and a switch from BRAF to CRAF dependency demonstrated in BRAF mutant melanoma cell lines that are resistant to RAF inhibition (Montagut et al., 2008). Importantly, sensitivity to MEK inhibition was maintained in these cell lines, supporting further novel drug combinations, such as a non-selective RAF inhibitor or selective CRAF inhibitor with a MEK or BRAF inhibitor to overcome this mechanism of resistance.

Amplification of the mutant BRAF allele has also been implicated in resistance via increased pMEK and subsequently pERK signalling, though the evidence for this lies in studies of BRAF mutant colorectal cancer cell lines. In three such cell lines, BRAF amplification was demonstrated as a mechanism of acquired resistance to MEK inhibitors with cross-resistance to BRAF inhibitors, although to a lesser degree (Corcoran et al., 2010; Little et al., 2011). Preclinical studies showed that increased concentrations of RAF or MEK inhibitors, as well as the combination of the two agents, could suppress ERK phosphorylation and downstream signalling (Corcoran et al., 2010).

Changes in signalling upstream of a target pathway as well as bypass signalling along alternate pathways have also been demonstrated as mechanisms of resistance (Figure 3). In this context the insulin-like growth factor 1 receptor (IGF1R) which signals upstream of the PI3K-AKT-mTOR and MAPK pathways has been found to contribute to resistance in a number of malignancies. For example, activity of trastuzumab was impaired in breast cancer cells that over-expressed both HER2 and IGF1R, but its activity could be restored when IGF1R activation was blocked (Lu et al., 2001). Moreover, in vitro models have demonstrated that IGF1R physically interacts with and induces phosphorylation of HER2 in trastuzumab-resistant cells, but not in trastuzumab-sensitive cells, with subsequent increased signalling through the PI3K-AKT-mTOR and MAPK pathways. Again, inhibition of IGF1R signalling either by antibody blockade or tyrosine kinase inhibition restored trastuzumab sensitivity, demonstrating another potential therapeutic mechanism to overcome secondary resistance to trastuzumab. Similar findings were also evident in BRAF V600E melanoma cell lines resistant to BRAF inhibition, providing early evidence for the combination of IGF1R and MEK inhibition in this setting. (Villanueva et al., 2010).

A number of other preclinical studies have also demonstrated aberrant activation of the PI3K-AKT pathway at other levels that contributes to both primary and secondary resistance in BRAF mutant cell lines (Jiang et al., 2011; Shao et al., 2010). Just as the combination of IGF1R inhibition with MEK inhibition is being investigated to overcome resistance mediated along the IGF1R and MAPK pathways, there may be a biologic rationale for the combination of PI3K and MEK inhibitors (Jiang et al., 2010). In such cases, phosphorylated AKT may act as a marker of activity of the PI3K-AKT-mTOR pathway and thus, may be used as a biomarker to select when the combination of PI3K inhibitors and BRAF/MEK inhibitors is appropriate to block both the PI3K and MAPK pathways respectively.

PTEN loss (PTEN-) and subsequent lack of inhibition on the PI3K-AKT-mTOR pathway has also been demonstrated to confer resistance to BRAF inhibition. Paraiso et al. (2011) showed that in cell lines with PTEN loss compared to cell lines with normal PTEN, BRAF inhibition with vemurafenib was associated with increased AKT signalling and decreased apoptosis. Dual treatment of PTEN- cell lines with both vemurafenib and a PI3K inhibitor could then restore increased levels of apoptosis (Paraiso et al., 2011).

Exemplified by preclinical and clinical examples in melanoma, signalling via the PI3K-AKT-mTOR pathway mediates an important MAPK-pathway independent mechanism of resistance in a variety of cancers and demonstrates a complex crosstalk between these pathways (Corcoran et al., 2011). Measurement of phosphorylated ERK and phosphorylated AKT to determine pathway activity may therefore help to guide therapeutic choices and combinations of selective BRAF, MEK or PI3K/AKT inhibitors. Thus, knowledge of secondary resistance mechanisms will increasingly influence decision making processes for further drug development and rational drug combinations.

Although mechanisms of secondary resistance are well described for several new targeted agents, challenges remain, particularly with anti-angiogenic or multitargeted agents such as bevacizumub, sunitinib and sorafenib. The complexity of resistance mechanisms to anti-angiogenic therapy reflects the difficulty in developing anti-angiogenic agents in parallel with corresponding biomarkers.

So far, two main resistance mechanisms for anti-angiogenic agents have been proposed: firstly, evasive resistance with adaptation to circumvent specific angiogenic blockade, and secondly, intrinsic or pre-existing indifference (Bergers & Hanahan., 2008). Evasion of anti-angiogenic therapy may occur via up-regulation of alternative pro-angiogenic signalling circuits or via a number of alterations in the micro-environment, including recruitment of vascular progenitor cells and pro-angiogenic monocytes from the bone marrow, increased and tight pericyte coverage protecting tumour blood vessels and increased capacity for invasion without angiogenesis.

Alternate pro-angiogenic signals that have been implicated in preclinical studies include fibroblast growth factor (FGF)-1 and -2, ephrin A1 and A2 and angiopoietin-1. To establish the significance of these up-regulated genes, preclinical studies used the combination of FGF signalling suppression with VEGFR inhibitors and demonstrated that the combination of these agents attenuated re-vascularisation and slowed tumour growth (Casanovas et al., 2005). These findings were also seen clinically in patients with glioblastoma treated with the VEGFR inhibitor cediranib (Batchelor et al., 2007). After initial response, peripheral blood levels of FGF2 increased when patients progressed, suggesting that signalling through FGF assists in restoring angiogenesis. Elevated levels of pro-angiogenic factors such as VEGF and placental growth factor (PGF) have been previously proposed as predictive biomarkers for tumour response (Bocci et al., 2004). However there is also evidence that the expression of pro-angiogenic growth factors such as FGF, PDGF and others increase in advanced stages of metastatic breast cancer, resulting in alternate pathway signalling (Relf et al., 1997). Thus, there is uncertainty regarding the significance of these factors; whether the presence of pro-angiogenic factors in peripheral blood are in fact markers of response or resistance, or neither. Understanding the complex regulatory networks, the interaction of pro- and anti-angiogenic factors and contributing components of the micro-environment, illustrates the difficulties to-date in target and biomarker development, as well as the potential mechanisms by which anti-angiogenic therapy can be optimised.

Malignancy and Drug	Target	Biomarker	Mechanisms of Resistance Under investigation
Breast cancer			
Tamoxifen	Estrogen receptor	ER/PR status on IHC	Loss of ER expression Epigenetic changes in ER gene Increased drug metabolism ER/HER2 cross-talk PI3K-AKT pathway activation Alterations in co-regulatory proteins (Ring et al., 2004)
Trastuzumab	HER2 receptor	HER2 expression on IHC and/or FISH	MUC4 binding to HER2 (Nagy et al.; 2005) HER2 & IGF1R crosstalk (Lu et al., 2001) PI3K-AKT pathway signalling and PTEN loss
Bevacizumab*	VEGF-A and VEGFR2	Nil currently validated Preliminary evidence on clinical, biochemical and radiological assessments	Alternate pro-angiogenic signalling circuits (eg. FGF) Bone marrow derived vascular progenitor cells & pro-angiogenic monocytes Increased pericyte coverage (Bergers & Hanahan, 2008)
Melanoma			
Sorafenib	RAF, VEGFR, PDGFRβ, cKIT, FLT3	Nil currently validated	Alternate pro-angiogenic signalling, PDGFR mt Glucose-regulated protein 78 (Chiou et al., 2010)
Vemurafenib/ GSK 2118436	BRAF V600E/K mt	BRAF mt status	Upstream: IGF1R, PDGF upregulation, NRAS mt (Nazarian et al., 2010; Villanueva et al., 2010)) Target level: BRAF amplification, CRAF activity (Corcoran et al., 2011; Montagut et al., 2008) Downstream: MEK mt (Corcoran et al., 2011) Alternate pathway signalling: PI3K-AKT-mTOR activation
Lung Cancer			
Erlotinib/ Gefitinib	EGFR	EGFR mt status	KRAS mt EGFR T790M mt (Pao et al., 2005) EGFR insertion mt in exon 20 (Hammerman et al., 2009) EGFR trafficking (Kwak et al., 2005)

Malignancy and Drug	Target	Biomarker	Mechanisms of Resistance Under investigation
Crizotinib	ALK and MET tyrosine kinases	EML4-ALK expression on IHC, ISH and/or RT PCR	EML4-ALK with C1156Y mt EML4-ALK with L1196M mt (Choi et al., 2010)
Colorectal Cancer			
Cetuximab	EGFR	KRAS mt (codon 12)	KRAS codon 61/146 mt BRAF mt (Loupakis et al., 2009) PIK3CA mt (Sartore-Bianchi et al., 2009) PTEN loss of expression (Frattini et al., 2007)
Haematologic malignancies			
Imatinib	BCR-ABL tyrosine kinase, cKIT	BCR-ABL mRNA on PCR (peripheral blood) Cytogenetic analysis on bone marrow aspirate	Drug efflux (Mahon et al., 2003) ATP binding site mt (Branford et al., 2003) KIT mutation (in GIST) (Tamborini et al.; 2004)
CAL-101	PI3K p110δ	pAkt and markers along the PI3K δ pathway	

*Evidence for bevacizumab also applies to colorectal cancer, NSCLC, renal cell carcinoma and other malignancies
ER: estrogen receptor, PR: progesterone receptor, HER2: human epidermal growth factor receptor 2; IHC: immunohistochemistry; mt: mutation
IGF1R: insulin growth factor-1 receptor; PDGF: platelet derived growth factor
EGFR: epidermal growth factor receptor; PI3K: phosphatidylinositol-3kinase
PTEN: phosphatise and tensin homologue

Fig. 3. Selected Examples of Molecularly Targeted Therapies and Mechanisms of Drug Resistance

5.2 The breakthroughs and dilemmas of recurrent tumour biopsies

Although many mechanisms of resistance can be identified through studies of cell lines and xenograft models, it is often through correlation with patients' tumour specimens that valid conclusions can be drawn about the significance of these resistance mechanisms in the clinical setting. To this end, access to longitudinal tumour biopsies and assessment of these in *'real-time'* may change the treatment paradigm for patients.

The need for longitudinal tumour biopsies is evidenced at a number of levels. Firstly, it assists in understanding and mapping the complex molecular networks, communication with the micro-environment, angiogenesis and other *'hallmarks'*. As technologies in tumour analysis improve, for example with high throughput genetic sequencing and unravelling the cancer genome, findings on the pre-clinical level can be investigated and explored clinically and changes in tissue can be correlated with therapeutic response.

Secondly, there are multiple variables that can affect the accuracy of mutational analysis on tumour tissue, not least that the tumour itself can develop new mutations and aberrations that drive tumorigenesis. Studies of concordance or lack thereof, between archival primary tissue and biopsies of metastatic disease have demonstrated this in breast, colorectal and other malignancies. Analyses of HER2 over-expression in primary breast cancer and metastatic sites demonstrate that up to 12% of patients may have HER2 negative primary breast cancers with HER2 positivity at the metastatic sites, and subsequent potential therapeutic benefit from trastuzumab (Zidan et al., 2005). Conversely, up to 30% of tumours could switch from HER2 positive status on primary tissue to HER2 negative status on metastatic tissue, again significantly impacting on future treatment decisions (Locatelli et al., 2010).

In patients with advanced colorectal cancer, retrospective analyses have assessed the concordance of KRAS mutation status and other alterations along the MAPK and PI3K-AKT-mTOR pathways between primary tumours and metastatic sites. Loupakis et al. (2008) assessed PTEN status which regulates the PI3K-AKT-mTOR pathway, and demonstrated that PTEN loss occurred in 37% of tumours with associated lack of response to cetuximab and irinotecan. Interestingly the reported PTEN concordance between primary tumours and metastases was 60% compared to 95% for KRAS mutations. In those patients who were KRAS wild-type and PTEN positive on metastases, there was evidence for improved RR and PFS indicating the importance of pathway profiling to predict clinical response.

These examples underline the importance of tumour assessment not only for patients who develop metastatic disease after resection of a primary cancer, but also for patients with progressive disease on treatment. Understanding of the *'driving'* pathway, receptor or network before treatment initiation, especially with new molecularly targeted agents, will become standard of care for several new treatments and guide us in the decision making algorithm even in advanced stages of disease.

This can be further evidenced by a recent study in a cohort of heavily pre-treated phase-I patients who were tested for aberrations in the MAPK and PI3K-AKT-mTOR pathways and then treated with drugs targeting these pathways (Tsimberidou et al., 2011). Impressively, those patients with molecular alterations treated with targeted therapy had a response rate of 29% (complete response or partial response) compared to 8% in the group without alterations. The proportion of patients with stable disease beyond 6 months and the median survival were also higher in this patient group.

Importantly the recent early phase-I melanoma studies with selective BRAF inhibitors have incorporated tumour biopsies at baseline, on-treatment and on-progression biopsies to analyse the changes in pathway signalling (McArthur et al., 2011; Nathanson et al., 2011). The tumour analyses included not only immunohistochemical staining, but also Sequenom MassARRAY of over 400 gene mutations, such as BRAF, RAS, PIK3CA, AKT1/2, CDK4 and others. Following this approach, patients were selected for the BRAF mutation at baseline and monitored during treatment with the measurement of phosphorylated MEK and ERK levels to confirm target inhibition. On progression, a number of potentially significant genetic alterations were identified, including NRAS and MEK1 mutations indicating continuing MAPK-pathway signalling. In addition PTEN loss and an increase in pAKT were observed, demonstrating activation of the PI3K-AKT-mTOR pathway as a possible alternate signalling pathway (Figure 2).

Clearly the risk-benefit of serial tumour biopsies needs to be well balanced and risks and disadvantages acknowledged. For example, in some cancers like NSCLC, access to tumour tissue is restricted by the site of disease with an increased potential risk of pneumothorax, bleeding and other complications secondary to a lung biopsy. Tissue biopsies also run the risk of sampling error, in part from tumour heterogeneity. As discussed with HER2 testing in gastric cancer, multiple biopsies may be required to minimise the chance of missing the alteration of interest, in this case HER2 amplification and protein over-expression. In addition sample handling, fixation, validation of assays, inter-observer variability and assessment, all contribute to the accuracy of the final result on which clinical decisions are made.

Finally, new technologies also need to be validated prior to routine introduction into clinical care. Although the ability to sequence the genome and perform genetic profiling on patients' tumours dramatically escalates the information available on an individual patient, the significance of this information is still, as yet, often unknown. The presence of a mutation does not determine its significance in tumorigenesis, such that inhibition of a given mutation will not correlate with clinical benefit, if the mutation was an incidental finding rather than an oncogenic mutation.

5.3 The role of circulating tumour cells and circulating free DNA

Detection of circulating tumour cells (CTCs), and circulating free DNA (cfDNA) in peripheral blood specimens potentially presents an easily accessible 'liquid biopsy' without the risk of tumour biopsies and further, may not only provide a predictive biomarker for a given treatment, but also contain information on molecular aberrations and changes in pathway signalling while on treatment.

There is increasing evidence that CTCs can be used as a surrogate endpoint for progression-free and overall survival and thus, allow an earlier assessment of the clinical benefit of a particular agent to streamline drug development and regulatory approval. Such 'surrogate endpoints' may accelerate drug development as long as adequate and well controlled clinical trials establish that the new drug has an effect on this surrogate, based on epidemiologic, therapeutic, pathophysiologic, or other evidence, and that this surrogate endpoint can predict clinical benefit and survival (Atkinson et al., 2001).

The enumeration of CTCs and their utility as a prognostic and predictive biomarker has been best characterised in breast, colorectal and prostate cancers with further evidence in other malignancies including melanoma and lung cancers. The most widely used and FDA approved method for CTC enumeration and molecular characterisation is the CellSearch system, which involves the immunomagnetic capture of CTCs using antibodies against the epithelial cell adhesion molecule (EpCAM), expressed on the cell surface of most epithelial malignancies. Additional cell identification includes the detection of pan-cytokeratin antibodies, DAPI nuclear staining (4,6-diamidino-2-phenylindole staining to detect nucleated cells) and CD45 negative selection to demonstrate the detected cell is not a leucocyte.

The presence of CTCs at baseline in metastatic breast cancer has not only been demonstrated to have prognostic significance but has also been shown to be the strongest predictor of overall survival when compared to age, hormone receptor status, HER2 status and metastatic site. It also maintains its prognostic value independent of line of treatment, site of recurrence and disease phenotype (Cristofanilli et al., 2005). Preliminary studies in breast cancer suggest that CTC enumeration may even be superior to radiological evaluation in predicting response to treatment and outcome. It may provide a more reproducible indication of disease status compared to current imaging methods, particularly in view of inter-reader variability in confirming radiological response which can vary by up to 15% compared to 1% variability for CTC counts (Budd et al., 2006).

In castrate resistant prostate cancer, the presence of CTCs at baseline and lack of a decline during treatment is also indicative of poor response and survival. In multivariate analyses, CTC counts and PSA doubling time have been demonstrated as the only independent predictors for clinical outcome as compared to PSA level, Gleason Score, bone metastases and age (De Bono et al., 2008). Additionally, there is now evidence that CTCs may be a potential surrogate biomaker in metastatic prostate cancer trials. The randomised, double-blind phase III trial in metastatic prostate cancer, in which abiraterone was compared to placebo, was the first of its kind to demonstrate the utility of CTCs in this setting. CTCs were measured at baseline and repeated at 4, 8 and 12 weeks post treatment. Pre-treatment CTCs were strongly correlated with OS, as was a fall in CTC count on treatment (Reid et al., 2010; Scher et al., 2011). Particularly in the setting of castrate resistant prostate cancer where there may be inter-observer variation regarding radiological progression, CTCs may provide an accurate and reproducible alternative.

In patients with metastatic colorectal cancer, higher baseline CTC counts correlate with shorter PFS and OS. Again, conversion of an unfavourable baseline CTC count to a favourable count at 3-5 weeks after starting treatment is associated with longer PFS and OS compared with patients with unfavourable counts at both time points. Baseline and follow-up CTC levels also remain strong predictors of PFS and OS after adjustment for clinically significant factors (Cohen et al., 2008).

Recent evaluation of CTCs in patients with NSCLC has also suggested prognostic significance (Krebs et al., 2011). CTCs in patients with NSCLC were found more commonly with stage IV (32%) compared to stage IIIB disease (7%) and in those patients with five or more CTCs detected, both PFS and OS were inferior. Particularly with the complexities in obtaining longitudinal tissue biopsies, further investigation of a prognostic 'liquid biopsy' and incorporation into early phase trials is of importance.

In patients with advanced melanoma, recent studies have demonstrated good correlation between CTC status and tumor-node-metastasis stage, underlining the prognostic role of CTCs (Mocellin et al., 2006). The predictive value of CTCs was so far limited by the fact that treatment options consisted of bio-chemotherapies with no effects on clinical outcomes. However, the presence of circulating melanoma cells after adjuvant treatment for stage III melanoma has been shown to correlate with inferior relapse-free and overall survival and may be a useful indicator of systemic subclinical disease (Koyanagi et al., 2005). Isolation and molecular characterisation of these cells, combined with analysis of cfDNA, presents an opportunity to obtain further information about the pathways driving tumorigenesis, invasion and metastasis. In addition to evaluating the role of CTCs in melanoma, one study found good correlation between CTCs and cfDNA suggesting both markers may be a useful determinant of disease status and treatment effect. Patients with measurable CTC or cfDNA showed poorer disease outcome compared with patients without these markers, and patients with both markers showed the most inferior disease outcome, despite the fact that the treatment regimens were heterogenous and consisted of bio-chemotherapies of limited clinical benefit (Koyanagi et al., 2006).

5.4 Optimising trial design

Given the diversity of novel compounds discovered over the last decade, clinical trial design for the evaluation of these targeted agents has evolved with the agents being tested. Many of these agents do not cause typical chemotherapy-induced side effects such as myelosupression around which early phase trial design has been based. Therefore design of clinical trials of novel agents has had to develop in order to evaluate these agents appropriately and efficiently.

In a standard dose escalation phase I trial, cohorts of three to six patients are treated at pre-defined dose levels, dose-limiting toxicity (DLT) is observed and the maximum tolerated dose (MTD) is defined as the dose level where >33% of patients treated have experienced a DLT. Dose levels are commonly defined using modification of the original Fibonacci design (increasing dose by fixed increments of 100%, 67%, 50%, 40% followed by 33% for all subsequent levels) but slow attainment of the MTD and exposure of significant numbers of patients to low doses have been criticisms of this approach (Rogatko et al, 2007). An accelerated trial design (Simon et al, 1997) is now a widely accepted alternative to the Fibonacci dose-definition model and many trials now allow individual patients to be dose-escalated within a study if safe to do so, aiming to minimise those being exposed to ineffective doses. Therefore there are many combinations of model-based and rule-based designs that allow flexibility of the recruitment structure in a trial and can be appropriately adapted to the agent under consideration (Ivy et al., 2010; Parulekar et al., 2004; Rogatko et al, 2005; Korn et al, 2001; Cannistra et al., 2008; Sleijfer et al., 2008; Bria et al., 2009).

The appropriateness of the primary endpoint of maximum tolerated dose (MTD) has been challenged for some of these agents and consideration has been given instead to the concept of optimal biological dose (OBD) (O'Reilly et al., 2010; Le Tourneau et al., 2009). Targeted biological agents are more commonly cystostatic rather than cytotoxic, therefore other endpoints should be considered when evaluating treatment efficacy (Rixe et al., 2007; Gelmon et al., 1999) including novel radiographic assessment and immunotherapy assessment (Wolchok et al., 2009).

There has also been an increasing realization that patients need to be appropriately selected for certain agents based on tumour biology and molecular characteristics. The question is whether patient selection should take place at the outset of drug development, as a targeted approach which is then diversified; or whether a broader recruitment strategy should prevail initially, followed by testing within a targeted population. There is therefore a critical need to integrate and validate novel biomarkers into drug development from the earliest stages of evaluation, incorporating tumour and non-tumour tissue samples to apply these biomarkers appropriately and guide patient selection.

Overall, in the era of development of molecularly targeted agents, appropriately designed hypothesis-testing trials should be conducted. Patients should be selected rationally according to tumour biology and molecular characteristics and above all, an element of flexibility should be allowed within the trial design to enable response to unexpected findings, whether that be toxicity or efficacy.

6. Conclusion

The increased understanding of tumour biology and genetics along with improvements in laboratory methodologies and IT-systems will continue to make a tremendous impact on oncology drug development. Critical to future oncology drug development is the incorporation of biomarkers from the earliest stages and supported by applied bioinformatics. In addition, the use of new preclinical models and novel clinical trial designs incorporating intermediate surrogate biomarker endpoints will be essential not only for the better understanding of mechanisms of action of new targeted drugs, but also in supporting confident *'go or no-go decisions'*. The *'personalised medicine'* approach involving molecular characterisation of the tumour and its context within the micro-environment and immune system, will help to define the right treatment, for the right patient at the right time. Increasing our understanding on how to combine established and novel therapeutics in an efficient timeframe is critical to improved outcomes for the treatment of solid malignancies.

7. Acknowledgments

Diagrams were designed with the assistance of Sabina Pasha, Sarah Cannon Research UK.

8. References

Albarello, L.; Pecciarini, L. & Doglioni, C. (2011) HER2 testing in gastric cancer. *Advances in Anatomic Pathology;* 18(1): 53-59.

Bang, Y-J.; Van Cutsem, E. ; Feyereislova, A. ; et al. (2010) Trastuzumab in combination with chemotherapy versus chemotherapy alone for treatment of HER2-positive advanced gastric or gastro-oesophageal junction cancer (ToGA): a phase 3, open-label, randomised controlled trial. *Lancet;* 376 (9742): 687-697.

Bartlett, M.S.; Going, J.J.; Mallon, E.A.; et al. (2001) Evaluating HER2 amplification and overexpression in breast cancer. *The Journal of Path;* 195 (4): 422-428.

Batchelor, T.T.; Sorensen, A.G.; di Tomasi, E.; et al. (2007) AZD2171, a pan-VEGF receptor tyrosine kinase inhibitor, normalizes tumor vasculature and alleviates edema in glioblastoma patients. *Cancer Cell;* 11: 83-95.

Bergers, G. & Hanahan, D. (2008) Modes of resistance to anti-angiogenic therapy. *Nature Reviews;* 8: 592-603.

Atkinson, A.J.; Colburn, W.A.; DeGruttola, V.G.; et al. (2001) Biomarkers and surrogate endpoints: preferred definitions and conception framework. *Clin Pharmacol Ther;* 69: 89-95.

Bocci, G.; Man, S.; Green, S.K.; et al. (2004) Increased plasma vascular endothelial growth factor (VEGF) as a surrogate marker for optimal therapeutic dosing of VEGF receptor-2 monoclonal antibodies. *Cancer Res;* 64: 6616-6625.

Branford, S. ; Rudzki, Z. ; Walsh, S. ; et al. (2003) Detection of BCR-ABL mutations in patients with CML treated with imatinib is virtually always accompanied by clinical resistance, and mutations in the ATP phosphate-binding loop (P-loop) are associated with poor prognosis. *Blood* ; 102 (1) : 276-283.

Bria, E.; Di Maio, M.; Carlini, P.; et al. (2009) Targeting targeted agents: Open issues for clinical trial design. *J Exp Clin Cancer Res;* 28: 66.

Budd, G.T. ; Cristofanilli, M. ; Ellis, M.J. ; et al. (2006) Circulating tumour cells versus imaging - predicting overall survival in metastatic breast cancer. *Clin Cancer Res;* 12: 6403-6409.

Cannistra, S.A. (2008) Challenges and pitfalls of combining targeted agents in phase i studies. *J Clin Oncol;* 26(22): 3665-3667.

Cappuzzo, F. ; Ciuleanu, T.; Stelmakh, L.; et al. (2010) Erlotinib as maintenance treatment in advanced non-small-cell lung cancer: a multicentre, randomised, placebo-controlled phase 3 study. *The Lancet Oncology;* 11(6): 521-529.

Carlson, B. (2008) HER2 Tests: How Do We Choose? *Biotechnology Healthcare*; Sept/Oct edition: 23-27.

Casanovas, O.; Hicklin, D.J.; Bergers, G. & Hanahan, D. (2005) Drug resistance by evasion of antiangiogenic targeting of VEGF signaling in late-stage pancreatic islet tumours. *Cancer Cell*; 8: 299-309.

Chapman, P.B.; Hauschild, A.; Robert, C.; et al. (2011) Improved survival with vemurafenib in melanoma with BRAF V600E mutation. *New Engl J Med*; June (10.1056/NEJMoa1103782).

Chiou, J-F.; Tai, C-J.; Huang, M-T. ; et al. (2010) Glucose-regulated proteint 78 is a novel contributor to acquisition of resistance to sorafenib in hepatocellular carcinoma. *Ann Surg Oncol*; 17(2): 603-612.

Choi, Y.L.; Soda, M.; Yamashita, Y.; et al. (2010) EML4-ALK mutations in lung cancer that confer resistance to ALK inhibitors. New Engl J Med; 363: 1734-1739.

Cohen, S.J.; Punt, C.J.; Iannotti, N.; et al (2008) Relationship of circulating tumor cells to tumor response, progression-free survival, and overall survival in patients with metastatic colorectal cancer. *J Clin Oncol*; 26(19): 3213-21.

Corcoran, R.B.; Dias-Santagata, D.; Bergethon, K.; et al. (2010) BRAF gene amplification can promote acquired resistance to MEK inhibitors in cancer cells harbouring the BRAF V600E mutation. *Sci Signal* 3: ra84.

Corcoran, R.B.; Settleman, J. & Engelman, J.A. (2011) Potential Therapetuic Strategies to overcome Acquired Resistance to BRAF or MEK inhibitors in BRAF mutant cancers. *Oncotarget* 2(4): 336-346.

Cristofanilli, M. ; Hayes, D.F. ; Budd, G.T. ; et al. (2005) Circulating Tumour cells : a novel prognostic factor for newly diagnosed metastic breast cancer. *J Clin Oncol*; 23(7): 1420-1430.

Cunningham, D.; Humblet, Y.; Siena, S.; et al. (2004) Cetuximab monotherapy and cetuximab plus irinotecan in irinotecan-refractory metastatic colorectal cancer. *New Engl J Med*; 351(4): 337-45.

Davies, H. ; Bignell, G.R. ; Cox, C. ; et al. (2002) Mutations of the BRAF gene in human cancer. *Nature* 417: 949-954.

De Bono, J.S.; Scher, H.I.; Montgomery, R.B.; et al. (2008) Circulating tumor cells predict survival benefit from treatment in metastatic castration-resistant prostate cancer. *Clin Cancer Res*; 14(9):6302-6309.

De Bono, J.S. & Ashworth, A. (2010) Translating cancer research into targeted therapeutics. *Nature*; 467: 543-549.

De Roock, W.; Jonker, D.J.; Di Nicolantonio, F.; et al. (2010) Association of KRAS p.G13D Mutation with outcome in patients with chemotherapy-refractory metastatic colorectal cancer treated with cetuximab. *JAMA*; 304(16): 1812-1820.

Eisen, T.; Ahmad, T.; Flaherty, K.T.; et al. (2006) Sorafenib in advanced melanoma : a Phase II randomised discontinuation trial analysis. *Br J of Cancer* 95: 581-586.

Emery, C.M.; Vijayendram, K.G.; Zipser, M.C.; et al. (2009) MEK1 mutations confer resistance to MEK and BRAF inhibition. *Proc Natl Acad Sci USA* 106(48): 20411-20416.

Escudier, B.; Szczylik, C.; Eisen, T.; et al. (2005) Randomized phase III trial of the multi-kinase inhibitor BAY 43-9006 in patients with advanced renal cell carcinoma. *Eur J Cancer Suppls*; 3: 226.

Flaherty, K.T.; Puzanov, I.; Kim, K.B.; et al. (2010) Inhibition of Mutated, Activated BRAF in Metastatic Melanoma. *New Engl J Med* 363(9): 809-819.

Flinn, I.W.; Byrd, J.C.; Furman, R.R.; et al. (2009) Preliminary evidence of clinical activity in a phase I study of CAL-101, a selective inhibitor of the p110δ isoform of phosphatidylinositol 3-kinase (PI3K), in patients with select haematologic malignancies. *J Clin Oncol*; 27: 15s (suppl; abstr 3543)

Frattini, M.; Saletti, P.; Romagnani, E.; et al. (2007) PTEN loss of expression predicts cetuximab efficacy in metastatic colorectal cancer patients. *Br J Cancer*; 97: 1139-1145.

Fukuoka, M.; Wu, Y-L.; Thongprasert, S. ; et al. (2011) Biomarker Analyses and Final Overall Survival Results from a phase III, randomised, open-label, first-line study of gefitinib versus carboplatin/paclitaxel in clinically selected patients with advanced non-small cell lung cancer in Asia (IPASS). *J Clin Oncol*, published online June 13: doi 10.1200/JCO.2010.33.4235.

Gelmon, K.A.; Eisenhauer, E.A.; Harris, A.L.; et al. (1999) Anticancer agents targeting signaling molecules and cancer cell environment: Challenges for drug development? *J Natl Cancer Inst*; 91(15): 1281-1287.

Gottesman, M.M. (2002) Mechanisms of Cancer Drug Resistance. Annu Rev Med; 53: 615-27.

Gysin, S.; Salt, M.; Young, A. & McCormick, F. (2011) Therapeutic Strategies for Targeting Ras proteins. *Genes & Cancer*; 2(3): 359-372.

Hammerman, P.S.; Jänne, P.A. & Johnson, B.E. (2009) Resistance to Epidermal Growth Factor Receptor Tyrosine Kinase Inhibitors in Non-Small Cell Lung Cancer. *Clin Can Res*; 15: 7502-7509.

Hanahan, D. & Folkman, J. (1996) Patterns and emerging mechanisms of the angiogenic switch during tumorigenesis. *Cell*: 86: 353-364.

Hanahan, D. & Weinberg, R.A. (2011) Hallmarks of Cancer: The Next Generation. Cell; 144: 646-669.

Hanahan, D. & Weinberg, R.A. (2000) The hallmarks of cancer. *Cell* 100; 57-70.

Hauschild, A., Agarwala, S.S.; Trefzer, U.; et al. (2009) Results of a phase III, randomized placebo-controlled study of sorafenib in combination with carboplatin and paclitaxel as second-line treatment in patients with unresectable stage III or IV melanoma. *J Clin Oncol* 27(17): 2823-2830.

Herman, S.E.M.; Gordon, A.L.; Wagner, A.J.; et al. (2010) Phosphatidylinositol 3-kinase- δ inhibitor CAL-101 shows promising preclinical activity in chronic lymphocytic leukaemia by antagonizing intrinsic and extrinsic cellular survival signals. *Blood*; 116(12): 2078-2088.

Hofmann, M.; Stoss, O.; Gaiser, T.; et al. (2008a) Central HER2 IHC and FISH analysis in a trastuzumab (Herceptin) phase II monotherapy study: assessment of test sensitivity and impact of chromosome 17 polysomy. *J Clin Pathol*; 61(1): 89-94.

Hofmann, M.; Stoss, O.; Shi, D.; et al. (2008b) Assessment of a HER2 scoring system for gastric cancer: results from a validation study. *Histopathology*; 52: 797–805

Houben, R.; Becker, J.C.; Kappel, A.; et al. (2004) Constitutive activation of the Ras-Raf signalling pathway in metastatic melanoma is associated with poor prognosis. *J of Carcinogenesis* 3 (1): 6.

Hurwitz, H; Fehrenbacher, L; Novotny, W; et al. (2004) Bevacizumab plus irinotecan, fluorouracil and leucovorin for metastatic colorectal cancer. *N Engl J Med*; 350(23): 2335-42.

Ivy, S.P.; Garrett-Mayer, E. & Rubinstein, L. (2010) Approaches to phase 1 clinical trial design focused on safety, efficiency, and selected patient populations: a report from the clinical trial design task force of the national cancer institute investigational drug steering committee. *Clin Cancer Res.*;16(6):1726-36.

Jakob, J.A.; Bassett, R.L.; Ng, C.S.; et al. (2011) Clinical characteristics and outcomes associated with BRAF and NRAS mutations in metastatic melanoma. *J Clin Oncol* 29 (suppl; abstr 8500)

Jiang, C.C. ; Lai, F. ; Thorne, R.F. ; et al. (2011) MEK-independent survival of B-RAF V600E melanoma cells selected for resistance to apoptosis induced by the RAF inhibitor PLX4720. *Clin Cancer Res* 17: 721-730.

Jubb, A.M.; Harris, A.L. (2010) Biomarkers to predict the clinical efficacy of bevacizumab in cancer. *Lancet Oncol*; 11: 1172-83.

Karapetis, C.S. ; Khambata-Ford, S. ; Jonker, D.J.; et al. (2008) K-ras mutations and benefit from cetuximab in advanced colorectal cancer. *New Engl J Med*; 359(17): 1757-65.

Karasarides, M.; Chiloeches, A.; Hayward, R.; et al. (2004) B-RAF is a therapeutic target in melanoma. *Oncogene* 23; 6292-6298.

Kefford, R.; Arkenau, H.; Brown, M.P.; et al. (2010) Phase I/II study of GSK2118436, a selective inhibitor of oncogenic mutant BRAF kinase, in patients with metastatic melanoma and other solid tumours. *J Clin Oncol* 28: 15s (suppl; abstr 8503).

Kobayashi, S. ; Ji, H. ; Yuza, Y. ; et al. (2005) An Alternative inhibitor overcomes resistance caused by a mutation of the epidermal growth factor receptor. *Cancer Res*; 65: 7096-7101.

Korn, E.L.; Arbuck, S.G.; Pluda, J.M.; et al. (2001) Clinical trial designs for cytostatic agents: Are new approaches needed? *J Clin Oncol*; 19(1): 265-272.

Koyanagi, K.; O'Day, S.J.; Gonzalez, R.; et al (2005) Serial Monitoring of circulating melanoma cells during neoadjuvant biochemotherapy for stage III melanoma: outcome prediction in a multicenter trial. *J Clin Oncol*; 23(31): 8057-8064.

Koyanagi, K. ; Mori, T. ; O'Day, S.; et al. (2006) Association of Circulating Tumour Cells with Serum Tumor-Related Methylated DNA in peripheral blood of melanoma patients. *Cancer Res*; 66: 6111-6117.

Krebs, M.G.; Sloane, R.; Priest, L.; et al. (2011) Evaluation and Prognostic Significance of Circulating Tumor cells in patients with non-small-cell lung cancer. *J Clin Oncol*; 29(12): 1556-1563.

Kwak, E.L.; Bang, Y-J.; Camidge, R.; et al. (2010) Anaplastic Lymphona Kinase inhibition in non-small-cell lung cancer. *N Engl J Med*, 363 (18): 1693-1703.

Kwak, E.L.; Sordella, R.; Bell, D.W.; et al. (2005) Irreversible inhibitors of the EGF receptor may circumvent acquired resistance to gefitinib. *Proc Nat Acad Sci*; 102 (21): 7665-7670

Lannutti, B.J.; Meadows, S.A.; Herman, S.E.M.; et al. (2011) CAL-101, a p110 δ selective phosphatidylinositol-3-kinase inhibitor for the treatment of B-cell malignancies inhibits PI3K signalling and cellular viability. *Blood*; 117(2): 591-594.

Le Tourneau, C.; Lee, J.J.; Siu, L.L. (2009) Dose escalation methods in phase I cancer clinical trials. *J Natl Cancer Inst*; 101(10): 708-720.

Lievre, A.; Bachet, J-B.; Le Corre, D. ; et al. (2006) KRAS mutation status is predictive of response to cetuximab therapy in colorectal cancer. *Cancer Res*; 66(8): 3992-3995.

Little, A.S.; Balmanno, K.; Sale, M.J.; et al. (2011) Amplification of the Driving Oncogene, KRAS or BRAF, Underpins Acquired Resistance to MEK1/2 Inhibitors in Colorectal Cancer Cells. *Sci Signal* 4: ra17.

Llovet, J.M.; Ricci, S.; Mazzaferro, V.; et al. Sorafenib in advanced hepatocellular carcinoma. *New Engl J Med*; 359: 378-380.

Locatelli, M.A.; Curigliano, G.; Fumagalli, L.; et al. (2010) Should liver metastases of breast cancer be biopsied to improve treatment choice? J Clin Onc; 28: 18s (suppl; abstr CRA1008)

Long, G.V.; Menzies, A.M.; Nagrial, A.M.; et al. (2011) Prognostic and clinicopathologic associations of oncogenic BRAF in metastatic melanoma. *J Clin Oncol* 29(10): 1239-1246.

Loupakis, F.; Pollina, L.; Stasi, I.; et al. (2008) Evaluation of PTEN expression in colorectal cancer (CRC) metastases (mets) and in primary tumors as predictors of activity of cetuximab plus irinotecan treatment. *J Clin Oncol*; 26: 15S (abstr 4003).

Loupakis, F. ; Ruzzo, A. ; Cremolini, C. ; et al. (2009) KRAS codon 61,146 and BRAF mutations predict resistance to cetuximab plus irinotecan in KRAS codon 12 and 13 wild-type metastatic colorectal cancer. *Br J Cancer*; 101: 715-721.

Lu, Y.H. ; Zi, X. ; Zhao, Y. ; et al. (2001) Insulin-like growth-factor-1 receptor signalling and resistance to trastuzumab (Herceptin). *J Natl Cancer Inst*; 93: 1852-1857.

Mahon, F.X. ; Belloc, F. ; Lagarde, V. ; et al. (2003) MDR1 gene overexpression confers resistance to imatinib mesylate in leukemia cell line models. *Blood*; 101: 2368–2373.

McArthur, G. ; Ribas, A. ; Chapman, P.B. ; et al. (2011) Molecular analyses from a Phase 1 trial of vemurafenib to study mechanism of action and resistance in repeated biopsies from BRAF mutation positive metastatic melanoma patients. *J Clin Oncol* 29 (suppl, abstr 8502).

Mocellin, S.; Hoon, D.; Ambrosi, A.; et al. (2006) The Prognostic Value of Circulating Tumor Cells in Patients with Melanoma: A Systematic Review and Meta-analysis. *Clin Cancer Res*, 12: 4605-4613

Montagut, C. ; Sharma, S.V. ; Shioda, T. ; et al. (2008) Elevated CRAF as a potential mechanism of acquired resistance to BRAF inhibition in melanoma. *Cancer Res* 68: 4853-4861.

Nagy, P. ; Friedlander, E. ; Tanner, M. ; et al. (2005) Decreased accessibility and lack of activation of ErbB2 in JIMT 1, a herceptin-resistant, MUC4-expressing breast cancer cell line. *Cancer Res*; 65: 473-482.

Nathanson, K.L. ; Martin, A. ; Letrero, R. ; et al. (2011) Tumor genetic analyses of patients with metastatic melanoma treated with the BRAF inhibitor GSK2118436 (GSK436). *J Clin Oncol* 29: (suppl; abstr 8501)

Nazarian, R.; Shi, H.; Wang, Q.; et al. (2010) Melanomas acquire resistance to B-RAF (V600E) inhibition by RTK or N-RAS upregulation. *Nature* 468: 973-977.

O'Reilly, T.; McSheehy, P.M.; Kawai, R.; et al. (2010) Comparative pharmacokinetics of RAD001 in normal and tumor-bearing rodents. Cancer Chemother Pharmacol; 65(4): 625-39.

Paik, S. ; Bryant, J. ; Tan-Chiu, E. ; et al. (2002) Real-world performance of HER2 testing-National Surgical Adjuvant Breast and Bowel Project experience. *J Natl Cancer Inst*; 94: 852-854.

Pao, W.; Miller, V.A.; Politi, K.A.; Riely, G.J.; Somwar, R.; et al. (2005) Acquired Resistance of Lung Adenocarcinomas to Gefitinib or Erlotinib Is Associated with a Second Mutation in the EGFR Kinase Domain. *PLoS Med* 2(3): e73. doi:10.1371/journal.pmed.0020073

Paraiso, K.H.T. ; Xiang, Y. ; Rebecca, V.W. ; et al. (2011) PTEN loss confers BRAF inhibitor resistance to melanoma cells through the suppression of BIM expression. *Cancer Res* 71(7): 2750-2760.

Parulekar, W.R. & Eisenhauer, E.A. (2004) Phase i trial design for solid tumor studies of targeted, non-cytotoxic agents: Theory and practice. *J Natl Cancer Inst;* 96(13): 990-997.

Platz, A.; Egyhazi, S.; Ringborg, U.; et al. (2008) Human cutaneous melanoma; a review of NRAS and BRAF mutation frequencies in relation to histogenic subclass and body site. *Mol Oncol* 1: 395-405.

Relf, M. ; LeJeune, S. ; Scott, P.A. ; et al. (1997) Expression of the angiogenic factors vascular endothelial cell growth factor, acidic and basic fibroblast growth factor, tumor growth factor beta-1, platelet-derived endothelial cell growth factor, placenta growth factor and pleiotrophin in human primary bresat cancer and its relation to angiogenesis. *Cancer Res;* 57: 963-969.

Reid, A.H.M.; Attard, G.; Danila, D.C.; et al (2010) Significant and Sustained antitumor activity in post-docetaxel, castration-resistant prostate cancer with the CYP17 inhibitor abiraterone acetate. *J Clin Onc;* 28(9): 1489-1495.

Ribas, A.; Kim, K.B.; Schuchter, L.M.; et al. (2011) BRIM-2: an open-label, multicenter phase II study of vemurafenib in previously treated patients with BRAFV600E mutation-positive melanoma. *J Clin Oncol* 29: Suppl:8509-8509.

Ring, A. & Dowsett, M. (2004) Mechanisms of tamoxifen resistance. *Endocr Relat Cancer;* 11: 643-658,

Rixe, O. & Fojo, T. (2007) Is cell death a critical end point for anticancer therapies or is cytostasis sufficient? *Clin Cancer Res:* 13(24): 7280-7287.

Robert, J. (1999) Multidrug resistance in oncology: diagnostic and therapeutic approaches. *Eur J of Clin Inv;* 29: 536-545.

Roche, P.C.; Suman, V.J.; Jenkins, R.B.; et al. (2002) Concordance between local and central laboratory HER2 testing in the breast intergroup trial N9831. *J Natl Cancer Inst ;* 94:855-857.

Rogatko, A.; Babb, J.S.; Tighiouart, M.; et al. (2005) New paradigm in dose-finding trials: Patient-specific dosing and beyond phase I. *Clin Cancer Res;* 11(15): 5342-5346.

Rogatko, A.; Schoeneck, D.; Jonas, W.; et al. (2007) Translation of innovative designs into phase i trials. *J Clin Oncol;* 25(31): 4982-4986.

Romond, E.H. ; Perez, E.A. ; Bryant, J. ; et al. (2005) Trastuzumab plus adjuvant chemotherapy for operable HER2-positive breast cancer. *N Engl J Med;*353:1673-1684

Rosell, R. ; Gervais, R. ; Vergnenegre, A. ; et al. (2011) Erlotinib versus chemotherapy in advanced non-small cell lung cancer (NSCLC) patients with epidermal growth factor receptor mutations: interim results of the European Erlotinib Versus Chemotherapy (EURTAC) phase III randomized trial. *J Clin Oncol;* 29: (suppl; abstr 7503).

Sartore-Bianchi, A.; Martini, M.; Molinari, F.; et al. (2009) PIK3CA mutations in colorectal cancer are associated with clinical resistance to EGFR-targeted monoclonal antibodies. *Cancer Res;* 69: 1851-1857.

Scher, H.I.; Heller, G.; Molina, A.; et al. (2011) Evaluation of circulating tumour cell (CTC) enumeration as an efficacy response biomarker of overall survival (OS) in metastatic castration-resistance prostate cancer (mCRPC): Planned final analysis (FA) of COU-AA-301, a randomized double-blind, placebo-controlled phase III study of abiraterone acetate (AA) plus low-dose prednisone (P) post docetaxel. *J Clin Oncol*; 29: suppl (abstr LBA4517)

Shao, Y.; Aplin, A.E. (2010) Akt3-mediated resistance to apoptosis in BRAF-targeted melanoma cells. *Cancer Res* 70(16): 6670-6681.

Shepherd, F.A. ; Pereira, J.R. ; Ciuleanu, T. ; et al. (2005) Erlotinib in Previouly Treated Non-Small-Cell Lung Cancer. *N Engl J Med*; 353: 123-132.

Simon, R.; Freedman, L.S.; (1997) Bayesian design and analysis of two x two factorial clinical trials. *Biometrics*; 53(2): 456-464.

Slamon, D.J.; Clark, G.M.; Wong, S.G.; et al. (1987) Human breast cancer : correlation of relapse and survival with amplification of the HER-2/neu oncogene. *Science (Wash DC)*; 235: 177-182.

Slamon, D.J. ; Godolphin, W. ; Jones, L.A. ; et al. (1989) Studies of the HER-2/neu proto-oncogene in human breast and ovarian cancer. *Science*; 244: 707-712.

Slamon, D.J.; Leyland-Jones, B.; Shak, S.; et al. (2001)Use of chemotherapy plus a monoclonal antibody against HER2 for metastatic breast cancer that overexpresses HER2. *N Engl J Med*; 344: 783-792

Sleijfer, S, & Wiemer, E. (2008) Dose selection in phase I studies: Why we should always go for the top. *J Clin Oncol*; 26(10): 1576-1578.

Szakacs, G.; Paterson, J.K.; Ludwig, J.A.; et al. (2006) Targeting multidrug resistance in cancer. *Nature Reviews*; 5: 219-234.

Tamborini, E.; Bonadiman, L.; Greco, A.; et al. (2004) A new mutation in the KIT ATP pocket causes acquired resistance to imatinib in a gastrointestinal stromal tumor patient. *Gastroenterology*; 127(1): 294-299.

Thatcher, N.; Chang, A.; Parikh, P.; et al. (2005) Gefitinib plus best supportive care in patients with refractory advanced non-small-cell lung cancer: results from a randomised, placebo-controlled, multicentre study (Iressa Survival Evaluation in Lung Cancer). *Lancet*; 366: 1527-1537.

Tsimberidou, A.M.; Iskander, N.G.; Hong, D.S.; et al. (2011) Personalized medicine in a phase 1 clinical trials program: The M.D. Anderson Cancer Center Initiative. *J Clin Oncol*; 29: (suppl; abstr CRA2500)

Villanueva, J. ; Vultur, A. ; Lee, J.T. ; et al. (2010) Acquired resistance to BRAF inhibitors mediated by a RAF kinase switch in melanoma can be overcome by targeting MEK and IGF-1R/PI3K. *Cancer Cell* 18: 683-695.

Wagle, N.; Emery, C.; Berger, M.F.; et al. (2011) Dissecting Therapeutic Resistance to RAF inhibition in melanoma by Tumor Genomic Profiling. *J Clin Oncol* published online on March 7, 2011 (DOI:10.1200/JCO.2010.33.2312).

Wiley, H.S. (2003) Trafficking of the ErbB receptors and its influence on signalling. *Exp Cell Res*; 284: 78-88.

Wilhelm, C.; Carter, C.; Lynch, M.; et al. (2006) Discovery and development of sorafenib: A multikinase inhibitor for treating cancer. *Nat Rev Drug Discov*; 5: 835-44.

Wolchok, J.D.; Hoos, A.; O'Day, S.; et al. (2009) Guidelines for the evaluation of immune therapy activity in solid tumors: immune-related response criteria. *Clin. Cancer Res*; 15(23): 7412–7420.

Wolff, A.C.; Hammond, E.H.; Schwartz, J.N.; et al. (2007) American Society of Clinical Oncology/College of American Pathologists Guideline Recommendations for Human Epidermal Growth Factor Receptor 2 Testing in Breast Cancer. *J Clin Oncol*; 25(1): 118-145.

Yano, T. ; Doi, T. ; Ohtsu, A. ; et al. (2006) Comparison of HER2 gene amplification assessed by fluorescence in situ hybridization and HER2 protein expression assessed by immunohistochemistry in gastric cancer. *Oncol Rep*; 15: 65-71.

Zidan, J.; Dashkovsky, I.; Stayerman, C.; et al. (2005) Comparison of HER2 overexpression in primary breast cancer and metastatic sites and its effect on biological targeting therapy of metastatic disease. *Br J Cancer*; 93: 552-556.

4

Drug Discovery into the 21st Century

Klaus Pors
Institute of Cancer Therapeutics, University of Bradford
UK

1. Introduction

Medicines discovery has come a long way since our ancient ancestors from the Neanderthals to the people of Mesopotamia, Egypt, Greece and China used herbal remedies to treat the sick people. In mediaeval times the quest for the *elixir of life* was pursued by alchemists, but it is the scientists of the past 100-150 years who have had success by translating laboratory-based discoveries into drugs that have literally saved countless millions of lives (Sneader, 2005). The German stock market collapsed in 1873 and it was during the recovery period that the upsurge in the economy lead to an expansion of chemical and electrical industries. The significant investment in the manufacture of synthetic dyes soon put Germany well ahead of all its competitors. As a consequence, German chemists did not only become very influential in the field of organic chemistry, but also led to the rise of the German pharmaceutical industry. Central to this industry were leading manufacturers including F. Bayer & Company and Farbenfabriken Hoechst who realised that their chemists researching and developing dyes also had the potential to produce new medicines (Sneader, 2005). One such scientist was Paul Ehrlich. Ehrlich was fascinated by colourful dyes and their capacity to interact with histological and cellular structures. Over several decades, he benefitted from chemical companies who provided hundreds to thousands of new dyes for his research. Given these dyes were biologically evaluated individually, the number of compounds probably exceeded the thousands or even millions of compounds being evaluated as a part of high-throughput screening (HTS) employed in academia and industry today. Ehrlich taught us that, in the broadest sense, the biological effect of a chemical compound such as a dye depends on its chemical composition and the cell on which it acts. He was able to establish a connection between chemistry, biology and medicine in an ingenious fashion; chemical dyes were the catalyst for this *revolutionary association* (Strebhardt & Ullrich, 2008). Simultaneous to his fascination of dyes, he also was inspired by his contemporaries carrying out research in immunology including Louis Pasteur, Robert Koch, Emil von Behring and Shibasaburo Kitasato. At the turn of the 20th century Ehrlich developed the receptor theory, which became instrumental to the understanding of how the binding of drugs to various types of receptors could occur due to structural differences in chemical compositions. He notably stated "Wir müssen chemisch zielen lernen" which translated to English equates "we have to learn how to aim chemically". Ehrlich's experiences with the treatment of infectious diseases with drugs derived from the German dye industry impelled him to look for ways of using organic chemistry to modify certain starting dyes in various ways to create new chemical structures with potential improved biological activity (Strebhardt & Ullrich, 2008). Erlich is often described as the founder of chemotherapy and his 'magic bullet concept' is still what today's scientists strive to aim for: to develop small molecules that attack pathogens yet remain harmless to healthy tissues.

During the two World Wars essential medicines normally supplied by Germany dried up and a gradual change in favour of synthetic drugs came about. Synthetic organic chemistry became an exceptional important discipline and is still one of the cornerstones of drug discovery. Synthetic organic chemistry has continually adapted to embrace innovative techniques and methodologies central to drug development. Much synthetic drug discovery emerged from cancer drug development and began with an observation that mustard gas, employed in chemical warfare during World Wars I and II, destroyed lymphatic tissue and bone marrow formation. The observations made by Drs. Gilman, Goodman and co-workers laid the foundation for conducting the first clinical trials with nitrogen mustards (β-chloroethylamines) in 1942 at Yale-New Haven Hospital, but a report of the clinical results was only made public four years later, due to the cloak of secrecy during World War II (Goodman *et al*, 1946; Hirsch, 2006). An array of DNA alkylating agents ensued, which paralleled an increased understanding of DNA in the 1950s. A number of other agents subsequently emerged, such as the vinca alkaloids and purine/pyrimidine synthesis inhibitors (Denny, 2002). These advances were, to a large extent, driven by the National Cancer Institute (NCI), enabling the assessment of primarily cytotoxic agents. By the 1970s, the importance of natural product-based early drug discovery had been realised (Denny, 2002). Unfortunately, the synthesis of many of these frequently promising, novel agents was often too complex and too expensive to allow progression into early stage clinical trials. This situation facilitated a paradigm shift whereby natural product screening was implemented into stage discovery initiatives, providing an opportunity to identify natural products as *bona fide* lead compounds. These leads were then subsequently developed into truncated molecules, which were more amenable to synthesis. More recently, advances in organic chemistry have successfully enabled the complete synthesis of many complex natural products, a milestone that has dramatically improved the ease with which chemists can now deal with the complexity of many of these naturally-derived architectural structures. Synthetic chemistry has also been instrumental in the development of drug delivery and prodrug strategies, which have focused on the development of selective therapeutics with reduced side-effect profiles (Brown & Wilson, 2004; Rooseboom *et al*, 2004). Although research in cancer medicines was the driver of much synthetic drug discovery it did run parallel with research against other diseases as illustrated in Figure 1.

Today, the emergence of the genomics era and the focus of events at the molecular level is changing the landscape of drug discovery. A wealth of convergent data that has caused many to not only speculate on an expanding druggable genome, but also given an optimism for grasping new opportunities to take drug discovery to the next level has become available (Billingsley, 2008). The number of gene products that are targets for existing drugs has been a topic for much debate and depends on the analysis performed, however, a valid estimate is in the region of 300-500 gene products (Overington *et al*, 2006). As the human genome is estimated to encode 20,000-25,000 human gene products, the number of drug targets is likely to increase. However, it will take some time to validate targets at the protein level, which has an added level of complexity. Both gene and protein expression profiling methodologies have been emerging over the last decade or so to monitor and catalogue changes in the expression of genes and their respective protein products. As such there are serious challenges ahead. Our understanding of human disease at the molecular level to elucidate changes in biochemical processes associated with disease phenotypes is of high significance. From a drug discovery point of view, the ultimate goal is to generate identifiable therapeutic targets while reducing drug development attrition.

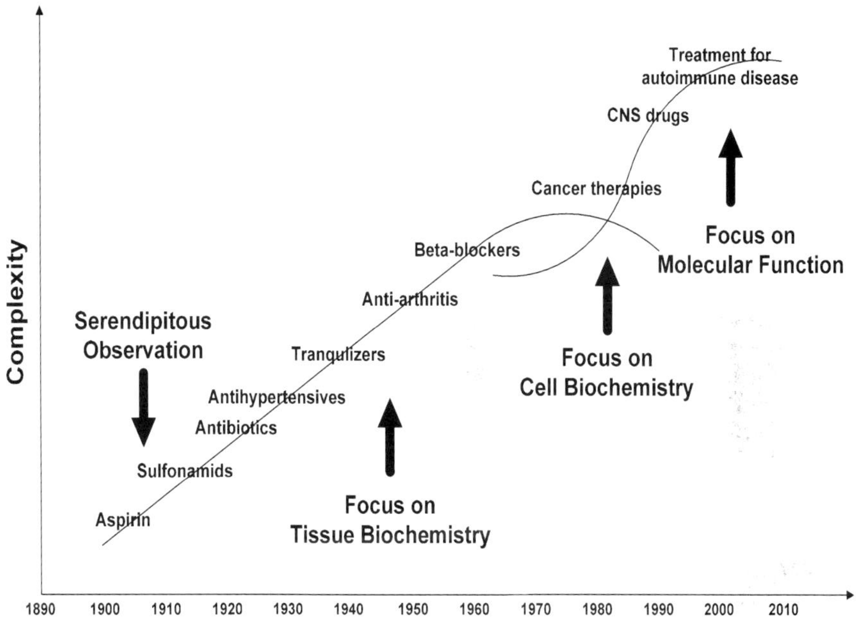

Fig. 1. Chronology of drug innovation. (Reprinted with permission from the Biopharmaceutical Industry Contributions to State and US Economics, available at www.milkeninstitute.org/pdf/biopharma_report.pdf, Milken Institute).

The mapping of the human genome was a gigantic landmark. Can scientists working at the interface of chemistry and biology in drug discovery utilise the data available to them to discover new ground-breaking drugs? Will the ever increasing cost of drug discovery halt the progression, especially in times of recession? Will research and development (R&D) in the emerging markets be an opportunity to climb to the next level of understanding in how to develop successful drugs? These are some of the questions that will be discussed in the following sections.

2. The evolution of modern drug discovery

At the beginning of the 20th century drug discovery was largely carried out by individuals such as Paul Ehrlich and his associates. This is now impossible, and requires teamwork encompassing members from various disciplines including chemistry, computational modelling, structural biology and pharmacology. This section outlines a general approach to drug discovery which has been dominant over the past couple of decades. The approach to drug design depends on the objectives of the design and investigational team, but will also depend to some extent on the disease that is targeted. The information available from the literature about a specific disease or target is used by the research team to decide what intervention would be most likely to bring about the desired result. The exact nature of the project progression depends on the resources available: for example, an academic group may not be as expansive as a large pharmaceutical company in terms of how to tackle the problems of validating a novel target or developing 'hit' and 'lead' compounds that will be able to modulate that target. The drug discovery process outlined in Figure 2 is, therefore, an approximate model which is employed by pharmaceutical companies, but one which a small biotech company or a university also can engage in through multiple collaborations. This discovery process can be instigated at several points and adapted to bring about the results needed to take a project to the next level. For a recent in-depth review of the early drug discovery process, see (Philpott *et al*, 2011).

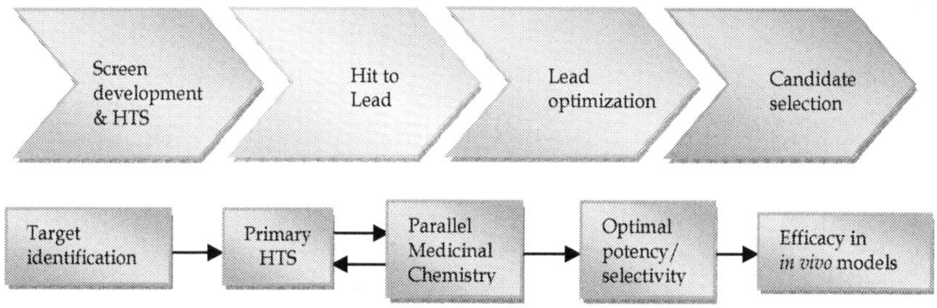

Fig. 2. The multi-faceted drug discovery process in the 21st Century.

Up until the mid 80s, drug discovery was focussed on isolation of natural products and medicinal chemistry was central for a research team to find more potent and selective compounds than the natural product or synthetic compound themselves. After isolation and characterisation of the natural products, structure-activity relationship (SAR) studies were and still are a vital tool in optimising a pharmacophore. Initially, a drug design process was an iterative course of action between the synthesis of new compounds by a synthetic/medicinal chemist and the screening of these for biological activity by a pharmacologist. The drug discovery process was chemistry-focussed rather than target-driven. As outlined in Figure 2, the discovery process of a drug now involves a multidisciplinary effort that is synergistic, which often encompasses HTS procedures. It is also one that often follows rules that are based on empirical findings from clinical investigations such as Lipinski's rule of 5 (Lipinski *et al*, 1997). 'Hit' compounds are progressed into a 'lead' compound, which undergoes thorough pharmacological and toxicological testing. The results of these tests enable a research team to decide whether it is profitable to continue with the progression of a specific project. The scenario is often to screen virtual or commercial libraries of compounds to identify hit molecules. The second stage is to prepare libraries of small molecules based around the hit molecule, measure their activity and correlate the results to determine the chemical structure with optimum activity. This analysis may make use of SARs, computational chemistry, combinatorial chemistry and enzymatic and cellular assays to help unravel biological activity derived from unique mechanism of action of a small molecule. The selection of a lead compound and the development of a synthetic pathway for its preparation on a large scale for preclinical and clinical investigations must also be considered at an early stage in the discovery process. If the lead molecule cannot be synthesised on a large scale progression to clinical evaluation will not be possible. Similarly, researchers must also devise suitable *in vitro* and *in vivo* tests to assess the activity and toxicity of the compounds produced. If there is no suitable way of testing a hit or lead molecule *in vivo* the project may come to a halt unless it is decided to spend resources on developing appropriate models.

Nowadays, hit and lead molecules with proven activity are assessed for susceptibility for phase I and II metabolism in the very early stages of the discovery process. For example, many HTS technologies are now available to detect cytochrome P450 (CYP) substrates or inhibitors, which should decrease the number of withdrawals of novel drugs from the market due to affinity for major CYP metabolising isozymes. HTS CYP data can be used to guide medicinal chemistry away from these interactions at an early stage and in certain cases might entirely solve the issue by targeted modification of the CYP interacting functionality (Zlokarnik *et al*, 2005).

HTS methodologies have been developed and have enabled research teams to generate vast numbers of compound variations of a desired pharmacophore. Combinatorial chemistry (combichem) was first applied to the generation of peptide arrays in 1984 and evolved rapidly into a new discipline that was hailed to revolutionise drug discovery (Lam & Renil, 2002). The early generations of combichem scientists captured the fascination of the industry, and coined or modified the common use of a number of buzzwords, phrases, and abbreviations that became widespread in the literature including deconvolution, diversomer, split-and-mix, multipin, SPOC or SPOS (solid-phase organic chemistry or synthesis), submonomer synthesis, T-bag (Teflon bag) to name a few (Moos *et al*, 2009). Interestingly, from the discovery point of view, the scientists working in the combichem environment require different management solutions to classical synthetic chemists. For example, chemists planning a traditional synthesis to obtain a target compound or a natural product typically conduct a retrosynthetic analysis to determine the best, and perhaps cheapest, way to obtain the target. In contrast, combinatorial chemists will primarily consider forward synthesis strategies that are founded in which building blocks are commercially available or indeed worth synthesising. Accordingly, chemical information systems that can be quickly accessed via updated databases of inventory and commercially available reagents are invaluable tools in reagent acquisition by the combinatorial chemists. While combichem matured from solid-phase synthesis to solid-supported synthesis, new synthetic strategies and techniques evolved. Some of these are now well integrated into the drug design process including microwave synthesis (Gedye *et al*, 1986), fluorous synthesis (Studer *et al*, 1997), click chemistry (Sharpless *et al*, 2001) and flow reactors (SalimiMoosavi *et al*, 1997). As with traditional drug design, combichem relies on organic synthesis methodologies and exploits automation and miniaturization to synthesize large libraries of compounds, which can accelerate the drug discovery process. The combinatorial approach is often systematic and repetitive, using sets of commercially available chemical reagents to form a diverse set of molecular entities. It is very powerful in early stage discovery and allows HTS to take place, combining rapid synthesis of chemical compounds to be screened using both enzymatic and cellular assays for evaluation. The quick turnaround of data allows a flow of information, which enables second and third generation of compounds to be generated in rapid fashion. Combichem mostly concerns "parallel" synthesis and "split-and-mix" synthesis (Figure 3).

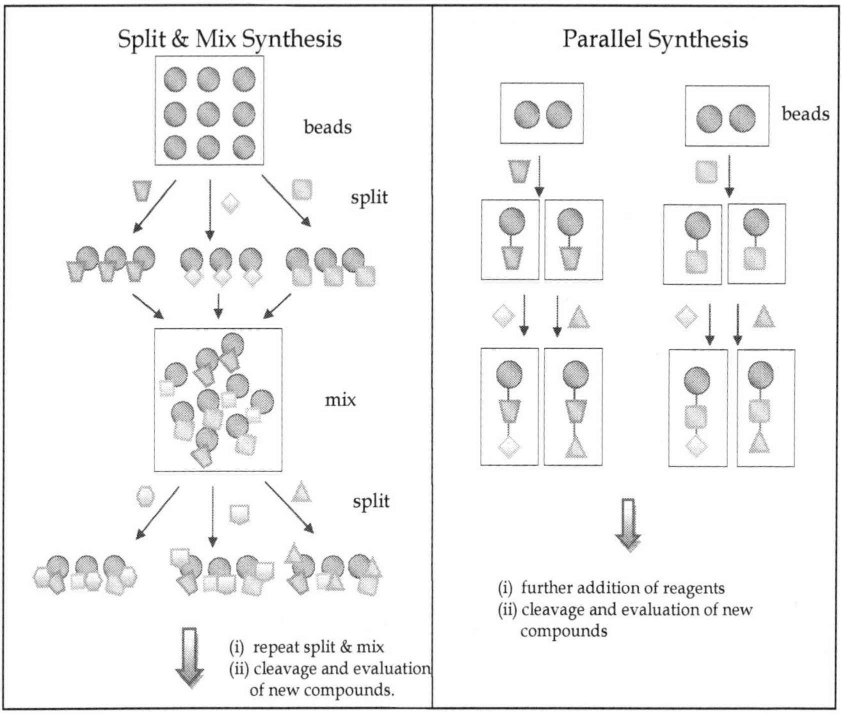

Fig. 3. Combinatorial chemistry approaches. The parallel synthesis is generally used to generate larger quantities of a small number of compounds and split and mix to generate smaller quantities of a larger number of molecules.

There is no doubt that combichem has become a mainstay tool of the drug discovery process. The strength of combinatorial techniques is based on the creation of large populations of molecules, or libraries that can be screened efficiently *en masse* in a short period of time. The vast amounts of money spent on development of combinatorial techniques have not yet resulted in many drug successes. The only real success story at present is the development of the multikinase inhibitor sorafenib, which now has been approved for clinical use by the *Food and Drug Administration (FDA)* for the treatment of advanced renal cancer (Wilhelm *et al*, 2006). However, combichem has spun out many exciting technologies that now occupy a central place in the biotech industry. The mapping of the human genome may have provided a new area of application of combichem in combination with other HTS methodologies including techniques and instruments developed for DNA microarrays. Indeed, high-density chemical microarrays can now be synthesized *in situ* on glass slides or be printed through covalent linkage or non-specific adsorption to the surface of the solid-support with fully automatic arrays. In conjunction with the one-bead one-compound combinatorial library method, chemical microarrays have proven to be very valuable in 'hit' identification and 'lead' optimization. HTS protein expression systems, robust high-density protein, peptide and small-molecule microarray systems, and automatic mass spectrometers are essential tools for the field of functional proteomics (Lam & Renil, 2002). In despite of this more focussed approach to drug discovery, combichem has been disappointing in delivering drugs to the market (Rydzewski, 2008). One of the main reasons is that combichem has been built on peptide chemistry that now has use in protein and nucleotide research, but which is not best suited to producing orally active drugs (Moos *et al.*, 2009). Another limitation of combichem is that small molecules developed via this technique do not cover broad *chemical space*. When comparing the properties of compounds in combichem libraries to those of approved drugs and natural products, it has been observed that combichem libraries suffer particularly from the lack of chirality, as well as structure rigidity, both of which are widely regarded as drug-like properties (Feher & Schmidt, 2003). Since the enormous success with natural products as drugs or use for drug development in the 70-80s, it has not been fashionable by the pharmaceutical industry to use these as leads for drug development. Often because of the complex structural architecture of natural products, which make them difficult to synthesise in the laboratory on a large scale basis. However, what cannot be disputed is that natural products cover much chemical diversity. As chirality and rigidity are the two most important features distinguishing approved drugs and natural products from compounds in combichem libraries, these are the two issues that are essential components of diversity-oriented synthesis (DOS) that aim at coverage of the chemical space, instead of libraries consisting of colossal numbers of compounds.

2.1 Discovery of small molecules to explore biological pathways and uncover new targets

The mapping of the human genome, the improved understanding of both pathological causes and function of biological targets and the development of HTS technologies ought to have resulted in a higher number of new chemical entities (NMEs) for medicinal use. So why has this not been the case? There may be several reasons, which will now be considered. Computational molecular modelling has provided scientists with an insight into biochemical events at the molecular level. An understanding of the binding process of small molecules to many macromolecules such as DNA is well understood, however the same cannot be said about other targets. Many stones are still left unturned, perhaps due to the lack of interest or belief that so-called "undruggable" proteins can be successfully targeted. It has been estimated that only 10–14% of the proteins encoded in the human genome are 'druggable' using existing 'drug-like' molecules (Hopkins & Groom, 2002). However, given that the *chemical space*, the complete set of all possible small molecules, has been calculated to comprise 10^{30}–10^{200} structures depending on the parameters used (Bauer *et al*, 2010) there are an incredible number of yet uncovered chemical structures. Considering the limitations of chemical libraries in addressing challenging targets, it is important to recognize that the vast majority of accessible libraries of small molecules are based on existing drugs (Moura-Letts *et al*, 2011). Drugging targets that are within our capacity to accept as targets and exercising principles such as Lipinski's "rule of five" that have yielded success in the past is safe territory, so it is perfectly understandable that we want to continue such lines of research. "Me too" compounds are likely to give pharmaceutical companies a financial return and academic scientists may obtain grant funding if the proposed research makes sense. Grant reviewers can appreciate the hypotheses and the scientific methodologies and may be inclined to fund projects that will give an outcome of sorts. However, it also appears that industry, research councils and other funding bodies want to keep an element of blue-sky research - they just don't want to fund it. Historically we know that serendipity has played a major part of most success stories. So to cut out funding that is not to support blue-sky but mainstream research is likely to have profound consequences. Although Lipinski's "rule of five" has merit and a place in drug discovery it may also be an Achilles heel in progressing new drug discovery projects (Abad-Zapatero, 2007). Why? A drawback is that the shape and size of drugs become limited. Unless carefully used, HTS technologies such as combichem will continue to only generate low hit rates, particularly when screening against challenging targets (Boehringer *et al*, 2000; Edwards *et al*, 2007). Additionally, optimisation of lead compounds can be problematic owing to the often large and relatively lipophilic nature of the screening hits (Chessari & Woodhead, 2009a). Wise men will always use experiences from the past and present, but discovery of NMEs must also entail trespassing new horizons or in the drug discovery world, new chemical space.

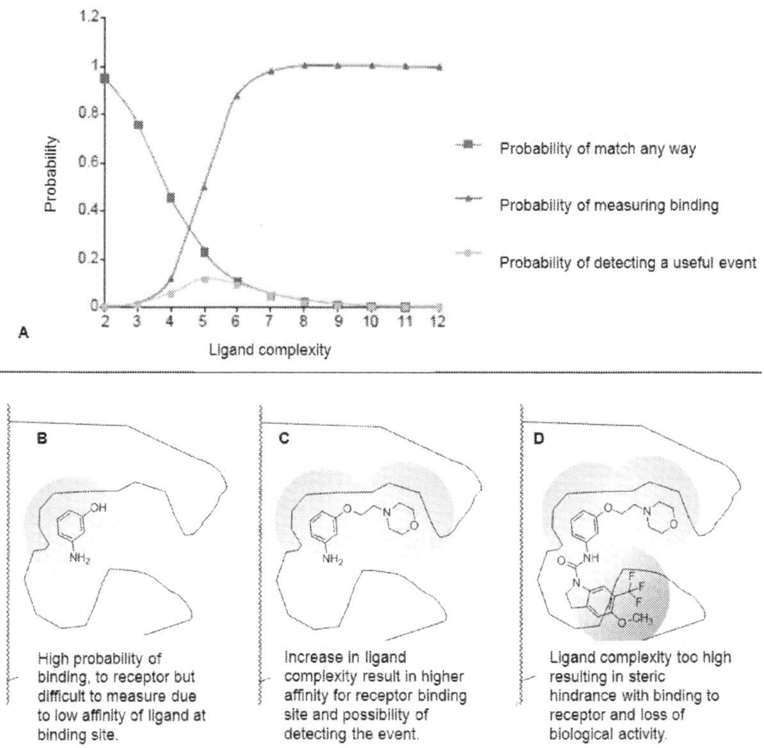

Fig. 4. (A) Success landscape for a binding site of ligands with increasing molecular complexity. (Reprinted with permission from Zartler & Shapiro, *Curr. Opin. Chem. Biol.* 2005, 9(4), 366-370, copyright (2005) Elsevier and *J.Chem. Inf. Comput. Sci.* 2001, 41, 856-864, copyright (2001), American Chemical Society). (B-D) An example of increase in ligand complexity using 3-aminophenol as starting material.

An insight into the difficulties in successful drug development is provided by Hann and co-workers who in their study suggest that if a drug discovery process starts with very simple chemical structures, then there is a better chance of finding both detectable binding and a

unique binding mode. Similarly, lead molecules that are simpler also give more available chemical space for optimization, especially in light of the properties that are needed for oral bioavailability (Zartler & Shapiro, 2005). Figure 4A shows the trade off between detecting binding and a unique match. Essentially, the chance of finding a detectable and unique binding mode is dependent on the chance of determining binding and the chance of having a distinctive binding mode or match. For example, if 3-aminphenol was a ligand in a screening collection, there would be a high probability of it binding, but due to low affinity and time of occupancy at the binding site, it would be difficult to detect any such binding (Figure 4B). If 3-aminophenol was further reacted to afford 3-(2-morpholinoethoxy)aniline, the complexity of this ligand would increase and the probability of the binding would increase as a result. However, if the aniline amine moiety was derivatised with a fluorinated indoline to generate a ligand of high complexity, steric hindrance would hamper any binding in this specific receptor model (Figure 4D). By increasing the molecular complexity of a ligand the chance of measuring the binding is enhanced, but at the same time such modifications may also augment the likelihood of negative interactions (Zartler & Shapiro, 2005).
One approach toward broadening our understanding of the relationship between structure and function of a target protein is to generate many new small molecules, simple in shape and size, which are in accordance with Hann's study, that modulate the proteins' functions. This enables the study of the interactions of ligand and protein. The past 10 years have seen the screening of specific components of small molecules evolve from a niche area of research to become an important tool known as fragment-based drug discovery (FBDD). Fragments are defined as low molecular weight (MW <300), moderately lipophilic (clogP < 3) and highly soluble organic molecules (Chessari & Woodhead, 2009a). As a consequence, medicinal chemists use hit compounds to probe new chemical space in a number of ways as illustrated in Figure 5.

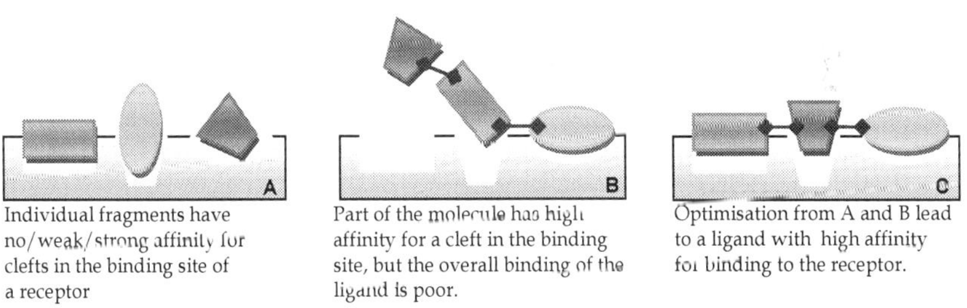

Fig. 5. Fragment-based drug discovery.

The first medicinal chemistry approaches employing FBDD as a key component of the discovery process can be traced back 15-20 years. In contrast to combichem, FBDD strategies have had a more rapid impact in terms of developing drugs with clinical potential. The wide variety of contexts in which FBDD is now being used (SAR-by-NMR, HTX, scaffold-hopping, selectivity mapping) illustrates its practical utility in mainstream medicinal chemistry. The promise of more resourceful technology has fuelled enthusiasm for FBDD, which is design intensive and enabled by structural biology. Indeed, screening fragments, particularly when using sensitive biophysical techniques may also allow scientists to tackle some of the more challenging drug discovery targets. Fragment libraries statistically cover

chemical space better than drug-like or lead-like libraries and as a consequence fewer compounds need to be screened. Also fragment-based screening tends to deliver high hit rates with the additional benefit of providing multiple start points for optimisation programmes (Chessari & Woodhead, 2009a).
FBDD's recent successes outlined in Table 1 (Chessari & Woodhead, 2009b) indicate that use of this design intensive drug discovery approach is delivering results that have paved the way to clinical evaluation and it may not be long before the first drug reaches the marketplace (de Kloe *et al*, 2009).

Compound	Company	Target	Progress	Detection method
ABT-263	Abbott	Bcl-X_L	Phase 2	NMR
AT9283	Astex	Aurora	Phase 2	X-ray
LY-517717	Lilly/Protherics	FXa	Phase 2	Computation/X-ray
NVP-AUY-922	Novartis/Vernalis	Hsp90	Phase 2	NMR
Indeglitazar	Plexxikon	PPAR antagonist	Phase 2	HCS/X-ray
ABT-518	Abbott	MMP-2 & 9	Phase 1	NMR
AT7519	Astex	CDK2	Phase 1	X-ray
AT13387	Astex	Hsp90	Phase 1	NMR/X-ray
IC-776	Lilly/ICOS	LFA-1	Phase 1	NMR
PLX-4032	Plexxikon	B-RafV^{600E}	Phase 1	HCS/X-ray
PLX-5568	Plexxikon	Kinase Inhibitor	Phase 1	HCS/X-ray
SGX-523	SGX Pharmaceuticals	Met	Phase 1	X-ray/HCS
SNS-314	Sunesis	Aurora	Phase 1	MS

Table 1. Fragment derived compounds and furthest stage of clinical development.
(Adapted with permission from Chessari & Woodhead, From fragment to clinical candidate-a historical perspective. *Drug Discov Today*, 2009, 14(13-14), 668-675, copyright (2009) Elsevier).

2.2 Exploring chemical space

Drug discovery today critically depends on HTS of compound libraries *in silico* and *in vitro*. Novel chemical structures (also known as chemotypes) are of particular interest since these might display different properties to drug-like small molecules and may be used to interrogate biological pathways. Unfortunately, most approaches to create new compounds rely on using commercially-available known starting materials or building blocks and utilise existing reactions to generate small molecules, which are not well-suited to uncover novel chemotypes (Reymond & Fink, 2007). A change to the discovery of small molecules that possess biological activity, but are under-represented in commercial screening collections may provide suitable fragments for further development. An analysis by Stoichet and co-workers (Shoichet *et al*, 2009) revealed amongst other things that currently commercially-available compounds and libraries have more in common with compounds derived from natural products and metabolites than with a virtual library of 26.4 million molecules (chemotypes containing of up to 11 atoms of C, N, O, and F comprising 110.9 million stereoisomers). Is this a surprise? Stoichet argued that the reason current libraries are effective at all in identifying new chemotypes is that they are based, albeit largely unintentionally, on structures in naturally occurring molecules, which have coevolved with proteins that bind them.

In a recent study, Tan and co-workers analysed 40 top-selling small molecule drugs (39 of which are orally bioavailable), a collection of 60 diverse natural products (including the 24 identified by Ganesan as having led to an approved drug from 1970 to 2006) and 20 drug-like compounds from ChemBridge and ChemDiv. Each compound was analyzed for 20 calculated structural and physicochemical parameters, and then principal component analysis was used to replot the data in a 2-dimensional format representing 73% of the information in the full 20-dimensional dataset (for full details, see (Bauer *et al*, 2010).

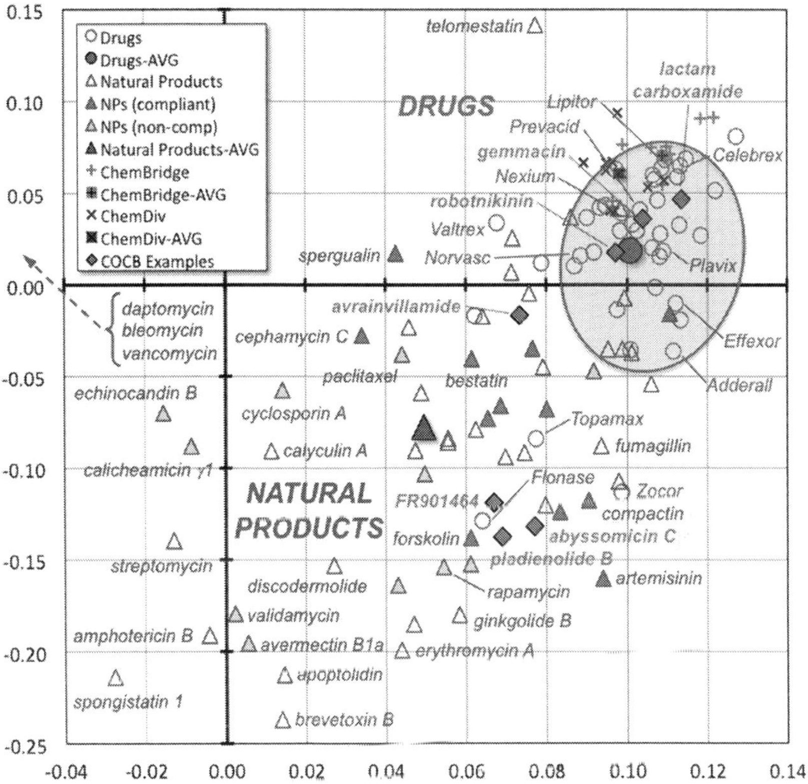

Fig. 6. Principal component analysis of 20 structural and physicochemical characteristics of 40 top-selling drugs (red circles), 60 natural products (blue triangles), including Ganesan's rule-of-five compliant (pink filled) and non-compliant (blue filled) subsets, and 20 compounds from commercial drug-like libraries (ChemBridge, pink plusses; Chem Div, maroon crosses). The two unitless, orthogonal axes represent 73% of the information in the full 20-dimensional dataset. Recent examples of natural products and library-derived probes that address challenging targets discussed herein are also shown (green diamonds). (Reprinted with permission from Bauer *et. al.*, Expanding the range of 'druggable' targets with natural product-based libraries: an academic perspective. *Curr. Opin. Chem. Biol.*, 2010, 14(3), 308-314, copyright (2009) Elsevier).

Putting the details aside, the key message from this data representation (Figure 6) is that the top-selling drugs are located as a cluster in a specific area of the plot with the drug-like libraries overlapping the same regional zone. Moreover, the few outlier drugs are natural products or derivatives, and these molecules, along with the 60 natural products, span a much broader range of chemical space. In part, this study points to natural products as chemical architectures that not only cover chemical space best but also are likely to be suitable for developing probe and drug-like molecules that can modulate macromolecular proteins in various ways.

Small molecules have great potential to aid the process of understanding and improving human health. Accordingly, there is much incentive for using small molecules to explore new chemical space by employing methodologies that are aimed at exploring unchartered waters and leaving well-researched areas behind, but by no means forgotten. As we have seen, FBDD is beginning to prove that developing technologies outside mainstream medicinal chemistry can be fruitful. Aware of the fact that bioactivity is not randomly dispersed in the vast chemical space, chemists have been cultivating hypotheses that can bring them closer to the islands of bioactivities. Natural products have always been a source of inspiration and their structural motifs provide biologically relevant starting points for library synthesis to generate new molecules integrating pharmacophores known to produce biological activity. In addition to FBDD, emerging tools to guide compound discovery include diversity-oriented synthesis and chemical genetics.

2.2.1 Diversity-oriented synthesis

Diversity-oriented synthesis (DOS) aims to synthesize small molecules that cover incongruent targets in a multidimensional descriptor space (Burke & Schreiber, 2004). Essentially what this means is that multiple regions in a confined chemical space are targeted with small molecules often comprising a fragment of a pharmacophore with proven biological activity. Such collections are also essential to chemical genetics, which is discussed further below (section 2.1.2.). DOS is built on a solid platform comprising traditional medicinal chemistry but can also incorporate HTS technologies such as combichem. Essentially, drug discovery of small molecules can be categorized into three approaches that cover chemical space differently: The first approach uses target-oriented synthesis (TOS) and resembles a well-trodden path that relies primarily on nature to discover molecules with useful, macromolecule-perturbing properties. After isolation and characterisation, natural products possessing biological activity become a target for chemical synthesis. Using conventional synthetic chemistry based on retrosynthetic planning, the aim of TOS is to populate a discrete point in chemical space that is known to yield biological activity (Figure 7A). The second approach uses either medicinal chemistry or combichem and aims to explore chemistry space that is in close vicinity to a precise region known to have useful properties (Figure 7B). The source of the starting or lead compounds can vary and may include a natural product, a known drug or pharmacophore, or a rationally designed structure derived from i.e. a crystal structure of a macromolecule of interest. The aim in this approach is to access diversity to some degree using diverse building blocks and usually involves synthesising analogues of a given target structure using retrosynthetic planning. The synthesis effort in DOS aims to create a broad distribution of compounds in chemistry space (Figure 7C), including currently poorly populated (or even vacuous) space, and in the future, space found empirically to correlate best with desired properties. Synthesis pathways employed in DOS are branched and divergent, and they are planned in the forward-synthetic direction (Bender *et al*, 2006; Burke & Schreiber, 2004; Spring *et al*, 2008).

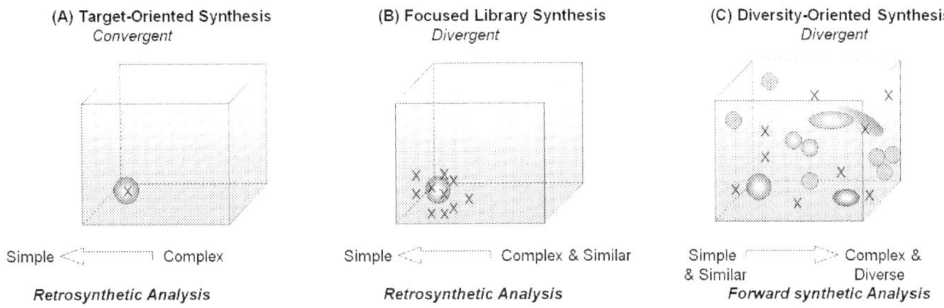

Fig. 7. TOS, focused library synthesis and DOS; a comparison of the planning strategies used (i.e. retrosynthetic or forward synthetic analysis and convergent or divergent synthesis) and the chemical space interrogated (i.e. focused point/area or diverse coverage). (Adapted with permission from Spring *et. al.* (2008) Diversity-oriented synthesis; a spectrum of approaches and results. *Organic & Biomolecular Chemistry*, 2008, 6(7), 1149-1158. Available at http://dx.doi.org/10.1039/B719372F, Copyright, The Royal Society of Chemistry (2008).

As described in two prominent reviews (Burke & Schreiber, 2004; Spring *et al*, 2008), skeletal diversity can be achieved principally in two ways. The first method involves the use of different reagents and a common building block as starting point. This 'reagent-based approach' is also known as a branching pathway. The second method or the 'substrate-based approach' uses different building blocks that contain pre-encoded information of desired architectural geometry which are subjected to a common set of conditions leading to a diverse set of small molecules (Figure 8). Although there are not many successes at this point in time, DOS is used increasingly as an attempt to probe biological pathways or develop NMEs. Conceptually, it is important to appreciate that it is the functional diversity and not the structural diversity of small molecules that is a key measure of success in the application of DOS. For specific chemical strategies of DOS application, see for example (Burke & Schreiber, 2004; Hanson *et al*, 2010; Nielsen & Schreiber, 2008b; Spandl *et al*, 2008).

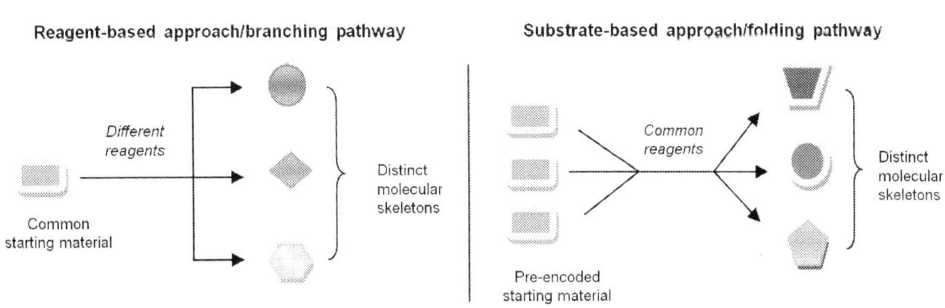

Fig. 8. Two common approaches for achieving skeletal diversity in DOS is "reagent-based approach/branching pathway" and "substrate-based approach/folding pathway".

2.2.2 Chemical genetics

In many ways, modern genetics began with the applied and theoretical work of the nature of inheritance in plants by German-Czech scientist Gregor Mendel in the mid-19th century. In comparison, the science in chemical genetics is only a couple of decades old, but has been gaining momentum in recent years. Chemical genetics has very much its origin in classical genetics and uses most of the methods and terminology already established. Genetic knockouts have been key to illustrating biological pathways and causations of pathological diseases and now the fields of chemical biology and related modern fields are enabling small molecules to be discovered and developed and used as chemical 'knockdowns'. To understand a system, you need to perturb it. This principle underlies most of the experimental sciences and explains why our depth of understanding of biological systems has been largely determined by the availability of tools that can be used to disrupt them (Stockwell, 2004). In order to close the genotype-phenotype gap, biological research has to reach beyond genomics, proteomics, and dissection of biological systems into their prime constituents (Bon & Waldmann, 2010). Protein function is regulated in complex networks with other biomacromolecules, small molecules and supramolecular structures like membranes (Zamir & Bastiaens, 2008). Whereas genetic manipulation results in a permanent alteration of the native structure of the network, chemical perturbations with small molecule modulators of protein function provides temporal control using dose-response explorations without fundamentally transforming the biological network (Stockwell, 2004). It is very attractive to use small molecules to perturb a biological system because of their dynamic nature, which offers many advantages: (i) ability to target a single domain of a multidomain protein, (ii) allows precise temporal control that is critical for rapidly acting processes, (iii) can target orthologous or paralogous proteins, enabling comparisons between species or redundant functions, and (iv) do not directly alter the concentrations of a targeted protein, thus avoiding indirect effects on multiprotein complexes (Lehar *et al*, 2008a).

The small molecules used to probe biological networks are ideally developed by mainstream medicinal chemistry and increasingly supported by modern methodologies such as DOS in order to encompass regions of chemical space that are not defined by existing screening collections as discussed previously. Essentially, chemical genetic studies can be designed to be either *forward* or *reverse* depending on the direction of learning that underlies their motivation (Nghiem & Kawasumi, 2007; Stockwell, 2004). *Forward* studies involve evaluating many chemical probes against one or a few phenotypes in order to identify active compounds, and reverse studies execute multiple phenotype measurements on a few related chemical probes to characterize their function. In both cases, the chemical probes can be analyzed across a panel of phenotypic assays to identify either broad activity or selectivity between the phenotypes (Lehar *et al*, 2008a). To elevate the complexity of the test system to reflect for example upon a diseased state of a cell combination chemical genetics (CCG) can be employed. CCG can be defined as the systematic testing of multiple perturbations involving chemical probes and can include either chemical combinations or mixed chemical and genetic perturbations. Classical and chemical genetics (Figure 9) are generally divided into *forward* screens, in which uncharacterized perturbers are tested against a selected phenotype to detect genes associated with that phenotype, and *reverse* studies, in which a specific gene or protein is modulated and multiple phenotypes are monitored to determine the effects of that specific target (Nghiem & Kawasumi, 2007; Stockwell, 2004). Studies involving combined perturbations can be similarly classified with the mechanistic focus shifted from individual targets to interactions between them (Lehar *et al*, 2008b).

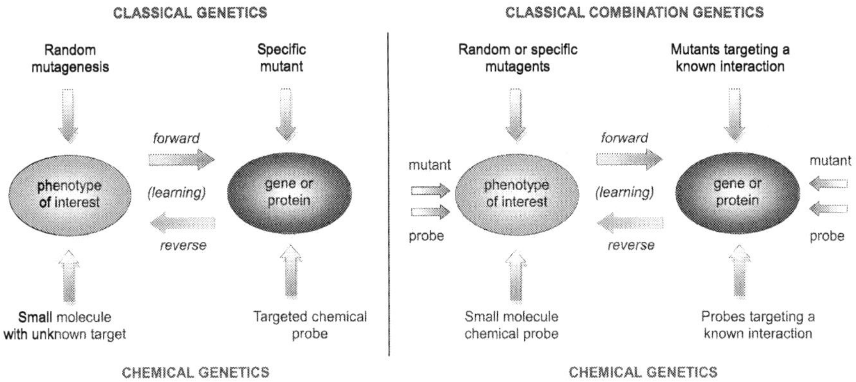

Fig. 9. Combined perturber studies in the context of forward and reverse genetics. The essence of classical and chemical genetics is to explore the function of individual genes or proteins. In combination chemical genetics, the focus of investigations shifts from individual targets to interactions between them or conditional target dependencies, and the perturbations are applied as combinations. (Adapted with permission from Lehar *et. al.* Combination chemical genetics. *Nat. Chem. Biol.* 2008, 4 (11), 674-681, copyright 2008, Macmillan Publishers Ltd).

Chemical biology has clearly made an impact in drug discovery and great strides towards offering new technologies that can progress our understanding of human health has been made. Given the temporal control offered by small molecules and the ability to use combinations of small molecule modulators, chemical genetics promises to complement the use of pure genetic analysis to study a wide range of biological systems. Chemical genetics aims to answer questions in complex test systems and may provide the field with commercial chemical probes that can be used to probe pathways and elucidate more about biological targets. The discovery of the potent and selective deacetylase inhibitors tubacin and histacin are examples of how powerful DOS and chemical genetics can be in combination with computational methods such as principal component analysis (Haggarty *et al*, 2003). However, good chemical probes for *in vitro* and especially *in vivo* perturbation are not easy to come by as small molecules are generally pleiotropic and they have multiple dose-dependent molecular targets that are often not fully characterized, which leads to unexpected activities. Obstacles and challenges are similar to those in drug development: small molecules often have inherent problems such as *in vitro* aggregation, poor solubility, difficulty in crossing biological membranes and reactive or toxic functionalities. At present, development of chemical probes for *in vivo* testing may be too ambitious a goal. As a result, evaluation of the effect of chemical 'knockdowns' in clinically relevant tissue should in the near future be in more complex assays that mimic for example malignant tissue. 3D cell culture technologies are increasingly becoming essential to *in vitro* screening. High content screening (HCS) has improved cell-based assays by combining high-resolution digital imaging with powerful software algorithms to increase the amount of data produced per well. 3D cell culture will not only empower HCS by supporting *in vivo* morphologies with current cell types, but also enable the use of primary and stem cells in drug discovery. Regardless of the challenges, primary and stem cells will become the focal point of 3D cell culture in the coming years (Justice *et al*, 2009), which could take chemical genetics to the next level. In summary the success of chemical genetics heavily relies on the availability of chemical libraries that offer structural diversity of small molecules that possess biological activity and complement libraries of compounds based on drugs and natural products (Lehar *et al*, 2008a). However, there is still a gap between developing commercial probes and inventing innovative drugs to treat illnesses.

3. R&D is moving global but will innovation increase?

"Trying to invent new drugs is no picnic." Sir James Black (1924-2010).

Only a small percentage of design and construction of scientific hypotheses that form the basis for a project actually yield exciting lead agents, let alone NMEs. Although the level of investment in pharmaceutical research and development (R&D) has increased dramatically since 1950 to US$50 billion per year at present, the number of new drugs that are approved annually is no greater now than it was in those days (Munos, 2009). From 1950 to 2008, the FDA approved 1,222 new drugs comprising of NMEs or new biologics (Figure 10). Historically, only approximately 1 out of 15–25 drug candidates survives the detailed safety and efficacy testing (in animals and humans) required for a drug to become a marketed product. As if these numbers were not disconcerting enough, from the industry's point of view, of the few drug candidates that successfully become marketed products, only one in three will become a major commercial product (Zhao & Guo, 2009). The discovery and development of a drug has often been quoted to take 10-15 years and cost in the region of $800 million to bring to market although the exact figure is probably much lower; i.e. the cost of NMEs is no doubt very high and close to $800 million but in contrast "me-too" drugs where most research has already been established the costs are nowhere near this figure (Angell, 2004). Regardless of the exact cost of developing a drug, the process of its development is a high-stakes, long-term and risky activity that has few peers in the commercial world, but the potential benefits to the millions of patients with serious diseases provide a constant motivating force for everybody involved in drug discovery.

A closer analysis reveals that 28 small-molecule first-in-class NMEs that entered the market between 1999 and 2008 were first discovered using phenotypic evaluation methods such as the employment of cell-based or whole-organism assays (Figure 11). Moreover, 17 NMEs were from target-based approaches and 5 NMEs were derived from natural substances. In contrast, 83 (51%) of the 164 follower drugs were discovered via target-based approaches. A possible contributing factor to this trend could have been a lag time between the introduction of new technologies and strategies, and their impact in terms of the number of approved first-in-class NMEs derived from such approaches. However, such a lag is not strongly apparent in a comparison of the cumulative number of NMEs from the two approaches during the period analysed (Swinney & Anthony, 2011).

3.1 Investment in education is vital to innovation

The investment in R&D has increased substantially in recent decades in efforts to obtain favourable market position and exclusivity in terms of IP position. The annual number of truly innovative new medicines approved by the FDA is not on the rise as highlighted in the previous section. Given the embracement of HTS technologies including combichem and FBDD combined with the improved understanding of disease pathogenesis, it is disappointing that there is no apparent evidence of an increase in the number of NMEs approved. An immediate answer is related to the accelerating costs of R&D which hampers progression of many research projects. Another deep-rooted answer may be related to education policies: how pupils in schools as well as both under- and postgraduate students in universities are being taught in the chemical, physical & biological sciences. Firstly, the development of HTS is costly and therefore largely inaccessible to academia that often carries out drug discovery on a shoe-string budget. One consequence is that academia, who historically has been the driver of much innovation, will feel not only compelled to lower

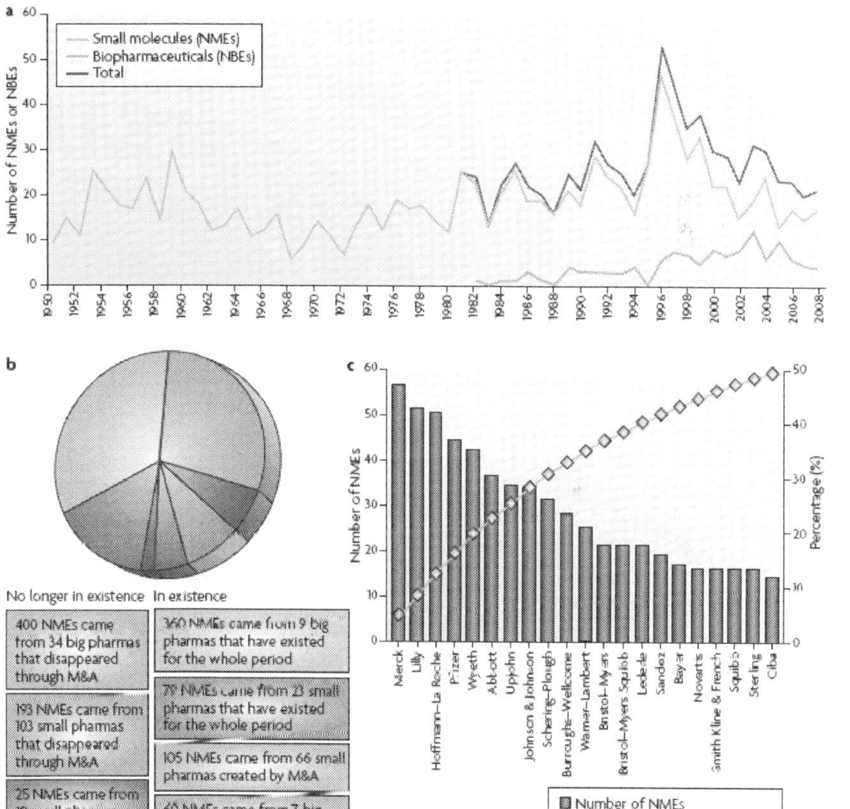

Fig. 10. Origins of new drugs. (a) Timeline of approvals of NMEs and new biological entities (NBEs) by the FDA between 1950 and 2008. (b) Characteristics of the 261 organizations that have produced the 1,222 NMEs approved since 1950. (c) 21 companies have produced half of all the NMEs that have been approved since 1950, although half of these companies no longer exist. In (b) and (c), both new small molecules and new biologics are grouped as NMEs for simplicity. M&A, mergers and acquisitions. (Reprinted with permission from Munos, B. Lessons from 60 years of pharmaceutical innovation. *Nature reviews*. 2009, *8* (12), 959-968, copyright 2009, Macmillan Publishers Ltd).

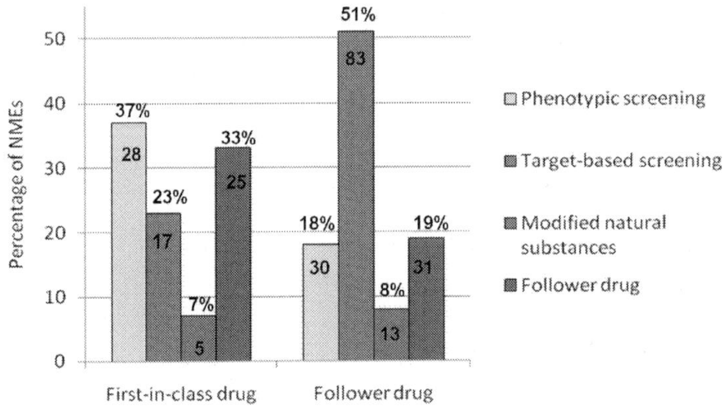

Fig. 11. The distribution of new drugs discovered between 1999 and 2008, according to the discovery strategy. The graph illustrates the number of NMEs in each category. (Adapted with permission from Swinney & Anthony. How were new medicines discovered? *Nature reviews*. 2011, 10(7), 507-519, copyright 2011, Macmillan Publishers Ltd).

their ambitions, but also hand over the baton to pharma- and biotech companies when it comes to innovative initiatives; that would be disastrous for many reasons. In particular, students would not be educated in using cutting-edge equipment and HTS technologies. Secondly, the approval of NMEs is also affected by the demonstration of adequate clinical safety and efficacy in humans which has become more complex, and ever-increasing amounts of data are now required by regulatory agencies (Lombardino & Lowe, 2004). Thirdly, it could also be argued that the dwindling supply of new drugs is related to a decrease in output by stifling the creativity of the scientists involved in drug discovery? This statement requires a more comprehensive discussion. In the western world the funding climate of academic institutions has changed and the pharmaceutical industry, in spite of scaling back on research operations and sizeable job cuts in 2010 (Mullin, 2010), is slowly returning to the funding levels available pre-recession and the international banking collapse in September 2008. For example, the UK funding landscape is having an impact on attracting and training students in synthetic organic chemistry. Many medicinal chemists working in the biotech and pharmaceutical industries received their PhDs in organic synthesis, a consequence of the view that excellence in organic synthesis is a prerequisite for a successful medicinal chemistry career (Frantz, 2003). However, the rise in small biotech companies has resulted in a demand for scientists that have research experience in multidisciplinary disciplines, and a broader education than in a single area such as synthetic organic chemistry (Pittman, 2010). Obtaining funding for chemical sciences may become more challenging in the future, due to a shift away from "responsive mode" applications; the success rate of EPSRC (the main British funding body for chemical sciences) applications has dropped from approx. 25% to 10% (Crow, 2008), and this coincided with a recent policy to limit applications from persistently unsuccessful academics (Lewcock, 2009). The EPSRC plans to cut research grant expenditure by £61 million to £372 million between 2010-2011 and 2014-2015. It will also stop accepting grant proposals regarding funding for PhD students by 2012, which instead will be supported exclusively through Centres for Doctoral Training Accounts (DTAs). Although, this shift provides a small £13 million rise in funding for studentships through to 2015 to offset the research grant decline it is potential very damaging for British universities that do not hold DTAs (Extance, 2011).

Restricting support is likely to result in a reduction of the pool of potential answers/solutions to critical problems, which arise from current and future challenges. This has led to concerns within industry that a reduced emphasis on organic synthesis would negatively impact the quality of future generations of scientists working at the interface of chemistry and biology (Pors *et al*, 2009). To balance these changes the EPSRC has initiated "grand challenges", where money is available to address key priorities for future collaborative research, such as in human health. These funding policy changes present opportunities for academics that can adapt, and a likely consequence is an increased degree of collaboration between organic synthesis and other disciplines. Ultimately this may result in the establishment of highly collaborative centres focused on chemical biology, drug discovery and other disciplines that support this important thematic initiative. One concern that industry has with such collaborative centres is that the students may find it more difficult to acquire highly specialised physical and synthetic organic chemistry skills and/or tools that would allow them to compete in a highly competitive job market. If, however, these centres do provide a thorough educational opportunity these PhD students may prove to be highly qualified for a career in medicinal chemistry and chemical biology, where success in projects frequently relies upon the successful collaboration and integration of multiple disciplines that are necessary for not only combating the major diseases, but also for becoming leaders in innovation (Pors *et al*, 2009).

Martin Schuurmann, the chairman of the European Institute of Innovation and Technology (EIT), has recently (Burke, 2011) opinionated that although Europe is a leader in research, it is not often in innovation. He believes that there are several reasons for this: a lack of education in entrepreneurship; too great a focus on research alone, rather than on the triangle' of education, research and business; a lack of focus on entrepreneurship as the key driver for innovation; and a weak leadership, typically embodied by committees. Although Schuurmann was talking broadly about innovation, there is no doubt that education and experience in entrepreneurship is vital to innovation in drug discovery too. Europe currently offers insufficient opportunities for young investigators to progress independent careers and to make the transition from assisting supervisors/projects leader to being independent researchers in their own right. As a consequence, highly talented research scientists are being hold back in their career progression and there is also a danger that these promising young scientists are encouraged to seek advancement outside the continent. In an attempt to maintain the best scientists of the future generations in Europe, the European Union has established *Starting Independent Researcher Grants* (ERC Starting Grants), which aim to support up-and-coming research leaders who are about to establish or consolidate a proper research team and to start conducting independent research in Europe. The budgets for the 2009 and 2010 calls were €325 and €580 million with a successful funding rate around 15% and 10% respectively for the two calls (European Research Council, 2011). The low success rate suggests high competition across Europe to obtain such prestigious grants, but is actually favourable to scientists working in *Life Sciences* where around 35% of the total funding was allocated in both 2009 and 2010. As such the European Union recognises the importance of research at the chemistry/biological interface, which in part underpins drug discovery.

While the system for funding students is slightly different in the USA, similar challenges and obstacles remain for principal investigators and the students in their laboratories. Take the example of cancer drug discovery, the National Cancer Institute, which is part of the National Institutes of Health (NIH) and the U.S. Department of Health and Human Services (DHHS), remains the principal agency for cancer research with other research grant support available from the Center for Disease Control (CDC) and Prevention and the Department of Defence (DOD) (National Cancer Institute, 2011a). The NCI is one of 27 Institutes and Centres that make up the NIH annual operating budget, which is allocated by the US Congress has remained flat at approximately $4.8 billion since 2004 (National Cancer Institute, 2011b); a number that has drastically lowered the funding payline with success rates for new Research Project Grants (better known as a RO1 grant) currently at or below 10% in year 2008 and 2009 (U.S. Department of Health & Human Services, 2010). While scientists earlier in their career are often supported for a period of 3-5 years through several financial mechanisms including foundations and academic departments, the current funding situation remains dichotomised given these significant federal budget constraints. While there is an appreciated need to support those in the earliest stage of their career the risk-reward equation from the viewpoint of many of these funding agencies is one that does not currently support innovative or highly translational research programs. Unfortunately, these programs are often the foundation of budding young scientists in drug discovery. With no or very little funding available to fund young academics there is a widespread concern in both the UK and US that innovative initiatives are stagnant or even on the decline. Indirectly, the tough financial times in Europe and the US may benefit the emerging countries such as China. Because of its traditional education philosophy and the "one-child" policy of the past 30 years, Chinese parents are eager to educate their child in the best possible institutions and invest between RMB 10,000-15,000 (USD 1,200-1,800) per year of study in higher education (Lian, 2005). This is a substantial amount of money that a lot of families have to borrow, but ensures a hard-working mentality and ability to survive that benefit project leaders in governmental and industrial research environments. These qualities coupled with a desire to learn from the West are central to education of the newer generations of students in China and ultimately to the establishment of the Pharma industry and rapid increase in the numbers of smaller biotech companies.

Whether in Europe, the US or in the emerging countries, new strategies are emerging as a result of re-focusing and restructuring of the drug discovery field, leading to a new 'front end' between pharma and academia which aims at more successfully taking new therapeutic entities through pre-clinical and clinical development to the market (Tralau-Stewart *et al*, 2009). By addressing "grand challenges" such as in healthcare and in setting up collaborative centres with a focus on drug discovery it may be that academia can benefit from advice and support from the pharmaceutical and biotech industries given their longstanding success in this field. During difficult economic times, however, many private sector companies are forced to reduce their R&D budgets. This is an opportunity for academics to fill an important innovation gap. In the business sector we are witnessing this change through the significant licensing as well as merger and acquisition activity that has been documented through numerous partnership deals between academic institutions and pharmaceutical companies. The goals of academia and industry may become more closely aligned if, as suggested by the research councils of the UK, there is a shift in academia from fundamental/basic research towards knowledge transfer and innovation. The EPSRC, for instance, encourages the formation of partnerships between academia and industry through its postgraduate CASE awards, which already serve to strengthen the ties between the two. Industry also contributes in a positive manner to undergraduate teaching of medicinal chemistry in many universities through educational tools, including industrial case histories as well as more traditional academic lecturers. However, some people in industry have the opinion that many of the key skills and novel techniques that are a part of modern drug discovery in industry are lacking at undergraduate level (Frantz, 2003). The challenge for universities is to ensure that the medicinal chemistry content of their chemistry courses is relevant to modern drug discovery and to address the opportunity for greater collaboration between industry and academia. Given the importance of the early stage knowledge transfer and the development of these core competencies, many institutions both in the UK and USA have developed or are developing both undergraduate and graduate curricula with a focus on bioinformatics, biotechnology and the interplay between the two. Whilst concerns over course content are, however, important for attracting and educating skilful chemists (Price & Hill, 2004), arguably the greater threat to medicinal and synthetic organic chemistry is funding. It is vital that both industry and academia work with public funding bodies to ensure that the core disciplines that will provide the next generation of innovative and skilled medicinal chemists are appropriately supported at the public, corporate and government level (Pors *et al*, 2009).

3.2 R&D in the emerging markets: An opportunity for collaboration and innovation?

The uncertainty of the funding climate and the lack of innovation (as measured by number of NMEs being approved for market) have naturally given cause for concern. In contrast to what has happened in the western countries after the recession, it appears that emerging markets are on the rise, partly because of heavy investment by the largest pharmaceutical companies in countries such as China over the past decade. Principally, the significantly lower cost of research in emerging economies has lead to a substantial increase in the outsourcing of the more routine activities such as compound synthesis and preclinical toxicity tests, but also outsourcing of R&D to augment internal capabilities of pharmaceutical companies are on the rise (Tremblay, 2010). Besides China, the pharmaceutical companies have used considerable efforts in establishing themselves in the emerging markets including China, India, Brazil, Russia, South Korea and Mexico. Given that 85% of the world's population lives in these countries combined with more open policies has meant that R&D has accelerated enormously in these countries. In 2004, China was the fastest-growing pharmaceutical market with growth rates of 28%. In 2015 Asia is expected to overtake Europe in pharmaceutical sales and become the second largest pharmaceutical market after the United States (Hughes, 2010). By 2050, Asia is projected to be the largest pharmaceutical market (Ward, 2008), which will have significant impact on drug discovery as a whole. The growth of the Chinese health-care market is largely being driven by the changing age profile of the population, its rapid economic development, and urbanization (Ward, 2008). As a consequence, the disease profile in China is changing. For example, type 2 diabetes was a rare disease in China 20 years ago, but its commonness has doubled in the past decade, with more than 55 million people affected today. A recent study conducted from June 2007 to May 2008 reported that 9.7% of the general adult population in China has diabetes and 15.5% have pre-diabetes, compared with 2.4% and 3.2%, respectively, in a similar study in 1994 (Yang *et al*, 2010). This increase in disease incidence has been ascribed to longer life expectancy and lifestyle changes that have occurred through rapid economic growth in especially Asia. As the emerging markets grow, an appreciation of population factors and changes associated with modernization is vital to dealing with and predicting how the Chinese health-care market will evolve (Ward, 2008). This is already starting to impact early-stage research aimed at specific medical needs of patients in these regions but also clinical trials are initiated with focus on enrolling enough patients from central as well as remote regions of China. Both early-stage research and clinical trials are of huge interest to the pharmaceutical industry that is investing heavily in Asia. Current discussion also concerns whether the focus of medical research is directly applicable for patient populations in Asia (Hughes, 2010). China has an estimated 100 million people suffering from hypertension and, with 62% of males being smokers, the country's lung cancer rates are among the highest in the world (Hughes, 2010). India, the second largest populated country in the world with over a billion citizens, has also seen an increase in lifestyle-associated diseases. By 2025, there will be more than 185 million people over the age of 60 years in India. As is often the case with an elderly population there is an increased risk of developing diabetes, cardiovascular disease and maybe also region specific diseases. As a result it is important to think of the medicines that will be available for these countries with regard to the types of disease, as well as their cost and accessibility (Hughes, 2010).

Despite of the investment in the emerging markets, recent data show that the US remains the single-largest location of pharmaceutical invention (Friedman, 2010). They also show that while the established pharmaceutical countries remain strong, there is little measurable innovative activity in terms of NMEs from India or China between 2001 and 2009. However, the factual situation is probably somewhat different due to a substantial time lag of 10 years or more between the initial discovery of a potential drug and its market approval. Indeed, China became the world leader in 2009 in terms of the number of chemistry patents published on an annual basis, according to Chemical Abstracts Service (CAS), a division of the American Chemical Society (Rovner, 2010). Accordingly, the recent nature of the increase in investment in innovative research in China and other emerging countries (Friedman, 2010) could facilitate an opportunity to innovate in a number of areas and as a result lead to a higher number of NMEs for market approval in the future. As such, the outlook for the patient is clearly very exciting. The next 50 years could see joint efforts between established and emerging markets in advancing many industries and technologies including drug discovery. The strategic planning and the vision by the pharmaceutical industry and American and European governments would facilitate a continuous input from established markets with R&D expertise that would maintain a high level of leadership in innovation, but also enable the emerging markets to be key players in future innovation.

4. Future directions

"Prediction is very difficult, especially about the future." Niels Bohr (1885 - 1962)

Drug discovery has come a long way since Paul Ehrlich's research into dyes for medicinal properties. Drug discovery now requires a multidisciplinary effort and the continuing need for the education of excellent scientists working at the interface of chemistry and biology is imperative, not only to successful drug development, but also to the exploration of new targets using small molecules to probe cellular and molecular mechanisms. Indeed, small molecules designed and synthesised in chemistry laboratories have been shown to be valuable for treating diseases and constitute many of the medicines marketed today (Nielsen & Schreiber, 2008a). Consequently, their effect on biomedical research during the past decade has been dramatic, providing both new tools for understanding living systems as

well as enabling a didactic transition from biology to medicine (Dobson, 2004; Nielsen & Schreiber, 2008a; Stockwell, 2004). The foundation of HTS technologies, the availability of chem- and bioinformatic databases coupled with emerging tools such as FBDD, DOS and chemical genetics has led drug discovery into the 21st century with optimism for further advancement and understanding of what is required for successful drug development. We know that there is no "magic bullet" around the corner, but through hard work and innovative thinking we are likely improve our knowledge and slowly but incrementally develop better drugs. There must also be an element of braveness and entrepreneurship if we are to solve challenging targets and there is a need for industry and governmental organisations to finance such ventures. For example, ventures into underexploited regions of chemical space is to expand the range of 'druggable' targets, such that the identification of new ligands for currently challenging targets such as protein-protein interaction (Fuller *et al*, 2009) ultimately becomes routine. Success in this endeavour is likely to have major positive impacts in medicinal chemistry, chemical biology and drug discovery (Moura-Letts *et al*, 2011). It is worth noting, however, that the commercial success of a drug is not related to the novelty of the mechanism upon which it is based, but the differentiation that it provides (Booth & Zemmel, 2003; Ma *et al*, 2008). Finding a new therapeutically relevant target is extremely difficult and pioneering drug discovery has become prohibitively expensive. Many validated targets should also be further exploited alongside innovative initiatives to provide better products with lower risk and cost (Zhao & Guo, 2009).
However, there is cause for concern. Declining government funding and reformed educational policies in the western world are likely to have serious implications for drug discovery educators and practitioners, which could widen the already significant gap between research scientists at the highest level and the education of students at undergraduate and postgraduate level. There is a real concern that the scientists of tomorrow will not possess the 'right' tools in the toolkit to be able to effectively interrogate and address the questions being asked by research scientists in academia and industry today. The challenges can only be met if the government agencies worldwide are willing to invest in the education of academics and students alike. The onus is also on academics to be able to adapt to the rapidly changing funding priorities (Pors *et al*, 2009). In addition, drug discovery is entering a period of uncertainty where it is vital that opportunities in the emerging markets are grasped by the horn. A close collaboration between the pharmaceutical industry, governments in US and Europe and the emerging markets is essential for adapting to ever-increasing costs of drug discovery. Accordingly, the recent nature of the increase in investment in innovative research in China and other emerging countries could facilitate an opportunity to innovate in a number of areas and as a result lead to a higher number of NMEs for market approval. The next 50 years could see joint efforts between established and emerging markets in advancing drug discovery. The strategic planning and the vision by the pharmaceutical industry and American and European governments would facilitate a continuous input from established markets with R&D expertise that would maintain a high level of leadership in innovation, but also enable the emerging markets to be key players in future innovation.

5. Acknowledgements

This work was supported by Yorkshire Cancer Research (U.K.). The author is grateful to Dr Robert A. Falconer for critical analysis and useful discussions during manuscript writing. Cheryl S. James is thanked for proofreading of manuscript.

6. References

Abad-Zapatero, C. (2007). A Sorcerer's apprentice and the rule of five: from rule-of-thumb to commandment and beyond. *Drug Discovery Today*, Vol. 12, pp. 995-997

Angell, M. (2004). The Truth About the Drug Companies: How They Deceive Us and What to Do About It pp. Random House Publishing, ISBN 0-37576094-37576096, New York, U.S.

Bauer, R. A.; Wurst J. M. & Tan D. S. (2010). Expanding the range of 'druggable' targets with natural product-based libraries: an academic perspective. *Current Opinion in Chemical Biology*, Vol. 14, pp. 308-314

Bender, A.; Fergus S.; Galloway W. R. J. D.; et al. (2006). Diversity oriented synthesis: A challenge for synthetic chemists. *Chemical Genomics: Small Molecule Probes to Study Cellular Function*, Vol. 58, pp. 47-60

Billingsley, M. L. (2008). Druggable targets and targeted drugs: enhancing the development of new therapeutics. *Pharmacology*, Vol. 82, pp. 239-244

Boehringer, M.; Boehm H. J.; Bur D.; et al. (2000). Novel inhibitors of DNA gyrase: 3D structure based biased needle screening, hit validation by biophysical methods, and 3D guided optimization. A promising alternative to random screening. *Journal of Medicinal Chemistry*, Vol. 43, pp. 2664-2674

Bon, R. S. & Waldmann H. (2010). Bioactivity-guided navigation of chemical space. *Account of Chemical Research*, Vol. 43, pp. 1103-1114

Booth, B. & Zemmel R. (2003). Opinion - Quest for best. *Nature Reviews Drug Discovery*, Vol. 2, pp. 838-841

Brown, J. M. & Wilson W. R. (2004). Exploiting tumour hypoxia in cancer treatment. *Nat Rev Cancer*, Vol. 4, pp. 437-447

Burke, M. (2011). Innovation: Europe must do better. *Chemistry World*, Vol. 8, pp. 12

Burke, M. D. & Schreiber S. L. (2004). A planning strategy for diversity-oriented synthesis. *Angewandte Chemie-International Edition*, Vol. 43, pp. 46-58

Chessari, G. & Woodhead A. J. (2009a). From fragment to clinical candidate--a historical perspective. *Drug Discov Today*, Vol. 14, pp. 668-675

Chessari, G. & Woodhead A. J. (2009b). From fragment to clinical candidate--a historical perspective. *Drug Discovery Today*, Vol. 14, pp. 668-675

Crow, J. M. (2008). UK chemists warn of funding crisis. *In: Chemistry World*, Vol. 5, pp. Available from http://www.rsc.org/chemistryworld/News/2008/October/20100801.asp

de Kloe, G. E.; Bailey D.; Leurs R.; et al. (2009). Transforming fragments into candidates: small becomes big in medicinal chemistry. *Drug Discov Today*, Vol. 14, pp. 630-646

Denny, W. A. (2002). The contribution of synthetic organic chemistry to anticancer drug development. *In Anticancer Drug Development, (Baguely B.C and Kerr D.J., eds)*, pp. 187-202, Academic Press

Dobson, C. M. (2004). Chemical space and biology. *Nature*, Vol. 432, pp. 824-828

Edwards, P. D.; Albert J. S.; Sylvester M.; et al. (2007). Application of fragment-based lead generation to the discovery of novel, cyclic amidine beta-secretase inhibitors with nanomolar potency, cellular activity, and high ligand efficiency. *Journal of Medicinal Chemistry*, Vol. 50, pp. 5912-5925

European Research Council (2011). ERC Starting Independent Researcher Grant pp. Available at http://erc.europa.eu/index.cfm?fuseaction=page.display&topicID=65

Extance, A. (2011). EPSRC plans represent 'huge change'. *Chemistry World*, Vol. 8, p. 8

Feher, M. & Schmidt J. M. (2003). Property distributions: Differences between drugs, natural products, and molecules from combinatorial chemistry. *Journal of Chemical Information and Computer Sciences*, Vol. 43, pp. 218-227

Frantz, S. (2003). Creating the right chemistry. *Nat Rev Drug Discov*, Vol. 2, p. 163

Friedman, Y. (2010). Location of pharmaceutical innovation: 2000-2009. *Nature Reviews Drug Discovery*, Vol. 9, pp. 835-836

Fuller, J. C.; Burgoyne N. J. & Jackson R. M. (2009). Predicting druggable binding sites at the protein-protein interface. *Drug Discovery Today*, Vol. 14, pp. 155-161

Gedye, R.; Smith F.; Westaway K.; et al. (1986). The Use of Microwave-Ovens for Rapid Organic-Synthesis. *Tetrahedron Letters*, Vol. 27, pp. 279-282

Goodman, L. S.; Wintrobe M. M.; Damescheck W.; et al. (1946). Nitrogen mustard therapy. Use of methyl-bis(β-chloroethyl)amine hydrochloride and tris-(β-chloroethyl)amine hydrochloride for Hodgkin's disease, lymphosarcoma, leukemia and certain allied and miscellaneous disorders. *J Am Med Assoc*, Vol. 132, pp. 126-132

Haggarty, S. J.; Koeller K. M.; Wong J. C.; et al. (2003). Multidimensional chemical genetic analysis of diversity-oriented synthesis-derived deacetylase inhibitors using cell-based assays. *Chemical Biology*, Vol. 10, pp. 383-396

Hanson, P. R.; Rolfe A. & Lushington G. H. (2010). Reagent based DOS: A "Click, Click, Cyclize" strategy to probe chemical space. *Organic & Biomolecular Chemistry*, Vol. 8, pp. 2198-2203

Hirsch, J. (2006). An anniversary for cancer chemotherapy. *JAMA*, Vol. 296, pp. 1518-1520

Hopkins, A. L. & Groom C. R. (2002). The druggable genome. *Nature Reviews Drug Discovery*, Vol. 1, pp. 727-730

Hughes, B. (2010). Evolving R&D for emerging markets. *Nature Reviews Drug Discovery*, Vol. 9, pp. 417-420

Justice, B. A.; Badr N. A. & Felder R. A. (2009). 3D cell culture opens new dimensions in cell-based assays. *Drug Discov Today*, Vol. 14, pp. 102-107

Lam, K. S. & Renil M. (2002). From combinatorial chemistry to chemical microarray. *Current Opinion in Chemical Biology*, Vol. 6, pp. 353-358

Lehar, J.; Stockwell B. R.; Giaever G.; et al. (2008a). Combination chemical genetics. *Nature Chemical Biology*, Vol. 4, pp. 674-681

Lehar, J.; Stockwell B. R.; Giaever G.; et al. (2008b). Combination chemical genetics. *Nat Chem Biol*, Vol. 4, pp. 674-681

Lewcock, A. (2009). EPSRC turnaround on blacklisting policy. *Chemistry World*, Vol. 6, pp. Available from http://www.rsc.org/chemistryworld/News/2009/May/05050904.asp

Lian, M. (2005). Chemistry education in china. *Nachrichten Aus Der Chemie*, Vol. 53, pp. 622-627

Lipinski, C. A.; Lombardo F.; Dominy B. W.; et al. (1997). Experimental and computational approaches to estimate solubility and permeability in drug discovery and development settings. *Advanced Drug Delivery Reviews*, Vol. 23, pp. 3-25

Lombardino, J. G. & Lowe J. A., 3rd (2004). The role of the medicinal chemist in drug discovery--then and now. *Nat Rev Drug Discov*, Vol. 3, pp. 853-862

Ma, P.; Gudiksen M.; Fleming E.; et al. (2008). Outlook - What drives success for specialty pharmaceuticals? *Nature Reviews Drug Discovery*, Vol. 7, pp. 563-567

Moos, W. H.; Hurt C. R. & Morales G. A. (2009). Combinatorial chemistry: oh what a decade or two can do. *Molecular Diversity*, Vol. 13, pp. 241-245

Moura-Letts, G.; Diblasi C. M.; Bauer R. A.; et al. (2011). Solid-phase synthesis and chemical space analysis of a 190-membered alkaloid/terpenoid-like library. *Proc Natl Acad Sci U S A*, Vol. 108, pp. 6745-6750

Mullin, R. (2010). Battening the Hatches. *Chemical & Engineering News*, Vol. 88, p. 14

Munos, B. (2009). Lessons from 60 years of pharmaceutical innovation. *Nature Reviews Drug Discovery*, Vol. 8, pp. 959-968

National Cancer Institute (2011a). Cancer Research Funding. pp. Available at http://www.cancer.gov/cancertopics/factsheet/NCI/research-funding

National Cancer Institute (2011b). The NCI Budget in Review. pp. Available at http://obf.cancer.gov/financial/factbook.htm

Nghiem, P. & Kawasumi M. (2007). Chemical genetics: Elucidating biological systems with small-molecule compounds. *Journal of Investigative Dermatology*, Vol. 127, pp. 1577-1584

Nielsen, T. E. & Schreiber S. L. (2008a). Towards the optimal screening collection: a synthesis strategy. *Angew Chem Int Ed Engl*, Vol. 47, pp. 48-56

Nielsen, T. E. & Schreiber S. L. (2008b). Towards the optimal screening collection: a synthesis strategy. *Angewandte Chemie-International Edition*, Vol. 47, pp. 48-56

Overington, J. P.; Al-Lazikani B. & Hopkins A. L. (2006). Opinion - How many drug targets are there? *Nature Reviews Drug Discovery*, Vol. 5, pp. 993-996

Philpott, K. L.; Hughes J. P.; Rees S.; et al. (2011). Principles of early drug discovery. *British Journal of Pharmacology*, Vol. 162, pp. 1239-1249

Pittman, D. (2010). Changing Their Ways. *Chemical & Engineering News*, Vol. 88, pp. 47-49

Pors, K.; Goldberg F. W.; Leamon C. P.; et al. (2009). The changing landscape of cancer drug discovery: a challenge to the medicinal chemist of tomorrow. *Drug Discovery Today*, Vol. 14, pp. 1045-1050

Price, W. S. & Hill J. O. (2004). Raising the Status of Chemistry Education. *The Royal Society of Chemistry*, pp. 13-20

Reymond, J. L. & Fink T. (2007). Virtual exploration of the chemical universe up to 11 atoms of C, N, O, F: Assembly of 26.4 million structures (110.9 million stereoisomers) and analysis for new ring systems, stereochemistry, physicochemical properties, compound classes, and drug discovery. *Journal of Chemical Information and Modeling*, Vol. 47, pp. 342-353

Rooseboom, M.; Commandeur J. N. & Vermeulen N. P. (2004). Enzyme-catalyzed activation of anticancer prodrugs. *Pharmacol Rev*, Vol. 56, pp. 53-102

Rovner, S. L. (2010). China Ascendant. *Chemical & Engineering News*, Vol. 88, pp. 35-37

Rydzewski, R. M. (2008). The Drug Discovery Busines to Date. *In: Real World Drug Discovery: A Chemist's Guide to Biotech and Pharmaceutical Research*, pp. 1-52, Elsevier, ISBN: 978-970-908-046617-046610, Amsterdam, The Netherlands.

SalimiMoosavi, H.; Tang T. & Harrison D. J. (1997). Electroosmotic pumping of organic solvents and reagents in microfabricated reactor chips. *Journal of the American Chemical Society*, Vol. 119, pp. 8716-8717

Sharpless, K. B.; Kolb H. C. & Finn M. G. (2001). Click chemistry: Diverse chemical function from a few good reactions. *Angewandte Chemie-International Edition*, Vol. 40, pp. 2004-2021

Shoichet, B. K.; Hert J.; Irwin J. J.; et al. (2009). Quantifying biogenic bias in screening libraries. *Nature Chemical Biology*, Vol. 5, pp. 479-483

Sneader, W. E. (2005). Legacy of the past. *Drug discovery: a history*, pp. John Wiley & Sons Ltd, ISBN-10 10-471-89979-89978, West Sussex (U.K.)

Spandl, R. J.; Bender A. & Spring D. R. (2008). Diversity-oriented synthesis; a spectrum of approaches and results. *Organic & Biomolecular Chemistry*, Vol. 6, pp. 1149-1158

Spring, D. R.; Spandl R. J. & Bender A. (2008). Diversity-oriented synthesis; a spectrum of approaches and results. *Organic & Biomolecular Chemistry*, Vol. 6, pp. 1149-1158

Stockwell, B. R. (2004). Exploring biology with small organic molecules. *Nature*, Vol. 432, pp. 846-854

Strebhardt, K. & Ullrich A. (2008). Paul Ehrlich's magic bullet concept: 100 years of progress. *Nature Reviews Cancer*, Vol. 8, pp. 473-480

Studer, A.; Hadida S.; Ferritto R.; et al. (1997). Fluorous synthesis: A fluorous-phase strategy for improving separation efficiency in organic synthesis. *Science*, Vol. 275, pp. 823-826

Swinney, D. C. & Anthony J. (2011). How were new medicines discovered? *Nature Reviews Drug Discovery*, Vol. 10, pp. 507-519

Tralau-Stewart, C. J.; Wyatt C. A.; Kleyn D. E.; et al. (2009). Drug discovery: new models for industry-academic partnerships. *Drug Discov Today*, Vol. 14, pp. 95-101

Tremblay, J. F. (2010). The Grand Experiment. *Chemical & Engineering News*, Vol. 88, p. 20

U.S. Department of Health & Human Services (2010). Research Project and R01-equivalent grants: success rates of new applications, by submission number. pp. Available at http://report.nih.gov/success_rates/index.aspx

Ward, S. (2008). Demographic factors in the Chinese health-care market. *Nature Reviews Drug Discovery*, Vol. 7, pp. 383-384

Wilhelm, S.; Carter C.; Lynch M.; et al. (2006). Discovery and development of sorafenib: a multikinase inhibitor for treating cancer. *Nature Reviews Drug Discovery*, Vol. 5, pp. 835-844

Yang, S. H.; Dou K. F. & Song W. J. (2010). Prevalence of diabetes among men and women in China. *New England Journal of Medicine*, Vol. 362, pp. 2425-2426; author reply 2426

Zamir, E. & Bastiaens P. I. H. (2008). Reverse engineering intracellular biochemical networks. *Nature Chemical Biology*, Vol. 4, pp. 643-647

Zartler, E. R. & Shapiro M. J. (2005). Fragonomics: fragment-based drug discovery. *Current Opinion in Chemical Biology*, Vol. 9, pp. 366-370

Zhao, H. & Guo Z. (2009). Medicinal chemistry strategies in follow-on drug discovery. *Drug Discov Today*, Vol. 14, pp. 516-522

Zlokarnik, G.; Grootenhuis P. D. & Watson J. B. (2005). High throughput P450 inhibition screens in early drug discovery. *Drug Discov Today*, Vol. 10, pp. 1443-1450

Part 2

Models

5

Genetically Engineered Mouse Models in Preclinical Anti-Cancer Drug Development

Sergio Y. Alcoser and Melinda G. Hollingshead
Biological Testing Branch, Developmental Therapeutics Program,
National Cancer Institute
USA

1. Introduction

According to the most recent American Cancer Society data, an estimated 569,490 Americans died from cancer in 2010 (American Cancer Society [ACS], 2010). The number of cancer-related deaths recently surpassed those from heart disease in Americans <85 yrs old (Kung et al., 2008). Developing new and more efficacious anti-cancer compounds is a paramount health care priority. At the Developmental Therapeutics Program of the U.S. National Cancer Institute, potential therapeutic agents are typically tested for activity in an *in vitro* 60-tumor cell line screen and subsequently by *in vivo* xenograft studies in rodents (Figure 1). Once selected for additional testing using established criteria (drugability, novelty of structure and/or mechanism of action, potency, cell panel selectivity, etc.), additional studies (pharmaocokinetics, pharmacodynamics, range finding toxicity, formulation, mechanism of action analysis, IND-directed toxicology, etc.) are initiated followed by the progression of a selected few candidate agents into human clinical trials. Efficacious drugs with tolerable toxicity are ushered into early phase clinical trials. However, most of the promising compounds identified in the multi-layered preclinical screenings are not as successful in human patients. Therefore, preclinical models that better predict drug efficacy and toxicity in humans are needed. Differences in drug absorption, distribution, metabolism and elimination (ADME), immune responses and over-interpretation of the preclinical efficacy data may contribute to clinical failures. However, a significant limitation is generating mouse models that histologically, genetically, and behaviorally recapitulate the human disease.

Over the past twenty years, researchers have identified many of the underlying genetic abnormalities that cause certain cancers and have genetically engineered them into mouse models to explore the oncogenic nature of those genes and related pathways. The resulting mouse models generate tumors that may better mimic those seen in humans. It is anticipated that therapeutic compounds which show efficacy and low toxicity in these more human-like genetically engineered mouse (GEM) models will be more successful in clinical trials and lead to increased cancer survivorship. Hundreds of GEM models currently exist that are associated with some form of human tumor development (see the eMICE website). It is well beyond the scope of this manuscript to adequately describe each of them. We instead briefly review some of the ground-breaking GEM models developed in the 1980s and 90s, describe more recent and sophisticated models, highlight some of the advantages and limitations for each, and explore the potential roles of molecular targeted therapies and GEM models in preclinical drug testing. For additional details on each model, we refer the reader to the original articles or prior in-depth reviews. While mice that develop genetically engineered tumors hold much promise, the relatively slow growth rate of these tumors and their low penetrance (regardless of genetics, some mice will not develop tumors during the time constraints of the experiment) makes them ill-suited to replace xenograft models as the primary *in vivo* screening tool. Instead, we envision GEM models as an additional screening mechanism that narrows and optimizes the field of therapeutic compounds before expensive and time-consuming human clinical trials are initiated.

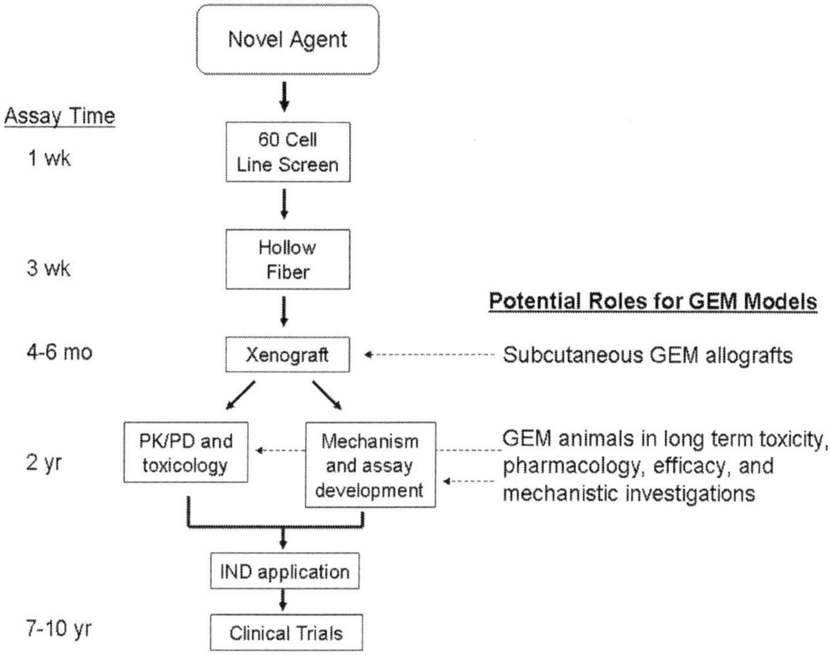

Fig. 1. Where GEMs Can Be Most Useful in the Preclinical Drug Development

Simplistic overview of preclinical drug development procedure in the NCI/DTP. Novel agents are introduced through the 60 Cell Line Screen (reviewed in Monks et al., 1991), which contains 60 human cultured tumor cell lines in a 96-well plate array. If anti-proliferative activity is observed in a number of cell lines, the agent is tested in a Hollow Fiber assay, which measures the anti-proliferative activity in cultured cells grown in hollow polyvinylidene fluoride (PVDF) fibers implanted intraperitoneally and subcutaneously in mice (reviewed in Decker et al., 2004). If active in Hollow Fiber assays, agents are administered to immunodeficient animals that possess human tumors generated from serially passaged human tumor cell lines (xenografts). Tolerable toxicity and activity measurable in xenograft models leads to simultaneous investigations into the agent's

PK/PD, mechanism of action and toxicology. Based on this data, where applicable an IND application is generated for FDA approval to initiate clinical trials. The agents may require further preclinical studies or can be approved for a small scale Phase 0 trial (reviewed in Murgo et al., 2008), or initial Phase I human clinical trials. Assay Time is a best case scenario for a single agent and does not include time for optimization and validation repetitions. PD = pharmacodynamics, PK = pharmacokinetics, GEM = genetically engineered mouse, IND = Investigational New Drug

2. Background: *in vivo* drug screening using the human tissue xenograft

After a potential therapeutic agent shows some activity in cultured tumor cell growth assays, its activity and toxicity are explored through *in vivo* xenograft models. Fragments of human tumors or cultured human tumor cells are implanted (often subcutaneously) into immunodeficient rodents. Once the tumors grow to a predetermined size, the potential anti-cancer agent is administered and the tumor response, generally assessed by tracking the tumor size, is measured over time. Drug doses and administration schedules are adjusted to optimize efficacy and to lower toxicity over several experimental cycles. This system generates valuable data and quickly returns a prediction on an agent's activity, often in several months. Unfortunately, promising anti-cancer compounds discovered through this route often fail in human clinical trials, commonly due to low efficacy (Kerbel et al., 2003; Sharpless & DePinho, 2006). The low predictive value of these xenograft models exemplifies the need for better *in vivo* mouse models for preclinical drug testing.

3. Birth of the transgenic "Oncomouse"

Transgenic mouse technology has evolved from the early 1980s (reviewed in Palmiter & Brinster, 1986) such that researchers can now conditionally and reversibly alter single gene expression. Thousands of publications have since supported the hypothesis that oncogene expression or tumor suppressor gene ablation in normal mammalian cells is sufficient to drive tumor development. The first report of a heritable tumor-prone transgenic mouse came in June 1984 (Brinster et al., 1984). These mice used the SV40 enhancer region to help drive expression of a construct consisting of the mouse metallothionein-1 gene promoter fused to the thymidine kinase gene from the herpes simplex virus (HSV). They included the whole SV40 upstream region, consisting of enhancer, promoter, and two T-antigen genes transcribed in the opposite direction. It was thought the T-antigen genes would be inactive in mice. Unexpectedly, they observed that the transgenic mice consistently developed brain tumors, as well as sporadic tumors in other tissues. Follow-up experiments showed that using only the SV40 enhancer/promoter region and the large T-antigen gene was sufficient to drive tumorigenesis (Palmiter et al., 1985). Subsequent reports have shown that expressing the large T-antigen in a specific cell type can promote tumor development. For example, Ornitz et al., (1985) demonstrated expression of the large T-antigen in acinar cells generated exocrine pancreatic tumors, whereas Hanahan (1985) used the insulin promoter driving the large T-antigen specifically in pancreatic beta-cells to produce endocrine pancreatic tumors.

Following the unexpected oncogenic ability of SV40, researchers tried to rationally design a tumor-generating transgenic mouse ("oncomouse"). In an effort to create a mouse model of a chromosomal translocation seen in some human B-cell lymphomas, Adams et al., (1985)

generated a transgene consisting of an immunoglobulin enhancer (Eμ) driving expression of the *Myc* gene. These mice heritably develop pre-B cell and mature B-cell lymphomas. Further studies by Strasser et al., (1990) showed that *Myc* required increased expression of the anti-apoptotic factor *Bcl-2* to drive tumorigenesis. Suppression of apoptosis is now understood to be a trademark of many cancer cells.

3.1 MMTV induced breast cancer

Using reciprocal matings between high tumor and low tumor mouse strains, Bittner (1936) reported tumor incidence in F1 females was dependent on the strain of the mother. Virologists demonstrated a virus (dubbed **M**urine **M**ammary **T**umor **V**irus, MMTV) was responsible for inducing tumors in mammary tissue and was passed from mother to offspring through her milk. Subsequent studies showed some mouse strains also had MMTV virus in their eggs and sperm (reviewed in Heston & Parks, 1977).

The utility of MMTV was expanded when it was shown that a short regulatory region (called long terminal repeat, LTR) was sufficient to confer hormone responsive and cell-specific expression *in vitro* (Huang et al., 1981). Stewart (1984) used the MMTV LTR to drive *Myc* expression in his transgenic mice that developed breast adenocarcinomas in mammary epithelial tissue. Since then the MMTV LTR has been fused with a variety of purported oncogenes to develop tumors in murine mammary tissue that are similar in morphology and gene expression profile to certain types of human breast cancers (reviewed in Robles & Varticovski, 2008). For example, the MMTV-driven **P**ol**y**oma **M**iddle-**T** antigen (*PyMT*) model develops tumors similar to a human breast cancer with luminal type morphology approximately 2-3 months after birth (Guy et al. 1992). A model expressing MMTV-driven *Wnt1* (wingless-type MMTV integration site family, member 1) generates mouse mammary tumors with characteristics similar to those of human basal type breast cancers (Huang et al., 2005). Several members of the *Wnt* gene family (encoding secretory glycoproteins that normally stimulate cell proliferation and differentiation) are expressed in the mouse mammary tissue during various stages of development. *Wnt-1* is not normally expressed in the mammary tissue; however, when driven ectopically by MMTV, it develops oncogenic properties. Like most of the other "first generation" transgenic oncomice, many of these models have a low tumor penetrance and widely variable latency period, making them difficult to use directly in large scale preclinical drug screenings. These limitations are partially overcome by resecting and transplanting transgenically induced tumors into many syngeneic recipient animals, generating a large cohort of tumor-bearing animals for drug-screening purposes (Maglione et al., 2004; Varticovski et al., 2007).

3.2 Activated kras

The KRAS2 gene encodes a G-protein that is a mammalian cellular homolog of a transforming gene isolated from the **K**irsten **RA**t **S**arcoma virus. This membrane-associated intracellular signal transducer plays a vital role in normal tissue signaling, proliferation, and differentiation (reviewed in Kranenburg, 2005). Several oncogenic point mutations interfere with the intrinsic GTPase activity of Kras, causing accumulation in a constitutively active GTP-bound state (Zenker et al., 2007). Expressing an activated *Kras* mutant transgene in acinar cells induces neoplasia in the fetal pancreas with large tumors developing only days after pancreatic differentiation (Quaife et al., 1987). Indeed, activating point mutations in the *Kras* gene have subsequently been shown to occur in 75 to 95% of spontaneous human pancreatic cancers (Almoguero et al., 1988) as well as > 90% of spontaneous and chemically induced mouse lung tumors (Malkinson 1998). Activated Kras expression in the mouse lung generates multiple tumors at an early age, so much so that the mice succumb quickly due to respiratory failure (Johnson et al., 2001). The varied penetrance and multi-focal primary tumor formation in addition to the short life span limits the use of this model in further studies of tumor development.

3.3 Knockout oncomice

The examples described thus far rely on the over expression of a nucleic acid sequence with purported oncogenic properties or mutations to drive tumorigenesis in mice. During the late 1980's the use of homologous recombination in mouse embryonic stem cells enabled researchers to inactivate ("knockout") single genes. This technology created a new wave of transgenic oncomice beginning with the heterozygous null retinoblastoma (Rb) mouse (Jacks et al., 1992). Rb inhibits the cell cycle by repressing expression of genes required for S phase progression (reviewed in Hanahan & Weiberg 2000). Mice lacking one Rb allele develop pituitary adenomas, whereas RB null offspring fail to develop beyond embryonic day 14 or 15, possibly due to excessive neuronal cell death.

The importance of tumor suppressor expression became evident from this and other knockout mouse models. Various cellular stresses prompt p53 to modulate expression of its target genes, many of which regulate cell cycle arrest, apoptosis, DNA repair, or cellular metabolism. Decreased or null expression of p53 has been observed in numerous human cancers (reviewed in Harris & Hollstein 1993). Mice lacking one or both p53 alleles are born normal but are predisposed to developing spontaneous lymphomas and sarcomas later in life (Donehower et al., 1992). Lacking a major tumor suppressor pathway, these p53 null mice became a useful background with which to elucidate the oncogenic potential of other genes. The Rb/p53 double knockout mice develop highly aggressive tumors in the cerebellum visible as early as 7 weeks of age (Marino et al., 2000). Mammary and skin tumors develop frequently in female mice carrying conditional null Brca2 and p53 alleles (Jonkers et al., 2001), suggesting synergistic inactivation of Brca2 and p53 can mediate mammary tumorigenesis.

Since these early transgenic and knockout mouse models have genetic alterations which are expressed in the germline and most, if not all, somatic cells, the models are more representative of human cancer predisposition syndromes. This is not the case for most human cancers, which develop spontaneously in a small number of cells in the adult. Many genes have distinct functions and expression patterns during embryonic development that are still poorly understood and different from those in the adult. In addition, these early transgenic models are notorious for their variable penetrance and tumor latency, making it nearly impossible to accumulate the number of animals with synchronous tumor development needed for large studies. While large scale production of transgenic mice is now possible with IVF and other high production methods (JAX® Speed Expansion Service; Charles River Laboratories Rapid Expansion Services), it does not obviate the issue of variable penetrance and tumor latency; it simply provides a large number of animals that can be held simultaneously to observe for tumor development. Early GEM models generated multiple primary lesions which far exceeded that observed in humans, limiting their predictive value and usefulness for preclinical studies. To better model most human cancers, genomic alterations should only occur in a small number of cells in the adult mouse tissue corresponding to the microenvironment in which the human cancer develops.

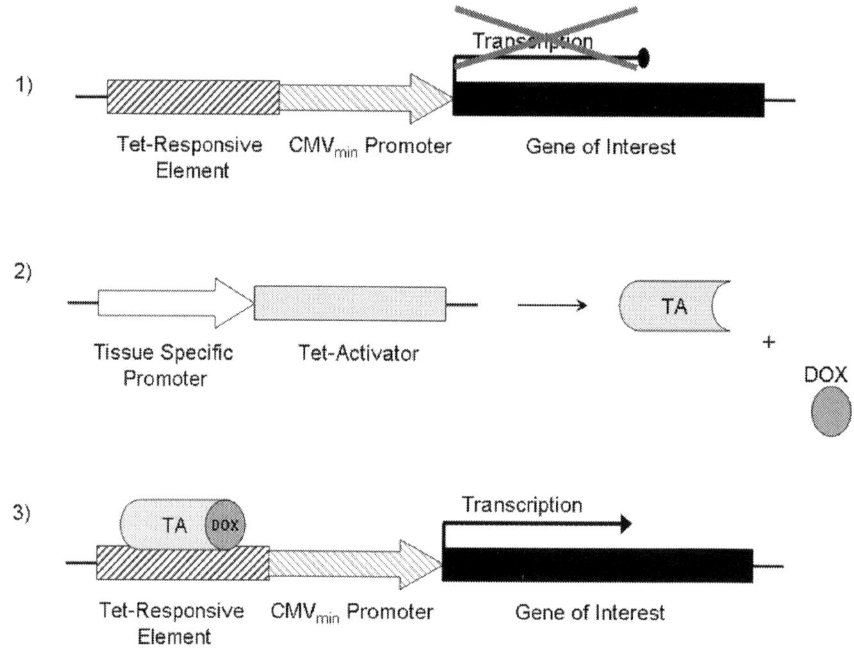

Fig. 2. Schematic Representation of the Tet-ON system; 1) Without the Tet-Activator (TA), the transgene consisting of the Gene-of-Interest (GOI) fused to the Tet-Responsive Element (TRE) will not be expressed. 2) Doxycycline can bind to the Tet-Activator protein, altering its protein structure such that TA can now bind to a TRE. 3) If both the Tet-Activator and the TRE-GOI transgenes are present in the same cell, upon doxycycline administration and TA activation, the GOI will be transcriptionally active.

4. Conditional and inducible oncogene expression

The ability to alter gene expression in a normal adult mouse overcomes many confounding factors gene manipulation might have in embryonic development and may better recapitulate human disease. A widely used inducible system is the Cre-Lox model (reviewed in Le & Sauer, 2001; Brault et al., 2007), where a segment of DNA is flanked by 34 base-pair (bp) LoxP sites (then referred to as floxed DNA). Co-expression of the Cre-recombinase (by crossbreeding with a tissue-specific Cre mouse (Nagy & Mar, 2001), or infecting with a virus carrying Cre) causes the region between the LoxP sequences to be spliced out (including all or part of the gene of interest) of the genome of that individual cell. Researchers have used this method to permanently silence genes in mice. There are two main limitations to the Cre-LoxP technology. The first obstacle is resolving how to administer Cre such that expression occurs only in the cells of interest. Crossing floxed mice with mice constitutively expressing Cre in a specific tissue often results in their offspring containing the deletion from the embryonic stage. It is difficult to administer Cre in the adult animal in a tissue-specific manner. The second limitation is the Cre-recombination event is irreversible and heritable.

To overcome some of these limitations, researchers have developed the Tet-ON/OFF system (reviewed in Sprengel & Hasan, 2007). It requires co-expression of two transgenes in a given cell, usually accomplished by cross-breeding. Driven by a user defined promoter, the first transgene generates the inactive Tetracycline Activator (TA). Doxycycline (a more potent isoform of the antibiotic tetracycline) can bind to and activate TA, which can bind the Tetracycline Response Element (TRE) on the second transgene and drive expression of its gene of interest (see Figure 2). Researchers use this system to initiate gene expression in adult animals through doxycycline administration in their chow. Since the oncogene expression is tied directly to the presence of doxycycline in their diet, the oncogene can be activated or silenced simply by adjusting an animal's diet. The main limitation to this procedure is the upfront time and labor needed to create mice that express the Tet-operator transgene and separate models expressing the tissue-specific Tet-activator transgene, then crossbreeding them to generate bi-transgenic offspring.

Both of these inducible expression systems can be used in reverse as well if the transgene constructs are designed accordingly. The Cre-recombinase can excise a multiple STOP cassette (Lox-STOP-Lox, LSL) integrated upstream of a transcription start site, enabling transcription of a previously silenced gene (see Figure 3). The Tet-ON/OFF system allows gene expression to be repeatedly induced or silenced in multiple cycles simply by providing or removing doxycycline from the animal's diet. However, the system was shown to be leaky in some early studies, resulting in incomplete expression inhibition or a low level of unregulated basal transcription. Adjunct technologies are continually being developed to obtain tighter gene expression control (reviewed in Freundlieb et al., 1999; Bockamp et al., 2007) which make these systems more robust, accurate, and thus more reliable as preclinical models. The following examples highlight the utility of inducible GEM tumor models.

4.1 Conditional cre-lox kras G12D system

Taking advantage of the Lox-Stop-Lox conditional transgene expression system, Jackson et al., (2001) created a transgenic mouse model which replaces one wild type *Kras* allele with a transcriptionally silent oncogenic Kras-G12D allele. Intranasally delivered adenovirus containing the Cre-recombinase (adeno Cre) splices out the LSL and enables expression of the activated Kras-G12D transgene in the lung. Small lesions can be seen 2 weeks post induction; by 12 weeks post induction, adenomas are observed, some with cytogenic characteristics of malignancy. By 16 weeks post induction, large adenomas and adenocarcinomas are present in many animals. Virus titrations in a number of animals demonstrate that the number of virus particle equivalents used for induction is directly related to the number of tumors that develop.

Around the same time, Fisher et al., (2001) created an activated Kras Tet-ON/OFF inducible model. Doxycycline (DOX) administration induces expression of the murine oncogenic Kras G12D allele in alveolar type II pneumocytes. Hyperplasia is observed after just seven days of DOX administration; at eight weeks post induction, adenomas and adenocarcinomas are observed in the lungs. Removal of DOX from their diet causes a rapid decrease in activated Kras expression (within seven days) and apoptotic regression of the tumors. One month after DOX withdrawal, lesions and tumors were no longer present in the lungs, implying expression of the mutant Kras gene product was required to maintain the viability of tumor cells. The requirement of continued oncogene expression (or constant inhibition of tumor suppressor) to maintain the induced tumors has given rise to the theory of "oncogene addiction" (reviewed in Weinstein, 2002).

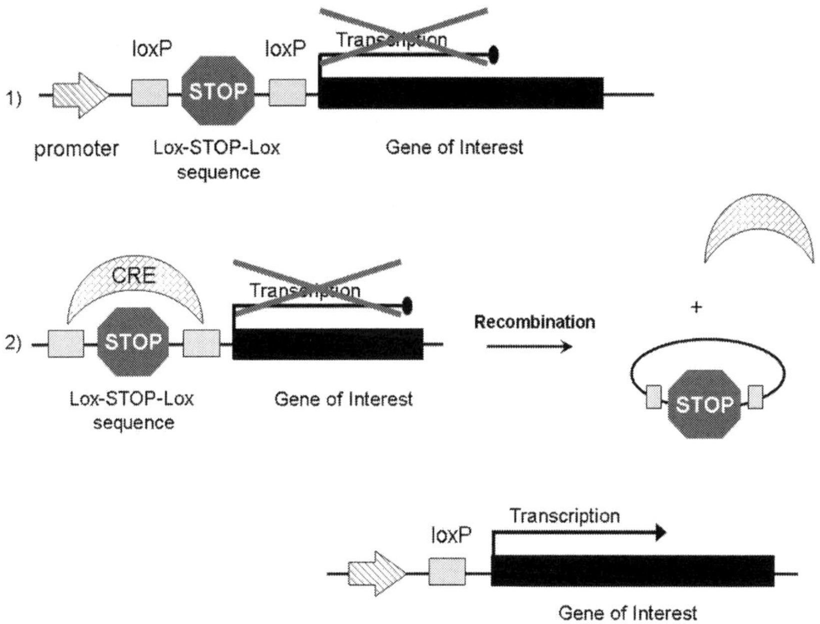

Fig. 3. CRE Recombination Mediates Lox-Stop-Lox Gene Activation. One popular method of inducing gene expression in adult mice is to use CRE recombination. 1) The transgenic mouse initially has the Lox-STOP-Lox sequence inserted upstream of the transcription start site for the gene of interest (GOI). This prevents GOI expression until acted upon by CRE. CRE recombinase is introduced to the appropriate cell population either by crossing with a second transgenic mouse expressing CRE recombinase using a tissue specific promoter, or by administering a virus expressing CRE recombinase in a tissue specific manner. 2) CRE recombinase splices out the STOP sequence between the two loxP sites from the transgenic DNA sequence, allowing GOI expression.

Sos et al., (2009) recently used computational genomic analysis to identify molecular and genetic predictors of therapeutic response to clinically relevant compounds in various NSCLC cancer cell lines which are highly representative of primary tumors. One of their findings was that cells expressing activated Kras also had enhanced Hsp90 dependency. They used the LSL-KrasG12D model to verify this observation. Mice were initially imaged by MRI 12-20 weeks post adeno-Cre administration, then split into placebo and 17-(Dimethylaminoethylamino)-17-demethoxygeldanamycin (17-DMAG a well-known Hsp90 inhibitor) groups. Mice were imaged by MRI after 1 week of drug treatment; tumor volume was decreased by 50% in 17-DMAG treated mice while tumor volume increased slightly in placebo treated animals. Prior to this study, there were no molecular targeted treatments for activated oncogenic Kras-driven lung tumors. But by combining the power of computational genomics and GEM models, researchers were able to rationally identify a possible therapeutic modality and evaluate its efficacy *in vivo*.

4.2 Inducible oncogenic mutations in the EGF receptor

The epidermal growth factor receptor (EGFr) is a transmembrane cell surface receptor which is mutated or alternatively expressed in a significant proportion of human gliomas and adenocarcinomas (especially of the head and neck, breast, colon, lung, and pancreas). EGFr is the human homolog of neu, a rat gene first identified in ethyl nitrosourea induced tumors (reviewed in Maguire & Greene, 1989), and is a member of the erythroblastic leukemia viral oncogene/human epidermal growth factor receptor (ERBB/HER) receptor tyrosine kinase family. Two of the most commonly observed EGFr mutations seen in lung adenocarcinomas include an in-frame deletion in exon 19 (eliminating an L-R-E-A [leucine-arginine-glutamic acid-alanine) amino acid motif that is conserved in all known vertebrate EGFr sequences) and a point mutation which results in a leucine to arginine substitution at position 858. These and other less common mutations in the kinase domain of EGFr are associated with increased therapeutic sensitivity to tyrosine kinase inhibitors such as gefitinib and erlotinib. Several studies demonstrated significantly extended survival and time to progression (TTP) in non-small-cell lung cancer (NSCLC) patients treated with gefitinib as their first line therapeutic (Han et al., 2005; Sequist et al., 2008; Yang et al., 2008). Erlotinib administration in patients who have had prior chemotherapy has an even greater survival benefit and is currently recommended by the FDA for second line therapy in new NSCLC patients (Shepherd et al., 2005). Inducible transgenic mouse models help to clarify this observation and provide a system to test other therapeutics that operate through the EGF receptor.

Politi et al., (2006) generated several Tet-ON/OFF mouse systems which overexpress various mutant EGFr alleles upon DOX administration. Lung adenocarcinomas were observed after two months post transgene induction in the exon 19 deletion and L858R transgenic EGFr mouse models. Similar to the Tet On/OFF activated Kras system, after one month of DOX withdrawal the observed tumor load in the EGFr transgene inducible models regressed to near pre-induction histology. To test the anti-tumor efficacy of an already clinically approved therapeutic in this model, the tyrosine kinase inhibitor erlotinib was administered to groups of transgenic EGFr mice maintained on DOX. After less than a week of erlotinib treatment, all of the animals which received at least 12 mg/kg/d showed partial or complete responses by magnetic resonance imaging (MRI). Longer lengths of treatment correlated with greater tumor regression. Ji et al., (2006) generated similar inducible EGFr transgenic mice (exon 19 in-frame deletion or L858R), but also added a luciferase fusion gene to the construct. This allows for the monitoring of lung tumor growth and regression *in vivo* using a non-invasive luciferase imaging system. The ability to non-invasively image tumor load repeatedly *in vivo* enables the effects of anti-cancer drug administration to be followed long term as the authors demonstrated with cetuximab.

4.3 GEMs possessing multiple genetic alterations

Patients with lung adenocarcinomas containing one of the common EGFr oncogenic mutations (deletion in exon 19 of the kinase domain [Del.ex19] and leucine 858 to arginine[L858R]) are sensitive to the EGFr-tyrosine kinase inhibitor (TKI) therapies (gefitinib and erlotinib). However, the TKI treated tumors invariably relapse within a year by developing resistance to the TKI therapy (reviewed in Morita et al., 2009), most commonly through one of the following mechanisms: EGFr-T790M point mutation (Kobayashi et al., 2005; Pao et al., 2005), MET proto-oncogene amplification (Engelman et al., 2007), or hyperphosphorylation and activation of insulin-like growth factor-I receptor (Guix et al., 2008). The EGFr-T790M mutation (observed in 50% of relapsed EGFr-mutant tumors) is thought to increase the ATP-binding affinity by an order of magnitude (Yun et al., 2008), thereby reducing the therapeutic ability of TKIs to out-compete ATP for receptor binding. MET amplification is thought to induce gefitinib resistance primarily by driving ERBB3 (HER3)-dependent activation of the PI3K and Erk pathways, which regulate cell survival and mitogenesis, respectively (reviewed in Kim & Salgia, 2009).

To overcome the acquired resistance of first generation TKIs, researchers have recently developed TKIs that bind EGFr irreversibly and are currently in or have completed phase II clinical trials (reviewed in Riely, 2008). The pan-ERBB inhibitor HKI-272 covalently binds to a cysteine in the EGFr kinase domain and regressed tumors at nanomolar concentrations in EGFR-L858R transgenic mice (Ji et al., 2006). The ability to inhibit ERBB2 (HER2) has led HKI-272 to be investigated primarily in breast cancer clinical trials (clinicaltrials.gov, 2011). However, other cancers driven by ErbB mutations may also be treated by HKI-272. Similarly, the irreversibly binding EGFr and HER2 inhibitor BIBW2992 is being tested in over 20 clinical trials of patients with advanced NSCLC, breast cancer, prostate cancer, malignant gliomas, and other solid tumors (clinicaltrials.gov, 2011). In addition to ERBB inhibitors, researchers are investigating other druggable targets related to the EGFr/HER2/ERK/AKT pathways. Shimamura et al., (2008) used an EGFR-L858R-T790M double transgenic GEM model to test the efficacy of an Hsp90 inhibitor, CL-387,785. Hsp90 is a chaperone thought to aid in the proper folding of EGFr; CL-387,785 binds irreversibly to Hsp90 thereby interfering with its chaperone function.

Cancer-related lethality in humans is often caused by the invasion of metastatic tumors in tissues far from the primary tumor. Yet few single transgene GEM models reliably develop metastatic lesions. By crossbreeding the pancreas-specific Cre-mediated activated Kras GEM (which alone generates only pre-malignant neoplasia) and the Ink4a/ARF conditional knockout models (does not induce neoplasia), Aguirre et al., (2003) generated mice that rapidly develop invasive, metastatic ductal pancreatic tumors which are lethal by 11 weeks. This tumor development is similar to the highly lethal human form of pancreatic ductal adenocarcinoma. Although the rapid murine mortality prevents long term studies, it may nevertheless be a useful model of a deadly human malignant cancer in short-term or cancer-prevention studies.

Similarly, Ji et al., (2007) crossed a lung-specific activated-Kras GEM with the following tumor suppressor knockout GEMs: Ink4a, p53, or the serine/threonine kinase 11 (Lkb1) knockout. Among the dual-knockout mice analyzed, the activated Kras x Lkb1 knockout had the most profound phenotype. These mice display a significantly increased lung tumor burden, rapid tumor onset, and <50% shorter survival when compared to the other double crosses or single knockout models examined. Regional lymph-node metastases were observed in 61% of the activated Kras x Lkb1 knockout mice, significantly more than the other models. The results from the previous few examples suggest an activating Kras mutation is responsible for initial neoplasia development, but a second mutated gene modulates the aggressiveness and metastatic behavior of the cancer. Accumulation of somatic mutations over time has long been a theory to explain the modulation and late onset of cancer in humans.

Winslow et al., (2011) expanded on this idea by administering a lentivirus expressing Cre recombinase to a double floxed GEM model. Upon CRE recombination, activated Kras would be expressed and p53 (flox/flox) would be silenced in certain cells of the adult lung. Because the lentivirus integrates randomly into the host cell's genome, the authors were able to use linkage-mediated PCR (LM-PCR) to generate a unique "fingerprint" for each primary tumor and monitor that "fingerprint" in any subsequent metastases. Although virus was delivered at a set time point and many primary foci seemed to successfully undergo the oncogenic double recombination event, only a few primary foci were responsible for generating macroscopic metastases outside the lung, suggesting other genetic or micro-environmental factors control a tumor's metastatic potential. This is an excellent example of using an inducible, double GEM to model genetic alterations seen in many human lung cancers and explore the genetics of malignant and non-malignant tumors.

Tp53 is not the only tumor suppressor being actively investigated using GEM models. The tumor suppressor phosphatase and tensin homologue (PTEN) is a lipid phosphatase which negatively regulates the PI3/AKT pathway, which is often upregulated in human malignancies. Sixty percent of primary human prostate cancers show a decrease/loss of PTEN expression; this gene also is deleteriously mutated in 70% of gliomas and in some forms of breast carcinomas and melanomas (Gray et al., 1998). To investigate the role of PTEN in prostate cancer, Trotman et al., (2003) created several PTEN GEM models, each with a different level of PTEN expression. Only the homozygous PTEN knockout show a significant phenotype (invasive prostate cancer develops after six months in all mice). However, none of the models generate metastases and the mice do not have decreased survival compared to wild type controls. A prostate-specific PTEN conditional knockout was created which also generated invasive prostate cancer; but in this case metastatic prostate tumors developed and were found in the lymph and lung (Wang et al., 2003). Concomitant inactivation of one or both Cdkn1b (encodes the tumor suppressor p27) alleles in a heterozygous PTEN knockout mouse accelerates spontaneous neoplasia formation which develop into prostate carcinoma at complete penetrance within three months from birth (Di Cristofano et al., 2001). When a conditional PTEN knockout mouse is crossed with a p53 knockout mouse the resulting offspring is a conditional double knockout GEM that develops aggressive, lethal prostate cancer with complete penetrance in seven months (Chen et al., 2005). The cancers observed in this new generation of GEM models recapitulate the progression and histopathologic features of some forms of prostate cancer observed in humans. These studies highlight the role of PTEN in tumorigenesis and the need for additional cooperative tumor suppressor inactivation to generate malignancies and lethal cancers.

The potential for drug discovery and validation using conditional GEM models is demonstrated with the Brca1/p53 mouse model. The majority of human BRCA1-associated tumors harbor mutations in both p53 and BRCA1. Poole et al., (2006) created such a Cre-LoxP conditional GEM model by inactivating both p53 and Brca1 specifically in the mouse mammary gland. The authors found that progesterone receptors are overexpressed in mutant mammary epithelial cells and presented a possible avenue of treatment. Administration of a progesterone agonist (mifepristone, RU 486) prevented mammary tumorigenesis in Brca1/p53-deficient mice. As the potential to genotype a patient's tumor to determine their status for EGFr, MET, p53, IGF, and other important neoplasia-associated targets becomes practical, it will be possible to better choose the optimal combination therapy to impact the relevant oncogenic pathways.

5. The predictive potential of GEMs

The potential predictive power of transgenic mice can be illustrated in the example of thiazolidinediones (TZDs). As an agonist of peroxisome proliferator-activated receptor-gamma (PPARγ), the TZD troglitazone had been an FDA-approved therapy for type-2 diabetes. TZD anti-tumor activity in cultured and xenografted human colon cancer cells prompted excitement in the scientific community that initiated its use in Phase II clinical trials in patients with colon cancer (Sarraf et al., 1998). However, in a study published a few pages after the xenograft study, troglitazone showed no anti-tumor activity in Min+/- mice; in fact, polyp formation increased with troglitazone administration in this model (Saez et al., 1998). This heterozygous knockout mouse model lacks one functional copy of the APC tumor suppresser gene, thus predisposing them to colon cancer. In the Phase II clinical trial patients treated with troglitazone actually showed disease progression within months of therapy initiation, correlating with the results predicted from the transgenic mouse model (Kulke et al., 2002).

5.1 Cautionary tale

Although many regard mice as "little fuzzy humans" in the analysis of preclinical data, there are vast and often unknown differences in drug metabolism, gene expression, and disease progression between the murine model and humans. One example of transgenic mouse models failing to accurately predict human clinical outcome is the Farnesyltransferase (FTase) story. FTase catalyzes the post-translational farnesylation of proteins containing a C-terminal CAAX motif, where C is the cysteine residue to be farnesylated, A represents an aliphatic amino acid, and X is any amino acid. When X is leucine, the protein is a preferred substrate for a similar enzyme named geranylgeranyltransferase I (GGTase).

Mendola & Backer, (1990) showed farnesylation of Ras proteins is critical for their transformation into potent oncogenes. This discovery ignited the hypothesis that interfering with prenylation using inhibitors of FTase (FTIs) or GGTase (GGTIs) could lead to tumor growth inhibition and a viable anti-cancer therapy. Although some data suggest an FTI and a GGTI need to be utilized simultaneously to achieve complete inhibition of Kras prenylation (Rowell et al., 1997), FTIs alone had been shown to inhibit growth of human tumor xenografts in nude mice (Sun et al., 1998). FTI monotherapy also demonstrates beneficial effects in transgenic mouse models: tumor regression in H-Ras mice (Kohl et al., 1995), tumor stasis in N-Ras mice (Mangues et al., 1998), and tumor growth inhibition in Ki-RasB mice (Omer et al., 2000). These results and others spurred excitement for FTI monotherapy in clinical trials. With the exception of a few trials in breast cancer and leukemia patients, FTIs used as single agents have not shown good efficacy against solid tumors (reviewed in Zhu et al., 2003). Thus, none of the various mouse models evaluated were able to predict drug efficacy in humans. However, many clinical trials are currently underway combining FTIs with other drugs including "classical" anticancer therapies (chemotherapy or radiotherapy) and molecular targeted therapeutics.

5.2 Targeted molecular therapeutics

For decades, cancer therapy has been one or a combination of the following three treatments: surgery, radiotherapy, and cytotoxic chemotherapy. However, all have their limitations and substantial side effects. Ideally, anti-cancer treatments would "target" cancer cells and minimize adverse effects to non-cancerous cells. Tumors often contain gene expression profiles and mutations that make them more or less sensitive to some targeted therapies than others. Identifying the tumor's gene expression profile and correlating it to the most successful therapies for that specific profile will keep therapeutic adverse side effects to a minimum and yield the best prognosis for the patient.

The two main types of targeted molecular therapies are monoclonal antibodies, which target the receptor's extracellular domain, and small molecule inhibitors, which target the intracellular signaling and kinase domains. Table 1 outlines some of the FDA-approved targeted therapeutics, their molecular targets, and the forms of cancer in which they have been proven to have a clinical benefit. Monoclonal antibodies (mabs) are generally administered no more than once weekly by intravenous injection, whereas small molecules (nibs) can generally be taken orally each day. Currently available targeted therapies may be administered as single agents, but many show greater benefits in combination with other agents or in addition to traditional therapies in those patient populations with tumors of susceptible genetic profiles. Tumors can be generated in genetically engineered mice which have these susceptible mutations and expression profiles, providing researchers with valuable preclinical drug screening opportunities.

Herceptin (HER2) is a transmembrane receptor that is over-expressed in 20-25% of breast cancers and is associated with aggressive tumor behavior and poor prognosis (reviewed in Nanda, 2007). Two early studies have shown the anti-HER2 monoclonal antibody trastuzumab plus chemotherapy significantly improves overall survival in HER2+ patients with metastatic breast cancer (Slamon et al., 2005). Antibody binding is thought to inhibit HER2 signaling, which disrupts DNA repair mechanisms and induces cytotoxicity. Resistance to trastuzumab commonly occurs and can render this treatment useless in subsequent relapses. A recent advance has been to conjugate the antibody with a toxin/drug, thereby creating a "guided missile" that targets a specific epitope over-expressed on cancer cells and delivers the toxic agent to those specific cells. Researchers at Genetech harvested mammary tumors from MMTV-HER2 transgenic mice, implanted them orthotopically into a large cohort of nude mice, staged the mice when mean tumor volumes were ~100-200 mm^3, and administered their trastuzumab-DM1 (T-DM1) conjugate at various time points and doses (Jumbe et al., 2010). DM1, also known as maytansine and derived from members of several tropical plant families, is a potent cytotoxin that irreversibly inhibits tubulin polymerization and arrests cells in M or G2 phase (Remillard et al., 1975; Rao et al., 1979). Because the toxin is specifically targeted to tumor cells, the authors saw no adverse events in the mice, with ~50% of the tumors showing complete regression at doses of 15 mg/kg given once every three weeks. PD/PK measures were obtained from the mice and this immunoconjugate therapy is now being evaluated in several clinical trials in patients with metastatic breast cancer.

Several therapeutics have been developed that target the EGFr receptor to treat non-small cell lung cancer and colorectal cancer, including cetuximab, panitumumab, erlotinib, and gefitinib. Tumors expressing EGFr with a deletion in exon 19 or sensitizing point mutation (L858R) in the ATP-binding pocket respond significantly better to gefitinib than patients with wild type EGFr (Lynch et al., 2008). Invariably, even the tumors with increased drug sensitivity relapse when resistance to gefitinib develops. Additional therapeutics need to be generated to overcome the inevitable drug resistance.

Targeted Therapy	Molecular Target	Approved Use
cetuximab (Erbitux®)	EGFr	Colorectal Cancer
erlotinib (Tarceva®)	EGFr	Non-Small Cell Lung Cancer Metastatic Pancreatic Cancer
gefitinib (Iressa®)	EGFr	Non-Small Cell Lung Cancer
panitumumab (Vectibix®)	EGFr	Colorectal Cancer
trastuzumab (Herceptin®)	HER2	Early and Metastatic Breast Cancer
lapatinib (Tykerb®)	HER2 and EGFr	Breast Cancer
bevacizumab (Avastin®)	VEGF	Metastatic Colorectal Cancer Metastatic Melanoma Non-Small Cell Lung Cancer
sunitinib (Sutent®)	VEGFr and PDGFr	Metastatic Renal Cell Carcinoma
sorafenib (Nexavar®)	Multi-Targeted Kinase Inhibitor	Metastatic Renal Cell Carcinoma
toceranib (Palladia®)	Multi-Targeted Kinase Inhibitor	Canine Specific Mastocytoma
pazopanib (Votrient®)	VEGFr, PDGFr, and cKIT	Advanced Renal Cell Carcinoma
imatinib (Gleevec®)	cKIT, ABL, and PDGFr2	Chronic Myeloid Leukemia and GIST
dasatinib (Sprycel®)	BCR/ABL and Src Family	Chronic Myeloid Leukemia with resistance to prior therapy
alemtuzumab (Campath®, MabCampath® or Campath-1H®)	CD52 on Mature Lymphocytes	Chronic Lymphocytic Leukemia (CLL) and Cutaneous T-cell Lymphoma (CTCL)
ofatumumab (Arzerra®)	CD20 on B-cells	Chronic Lymphocytic Leukemia (CLL)
rituximab (MabThera® and Rituxan®)	CD20 on B-cells	B-cell Non-Hodgkin's Lymphoma
nilotinib (Tasigna®)	BCR/ABL kinase inhibitor	Philadelphia chromosome positive chronic myeloid leukemia (CML)
vandetanib (Zactima®)	VEGFr, EGFr, RET	Metastatic Medullary Thyroid Cancer

EGFr: Epidermal growth factor receptor;erythroblastic leukemia viral (v-erb-b) oncogene homolog 1
VEGFr: Vascular endothelial growth factor receptor
PDGFr2: Platelet-derived growth factor receptor-alpha
BCR/ABL: c-abl oncogene 1, receptor tyrosine kinase
cKIT: v-kit Hardy-Zuckerman 4 feline sarcoma viral oncogene homolog
Her2: Herceptin receptor; v-erb-b2 erythroblastic leukemia viral oncogene homolog 2
RET: "Rearranged during transfection" proto oncogene

Table 1. An overview of the currently FDA approved targeted therapy compounds.

Since vascularization is required for growth and health of a tumor, the angiogenesis associated factor VEGF became a desired target for therapy. Bevacizumab is an anti-VEGF antibody which has been shown to bind and inhibit VEGF, slowing angiogenesis and aiding in solid tumor starvation and elimination (Brekken et al., 2000). When used as single agents in unsorted cancer patients, anti-angiogenic therapeutics do not show significant activity. However, when used in combination with other therapies (especially cytotoxic chemotherapy), subgroups of patients show promise (reviewed in Cabebe, 2007). Bevacizumab, in addition to paclitaxel and a platinum cytotoxic agent, is now part of a first line therapy for newly diagnosed non-small cell lung cancer. Hundreds of Phase II and Phase III trials using bevacizumab in combination with other therapies in many other cancers are currently ongoing (clinicaltrials.gov, 2011).

5.3 GEM oncomice in cancer prevention

GEM models are beginning to realize their potential as preclinical models of cancer prevention (briefly reviewed in Abate-Shen et al., 2008). In a recent example, Ohashi et al., (2009) used the EGFR-L858R-FLAG transgenic mouse to test the cancer preventative potential of gefitinib administration. Twenty-five 3-week old transgenic mice were administered gefitinib, with 5, 5, and 15 mice euthanized at weeks 8, 13, and 18, respectively. At termination the lungs tumors were counted and measured macroscopically and histologically. Those receiving gefitinib failed to develop adenocarcinomas, whereas the groups given vehicle control developed hyperplastic regions at 5 weeks and large adenocarcinomas by 15 weeks. One week after cessation of the 15-week gefitinib administration period, the transgenic mice showed signs of hyperplastic cell expansion in the lung (by PCNA staining), suggesting gefitinib was the lone factor preventing EGFr-L858R tumor development in these mice. Longer term studies are needed to see if the EGFr-L858R transgenic mice eventually develop gefitinib resistance, as is seen in human NCSLC patients with EGFr-L858R driven lung tumors. Similar studies with erlotinib, other tyrosine kinase inhibitors, and novel anti-cancer agents should be performed on this and other informative GEM models to further investigate the tumor-preventative aspects of these agents.

5.4 Cancer vaccine

It is conceivable that patients with a high risk (family history, environmental exposure, or heritable mutations) associated with a specific cancer subtype might benefit from being immunized at a young age. Vaccine development depends on the identification of antigens specific for a given cancer subtype or tumor-inducing biological agent. The heterogeneity and unstable genome in most cancers suggests resistant mutant cells might accumulate quickly and overcome the immunotherapy. However, vaccines against oncogenic strains of viruses have proven to be very beneficial and often lean on the preclinical use of GEM models to show the oncogenic potential of viral genes.

In 1993, two studies using transgenic mice emerged clearly showing the oncogenic potential of the human papillomavirus (HPV) early genes E6 and E7 (Lambert et al., 1993; Arbeit et al., 1993). HPV DNA has also been found in and hypothesized by some to induce a subset of tongue and other oropharyngeal carcinomas (reviewed in Syrjänen, 2005). Transgenic mice expressing HPV early genes have been used to demonstrate the oncogenic potential of HPV in certain skin cancers [HPV 8 (Schaper et al., 2005) and HPV 20 (Michel et al., 2006)]. Spurred by these and many studies elucidating the relationship between HPV and cervical cancer, the FDA approved the HPV vaccine Gardasil (Merck) for preventing the most common forms of human papillomavirus (HPV)-induced cervical cancer (reviewed in McLemore, 2006). Feng et al., (2008) recently discovered a novel polyomavirus (similar to SV40) that integrated itself into the genome of 80% of the Merkel cell carcinomas they examined. Though a rare cancer, this is another example of a virus-associated cancer which could be a target for cancer-preventing vaccines and could be tested preclinically in GEM models.

5.5 Legal obstacles of preclinical testing in GEM models

In 1988 Harvard University filed the first of three exceptionally broad U.S. patents regarding the development and use of transgenic animals. Dupont (a sponsor of one of the Harvard investigators developing transgenic mice) became the exclusive licensee of transgenic patents and merely sublicensed the patent rights (imposing large fees and restrictions) to industry and academia. This arrangement severely constrained use of transgenic mice beyond basic discovery applications (reviewed in Sharpless & Depinho, 2006). Fortunately for the greater scientific community, the first of these patents expired in 2005 and the second expired in February 2009; the third patent covering testing methods using transgenic oncomice is still in force through 2016. Hundreds of oncomice have been developed (primarily in academia), but have yet to be thoroughly studied and used on a large scale to test the growing number of possible anti-cancer therapies. Once the final restriction is lifted, researchers in industry, academia, and government alike will undoubtedly expand their use of transgenic models for preclinical drug studies.

6. Conclusion: Role GEMs can play in preclinical studies

To process the thousands of novel natural product and synthetic purported anti-cancer compounds that arise each year, preclinical drug screens must be as quick and comprehensive as resources allow. This can best be accomplished by *in vitro* screens using cultured cell lines that have oncogenic gene expression profiles similar to those seen in human patients. Compounds which show activity can then be moved to xenograft studies, which test toxicity and tumor regression potential. Although we have reviewed the power of GEM models in verifying drug efficacy and pathway mechanism analysis, GEM models as they exist today have fundamental flaws that preclude their use as high-throughput drug-screening tools.

GEMs require several months to develop tumors, and the penetrance is often far less than 100%. Tumors arise and grow at different rates in each individual mouse in a given study. Except for melanoma, breast cancer, and some prostate cancer models where palpable tumors develop, identifying which animals have developed tumors at any given moment becomes a nearly insurmountable task. Many published studies use MRI images to follow tumor progression. Considering imaging the thorax of one mouse in an MRI can take up to one hour, this method is incompatible with large, high throughput studies. Small animal in vivo imaging (SAIVI) using fluorescent or bioluminescent tagged agents targeting tumors is a promising alternative, but the technology is still in its infancy, lacks appropriate inducible GEM models for most forms of cancer, and often requires purchase of expensive, photosensitive probes and detection systems. Computed Tomography (CT) Imaging with clinical-size instruments cannot be used because the dose of radiation used during imaging may have therapeutic effects on the tumors, especially when GEM models will require multiple imaging sessions over their lifetime to first identify a tumor and then to monitor therapeutic drug effects. However as smaller, less powerful, rodent-specific CT imagers become available to researchers, this may prove to be a useful method to measure tumor size in deep tissue. To best utilize current GEM models in preclinical drug trials, traditional tumor staging strategies must be revised so that each mouse is treated as a patient in a clinical trial. Therapeutic agents must not be administered en mass to all individuals in a treatment group at a given time point, but tailored to each mouse reflecting the date the tumor was recognized by whatever modality the researcher has developed. This can create a logistical nightmare, especially if large combination therapy treatment trials testing multiple vehicles, routes of administration, dosing schedules, and multiple dose concentrations are attempted. Day 0 should be marked at the time an animal's measured tumor size or total "tumor burden" (if the GEM generates multiple foci simultaneously) crosses a pre-determined threshold quantity.

Therefore, we cannot envision GEM models replacing *in vitro* and xenograft models for the high throughput efficacy screens of novel agents. However, we do believe GEM models can be of great value during three steps in the preclinical process (Figure 1). First, if GEM tumors are harvested and fragments successfully implanted subcutaneously (SC) or orthotopically into syngeneic, immune competent mice, enough animals can be amassed to perform traditional xenograft-like screens with genetically desirable murine tumors (allografts). Varticovski et al., (2007) provide an example of this approach, harvesting MMTV-PyMT breast tumors from a few mice and passing them as fragments or cell suspensions into numerous host animals for subsequent drug studies. DNA microarrays were used to verify only slight changes in gene expression after two serial passages from the original tumor. Second passage tumors exhibited similar sensitivity to paclitaxel and cyclophosphamide compared to the original tumor material.

Once an agent shows activity *in vitro* and in tumor transplants, GEM models can be used to explore the drug mechanism and further optimize *in vivo* dosing before an agent heads into the much more expensive and laborious clinical trials (Figure 1). These optimization studies need not be high throughput and may take a year or more to complete. Thus, fewer anti-cancer agents will successfully pass through these additional preclinical evaluations than do currently advance to clinical trial. Currently, only ~5% of novel anti-cancer agents entering clinical trials achieve FDA approval (Kola & Landis, 2004); most of the cost and attrition occurs during Phase II and Phase III clinical trials. Therefore any extra time GEM-based drug screening would add to the preclinical drug development pipeline should be financially worthwhile to the drug sponsors and ethically beneficial for the volunteers participating in clinical trials if more efficacious therapies are discovered.

GEM models may ultimately have a fourth role in preclinical drug testing if researchers can effectively "humanize" them for use in toxicology and pharmacology studies. The cytochrome P450 (CYP) family of enzymes are expressed primarily in the liver and are involved in the metabolism of a diverse range of therapeutic compounds, toxins, carcinogens, hormones, and xenobiotic agents we may encounter. The seven main CYP gene clusters found in humans are present and expanded in mice (57 putative human CYP genes versus 102 putative functional genes in mice) (Nelson et al., 2004). But studies have shown that many individual CYPs are differentially expressed or differentially active between the mouse and human (Bogaards et al., 2000). This explains why drug metabolism in the mouse does not always reflect and predict drug metabolism and toxicity in the human clinical trials. Several GEM models have been generated in which the endogenous mouse CYPs or other xenobiotic-related metabolism genes are deleted and replaced with their human orthologues, or simply over express the human orthologue in addition to the mouse CYP (reviewed in Cheung & Gonzalez, 2008). Expression of one or two human genes certainly is not enough to declare a potential GEM model as functionally "humanized" and ready for high throughput toxicity and pharmacology studies. But as transgenic technology evolves and these mice express numerous human orthologues, they may indeed be able to better predict human drug activity and toxicity, and be of vital importance in preclinical therapeutic drug development.

7. References

Abate-Shen C, Brown PH, Colburn NH, Gerner EW, Green JE, Lipkin M, Nelson WG, Threadgill D. (2008). The untapped potential of genetically engineered mouse models in chemoprevention research: opportunities and challenges. *Cancer Prev Res (Phila Pa).* 1(3):161-6.

Adams JM, Harris AW, Pinkert CA, Corcoran LM, Alexander WS, Cory S, Palmiter RD, Brinster RL. (1985). The c-myc oncogene driven by immunoglobulin enhancers induces lymphoid malignancy in transgenic mice. *Nature.* 318(6046):533-8.

Aguirre AJ, Bardeesy N, Sinha M, Lopez L, Tuveson DA, Horner J, Redston MS, DePinho RA. (2003). Activated Kras and Ink4a/Arf deficiency cooperate to produce metastatic pancreatic ductal adenocarcinoma. *Genes Dev.* 17(24):3112-26.

Almoguera, C.; Shibata, D.; Forrester, K.; Martin, J.; Arnheim, N.; Perucho, M. (1988). Most human carcinomas of the exocrine pancreas contain mutant c-K-ras genes. *Cell.* 53: 549-554.

American Cancer Society (ACS). (2010). Cancer Facts & Figures 2010. Atlanta: American Cancer Society.

Arbeit JM, Münger K, Howley PM, Hanahan D. (1993). Neuroepithelial carcinomas in mice transgenic with human papillomavirus type 16 E6/E7 ORFs. *Am J Pathol.* 142(4):1187-97.

Bittner JJ. Some possible effects of nursing on the mammary gland tumor incidence in mice. *Science.* 1936; 84:162.

Bockamp E, Christel C, Hameyer D, Khobta A, Maringer M, Reis M, Heck R, Cabezas-Wallscheid N, Epe B, Oesch-Bartlomowicz B, Kaina B, Schmitt S, Eshkind L. (2007). Generation and characterization of tTS-H4: a novel transcriptional repressor that is compatible with the reverse tetracycline-controlled TET-ON system. *J Gene Med.* 9(4):308-18.

Bogaards JJ, Bertrand M, Jackson P, Oudshoorn MJ, Weaver RJ, van Bladeren PJ, Walther B. (2000). Determining the best animal model for human cytochrome P450 activities: a comparison of mouse, rat, rabbit, dog, micropig, monkey and man. *Xenobiotica.* 30(12):1131-52.

Brault V, Besson V, Magnol L, Duchon A, Hérault Y. (2007). Cre/loxP-mediated chromosome engineering of the mouse genome. *Handb Exp Pharmacol.* (178):29-48.

Brekken RA, Overholser JP, Stastny VA, Waltenberger J, Minna JD, Thorpe PE. (2000). Selective inhibition of vascular endothelial growth factor (VEGF) receptor 2

(KDR/Flk-1) activity by a monoclonal anti-VEGF antibody blocks tumor growth in mice. *Cancer Res*. 60(18):5117-24.

Brinster RL, Chen HY, Messing A, van Dyke T, Levine AJ, Palmiter RD. (1984). Transgenic mice harboring SV40 T-antigen genes develop characteristic brain tumors. *Cell*. 37(2):367-79.

Cabebe E and Wakelee H. (2007). Role of anti-angiogenesis agents in treating NSCLC: focus on bevacizumab and VEGFR tyrosine kinase inhibitors. *Curr Treat Options Oncol*. 8(1):15-27.

Charles River Laboratories Rapid Expansion Services. (2006). In: *Assisted Reproductive Technologies*. Charles River Laboratories. 1 July 2011. Available from: <http://www.criver.com/sitecollectiondocuments/rm_tg_d_sperm_ovarian_cryopreservation.pdf>

Chen Z, Trotman LC, Shaffer D, Lin HK, Dotan ZA, Niki M, Koutcher JA, Scher HI, Ludwig T, Gerald W, Cordon-Cardo C, Pandolfi PP. (2005). Crucial role of p53-dependent cellular senescence in suppression of Pten-deficient tumorigenesis. *Nature*. 436(7051):725-30.

Cheung C, Gonzalez FJ. (2008). Humanized mouse lines and their application for prediction of human drug metabolism and toxicological risk assessment. *J Pharmacol Exp Ther*. 327(2):288-99.

Clinicaltrials.gov. n.d. *U.S. National Institutes of Health*. 1 July 2011. Available from: <http://www.clinicaltrials.gov/ct2/home>

Decker S, Hollingshead M, Bonomi CA, Carter JP, Sausville EA. (2004). The hollow fibre model in cancer drug screening: the NCI experience. *Eur J Cancer*. 40(6):821-6.

Di Cristofano A, De Acetis M, Koff A, Cordon-Cardo C, Pandolfi PP. (2001). Pten and p27KIP1 cooperate in prostate cancer tumor suppression in the mouse. *Nat Genet*. 27(2):222-4.

Donehower LA, Harvey M, Slagle BL, McArthur MJ, Montgomery CA Jr, Butel JS, Bradley A. (1992). Mice deficient for p53 are developmentally normal but susceptible to spontaneous tumours. *Nature*. 356(6366):215-21.

eMICE. electronic Models Information, Communication, and Education. n.d. National Cancer Institute. 1 July 2011. Available from: <http://emice.nci.nih.gov/acquiring-models/Mice>

Engelman JA, Zejnullahu K, Mitsudomi T, Song Y, Hyland C, Park JO, Lindeman N, Gale CM, Zhao X, Christensen J, Kosaka T, Holmes AJ, Rogers AM, Cappuzzo F, Mok T, Lee C, Johnson BE, Cantley LC, Jänne PA. (2007). MET amplification leads to gefitinib resistance in lung cancer by activating ERBB3 signaling. *Science*. 316(5827):1039-43.

Feng H, Shuda M, Chang Y, Moore PS. (2008). Clonal integration of a polyomavirus in human Merkel cell carcinoma. Science. 319(5866):1096-100.

Fisher GH, Wellen SL, Klimstra D, Lenczowski JM, Tichelaar JW, Lizak MJ, Whitsett JA, Koretsky A, Varmus HE. (2001). Induction and apoptotic regression of lung adenocarcinomas by regulation of a K-Ras transgene in the presence and absence of tumor suppressor genes. *Genes Dev*. 15(24):3249-62.

Freundlieb S, Schirra-Müller C, Bujard H. (1999). A tetracycline controlled activation/repression system with increased potential for gene transfer into mammalian cells. *J Gene Med.* 1(1):4-12.

Gray IC, Stewart LM, Phillips SM, Hamilton JA, Gray NE, Watson GJ, Spurr NK, Snary D. (1998). Mutation and expression analysis of the putative prostate tumour-suppressor gene PTEN. *Br J Cancer.* 78(10):1296-300.

Guix M, Faber AC, Wang SE, Olivares MG, Song Y, Qu S, Rinehart C, Seidel B, Yee D, Arteaga CL, Engelman JA. (2008). Acquired resistance to EGFR tyrosine kinase inhibitors in cancer cells is mediated by loss of IGF-binding proteins. *J Clin Invest.* 118(7):2609-19.

Guy CT, Cardiff RD, Muller WJ. (1992). Induction of mammary tumors by expression of polyomavirus middle T oncogene: a transgenic mouse model for metastatic disease. *Mol Cell Biol.* 12(3):954-61.

Han SW, Kim TY, Hwang PG, Jeong S, Kim J, Choi IS, Oh DY, Kim JH, Kim DW, Chung DH, Im SA, Kim YT, Lee JS, Heo DS, Bang YJ, Kim NK. (2005). Predictive and prognostic impact of epidermal growth factor receptor mutation in non-small-cell lung cancer patients treated with gefitinib. *J Clin Oncol.* 23(11):2493-501.

Hanahan D. (1985). Heritable formation of pancreatic beta-cell tumours in transgenic mice expressing recombinant insulin/simian virus 40 oncogenes. *Nature.* 315(6015):115-22.

Hanahan D and Weinberg RA. (2000). The hallmarks of cancer. *Cell.* 100: 57-70.

Harris CC and Hollstein M. (1993). Clinical implications of the p53 tumor-suppressor gene. *New Eng. J. Med.* 329: 1318-1327.

Heston WE and Parks WP. (1977). Mammary tumors and mammary tumor virus expression in hybrid mice of strains C57BL and GR. *J. Exp. Med.* 146: 1206-1220.

Huang AL, Ostrowski MC, Berard D, Hager GL. (1981). Glucocorticoid regulation of the Ha-MuSV p21 gene conferred by sequences from mouse mammary tumor virus. *Cell.* 27(2 Pt 1):245-55.

Huang S, Li Y, Chen Y, Podsypanina K, Chamorro M, Olshen AB, Desai KV, Tann A, Petersen D, Green JE, Varmus HE. (2005). Changes in gene expression during the development of mammary tumors in MMTV-Wnt-1 transgenic mice. *Genome Biol.* 6(10):R84.

Jacks T, Fazeli A, Schmitt EM, Bronson RT, Goodell MA, Weinberg RA. (1992). Effects of an Rb mutation in the mouse. *Nature.* 359(6393):295-300.

Jackson EL, Willis N, Mercer K, Bronson RT, Crowley D, Montoya R, Jacks T, Tuveson DA. (2001). Analysis of lung tumor initiation and progression using conditional expression of oncogenic K-ras. *Genes Dev.* 15(24):3243-8.

JAX® Speed Expansion Service. n.d. *The Jackson Laboratory.* 1 July 2011. Available from: <http://jaxservices.jax.org/breeding/speed-expansion.html>

Ji H, Li D, Chen L, Shimamura T, Kobayashi S, McNamara K, Mahmood U, Mitchell A, Sun Y, Al-Hashem R, Chirieac LR, Padera R, Bronson RT, Kim W, Jänne PA, Shapiro GI, Tenen D, Johnson BE, Weissleder R, Sharpless NE, Wong KK. (2006). The impact of human EGFR kinase domain mutations on lung tumorigenesis and in vivo sensitivity to EGFR-targeted therapies. *Cancer Cell.* 9(6):485-95.

Ji H, Ramsey MR, Hayes DN, Fan C, McNamara K, Kozlowski P, Torrice C, Wu MC, Shimamura T, Perera SA, Liang MC, Cai D, Naumov GN, Bao L, Contreras CM, Li D, Chen L, Krishnamurthy J, Koivunen J, Chirieac LR, Padera RF, Bronson RT, Lindeman NI, Christiani DC, Lin X, Shapiro GI, Jänne PA, Johnson BE, Meyerson M, Kwiatkowski DJ, Castrillon DH, Bardeesy N, Sharpless NE, Wong KK. (2007). LKB1 modulates lung cancer differentiation and metastasis. *Nature.* 448(7155): 807-10.

Johnson L, Mercer K, Greenbaum D, Bronson RT, Crowley D, Tuveson DA, and Jacks T. (2001). Somatic activation of the K-ras oncogene causes early onset lung cancer in mice. *Nature.* 410: 1111–1116.

Jonkers J, Meuwissen R, van der Gulden H, Peterse H, van der Valk M, Berns A. (2001). Synergistic tumor suppressor activity of BRCA2 and p53 in a conditional mouse model for breast cancer. *Nature Genet.* 29: 418-425.

Jumbe NL, Xin Y, Leipold DD, Crocker L, Dugger D, Mai E, Sliwkowski MX, Fielder PJ, Tibbitts J. (2010). Modeling the efficacy of trastuzumab-DM1, an antibody drug conjugate, in mice. *J Pharmacokinet Pharmacodyn.* 37(3):221-42.

Kerbel RS. (2003). Human tumor xenografts as predictive preclinical models for anticancer drug activity in humans: better than commonly perceived-but they can be improved. *Cancer Biol Ther.* 2(4 Suppl 1):S134-9.

Kim ES and Salgia R. (2009). MET pathway as a therapeutic target. *J Thorac Oncol.* 4(4): 444-7.

Kobayashi S, Boggon TJ, Dayaram T, Jänne PA, Kocher O, Meyerson M, Johnson BE, Eck MJ, Tenen DG, Halmos B. (2005). EGFR mutation and resistance of non-small-cell lung cancer to gefitinib. *N Engl J Med.* 352:786–792.

Kohl NE, Omer CA, Conner MW, Anthony NJ, Davide JP, deSolms SJ, Giuliani EA, Gomez RP, Graham SL, Hamilton K, Handt LK, Hartman GE, Koblan KS, Kral AM, Miller PJ, Mosser SD, O'Neil TJ, Rands E, Schaber MD, Gibbs JB, Oliff A. (1995). Inhibition of farnesyltransferase induces regression of mammary and salivary carcinomas in ras transgenic mice. *Nat Med.* 1(8):792-797.

Kola I and Landis J. (2004). Can the pharmaceutical industry reduce attrition rates? *Nat Rev Drug Discov.* 3(8):711-5.

Kranenburg O. (2005) The KRAS oncogene: past, present, and future. *Biochim. Biophys. Acta.* 1756: 81-82.

Kulke MH, Demetri GD, Sharpless NE, Ryan DP, Shivdasani R, Clark JS, Spiegelman BM, Kim H, Mayer RJ, Fuchs CS. (2002). A phase II study of troglitazone, an activator of the PPARgamma receptor, in patients with chemotherapy-resistant metastatic colorectal cancer. *Cancer J.* 8(5):395-9.

Kung HC, Hoyert D, Xu J, and Murphy SL. (2008). Deaths: Final Data for 2005. *National Vital Statistics Reports.* 56(10):5.

Lambert PF, Pan H, Pitot HC, Liem A, Jackson M, Griep AE. (1993). Epidermal cancer associated with expression of human papillomavirus type 16 E6 and E7 oncogenes in the skin of transgenic mice. *Proc Natl Acad Sci USA.* 90(12):5583-7.

Le Y and Sauer B. (2001). Conditional Gene Knockout Using Cre Recombinase. *Molecular Biotechnology.* 17: 269-275.

Lynch TJ, Bell DW, Sordella R, Gurubhagavatula S, Okimoto RA, Brannigan BW, Harris PL, Haserlat SM, Supko JG, Haluska FG, Louis DN, Christiani DC, Settleman J, Haber DA. (2004). Activating mutations in the epidermal growth factor receptor underlying responsiveness of non-small-cell lung cancer to gefitinib. *N Engl J Med* 350:2129–2139.

Maglione JE, McGoldrick ET, Young LJ, Namba R, Gregg JP, Liu L, Moghanaki D, Ellies LG, Borowsky AD, Cardiff RD, MacLeod CL. (2004). Polyomavirus middle T-induced mammary intraepithelial neoplasia outgrowths: single origin, divergent evolution, and multiple outcomes. *Mol Cancer Ther.* 3(8):941-53.

Maguire HC Jr and Greene MI. (1989). The neu (c-erbB-2) oncogene. *Semin Oncol.*16(2):148-55.

Malkinson AM. (1998). Molecular comparison of human and mouse pulmonary adenocarcinomas. *Exp Lung Res.* 24(4):541-55.

Mangues R, Corral T, Kohl NE, Symmans WF, Lu S, Malumbres M, Gibbs JB, Oliff A, Pellicer A. (1998). Antitumor effect of a farnesyl protein transferase inhibitor in mammary and lymphoid tumors overexpressing N-Ras in transgenic mice. *Cancer Res.* 58(6):1253-1259.

Marino S, Vooijs M, van der Gulden H, Jonker J, Berns A. (2000). Induction of medulloblastomas in p53-null mutant mice by somatic inactivation of Rb in the external granular layer cells of the cerebellum. *Genes Dev.* 14: 994-1004.

Marty M, Cognetti F, Maraninchi D, Snyder R, Mauriac L, Tubiana-Hulin M, Chan S, Grimes D, Antón A, Lluch A, Kennedy J, O'Byrne K, Conte P, Green M, Ward C, Mayne K, Extra JM. (2005). Randomized phase II trial of the efficacy and safety of trastuzumab combined with docetaxel in patients with human epidermal growth factor receptor 2-positive metastatic breast cancer administered as first-line treatment: the M77001 study group. *J Clin Oncol.* 23(19):4265-74.

McLemore MR. (2006). Gardasil: Introducing the new human papillomavirus vaccine. *Clin J Oncol Nurs.* 10(5):559-60.

Mendola CE, Backer JM. (1990). Lovastatin blocks N-ras oncogene-induced neuronal differentiation. *Cell Growth Differ.* 1(10):499-502.

Michel A, Kopp-Schneider A, Zentgraf H, Gruber AD, de Villiers EM. (2006). E6/E7 expression of human papillomavirus type 20 (HPV-20) and HPV-27 influences proliferation and differentiation of the skin in UV-irradiated SKH-hr1 transgenic mice. *J Virol.* 80(22):11153-64.

Monks A, Scudiero D, Skehan P, Shoemaker R, Paull K, Vistica D, Hose C, Langley J, Cronise P, Vaigro-Wolff A, Gray-Goodrich M, Campbell H, Mayo J, Boyd M. (1991). Feasibility of a high-flux anticancer drug screen using a diverse panel of cultured human tumor cell lines. *J Natl Cancer Inst.* 83(11):757-66.

Morita S, Okamoto I, Kobayashi K, Yamazaki K, Asahina H, Inoue A, Hagiwara K, Sunaga N, Yanagitani N, Hida T, Yoshida K, Hirashima T, Yasumoto K, Sugio K, Mitsudomi T, Fukuoka M, Nukiwa T. (2009). Combined survival analysis of prospective clinical trials of gefitinib for non-small cell lung cancer with EGFR mutations. *Clin Cancer Res.* 15(13):4493-8.

Murgo AJ, Kummar S, Rubinstein L, Gutierrez M, Collins J, Kinders R, Parchment RE, Ji J, Steinberg SM, Yang SX, Hollingshead M, Chen A, Helman L, Wiltrout R,

Tomaszewski JE, Doroshow JH. (2008). Designing phase 0 cancer clinical trials. *Clin Cancer Res.* 14(12):3675-82.

Nagy A and Mar L. (2001). Creation and Use of a Cre Recombinase Transgenic Database. *Methods Mol Biol* 158:95-106. Database available from: <http://nagy.mshri.on.ca/cre/index.php>

Nanda R. (2007). Targeting the human epidermal growth factor receptor 2 (HER2) in the treatment of breast cancer: recent advances and future directions. *Rev Recent Clin Trials.* 2(2):111-6.

Nelson DR, Zeldin DC, Hoffman SM, Maltais LJ, Wain HM, Nebert DW. (2004). Comparison of cytochrome P450 (CYP) genes from the mouse and human genomes, including nomenclature recommendations for genes, pseudogenes and alternative-splice variants. *Pharmacogenetics.* 14(1):1-18.

Ohashi K, Takigawa N, Osawa M, Ichihara E, Takeda H, Kubo T, Hirano S, Yoshino T, Takata M, Tanimoto M, Kiura K. (2009). Chemopreventive Effects of Gefitinib on Nonsmoking-Related Lung Tumorigenesis in Activating Epidermal Growth Factor Receptor Transgenic Mice. *Cancer Res.* 69(17):7088-7095.

Omer CA, Chen Z, Diehl RE, Conner MW, Chen HY, Trumbauer ME, Gopal-Truter S, Seeburger G, Bhimnathwala H, Abrams MT, Davide JP, Ellis MS, Gibbs JB, et al. (2000). Mouse mammary tumor virus-Ki-rasB transgenic mice develop mammary carcinomas that can be growth-inhibited by a farnesyl:protein transferase inhibitor. *Cancer Res.* 60(10):2680-2688.

Ornitz DM, Palmiter RD, Messing A, Hammer RE, Pinkert CA, Brinster RL. (1985). Elastase I promoter directs expression of human growth hormone and SV40 T antigen genes to pancreatic acinar cells in transgenic mice. *Cold Spring Harb Symp Quant Biol.* 50:399-409.

Paez JG, Jänne PA, Lee JC, Tracy S, Greulich H, Gabriel S, Herman P, Kaye FJ, Lindeman N, Boggon TJ, Naoki K, Sasaki H, Fujii Y, Eck MJ, Sellers WR, Johnson BE, Meyerson M. (2004). EGFR mutations in lung cancer: correlation with clinical response to gefitinib therapy. *Science.* 304(5676):1497-500.

Palmiter RD, Chen HY, Messing A, Brinster RL. (1985). SV40 enhancer and large-T antigen are instrumental in development of choroid plexus tumours in transgenic mice. *Nature.* 316(6027):457-60.

Palmiter RD, Brinster RL. (1986). Germ-line transformation of mice. *Annu Rev Genet.* 20:465-99.

Pao W, Miller VA, Politi KA, Riely GJ, Somwar R, Zakowski MF, Kris MG, Varmus H. (2005). Acquired resistance of lung adenocarcinomas to gefitinib or erlotinib is associated with a second mutation in the EGFR kinase domain. *PLoS Med.* 2(3):e73.

Politi K, Zakowski MF, Fan PD, Schonfeld EA, Pao W, Varmus HE. (2006). Lung adenocarcinomas induced in mice by mutant EGF receptors found in human lung cancers respond to a tyrosine kinase inhibitor or to down-regulation of the receptors. *Genes Dev.* 20(11):1496-510.

Poole AJ, Li Y, Kim Y, Lin SC, Lee WH, Lee EY. (2006). Prevention of Brca1-mediated mammary tumorigenesis in mice by a progesterone antagonist. *Science.* 314: 1467-1470.

Quaife CJ, Pinkert CA, Ornitz DM, Palmiter RD, Brinster RL (1987). Pancreatic neoplasia induced by ras expression in acinar cells of transgenic mice. *Cell.* 48(6):1023-34.

Rao PN, Freireich EJ, Smith ML, Loo TL. (1979). Cell cycle phase-specific cytotoxicity of the antitumor agent maytansine. Cancer Res. 39(8):3152-5.

Remillard S, Rebhun LI, Howie GA, Kupchan SM. (1975). Antimitotic activity of the potent tumor inhibitor maytansine. Science. 189(4207):1002-5.

Riely GJ. (2008). Second-generation epidermal growth factor receptor tyrosine kinase inhibitors in non-small cell lung cancer. *J Thorac Oncol.* 3(6 Suppl 2):S146-9.

Robles AI and Varticovski L. (2008). Harnessing genetically engineered mouse models for preclinical testing. *Chem Biol Interact.* 171(2):159-64.

Rowell CA, Kowalczyk JJ, Lewis MD, Garcia AM. (1997). Direct demonstration of geranylgeranylation and farnesylation of Ki-Ras in vivo. *J Biol Chem.* 272 (22):14093-14097.

Saez E, Tontonoz P, Nelson MC, Alvarez JG, Ming UT, Baird SM, Thomazy VA, Evans RM. (1998). Activators of the nuclear receptor PPARgamma enhance colon polyp formation. *Nat Med.* 4(9):1058-61.

Sarraf P, Mueller E, Jones D, King FJ, DeAngelo DJ, Partridge JB, Holden SA, Chen LB, Singer S, Fletcher C, Spiegelman BM. (1998). Differentiation and reversal of malignant changes in colon cancer through PPARgamma. *Nat Med.* 4(9):1046-52.

Schaper ID, Marcuzzi GP, Weissenborn SJ, Kasper HU, Dries V, Smyth N, Fuchs P, Pfister H. (2005). Development of skin tumors in mice transgenic for early genes of human papillomavirus type 8. *Cancer Res.* 65(4):1394-400.

Sequist LV, Martins RG, Spigel D, Grunberg SM, Spira A, Jänne PA, Joshi VA, McCollum D, Evans TL, Muzikansky A, Kuhlmann GL, Han M, Goldberg JS, Settleman J, Iafrate AJ, Engelman JA, Haber DA, Johnson BE, Lynch TJ. (2008). First-line gefitinib in patients with advanced non-small-cell lung cancer harboring somatic EGFR mutations. *J Clin Oncol.* 26(15):2442-9.

Sharpless NE and Depinho RA. (2006). The mighty mouse: genetically engineered mouse models in cancer drug development. *Nat Rev Drug Discov.* 5(9):741-54.

Shepherd FA, Rodrigues Pereira J, Ciuleanu T, Tan EH, Hirsh V, Thongprasert S, Campos D, Maoleekoonpiroj S, Smylie M, Martins R, van Kooten M, Dediu M, Findlay B, Tu D, Johnston D, Bezjak A, Clark G, Santabárbara P, Seymour L; National Cancer Institute of Canada Clinical Trials Group. (2005). Erlotinib in previously treated non-small-cell lung cancer. *N Engl J Med.* 353(2):123-32.

Shimamura T, Li D, Ji H, Haringsma HJ, Liniker E, Borgman CL, Lowell AM, Minami Y, McNamara K, Perera SA, Zaghlul S, Thomas RK, Greulich H, Kobayashi S, Chirieac LR, Padera RF, Kubo S, Takahashi M, Tenen DG, Meyerson M, Wong KK, Shapiro GI. (2008). Hsp90 inhibition suppresses mutant EGFR-T790M signaling and overcomes kinase inhibitor resistance. *Cancer Res.* 68(14):5827-38.

Slamon DJ, Leyland-Jones B, Shak S, Fuchs H, Paton V, Bajamonde A, Fleming T, Eiermann W, Wolter J, Pegram M, Baselga J, Norton L. (2001). Use of chemotherapy plus a monoclonal antibody against HER2 for metastatic breast cancer that overexpresses HER2. *N Engl J Med.* 2001 Mar 15; 344(11):783-92.

Sos ML, Michel K, Zander T, Weiss J, Frommolt P, Peifer M, Li D, Ullrich R, Koker M, Fischer F, Shimamura T, Rauh D, Mermel C, Fischer S, Stückrath I, Heynck S, et al. (2009). Predicting drug susceptibility of non-small cell lung cancers based on genetic lesions. *J Clin Invest.* 119(6):1727-40.

Sprengel R, Hasan MT. (2007). Tetracycline-controlled genetic switches. *Handb Exp Pharmacol.* (178):49-72.

Stewart TA, Pattengale PK, Leder P. (1984). Spontaneous mammary adenocarcinomas in transgenic mice that carry and express MTV/myc fusion genes. *Cell.* 38(3):627-37.

Strasser A, Harris AW, Bath ML, Cory S. (1990). Novel primitive lymphoid tumours induced in transgenic mice by cooperation between myc and bcl-2. *Nature.* 348(6299):331-3.

Sun J, Qian Y, Hamilton AD, Sebti SM. (1998). Both farnesyltransferase and geranylgeranyltransferase I inhibitors are required for inhibition of oncogenic K-Ras prenylation but each alone is sufficient to suppress human tumor growth in nude mouse xenografts. *Oncogene.* 16(11):1467-1473.

Syrjänen S. (2005). Human papillomavirus (HPV) in head and neck cancer. *J Clin Virol.* 32 Suppl 1:S59-66.

Trotman LC, Niki M, Dotan ZA, Koutcher JA, Di Cristofano A, Xiao A, Khoo AS, Roy-Burman P, Greenberg NM, Van Dyke T, Cordon-Cardo C, Pandolfi PP. (2003). Pten dose dictates cancer progression in the prostate. *PLoS Biol.* 1(3):E59.

Varticovski L, Hollingshead MG, Robles AI, Wu X, Cherry J, Munroe DJ, Lukes L, Anver MR, Carter JP, Borgel SD, Stotler H, Bonomi CA, Nunez NP, Hursting SD, Qiao W, Deng CX, Green JE, Hunter KW, Merlino G, Steeg PS, Wakefield LM, Barrett JC. (2007). Accelerated preclinical testing using transplanted tumors from genetically engineered mouse breast cancer models. *Clin Cancer Res.* 13(7):2168-77.

Ventura A, Kirsch DG, McLaughlin ME, Tuveson DA, Grimm J, Lintault L, Newman J, Reczek EE, Weissleder R, Jacks T. (2007). Restoration of p53 function leads to tumour regression in vivo. *Nature.* 445(7128):661-5.

Wang S, Gao J, Lei Q, Rozengurt N, Pritchard C, Jiao J, Thomas GV, Li G, Roy-Burman P, Nelson PS, Liu X, Wu H. (2003). Prostate-specific deletion of the murine Pten tumor suppressor gene leads to metastatic prostate cancer. *Cancer Cell.* 4(3):209-21.

Weinstein IB. (2002). Addiction to oncogenes--the Achilles heal of cancer. *Science.* 297(5578): 63-4.

Winslow MM, Dayton TL, Verhaak RG, Kim-Kiselak C, Snyder EL, Feldser DM, Hubbard DD, Dupage MJ, Whittaker CA, Hoersch S, Yoon S, Crowley D, Bronson RT, Chiang DY, Meyerson M, Jacks T. (2011). Suppression of lung adenocarcinoma progression by Nkx2-1. *Nature.* 473(7345):101-4.

Yang CH, Yu CJ, Shih JY, Chang YC, Hu FC, Tsai MC, Chen KY, Lin ZZ, Huang CJ, Shun CT, Huang CL, Bean J, Cheng AL, Pao W, Yang PC. (2008). Specific EGFR mutations predict treatment outcome of stage IIIB/IV patients with chemotherapy-naive non-small-cell lung cancer receiving first-line gefitinib monotherapy. *J Clin Oncol.* 26(16):2745-53.

Yun CH, Mengwasser KE, Toms AV, Woo MS, Greulich H, Wong KK, Meyerson M, Eck MJ. (2008). The T790M mutation in EGFR kinase causes drug resistance by increasing the affinity for ATP. *Proc Natl Acad Sci USA*. 105(6):2070-5.

Zenker M, Lehmann K, Schulz AL, Barth H, Hansmann D, Koenig R, Korinthenberg R, Kreiss-Nachtsheim M, Meinecke P, Morlot S, Mundlos S, Quante AS, Raskin S, Schnabel D, Wehner LE, Kratz CP, Horn D, Kutsche K. (2007). Expansion of the genotypic and phenotypic spectrum in patients with KRAS germline mutations. *J. Med. Genet.* 44:131-135.

Zhu K, Hamilton AD, Sebti SM. (2003). Farnesyltransferase inhibitors as anticancer agents: current status. *Curr Opin Investig Drugs*. 4(12):1428-35.

6

Genetic Pharmacotherapy

Celia Gellman[1,2], Susana Mingote[1,2], Yvonne Wang[1,2],
Inna Gaisler-Salomon[1,3] and Stephen Rayport[1,2]
[1]*Department of Psychiatry, Columbia University*
[2]*Department of Molecular Therapeutics, New York State Psychiatric Institute*
[3]*Department of Psychology, University of Haifa*
USA

1. Introduction

In current drug development, *proof-of-concept*—determining whether a ligand engaging its target is likely to be therapeutic—requires specific ligands. This presents a catch-22, as the motivation to develop ligands requires proof-of-concept studies that cannot be conducted without ligands. A strategy we term *genetic pharmacotherapy*—a refinement of genetic blockade focused on druggable targets—obviates the catch-22 by enabling proof-of-concept studies *prior* to the development of specific ligands via genetic means in mouse models. In this strategy, which could help avert investment in molecular entities that will ultimately prove therapeutically inefficacious, a gene is conditionally down-regulated via a molecular *switch* in adult mice. Both the precise temporal control of the intervention and the consequent change in target protein function parallel the administration of drugs, with the additional advantage of perfect specificity. Moreover genetic pharmacotherapy overcomes the impediment of the blood-brain barrier, which makes developing ligands for psychiatric disorders particularly challenging. Here, we describe the transgenic technologies that form the basis for the strategy, discuss the advantages and limitations in juxtaposition with other gene expression modification approaches, contrast examples of prior implementation, address the feasibility for systematic use, and illustrate past and future opportunities. Although the molecular tools are widely available, genetic pharmacotherapy has only been implemented outside the central nervous system (CNS), despite its particular utility for CNS disorders. The systematic application of this strategy should foster the development of new, innovative molecular therapies.

2. The conceptual basis and requisite components of genetic pharmacotherapy

We define genetic pharmacotherapy as the use of a genetic intervention to achieve a pharmacological effect. Genetic pharmacotherapy has two requirements. First, genetic blockade must be universal – reaching all cells in the body, including the brain – to simulate organism-wide drug distribution. Second, induction of gene-modulation must be temporally controllable, as opposed to originating during embryogenesis, so that target modulation occurs as it would with drug administration. While traditional knockout strategies have been used extensively to study the roles of proteins in a broad range of disorders, constitutive mutations are often lethal in early life precluding study of target gene function in adulthood (Lewandoski, 2001). Moreover, many non-lethal knockouts of genes of interest elicit paradoxical phenotypes – phenotypes that are opposite to the effects of pharmacologic blockade of the same target in adulthood – as a result of developmental compensations (Gingrich & Hen, 2000). The genetic strategy that satisfies these two requirements is a refinement of Cre-lox recombination, in which two individually silent mutations are introduced. One mutation drives a ligand-inducible effector enzyme that enables target-modulation, and the other mutation makes the target gene of interest susceptible to inactivation by the effector enzyme. This involves breeding a mouse carrying the inducible effector – CreERT – with an animal carrying the effector-sensitized *floxed* gene-of-interest. In the resulting progeny, inducing the CreERT produces irreversible target modulation paralleling the institution of pharmacotherapy.

2.1 Origins of the inducible-Cre strategy

In Cre-lox recombination, Cre recombinase – from P1 bacteriophage – recognizes two closely spaced 34-base pair loxP sequences, excises the intervening sequence, and recombines the flanking strands. When placed strategically by homologous recombination, the excision inactivates the so-called floxed gene (Nagy, 2000; Sternberg & Hamilton, 1981) (**Figure 1a**). To inactivate the target gene, a mouse that carries the Cre transgene is bred with a mouse carrying loxP sites flanking a portion of the gene of interest (the floxed gene); in the resulting F_1 progeny the floxed gene is inactivated in all cells where Cre is expressed (**Figure 1b**).

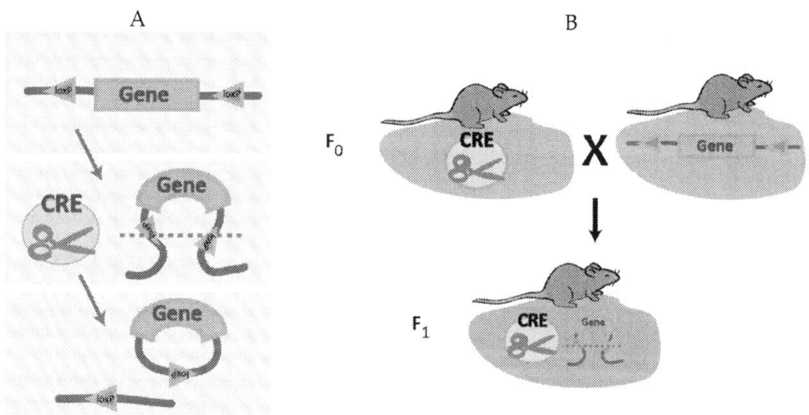

Fig. 1. Removal of targeted DNA sequences by Cre-lox recombination. A. Cre recombinase excises the portion of DNA between the loxP recognition sites (the floxed gene), recombining the flanking strands. B. To accomplish this in mice, a mouse carrying the Cre transgene is bred with a mouse carrying the floxed gene (F_0 generation). In the progeny (F_1), the floxed gene will be recombined in all Cre-expressing cells. If Cre is driven by a cell-specific promoter, recombination will be restricted to just those cells; if Cre is driven by a universally-expressed promoter, recombination will be universal.

In 1992, two groups (Lakso et al., 1992; Orban et al., 1992) reported the first use of Cre in mice to achieve tissue-specific expression. In 1994, Rajewsky and colleagues (Gu et al., 1994) employed Cre as a conditional gene-targeting tool to circumvent the pleiotropic embryonic lethality of the same null mutation. Tissue-specific Cre-mediated conditional gene inactivation has enabled investigators to address questions that would be otherwise intractable in global knockouts (Lewandoski, 2001). However, as mentioned, to best simulate treatment with a drug, which permeates the entire body, inactivation of the target gene should take place in every tissue type – and thus Cre expression should be driven by a universally-expressed promoter such as the hybrid chicken beta-actin promoter and cytomegalovirus enhancer (CAG) promoter. This promoter was dramatically shown to drive expression of enhanced green fluorescent protein (EGFP) in virtually every cell type to produce green mice (Okabe et al., 1997) (**Figure 2**).

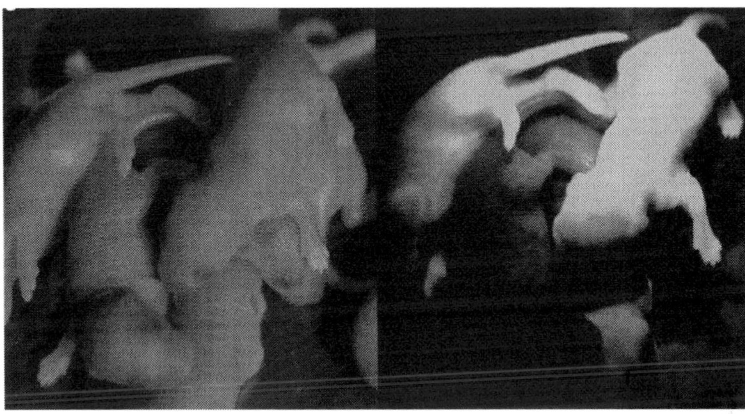

Fig. 2. The transgenic CAG promoter drives expression universally. Five mouse pups are seen under normal light (left); under blue light excitation (right), two of the pups fluoresce green as a result of expression of the ubiquitous CAG promoter that drives EGFP expression in all cell types (in the mice, only red blood cells and hair are not green) (From: Okabe et al., 1997, with permission).

2.1 Modified, ligand-activated CreERT enables temporal control over target gene modulation

To achieve temporal control of Cre recombination, Chambon and colleagues (Feil et al., 1996; Metzger & Chambon, 2001; Metzger et al., 1995) created a ligand-dependent version of Cre, the chimeric protein CreERT, which mediates recombination only in the presence of the drug tamoxifen or its derivatives. In CreERT, Cre is fused to the mutated ligand-binding domain of the estrogen receptor, which recognizes tamoxifen and 4OH-tamoxifen, but not endogenous estrogen (**Figure 3a**). As a steroid receptor of the nuclear receptor family, the estrogen receptor in its inactive form is restricted to the cytoplasm via association with chaperone proteins (Giguère, 2003). As with estrogen activation of the native steroid receptor, tamoxifen releases CreERT from chaperone proteins, enabling the recombinase to diffuse into the nucleus to mediate site-specific recombination (**Figure 3b**). Consequently, target gene-inactivation is temporally controlled and tamoxifen-dependent, as CreERT remains in the cytoplasm until tamoxifen-administration, and returns to the cytoplasm once tamoxifen is no longer in the system.

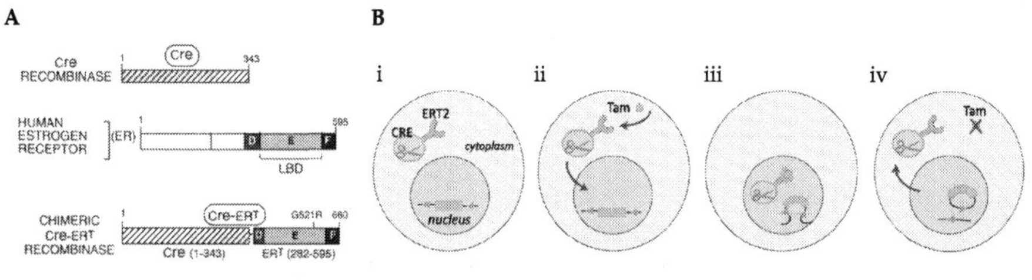

Fig. 3. Temporally controlled, ligand-dependent Cre-lox recombination. A. A mutated version (Gly521→Arg) of the estrogen receptor ligand binding domain (LBD) that recognizes tamoxifen but not estrogen was fused to the Cre protein, resulting in the chimeric protein CreERT (From Metzger & Chambon, 2001, with permission). B. In the absence of tamoxifen or derivatives, the location of CreERT is restricted to the cytoplasm by association with chaperone proteins (i). When engaged by its high-affinity, high-specificity ligand tamoxifen, CreERT is released from the chaperone proteins and diffuses into the nucleus (ii), only then allowing Cre access to recombine genomic DNA irreversibly (iii & iv). After tamoxifen clearance, CreERT will again become sequestered in the cytoplasm (iv).

An enhanced version, CreERT2, is now generally used as it has about a 4-fold greater induction efficiency over CreERT (Indra et al., 1999; Lewandoski, 2001 citations 112-115). For some transgene combinations, there may be some recombination in the absence of tamoxifen (**Figure 4**) (Hayashi, 2002), so evaluation of the magnitude of pre-tamoxifen recombination will therefore be a necessary control. Several ubiquitous inducible Cre lines are available (**Table 1**). An alternate strategy employs a modified progesterone receptor that is activated by RU486 (Kellendonk et al., 1999).

Cre line	Strain name	Stock Number
CagCreERT1	B6.Cg-Tg(CAG-cre/Esr1*)5Amc/J	004682
RosaCreERT2	B6.129-Gt(ROSA)26Sortm1(cre/ERT2)Tyj/J	008463
UBC-CreERT2	B6.Cg-Tg(UBC-cre/ERT2)1Ejb/J	008085

Table 1. Ubiquitously expressed inducible Cre lines. Mice are readily available (jaxmice.jax.org).

Until recently, mice with floxed alleles were generated in individual laboratories and the range of commercially available lines of mice with floxed alleles was limited. Now, floxed mice are being made systematically through a multinational consortium, the Knockout Mouse Project (www.komp.org) (Skarnes et al., 2011). The goal of KOMP is to produce conditional alleles of all expressed mouse genes. So far, 9,000 floxed alleles are or will soon be available, and floxed alleles for the remainder of mouse genes should be accessible in the near term. This comprehensive resource provides the basis for systematic target evaluation using genetic pharmacotherapy.

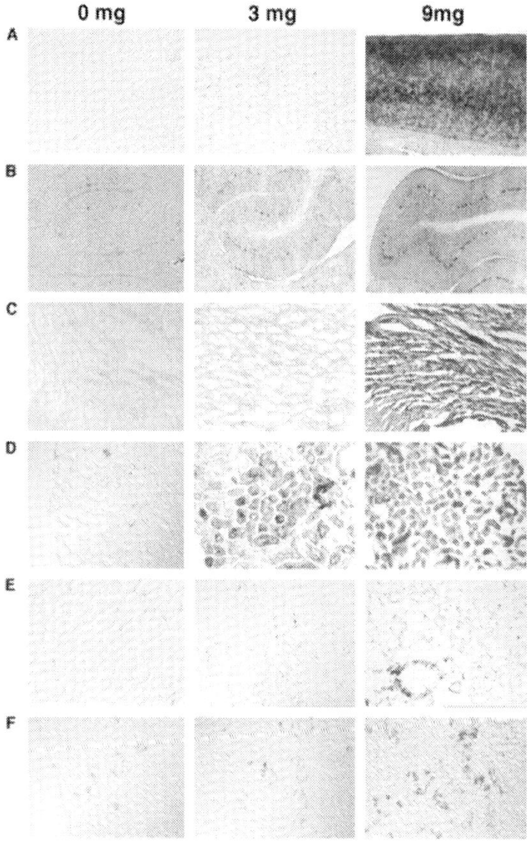

Fig. 4. CreERT2-mediated recombination prior to tamoxifen induction. In a small percentage of cells, recombination occurs in (A) cerebral cortex, (B) cerebellum, (C) heart, (D) kidney, (E) lung, and (F) liver in the absence of tamoxifen (left-most column), as shown by β-galactosidase expression, with the CagCreERT2 mouse line. After tamoxifen (doses shown on top) there is a massive induction of expression (From: Hayashi, 2002, with permission).

3. Comparability to target-specific drugs, with advantages and limitations

Using inducible Cre-lox recombination to inhibit target gene expression offers comparability to, as well as many advantages over, ligand-based inhibition for proof-of-concept studies. Comparable to pharmacologic treatment, genetic pharmacotherapy enables control over the degree of target modulation, analogous to adjustments in drug dose, to assess dose-response; and it also mimics the global, organism-wide action of drug intervention, which enables assessment of possible side effects due to pleiotropic target expression. The strategy's advantages include preclusion of off-target effects via perfect target-specificity, and access to targets in the CNS via permeation of the blood-brain-barrier, which stymies the evaluation of many drug candidates for CNS disorders. There are limitations; these include relative difficulty in targeting splice variants (protein isoforms from the same gene), as the strategy works at the DNA level, and an inability to capture the subtleties of drug action at targets that exhibit functional heterogeneity, i.e. differential structural conformations, drug affinities, and function of a single gene product. We examine each of these points in further illustration below.

3.1 Relative change induced in target-protein function is commensurate to agonism and antagonism

Often, in order to evoke a response in the host cell system, a drug need occupy only a fraction of the total receptors available—a function of both the drug's affinity and the intrinsic ability of the drug-receptor interaction to induce cellular change. This causes the dose-response curve to shift to the left of the receptor occupancy curve, so that a drug dose that elicits maximal tissue response may cause only partial occupation of the available receptors (**Figure 5**).

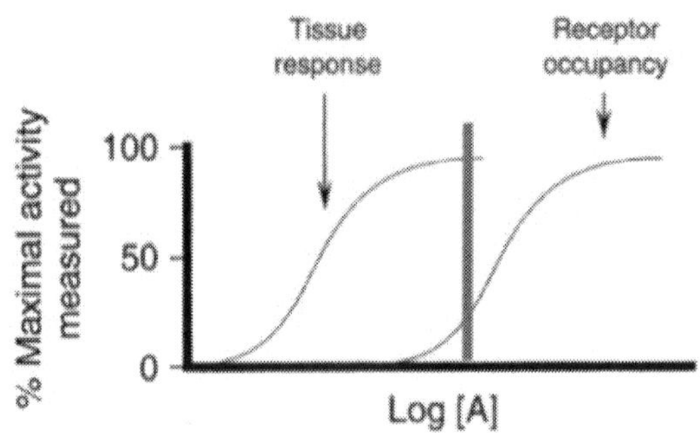

Fig. 5. Maximal tissue response at sub-maximal receptor occupancy. Based on efficacy, drug doses generally need to activate only a fraction of the total available receptors to induce a maximal tissue response. In this illustration, the drug dose that induces maximal tissue response (red line) activates only a fraction of the total available receptors. (Modified from: Ross & Kenakin, 2001, with permission from the McGraw-Hill Companies, Inc.)

For example, opiate agonists etorphine and sufentanil have significant analgesic activity at very low receptor occupancy – approximately 2% at the ED_{50} (Rosenbaum et al., 1984); and in another example, only 22% receptor occupancy is needed for half-maximal stimulation by PEG-TPOm, a mimetic peptide agonist in development for protection against chemotherapy-induced thrombocytopenia (loss of blood platelets) (Samtani et al., 2009). The antipsychotic dopamine D2 receptor antagonist olanzapine achieves optimal clinical efficacy at about 60% receptor occupancy (Mamo et al., 2007).

Similarly, genetic pharmacotherapy need not produce full target inhibition in order to elicit a response. Quantitative gradation in target protein expression (in analogy to a drug dose range) can be controlled by floxing one or both alleles of the gene of interest, and by tamoxifen dose (**Figure 6**) and frequency of administration; in adult mice, tamoxifen is generally administered once daily for 5 days to achieve full recombination. Varying tamoxifen dosing can then mimic the range of drug action.

While the Cre-lox strategy can also be used to simulate agonism, as discussed in later sections, we focus mainly on its application to simulate target antagonism, as the majority of drugs are inhibitors (Copeland et al., 2007; Li et al., 2007) and the accessibility of both ubiquitous CreERT2 mice and the floxed target of choice should now enable systematic *in vivo* target evaluation.

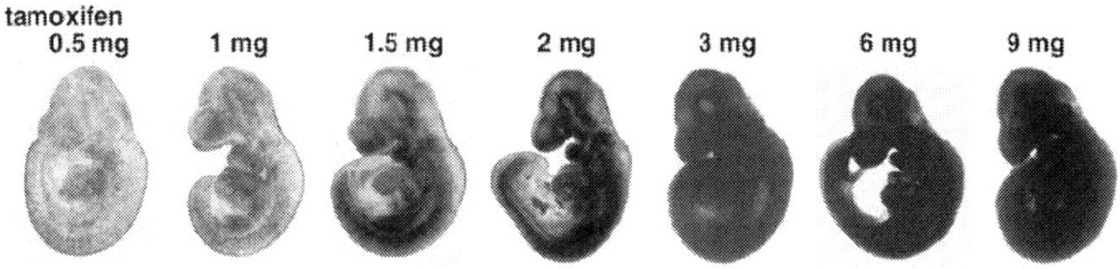

Fig. 6. Tamoxifen dose-dependent recombination in embryos with CreERT driven by a universally expressed promoter. Although Cre-mediated gene modulation is irreversible, "dosing" as a percentage of cells undergoing recombination can still be controlled. Whole-mount transgenic embryos were assayed 9.5 days post-coitum for activity of target gene, β-galactosidase, whose expression had been induced by tamoxifen at the indicated doses (per 40 kg mouse weight) 24 hours prior via intraperitoneal injection of the pregnant dam. (From: Hayashi, 2002, with permission).

To evaluate potential therapeutic efficacy of target modulation, biomarkers or surrogate endpoints specific to the disease model can be used as a response measure—for example, the lowering of blood glucose for genetic pharmacotherapy interventions in diabetes models, LDL cholesterol levels in dyslipidemia models, or PET imaging of ligand binding in CNS models.

3.2 Ubiquitously expressed effector simulates organism-wide pharmacologic actions

In this gene expression modulation system, the effector protein CreERT2 controls the expression of the target gene (for the candidate drug target). In order to achieve the closest simulation of a pharmacologic agent, which has organism-wide effects, it is paramount that a ubiquitously expressed locus such as Rosa26 (Soriano, 1999; Ventura et al., 2007) be used to drive the effector protein expression (**Table 1**). This way it is possible to assess the phenotypic consequences of pleiotropy occurring in targets – that is, the side effects arising from inhibiting a gene product that participates in multiple signaling or metabolic pathways or in different tissues (for further discussion of the relevance of pleiotropics to pharmacotherapy, see Hodgkin, 1998; Searls, 2003). While small interfering RNA (siRNA) has been used extensively for controlled gene inhibition in proof-of-concept studies, siRNA is not drug-like, as it must be delivered to the tissue of interest (Davidson & McCray, 2011).

3.3 Superiority over pharmacologics: preclusion of off-target effects via perfect target-specificity

Since Paul Ehrlich, drug design has aspired to the ideal of "magic bullet" drugs that seek out only "enemy targets" involved in pathology while leaving the body unharmed (Parascandola, 1981). Lack of target specificity not only severely limits the use of small molecules as therapeutics – for example, the clinical use of anti-Parkinsonian drugs pergolide and cabergoline has been greatly limited because their off-target effects cause valvular heart disease (Keiser et al., 2009) – but also restricts their use as experimental tools in proof-of-concept evaluation (Peterson, 2008). Although promiscuous targeting and multi-receptor activity do produce therapeutic benefits when single-receptor action does not – for example, in the case of statins and psychotropic medications (Keiser et al., 2009; Peterson, 2008) – it is nonetheless preferable that well-defined functional outcomes be understood through well-delineated biochemical actions. Even a drug with high specificity that achieves a desirable outcome in an animal model or clinically still cannot be concluded to work only via the pathway assumed. Genetic pharmacotherapy, on the other hand, enables demonstration of precise, controlled causality in *in vivo* studies.

This is not to say that benefits of polypharmacy cannot be addressed with genetic pharmacotherapy; indeed, the synergy of inhibiting multiple targets simultaneously could be assessed in mice with multiple floxed alleles or by combining genetic pharmacotherapy with traditional pharmacotherapy. It may be impractical to translate findings from such an experiment into a ligand that accomplishes the same synergistic inhibition, but it would enable investigators to parse precisely which targets mediate the desired results, and could guide drug optimization efforts.

Along these lines, genetic pharmacotherapy raises the possibility of validating previously established targets. For example, every antipsychotic drug approved so far has dopamine D2 receptor-blocking activity based on the presumed mode of action of first-generation antipsychotics, which was an entirely serendipitous discovery. However, it likely that their therapeutic efficacy involves interaction with other targets; for instance, antipsychotics inhibit *KCNH2*, a recently described potassium channel, found to be overexpressed in the brains of patients with schizophrenia (Huffaker et al., 2009). The authors state:

> "Whereas D2 receptor affinity is thought to account for the therapeutic effects of antipsychotics, KCNH2 binding is responsible at least for side effects such as altered QT interval or even sudden cardiac failure. Given that KCNH2 controls neuronal excitability and firing patterns, could the therapeutic effects of antipsychotic drugs also be related to their affinities for the brain-specific isoforms of KCNH2? (Huffaker et al., 2009)"

With the present lack of specific KCNH2 ligands, genetic pharmacotherapy could enable further dissection of this possibility and resolve the conceptual justifications guiding the development of compounds with similarly intended actions, pharmacologic or therapeutic.

3.4 Specific advantages with regard to CNS targets

Genetic pharmacotherapy offers particular advantages for proof-of-concept studies for CNS disorders. Such studies face not only the obstacle of designing high-affinity, high-specificity ligands, as in evaluation of targets in other tissues, but also the blood-brain barrier – the superfine filter composed of endothelial cells lining brain capillaries and astrocytes – that either blocks or actively transports out more than 98% of candidate drugs (Miller, 2002). Genetic pharmacotherapy circumvents this obstacle because tamoxifen permeates the blood-brain barrier freely.

3.5 Limitations of achieving target inhibition via DNA modification

While drugs can distinguish between different protein isoforms arising from RNA splice variants (Thompson et al., 2011) that may have different anatomical and functional specificities (Huffaker et al., 2009), genetic pharmacotherapy cannot make such a distinction easily, as target inhibition is mediated via changes at the DNA level. Similarly, a drug may interact differentially with receptors exhibiting functional heterogeneity – e.g. a receptor with distinct allosteric conformations and signaling complexes, varying by anatomical distribution (Mailman, 2007; Mailman & Murthy, 2010) – a subtlety less amenable to simulation with genetic pharmacotherapy but achievable in some cases with pharmacology. The D2 dopamine receptor provides a classic example: agonist stimulation of presynaptic D2 dopamine autoreceptors diminishes dopamine synthesis and release, which may achieve a dopamine antagonist-like effect post-synaptically via decreased dopamine neurotransmission -- whereas preferential agonism of post-synaptic D2 dopamine receptors would achieve the opposite effect. Selective targeting of distinct cell-type D2 receptors cannot be achieved with a universal CreERT line, but the D2 receptor partial agonist aripiprazole appears to exhibit such functional selectivity. Nevertheless, a judiciously chosen tissue-specific inducible CreERT2 strategy may allow such issues to be addressed with better precision than with pharmacology. For instance, presynaptic dopamine D2 receptors have been selectively targeted using a DAT-Cre driver (Bello et al., 2011), and DAT-CreERT2 mice have been reported (Engblom et al., 2008), so that such changes could be induced in adulthood to model an autoreceptor selective dopamine D2 receptor antagonist.

4. Evolution of genetic pharmacotherapy

Genetic pharmacotherapy builds on molecular developments of the last two decades. Below we describe seminal applications of aspects of the genetic pharmacotherapy strategy, and, in certain instances, the molecular entities with actions mirroring the corresponding genetic intervention. Where we wish to build on these foundations is in illustrating the feasibility and advantages of applying this concept – specifically, by employing inducible Cre-lox technology – to evaluate new potential therapeutic drug targets systematically, particularly in the CNS, a possibility that has not yet been articulated until now.

4.1 Genetic blockade *In lieu* or absence of pharmacologic blockade

The potential advantages of using genetic blockade in place of a pharmacologic blockade for CNS studies were described in 1996 in studies reporting the first transgenic expression of Cre in the mouse nervous system (Tsien et al., 1996):

> "Studies of ... mechanisms underlying ... vertebrate animal [behavior] have traditionally been carried out using pharmacological blockades.... gene knockouts provide an alternative means. While the two methods are complementary, genetic deletion is generally superior to pharmacological blockade with respect to molecular and anatomical specificities and animal-to-animal reproducibility. For instance, while many antagonists cannot distinguish receptor isoforms, genetic blockade can make that distinction. Likewise... a genetic blockade can be highly confined and reproducible."

The juxtaposition of genetic and pharmacologic blockade, in this instance, pertains to their relative merits as experimental tools for addressing questions regarding memory formation as opposed to new therapeutic targets. In a related, concurrent study, the tetracycline transactivator system (described below) was used for regional and temporal control over calcium-calmodulin-dependent kinase II (CamKII) expression to demonstrate the requirement of CamKII for both implicit and explicit memory formation (Mayford et al., 1996).

4.1.1 Tetracycline-regulatable gene expression

The tetracycline transactivator system (Gossen & Bujard, 1992) offers another ligand-controlled gene expression system, in which the targeted gene is turned off or on by the administration of tetracycline or (more commonly) doxycycline (**Figure 7a**). In this system, the *E. coli*-derived tetracycline-controlled transactivator (tTA) drives target-gene transcription by binding to a modified *tet* operator (*tet*O) sequence, and this activity can be diminished and switched off depending on varying concentrations of doxycycline. This strategy is adapted from the *E. coli* tetracycline-resistance operon, in which transcription of tetracycline resistance-mediating genes is negatively regulated by the tetracycline repressor (*tet*R). The presence of tetracycline causes the dissociation of *tet*R from the promoter region of the operon and enables transcription of resistance genes. In contrast, as just mentioned, the modified transactivator tTA, based on *tet*R, *stimulates* (as opposed to repressing) transcription when bound to minimal promoters fused to *tet*O sequences, and the presence of low concentrations of tetracycline (<100 nM) or doxycycline prevents the binding of tTA to the tetO sequences and thereby halts transcription. In the modified tet-on version of this system (Kistner et al., 1996), doxycycline turns on target gene expression via a reverse tTA (rtTA). In this case, rtTA will bind tetO to activate transcription only in the presence of doxycycline (**Figure 7b**).

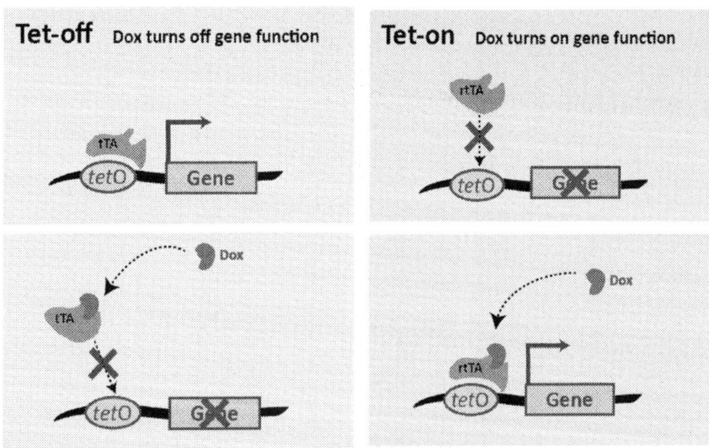

Fig. 7. Tetracycline transactivator (tTA)-controlled gene expression. (a) In tet-off gene regulation, the effector protein tTA binds to the *tet*O promoter, which activates transcription of the target gene. Upon the administration of doxycycline, tTA changes conformation and ceases to activate the target gene's transcription. (b) In the tet-on system, a modified *reverse* tTA (rtTA) binds *tet*O only in the presence of doxycycline.

While the tet-regulatable strategy is appealing for the reversibility of target modulation (with the addition or removal of doxycycline administration) in inhibition studies, it is impossible to produce a silent mutation in the target gene, such as the introduction of loxP sites. In order to control the gene of interest, the *tet*O promoter must be substituted for the native promoter on one allele of the target gene, and the native promoter on the other allele, in turn, used to drive tTA. A study employed this strategy (**Figure 8**) to examine the role of the dopamine transporter (DAT) in scaling learning (Cagniard et al., 2006).

In this tandem design, tissue specificity of target gene expression is maintained, but pre-doxycycline expression levels vary considerably; this is problematic for genetic pharmacotherapy because target gene function should be at basal levels prior to induction. In the strategy illustrated in **Figure 8**, the mutant mice expressed modestly reduced levels of DAT, and it took several weeks of doxycycline administration to achieve significant suppression of DAT expression (Cagniard et al., 2006). In another study examining the role of potassium SK3 channels, SK3 expression was several fold higher than control, and was suppressed with doxycycline (Bond et al., 2000).

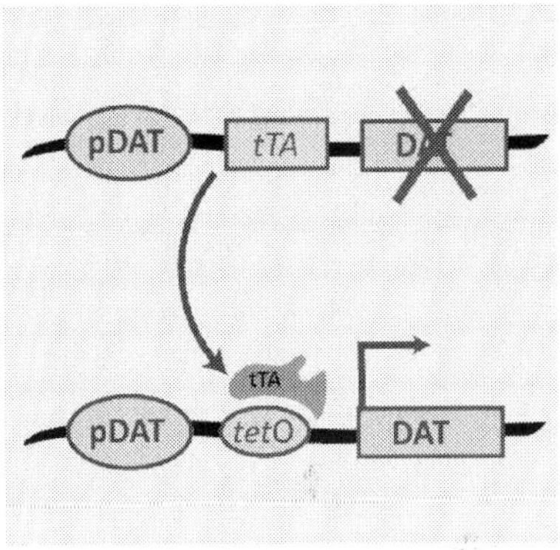

Fig. 8. Target inhibition with tet-off system. For doxycycline-induced knockdown of the targeted dopamine transporter (DAT) function, tTA is expressed under the control of the DAT promoter pDAT on one allele, abrogating DAT expression at that locus; endogenous DAT expression at the other allele is also disrupted by placement of the *tet*O promoter ahead of the gene—but in cells with endogenous pDAT promoter activity driving tTA expression, DAT will be expressed via the *tet*O promoter. Thus tissue specificity of target expression is maintained. Doxycycline then blocks tTA action and so inhibits all DAT expression.

Though less ideal for systematic target evaluation when compared to CreERT2, the tetracycline-transactivator system has nevertheless been particularly powerful in modeling a disease state and subsequently assaying the proof-of-concept of its reversibility via doxycycline administration. In a landmark paper, Yamamoto and colleagues (2000) created a mouse model of Huntington's disease (HD) by *tet*O-driven, striatum-restricted expression of a pathogenic version of the Huntingtin protein. By 4 weeks of age, the mice began to exhibit choreic movements and dystonia, and by 8 weeks showed striatal Huntingtin aggregates – both hallmarks of HD. HD is progressive, without a specific treatment or cure, and prior to this study was assumed to be inexorable in its course. However, abolishing the expression of mutant Huntingtin by doxycycline administration in symptomatic mice not only halted but also *reversed* the accumulation of protein aggregates and progressive motor decline. Although developing a pharmacologic intervention for HD has yet to be achieved, this study demonstrated that blocking expression of pathogenic Huntingtin in symptomatic subjects reversed manifestations of the disease, and indeed could be viewed as having achieved *a cure*. This proof-of-concept clearly motivates a search for drugs that would reverse or prevent Huntingtin protein aggregate formation.

Kellendonk and colleagues (2006) used the tetracycline-transactivator system to address the possibility of reversing schizophrenia-like abnormalities induced by dopamine D2 receptor overexpression (D2OE) in the striatum. Imaging studies have shown that dopamine transmission is increased in patients with schizophrenia, involving both increased dopamine release and increased dopamine D2 receptor binding (Guillin et al., 2007). The D2OE mice, in which tTA drove striatally restricted expression of an extra human D2R allele, exhibited elevated receptor binding capacity – 15% higher than control littermates. The pivotal finding was that dopamine dysfunction – previously thought only to account for the positive symptoms, such as hallucinations and delusions – could be causally linked to cognitive deficits (Simpson et al., 2010). D2OE mice showed altered dopamine transmission in the prefrontal cortex as well as selective cognitive impairment in working memory tasks, a prefrontal cortex-dependent process, without more general cognitive deficits – similar to cognitive impairments in patients with schizophrenia. Administering doxycycline to reverse the D2OE did not reverse the working memory impairment, suggesting that the cognitive deficits in these mice arose not from continued D2OE but as a consequence of D2OE during development. Whether D2OE occurs prior to the onset of schizophrenia in patients is not known; however, dopamine release is increased (Howes et al., 2008), so there is clear evidence for increased dopamine transmission prior to the onset of schizophrenic symptoms. The earlier consequences of increased dopamine transmission in the D2OE mice are consistent with the well-recognized inability of dopamine D2 receptor antagonists to ameliorate cognitive impairments. It must also be noted that while genetic blockade of transgene expression accomplished down-regulation of D2 receptor overexpression, it did not mimic actual D2 receptor antagonist pharmacotherapy fully, as doxycycline inhibited only the transgenic D2 receptors while D2 antagonists would block both the transgenic as well as native D2 receptors.

In these studies, the tetracycline-transactivator system was used to model a disease, and subsequently doxycycline administration was used to turn off pathogenic protein expression to establish causality between protein and disease. In genetic pharmacotherapy studies, introduction of an extra tet-regulatable allele could be used to test the effects of increasing target expression, mimicking the actions of a target agonist. One benefit of this strategy, as mentioned, is reversibility of the target modulation; however, the transgenic mice would need to be engineered on a per-target basis, as there is no repository analogous to KOMP for tet-regulatable alleles. Using the tet-off system in inhibition studies, as in the DAT study, disadvantageously requires engineering two transgenic mice (for both the *tet*O and tTA alleles).

4.2 Genetic blockade techniques beyond inducible Cre and tTA

Genetic blockade as a proof-of-concept tool has also been used in a number of oncogenic signaling pathway studies. Although the blockade in the following two examples was accomplished via methods difficult to translate to other druggable targets, the studies successfully established a therapeutic proof-of-concept via genetic means in the absence of a high-specificity ligand against the endogenous target. In one study, a silent mutation engineered into an oncogenic kinase allowed for its selective inhibition, whereas kinase inhibitor non-specificity had previously deterred such an investigation (Fan et al., 2002). In a second study, tumorigenic expression of an endocrine receptor was suppressed by a truncated version of the same receptor (delivered via an adenovirus) that acted as a dominant-negative inhibitor (Min et al., 2003). In both cases, the subsequently developed pharmacologic inhibitors produced the same effect as the genetic blockade, corroborating the parallel between genetic and pharmacologic target blockade.

4.2.1 Engineering a kinase for selective inhibition to determine its role in oncogenic signaling

To overcome the lack of specific kinase inhibitors, Fan and colleagues engineered a silent mutation into a target kinase gene that allowed selective inhibition while retaining kinase activity prior to administration of the mutant kinase-specific antagonist, NaPP1 (Fan et al., 2002). Mice subcutaneously injected with cancer cells containing endogenous or NaPP1-sensitized versions of the epithelial growth factor receptor (EGFP) oncogene v-erbB grew tumors of similar size and with similar latencies – but the inhibitor NaPP1 suppressed growth only in tumors with the sensitized allele (**Figure 9**).

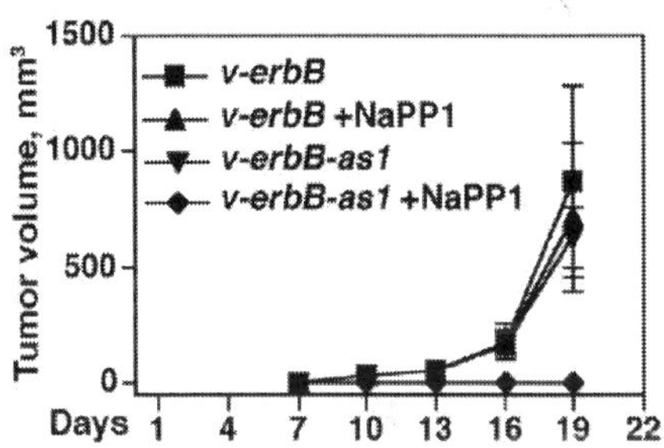

Fig. 9. Chemical genetic blockade in a proof-of-concept study. Assay of tumor growth inhibition in nude mice injected with *v-erbB-* or *v-erbB-as1*-transformed cells. NaPP1 blocks tumor growth only in the mice with the mutagenized *v-erbB-as1* allele that renders the kinase susceptible to selective inhibition by NaPP1 (From: Fan et al., 2002, with permission)

Fan and colleagues (2002) concluded that selective inhibitors of EGFR may effectively arrest cancer cell proliferation at a favorable therapeutic index, as basal signaling in normal cells is unlikely to be affected. Although inhibitors selective for the ErbB EGFR were not available at the time of this chemical-genetic blockade study, genetically engineering inhibitor sensitivity demonstrated the target's proof-of-concept. This incentivized further efforts to develop ligands specific for EGFR subtypes such as ErbB. Indeed, initial marketing of Gefitinib, an EGFR tyrosine kinase inhibitor, was approved in 2003 for patients with non-small cell lung cancer, and Erlotinib, another EGFR tyrosine kinase inhibitor, was approved for the same indication in 2004 and for pancreatic cancer in 2005 (National Cancer Institute Online Drug Information, Pao, 2005).

4.2.2 Virally delivered truncated IGF-I receptor as dominant-negative inhibitor of tumorigenesis

Like EGFR, the insulin-like growth factor I receptor (IGF-Ir) is a mitotic growth factor that stimulates cell growth and is implicated in tumorigenesis (Prager et al., 1994). In certain tumors, IGF-Ir appears to be essential for both malignant transformation and maintenance of the malignant state (Baserga, 1995; Sell et al., 1993). Additionally, initial studies indicated potential tumor selectivity in targeting IGF-Ir for therapeutic applications: reduction of IGF-Ir function induced apoptosis in tumor cells but produced only growth arrest in untransformed cells; and IGF-Ir knockout mice are viable, indicating it is not indispensable for relatively normal development (Min et al., 2003). Prior to the availability of selective ligands, blocking receptor function was accomplished by introducing into tumor cells a recombinant, truncated version of the IGF-Ir with a deleted intracellular tyrosine kinase domain, enabling non-functional heterodimerization. Genetic blockade via dominant-negative receptor expression prevented the formation of sarcomas in nude mice (Prager et al., 1994) and was successful in treating lung, colorectal, and pancreatic xenograft models (Min et al., 2003). Since then, a number of small-molecule IGF-Ir inhibitors have been discovered, with anti-neoplastic action in a wide range of cancers (Carboni et al., 2009; Flanigan et al., 2010; García-Echeverría et al., 2004; He et al., 2010; Iwasa et al., 2009; Kurio et al., 2011), including several that have now moved into clinical trials (Carboni et al., 2009; Iwasa et al., 2009).

4.3 Genetic pharmacotherapy simulates ligand-mediated restoration of p53 anti-tumor activity

Ventura and colleagues did the study — outside the CNS — that most closely embodies our vision of genetic pharmacotherapy (Ventura et al., 2007). They restored function of the transcription factor p53, which has tumor suppressor activity, via a global inducible Cre strategy. p53 was shown in 1991 to be the most frequently inactivated protein in human cancer (Hollstein et al., 1991) so its pathway has been of longstanding interest, and has been the subject of molecular therapeutic development efforts (Vassilev, 2004). Pharmacological restoration of p53 protein function to achieve tumor regression was achieved indirectly by disrupting its interaction with its suppressor protein, MDM2. Indeed, a series of small molecules named Nutlins were discovered that are active in the mid-nanomolar range (Vassilev, 2004).

Ventura and colleagues sought to determine whether rescuing p53 function directly would induce apoptosis and tumor regression. They made p53-LSL mice in which p53 is knocked out due to the insertion of a floxed-Stop (lox-Stop-lox, "LSL") cassette — which stops transcription ahead of the p53 gene — but can be restored by Cre-mediated removal of the cassette. These mice were bred with global ROSA26-CreERT2 mice to produce p53 knockout mice in which tamoxifen could restore p53 function. After irradiating double mutant progeny shortly after birth to accelerate tumor formation, they then showed that tamoxifen treatment of the CreERT2-bearing p53-LSL mice resulted in regression of autochthonous lymphomas and sarcomas, without affecting normal tissues (**Figure 10**).

4.4 Contrasting inducible Cre-lox genetic pharmacotherapy with other modes of genetic blockade

For each of the three targets discussed above for cancer therapy — EGFR, IGF-Ir, and p53 — the drug effects mirror those of the genetic pharmacotherapy intervention, corroborating the technique's comparability as a means of testing a pharmacologic proof-of-concept. Although the Nutlin molecules increase p53 activity indirectly via MDM2 inhibition, and a genetic intervention more directly analogous to the corresponding drug might have targeted a floxed-MDM2 allele, the two studies nonetheless demonstrate the anti-tumor effects (proof-of-concept) of p53-up-regulation (**Figure 11**).

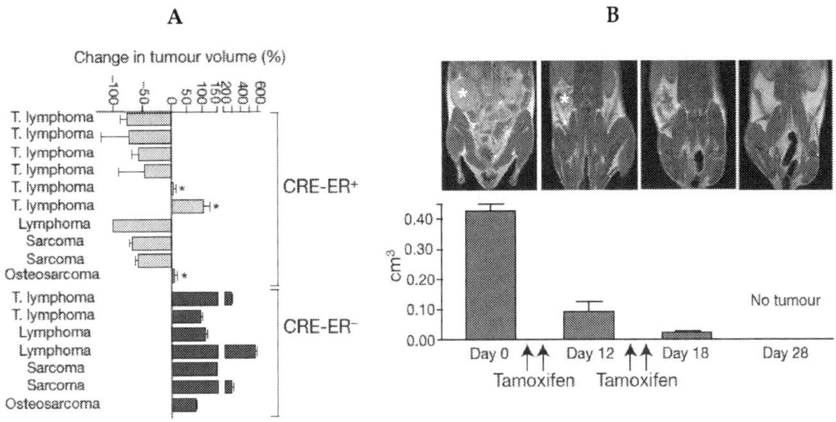

Fig. 10. Genetic pharmacotherapy mediates up-regulation of p53 expression and causes regression of autochthonous sarcomas and lymphomas. A. Tamoxifen administration caused tumor regression in p53-LSL mice expressing tamoxifen-inducible CreERT2, but not in CreERT2-negative p53-LSL mice. B. A series of MRI images (top) shows the regression of an abdominal lymphoma (indicated by the white asterisk) after the administration of tamoxifen. Below, the tumor volume at the time point of each corresponding MRI image. (From: Ventura et al., 2007, with permission)

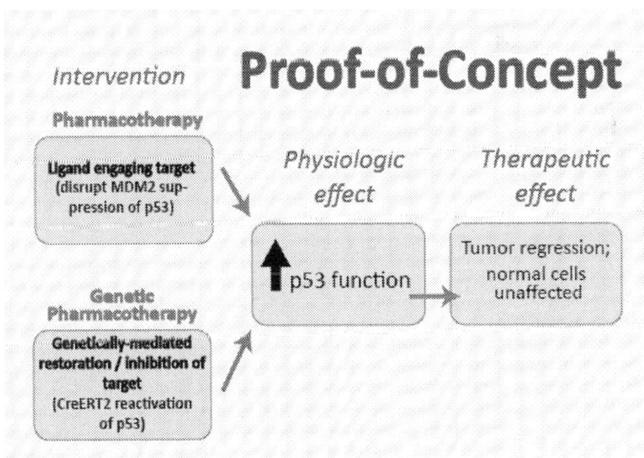

Fig. 11. Parallels in proof-of-concept studies for drug development between ligand-based pharmacotherapy and genetic pharmacotherapy, as exemplified by p53 up-regulation for cancer pharmacotherapy (Vassilev, 2004; Ventura et al., 2007). Both ligand inhibition of MDM2 and tamoxifen-inducible Cre-mediated rescue of homozygous null p53 alleles result in an up-regulation of p53 function that halts tumor cell growth and causes apoptosis, leading to tumor reduction in mice.

schizophrenia. They showed diminished sensitization to amphetamine (Gaisler-Salomon et al., unpublished) – sensitization is thought to be a key process involved in the progression of schizophrenia (Duncan et al., 1999), and in contrast to patients with schizophrenia, *Gls1* hets showed diminished ketamine-induced frontal cortex activation. The mice showed enhanced latent inhibition, a behavioral measure typically diminished in schizophrenia and enhanced by administration of antipsychotic drugs (Weiner & Arad, 2009). Other measures affected in schizophrenia, including pre-pulse inhibition and working memory, were unaffected. Thus, reduction in *Gls1* function engendered endophenotypic changes suggestive of potential resilience to schizophrenia. Moreover, the global glutaminase deficiency seen in *Gls1* hets had its strongest impact in the hippocampus, suggesting that systemic *Gls1* inhibitors should have a similar focal action. Lacking CNS-active glutaminase inhibiters, genetic pharmacotherapy offers a way to test the therapeutic potential of glutaminase inhibition (Gellman et al., 2011).

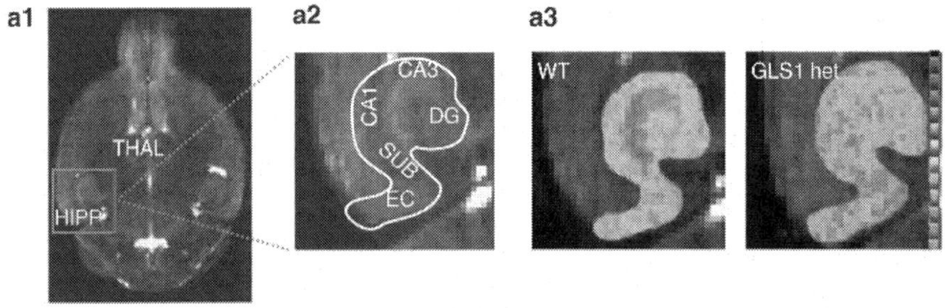

Fig. 13. Cerebral blood volume (CBV) imaging in the hippocampus of *GLs1* het mice. The hippocampal formation (a1, a2) is color-coded in an individual CBV map (a3) such that warmer colors reflect higher CBV values. Regional CBV is fairly uniform across hippocampal subregions in WT mice, but *Gls1* het mice show a selective reduction in the subiculum and CA1. (From: Gaisler-Salomon *et al.* (2009), with permission of the authors).

6. Feasibility and recommendations for systematic use

For disorders with well-defined molecular targets, genetic pharmacotherapy offers a direct way to test the therapeutic potential of inhibiting the target in advance of ligand development. The investigator administers tamoxifen to a disease-modeling mouse carrying both the global-inducible CreERT2 allele and the floxed version of the targeted allele. The resulting DNA recombination event and ensuing change in target expression levels simulates pharmacologic target-modulation. The Knockout Mouse Project (www.komp.org) (Skarnes et al., 2011) now makes available floxed alleles of genes of interest so that the requisite tools are readily or will shortly be available.

While the Cre-ERT2 approach is most directly applicable to antagonism studies, it can also be used for tests of agonism with transgenic mice bearing flox-Stop alleles so that tamoxifen administration would turn on an additional allele or alleles; however, such mice are not widely available. The tTA-tetO system is similarly useful for studies of agonism, which could be most straightforwardly accomplished in transgenic mice bearing the promoter for the target gene driving tTA in tandem with tetO driving the target gene. In contrast, antagonism with tTA-tetO, as noted above, is inherently limited by the inability to design mutant mice in which the target gene is unperturbed. The utility of these approaches is summarized in **Table 2**.

In psychiatric disorders such as schizophrenia, molecular targets are less well defined. Diagnosis remains symptom-based due to lack of specific biomarkers or objective diagnostic tests. Mouse models capture many dimensions of the disorder but cannot be said to be models of the disorder (Arguello & Gogos, 2006; Nestler & Hyman, 2010). As such, for psychiatric disorders, the search for therapeutics is conducted in two stages. In the first stage, recognized behavioral dimensions are evaluated for desired effects of target modulation. For schizophrenia, these dimensions include reduction in correlates of positive symptoms (Carpenter & Koenig, 2008) and negative symptoms (O'Tuathaigh et al., 2010). In the second stage, a mouse model with construct validity – that is, a mouse carrying a mutation known to be implicated in the disease state, or that has been exposed to exogenous agents known to elicit the disorder – is subjected to the same genetic pharmacotherapy and phenomenological assays. Many genetic mouse models have been developed for schizophrenia based on genetic mutations that have been associated with the disorder, both constitutive (Carpenter & Koenig, 2008) and inducible (Pletnikov, 2009). Models based on exogenous agents include *in utero* challenges (Lodge & Grace, 2009), perinatal lesions (Tseng et al., 2009) and drug-induced states (Bickel & Javitt, 2009; Gonzalez-Maeso & Sealfon, 2009).

	CreERT2	tTA-tetO
Antagonism	Ubiquitous CreERT2 :: flox-Target	*(unperturbed control impossible)*
Agonism	Ubiquitous CreERT2:: flox-Stop-Target	pTarget-tTA :: tetO-Target

Table 2. Mouse genetic strategies for genetic pharmacotherapy. Genetic pharmacotherapy can mimic pharmacotherapy for both inhibition (target antagonism) or stimulation (target agonism). CreERT2 is most practical for inhibition studies as the requisite mouse lines (ubiquitous inducible Cre mice, and komp.com-accessible floxed-target mice) are widely available. tTA-tetO cannot be used for inhibition as it is impossible to make a doxycycline-regulatable line without perturbing control expression. Both CreERT2 and tTA-tetO strategies are suitable for stimulation studies, limited by the need to make the requisite mouse lines.

7. Conclusions

The genetic pharmacotherapy strategy enables testing the therapeutic proof-of-concept of target modulation in the absence of specific ligands. It allows circumvention of the proof-of-concept catch-22 in drug development, where the risk of investing in targets with limited validation often impedes the pursuit of specific ligands that would eventually be validated. It also minimizes the complementary problem of investment in selective ligands that would ultimately fail in clinical proof-of-concept studies (**Figure 14**). The recently announced conditional allele library resource (Skarnes et al., 2011) will facilitate efforts to test multiple targets with the inducible Cre strategy. Druggable targets that are likely to be disease modifying have now been identified (Hajduk et al., 2005; Knox et al., 2011; Zhu et al., 2010). The concept and tools of genetic pharmacotherapy have been well established for some time, but their potential for systematic application to proof-of-concept evaluation for drug development efforts has not been fully appreciated. Genetic pharmacotherapy should prove to be a powerful orthogonal tool (Hardy & Peet, 2004) for drug development.

The lack of investment in truly innovative psychiatric drugs over the past decades underpins the vastly unmet need for better treatments, as the burden of psychiatric illness remains high and current treatments remain ineffective or nonexistent (Brundtland, 2001; Miller, 2010). Critics of psychiatric drug development argue that because the etiology of major mental illnesses remains so poorly understood, adequate treatments cannot be developed (Conn & Roth, 2008). However, applying genetic pharmacotherapy in increasingly sophisticated mouse models of psychiatric disorders promises to make the full mouse genome accessible to drug discovery and so expand greatly the accessibility of molecular targets for pharmacotherapies. We believe that this strategy will expedite the development of innovative new molecular therapies, particularly for CNS disorders.

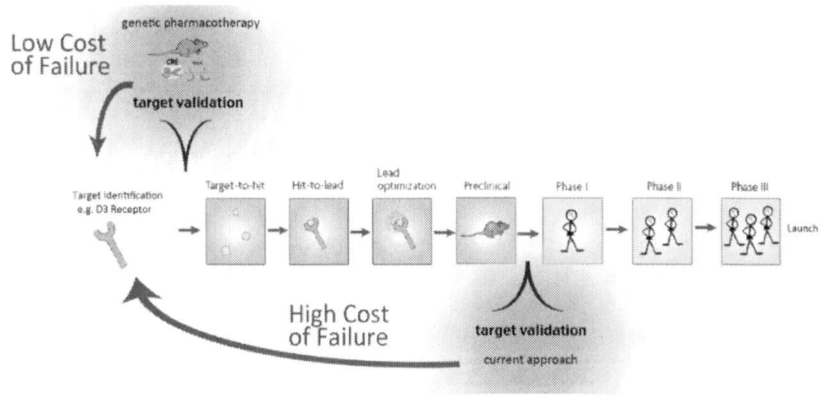

Fig. 14. Role for genetic pharmacotherapy in early stages of the drug development pipeline. Genetic pharmacotherapy (low cost of failure) bypasses ligand development (high cost of failure) in enabling target validation; ligand development (tan shading) can then be implemented for the most promising targets for which proof-of-concept studies demonstrate higher likelihood of success in clinical development (blue shading).

8. Acknowledgements

We are grateful to Anissa Abi-Dargham, Peter Balsam, Laura Bradley, Jay Gingrich, René Hen, Jonathan Javitch, Daniel Javitt, Christoph Kellendonk, Jerry Kokoshka, Jeffrey Lieberman, Holly Moore, Scott Schobel, Scott Small and members of our laboratory for their input and advice on the development of the Genetic Pharmacotherapy strategy. Our research on glutaminase deficient mice is supported by Lieber Center for Schizophrenia Research and Treatment, NIMH Silvio O. Conte Center for Schizophrenia Research (P50 MH066171), and R01 MH087758.

9. References

Arguello, P.A. and Gogos, J.A. (2006) Modeling madness in mice: one piece at a time. *Neuron*, Vol. 52, No. 1, pp. 179-196

Baserga, R. (1995) The insulin-like growth factor I receptor: a key to tumor growth? *Cancer Res.*, Vol. 55, No. 2, pp. 249-252

Bello, E.P., Mateo, Y., Gelman, D.M., Noaín, D., Shin, J.H., Low, M.J., Alvarez, V.A., Lovinger, D.M. and Rubinstein, M. (2011) Cocaine supersensitivity and enhanced motivation for reward in mice lacking dopamine D2 autoreceptors. *Nat. Neurosci.*, Vol. 14, No. 8, pp. 1033-1038

Bickel, S. and Javitt, D. (2009) Neurophysiological and neurochemical animal models of schizophrenia: focus on glutamate. *Behav. Brain Res.*, Vol. 204, No. 2, pp. 352-362

Bond, C.T., Sprengel, R., Bissonnette, J.M., Kaufmann, W.A., Pribnow, D., Neelands, T., Storck, T., Baetscher, M., Jerecic, J., Maylie, J., Knaus, H.G., Seeburg, P.H. and Adelman, J.P. (2000) Respiration and parturition affected by conditional overexpression of the Ca2+-activated K+ channel subunit, SK3. *Science*, Vol. 289, No. 5486, pp. 1942-1946

Brundtland, G.H. (2001) From the World Health Organization. Mental health: new understanding, new hope. *JAMA*, Vol. 286, No. 19, pp. 2391

Cagniard, B., Beeler, J.A., Britt, J.P., McGehee, D.S., Marinelli, M. and Zhuang, X. (2006) Dopamine scales performance in the absence of new learning. *Neuron*, Vol. 51, No. 5, pp. 541-547

Carboni, J.M., Wittman, M., Yang, Z., Lee, F., Greer, A., Hurlburt, W., Hillerman, S., Cao, C., Cantor, G.H., Dell-John, J., Chen, C., Discenza, L., Menard, K., Li, A., Trainor, G., Vyas, D., Kramer, R., Attar, R.M. and Gottardis, M.M. (2009) BMS-754807, a small molecule inhibitor of insulin-like growth factor-1R/IR. *Molecular Cancer Therapeutics*, Vol. 8, No. 12, pp. 3341-3349

Carpenter, W.T. and Koenig, J. (2008) The evolution of drug development in schizophrenia: past issues and future opportunities. *Neuropsychopharmacology*, Vol. 33, No. 9, pp. 2061-2079

Chien, E.Y.T., Liu, W., Zhao, Q., Katritch, V., Han, G.W., Hanson, M.A., Shi, L., Newman, A.H., Javitch, J.A., Cherezov, V. and Stevens, R.C. (2010) Structure of the human dopamine D3 receptor in complex with a D2/D3 selective antagonist. *Science*, Vol. 330, No. 6007, pp. 1091-1095

Conn, P.J. and Roth, B.L. (2008) Opportunities and Challenges of Psychiatric Drug Discovery: Roles for Scientists in Academic, Industry, and Government Settings. *Neuropsychopharmacology*, Vol. 33, No. 9, pp. 2048-2060

Copeland, R.A., Harpel, M.R. and Tummino, P.J. (2007) Targeting enzyme inhibitors in drug discovery. *Expert Opin Ther Targets*, Vol. 11, No. 7, pp. 967-978

Davidson, B.L. and McCray, P.B. (2011) Current prospects for RNA interference-based therapies. *Nature Publishing Group*, Vol. 12, No. 5, pp. 329-340

Di Chiara, G. and Imperato, A. (1988) Drugs abused by humans preferentially increase synaptic dopamine concentrations in the mesolimbic system of freely moving rats. *PNAS*, Vol. 85, No. 14, pp. 5274-5278

Duncan, G.E., Sheitman, B.B. and Lieberman, J.A. (1999) An integrated view of pathophysiological models of schizophrenia. *Brain Res. Brain Res. Rev.*, Vol. 29, No. 2-3, pp. 250-264

Engblom, D., Bilbao, A., Sanchis-Segura, C., Dahan, L., Perreau-Lenz, S., Balland, B., Parkitna, J.R., Luján, R., Halbout, B., Mameli, M., Parlato, R., Sprengel, R., Lüscher, C., Schütz, G. and Spanagel, R. (2008) Glutamate receptors on dopamine neurons control the persistence of cocaine seeking. *Neuron*, Vol. 59, No. 3, pp. 497-508

Fan, Q.-W., Zhang, C., Shokat, K.M. and Weiss, W.A. (2002) Chemical genetic blockade of transformation reveals dependence on aberrant oncogenic signaling. *Curr. Biol.*, Vol. 12, No. 16, pp. 1386-1394

Feil, R., Brocard, J., Mascrez, B., LeMeur, M., Metzger, D. and Chambon, P. (1996) Ligand-activated site-specific recombination in mice. *PNAS*, Vol. 93, No. 20, pp. 10887-10890

Flanigan, S.A., Pitts, T.M., Eckhardt, S.G., Tentler, J.J., Tan, A.C., Thorburn, A. and Leong, S. (2010) The Insulin-like Growth Factor I Receptor/Insulin Receptor Tyrosine Kinase Inhibitor PQIP Exhibits Enhanced Antitumor Effects in Combination with Chemotherapy Against Colorectal Cancer Models. *Clin. Cancer Res.*, Vol. 16, No. 22, pp. 5436-5446

Gaisler-Salomon, I., Miller, G.M., Chuhma, N., Lee, S., Zhang, H., Ghoddoussi, F., Lewandowski, N., Fairhurst, S., Wang, Y., Conjard-Duplany, A., Masson, J., Balsam, P., Hen, R., Arancio, O., Galloway, M.P., Moore, H.M., Small, S.A. and Rayport, S. (2009) Glutaminase-deficient mice display hippocampal hypoactivity, insensitivity to pro-psychotic drugs and potentiated latent inhibition: relevance to schizophrenia. *Neuropsychopharmacology*, Vol. 34, No. 10, pp. 2305-2322

García-Echeverría, C., Pearson, M.A., Marti, A., Meyer, T., Mestan, J., Zimmermann, J., Gao, J., Brueggen, J., Capraro, H.-G., Cozens, R., Evans, D.B., Fabbro, D., Furet, P., Porta, D.G., Liebetanz, J., Martiny-Baron, G., Ruetz, S. and Hofmann, F. (2004) In vivo antitumor activity of NVP-AEW541-A novel, potent, and selective inhibitor of the IGF-IR kinase. *Cancer Cell*, Vol. 5, No. 3, pp. 231-239

Gellman, C., Mingote, S., Wang, Y., Gaisler-Salomon, I. and Rayport, S. (2011) Genetic pharmacotherapy: A new approach to drug development for schizophrenia. *Advancing Drug Discovery for Schizophrenia, NY Academy of Sciences,* New York, NY, 03/18/11

Giguère, V. (2003) In Bradshaw, R. A. and Dennis, E. A. (eds.), *Handbook of Cell Signaling, Volume* 3. Academic Press, Amsterdam, Vol. 3, pp. 35-38.

Gingrich, J.A. and Hen, R. (2000) The broken mouse: the role of development, plasticity and environment in the interpretation of phenotypic changes in knockout mice. *Curr. Opin. Neurobiol.*, Vol. 10, No. 1, pp. 146-152

Gonzalez-Maeso, J. and Sealfon, S.C. (2009) Psychedelics and schizophrenia. *Trends Neurosci.*, Vol. 32, No. 4, pp. 225-232

Gossen, M. and Bujard, H. (1992) Tight control of gene expression in mammalian cells by tetracycline-responsive promoters. *PNAS*, Vol. 89, No. 12, pp. 5547-5551

Grace, A.A. and Bunney, B.S. (1986) Induction of depolarization block in midbrain dopamine neurons by repeated administration of haloperidol: analysis using in vivo intracellular recording. *J. Pharmacol. Exp. Ther.*, Vol. 238, No. 3, pp. 1092-1100

Gu, H., Marth, J.D., Orban, P.C., Mossmann, H. and Rajewsky, K. (1994) Deletion of a DNA polymerase beta gene segment in T cells using cell type-specific gene targeting. *Science*, Vol. 265, No. 5168, pp. 103-106

Guillin, O., Abi-Dargham, A. and Laruelle, M. (2007) Neurobiology of dopamine in schizophrenia. *Int. Rev. Neurobiol.*, Vol. 78, pp. 1-39

Hajduk, P.J., Huth, J.R. and Tse, C. (2005) Predicting protein druggability. *Drug Discovery Today*, Vol. 10, No. 23-24, pp. 1675-1682

Hardy, L.W. and Peet, N.P. (2004) The multiple orthogonal tools approach to define molecular causation in the validation of druggable targets. *Drug Discovery Today*, Vol. 9, No. 3, pp. 117-126

Hayashi, S. (2002) Efficient Recombination in Diverse Tissues by a Tamoxifen-Inducible Form of Cre: A Tool for Temporally Regulated Gene Activation/Inactivation in the Mouse. *Dev. Biol.*, Vol. 244, No. 2, pp. 305-318

He, Y., Zhang, J., Zheng, J., Du, W., Xiao, H., Liu, W., Li, X., Chen, X., Yang, L. and Huang, S. (2010) The insulin-like growth factor-1 receptor kinase inhibitor, NVP-ADW742, suppresses survival and resistance to chemotherapy in acute myeloid leukemia cells. *Oncol. Res.*, Vol. 19, No. 1, pp. 35-43

Hodgkin, J. (1998) Seven types of pleiotropy. *Int. J. Dev. Biol.*, Vol. 42, No. 3, pp. 501-505

Hollstein, M., Sidransky, D., Vogelstein, B. and Harris, C.C. (1991) p53 mutations in human cancers. *Science*, Vol. 253, No. 5015, pp. 49-53

Howes, O., Montgomery, A., Valli, I., Asselin, M., Murray, R., Grasby, P. and Mcguire, P. (2008) Striatal dopamine dysfunction predates the onset of schizophrenia and is linked to prodromal symptoms and neurocognitive function. *Schizophr. Res.*, Vol. 102, No. 1-3, pp. 30-30

Huffaker, S.J., Chen, J., Nicodemus, K.K., Sambataro, F., Yang, F., Mattay, V., Lipska, B.K., Hyde, T.M., Song, J., Rujescu, D., Giegling, I., Mayilyan, K., Proust, M.J., Soghoyan, A., Caforio, G., Callicott, J.H., Bertolino, A., Meyer-Lindenberg, A., Chang, J., Ji, Y., Egan, M.F., Goldberg, T.E., Kleinman, J.E., Lu, B. and Weinberger, D.R. (2009) A primate-specific, brain isoform of KCNH2 affects cortical physiology, cognition, neuronal repolarization and risk of schizophrenia. *Nat. Med.*, Vol. 15, No. 5, pp. 509-518

Indra, A.K., Warot, X., Brocard, J., Bornert, J.M., Xiao, J.H., Chambon, P. and Metzger, D. (1999) Temporally-controlled site-specific mutagenesis in the basal layer of the epidermis: comparison of the recombinase activity of the tamoxifen-inducible Cre-ER(T) and Cre-ER(T2) recombinases. *Nucleic Acids Res.*, Vol. 27, No. 22, pp. 4324-4327

Iwasa, T., Okamoto, I., Suzuki, M., Hatashita, E., Yamada, Y., Fukuoka, M., Ono, K. and Nakagawa, K. (2009) Inhibition of Insulin-Like Growth Factor 1 Receptor by CP-751,871 Radiosensitizes Non-Small Cell Lung Cancer Cells. *Clin. Cancer Res.*, Vol. 15, No. 16, pp. 5117-5125

Javitt, D.C. (2007) Glutamate and schizophrenia: Phencyclidine, n-methyl-d-aspartate receptors, and dopamine-glutamate interactions. *Int. Rev. Neurobiol.*, Vol. 78, pp. 69-108

Javitt, D.C. (2010) Glutamatergic theories of schizophrenia. *Isr. J. Psychiatry Relat. Sci.*, Vol. 47, No. 1, pp. 4-16

Keiser, M.J., Setola, V., Irwin, J.J., Laggner, C., Abbas, A.I., Hufeisen, S.J., Jensen, N.H., Kuijer, M.B., Matos, R.C., Tran, T.B., Whaley, R., Glennon, R.A., Hert, J., Thomas, K.L.H., Edwards, D.D., Shoichet, B.K. and Roth, B.L. (2009) Predicting new molecular targets for known drugs. *Nature*, Vol. 462, No. 7270, pp. 175-181

Kellendonk, C., Simpson, E.H., Polan, H.J., Malleret, G., Vronskaya, S., Winiger, V., Moore, H. and Kandel, E.R. (2006) Transient and selective overexpression of dopamine D2 receptors in the striatum causes persistent abnormalities in prefrontal cortex functioning. *Neuron*, Vol. 49, No. 4, pp. 603-615

Kellendonk, C., Tronche, F., Casanova, E., Anlag, K., Opherk, C. and Schutz, G. (1999) Inducible site-specific recombination in the brain. *J. Mol. Biol.*, Vol. 285, No. 1, pp. 175-182

Kistner, A., Gossen, M., Zimmermann, F., Jerecic, J., Ullmer, C., Lübbert, H. and Bujard, H. (1996) Doxycycline-mediated quantitative and tissue-specific control of gene expression in transgenic mice. *PNAS*, Vol. 93, No. 20, pp. 10933-10938

Knox, C., Law, V., Jewison, T., Liu, P., Ly, S., Frolkis, A., Pon, A., Banco, K., Mak, C., Neveu, V., Djoumbou, Y., Eisner, R., Guo, A.C. and Wishart, D.S. (2011) DrugBank 3.0: a comprehensive resource for 'omics' research on drugs. *Nucleic Acids Res*, Vol. 39, Database issue, pp. D1035-1041

Kurio, N., Shimo, T., Fukazawa, T., Takaoka, M., Okui, T., Hassan, N.M.M., Honami, T., Hatakeyama, S., Ikeda, M., Naomoto, Y. and Sasaki, A. (2011) Anti-tumor effect in human breast cancer by TAE226, a dual inhibitor for FAK and IGF-IR in vitro and in vivo. *Exp. Cell Res.*, Vol. 317, No. 8, pp. 1134-1146

Kvamme, E., Torgner, I.A. and Roberg, B.A. (2001) Kinetics and localization of brain phosphate activated glutaminase. *J. Neurosci. Res.*, Vol. 66, No. 5, pp. 951-958

Lã Ber, S., Hübner, H., Tschammer, N. and Gmeiner, P. (2011) Recent advances in the search for D3- and D4-selective drugs: probes, models and candidates. *Trends Pharmacol. Sci.*, Vol. 32, No. 3, pp. 148-157

Lakso, M., Sauer, B., Mosinger, B., Jr., Lee, E.J., Manning, R.W., Yu, S.H., Mulder, K.L. and Westphal, H. (1992) Targeted oncogene activation by site-specific recombination in transgenic mice. *PNAS*, Vol. 89, No. 14, pp. 6232-6236

Lewandoski, M. (2001) Conditional control of gene expression in the mouse. *Nature Rev Genet*, Vol. 2, No. 10, pp. 743-755

Li, Q.-X., Tan, P., Ke, N. and Wong-Staal, F. (2007) Ribozyme technology for cancer gene target identification and validation. *Adv. Cancer Res.*, Vol. 96, pp. 103-143

Lieberman, J.A., Stroup, T.S., McEvoy, J.P., Swartz, M.S., Rosenheck, R.A., Perkins, D.O., Keefe, R.S., Davis, S.M., Davis, C.E., Lebowitz, B.D., Severe, J. and Hsiao, J.K. (2005) Effectiveness of antipsychotic drugs in patients with chronic schizophrenia. *N. Engl. J. Med.*, Vol. 353, No. 12, pp. 1209-1223

Lisman, J.E., Pi, H.J., Zhang, Y. and Otmakhova, N.A. (2010) A thalamo-hippocampal-ventral tegmental area loop may produce the positive feedback that underlies the psychotic break in schizophrenia. *Biol. Psychiatry*, Vol. 68, No. 1, pp. 17-24

Lodge, D.J. and Grace, A.A. (2009) Gestational methylazoxymethanol acetate administration: a developmental disruption model of schizophrenia. *Behav. Brain Res.*, Vol. 204, No. 2, pp. 306-312

Lodge, D.J. and Grace, A.A. (2011) Hippocampal dysregulation of dopamine system function and the pathophysiology of schizophrenia. *Trends Pharmacol. Sci.*, Vol. 32, No. 9, pp. 507-513

Mailman. (2007) GPCR functional selectivity has therapeutic impact. *Trends Pharmacol. Sci.*, Vol. 28, No. 8, pp. 390-396

Mailman, R.B. and Murthy, V. (2010) Ligand functional selectivity advances our understanding of drug mechanisms and drug discovery. *Neuropsychopharmacology*, Vol. 35, No. 1, pp. 345-346

Mamo, D., Kapur, S., Keshavan, M., Laruelle, M., Taylor, C.C., Kothare, P.A., Barsoum, P. and McDonnell, D. (2007) D2 Receptor Occupancy of Olanzapine Pamoate Depot Using Positron Emission Tomography: An Open-label Study in Patients with Schizophrenia. *Neuropsychopharmacology*, Vol. 33, No. 2, pp. 298-304

Mayford, M., Bach, M.E., Huang, Y.Y., Wang, L., Hawkins, R.D. and Kandel, E.R. (1996) Control of memory formation through regulated expression of a CaMKII transgene. *Science*, Vol. 274, No. 5293, pp. 1678-1683

Metzger, D. and Chambon, P. (2001) Site- and time-specific gene targeting in the mouse. *Methods*, Vol. 24, No. 1, pp. 71-80

Metzger, D., Clifford, J., Chiba, H. and Chambon, P. (1995) Conditional site-specific recombination in mammalian cells using a ligand-dependent chimeric Cre recombinase. *PNAS*, Vol. 92, No. 15, pp. 6991-6995

Miller, G. (2002), *Science*, Vol. 297, pp. 1116-1118.
Miller, G. (2010), *Science*, Vol. 329, pp. 502-504.
Min, Y., Adachi, Y., Yamamoto, H., Ito, H., Itoh, F., Lee, C.-T., Nadaf, S., Carbone, D.P. and Imai, K. (2003) Genetic blockade of the insulin-like growth factor-I receptor: a promising strategy for human pancreatic cancer. *Cancer Res.*, Vol. 63, No. 19, pp. 6432-6441
Moghaddam, B. (2003) Bringing order to the glutamate chaos in schizophrenia. *Neuron*, Vol. 40, No. 5, pp. 881-884
Moghaddam, B. and Adams, B.W. (1998) Reversal of phencyclidine effects by a group II metabotropic glutamate receptor agonist in rats. *Science*, Vol. 281, No. 5381, pp. 1349-1352
Nagy, A. (2000) Cre recombinase: the universal reagent for genome tailoring. *Genesis*, Vol. 26, No. 2, pp. 99-109
Nestler, E.J. and Hyman, S.E. (2010) Animal models of neuropsychiatric disorders. *Nat. Neurosci.*, Vol. 13, No. 10, pp. 1161-1169
O'Tuathaigh, C., Kirby, B., Moran, P. and Waddington, J. (2010) Mutant Mouse Models: Genotype-Phenotype Relationships to Negative Symptoms in Schizophrenia. *Schizophr. Bull.*, Vol. 36, No. 2, pp. 271-288
Okabe, M., Ikawa, M., Kominami, K., Nakanishi, T. and Nishimune, Y. (1997) 'Green mice' as a source of ubiquitous green cells. *FEBS Lett.*, Vol. 407, No. 3, pp. 313-319
Orban, P.C., Chui, D. and Marth, J.D. (1992) Tissue- and site-specific DNA recombination in transgenic mice. *PNAS*, Vol. 89, No. 15, pp. 6861-6865
Pao, W. (2005) Epidermal Growth Factor Receptor Mutations, Small-Molecule Kinase Inhibitors, and Non-Small-Cell Lung Cancer: Current Knowledge and Future Directions. *J. Clin. Oncol.*, Vol. 23, No. 11, pp. 2556-2568
Parascandola, J. (1981) *The theoretical basis of Paul Ehrlich' chemotherapy.*
Patil, S.T., Zhang, L., Martenyi, F., Lowe, S.L., Jackson, K.A., Andreev, B.V., Avedisova, A.S., Bardenstein, L.M., Gurovich, I.Y., Morozova, M.A., Mosolov, S.N., Neznanov, N.G., Reznik, A.M., Smulevich, A.B., Tochilov, V.A., Johnson, B.G., Monn, J.A. and Schoepp, D.D. (2007) Activation of mGlu2/3 receptors as a new approach to treat schizophrenia: a randomized Phase 2 clinical trial. *Nat. Med.*, Vol. 13, No. 9, pp. 1102-1107
Peterson, R.T. (2008) Chemical biology and the limits of reductionism. *Nat. Chem. Biol.*, Vol. 4, No. 11, pp. 635-638
Pletnikov, M.V. (2009) Inducible and conditional transgenic mouse models of schizophrenia. *Prog. Brain Res.*, Vol. 179, pp. 35-47
Prager, D., Li, H.L., Asa, S. and Melmed, S. (1994) Dominant negative inhibition of tumorigenesis in vivo by human insulin-like growth factor I receptor mutant. *PNAS*, Vol. 91, No. 6, pp. 2181-2185
Rosenbaum, J.S., Holford, N.H. and Sadée, W. (1984) Opiate receptor binding-effect relationship: sufentanil and etorphine produce analgesia at the mu-site with low fractional receptor occupancy. *Brain Res.*, Vol. 291, No. 2, pp. 317-324
Ross, E.M. and Kenakin, T.P. (2001) In Goodman, L. S., Hardman, J. G., Limbird, L. E. and Gilman, A. G. (eds.), *Goodman & Gilman's The Pharmacological Basis of Therapeutics.* 10th ed. McGraw-Hill Medical Pub. Division, New York, pp. 31-43.
Samtani, M.N., Perez-Ruixo, J.J., Brown, K.H., Cerneus, D. and Molloy, C.J. (2009) Pharmacokinetic and pharmacodynamic modeling of pegylated thrombopoietin mimetic peptide (PEG-TPOm) after single intravenous dose administration in healthy subjects. *J Clin Pharmacol*, Vol. 49, No. 3, pp. 336-350

Schobel, S.A., Lewandowski, N.M., Corcoran, C.M., Moore, H., Brown, T., Malaspina, D. and Small, S.A. (2009) Differential targeting of the CA1 subfield of the hippocampal formation by schizophrenia and related psychotic disorders. *Arch. Gen. Psychiatry*, Vol. 66, No. 9, pp. 938-946

Searls, D.B. (2003) Pharmacophylogenomics: genes, evolution and drug targets. *Nat Rev Drug Discov*, Vol. 2, No. 8, pp. 613-623

Sell, C., Rubini, M., Rubin, R., Liu, J.P., Efstratiadis, A. and Baserga, R. (1993) Simian virus 40 large tumor antigen is unable to transform mouse embryonic fibroblasts lacking type 1 insulin-like growth factor receptor. *PNAS*, Vol. 90, No. 23, pp. 11217-11221

Simpson, E.H., Kellendonk, C. and Kandel, E. (2010) A possible role for the striatum in the pathogenesis of the cognitive symptoms of schizophrenia. *Neuron*, Vol. 65, No. 5, pp. 585-596

Skarnes, W.C., Rosen, B., West, A.P., Koutsourakis, M., Bushell, W., Iyer, V., Mujica, A.O., Thomas, M., Harrow, J., Cox, T., Jackson, D., Severin, J., Biggs, P., Fu, J., Nefedov, M., de Jong, P.J., Stewart, A.F. and Bradley, A. (2011) A conditional knockout resource for the genome-wide study of mouse gene function. *Nature*, Vol. 474, No. 7351, pp. 337-342

Sokoloff, P., Giros, B., Martres, M.P., Bouthenet, M.L. and Schwartz, J.C. (1990) Molecular cloning and characterization of a novel dopamine receptor (D3) as a target for neuroleptics. *Nature*, Vol. 347, No. 6289, pp. 146-151

Soriano, P. (1999) Generalized lacZ expression with the ROSA26 Cre reporter strain. *Nat. Genet.*, Vol. 21, No. 1, pp. 70-71

Sternberg, N. and Hamilton, D. (1981) Bacteriophage P1 site-specific recombination. I. Recombination between loxP sites. *J. Mol. Biol.*, Vol. 150, No. 4, pp. 467-486

Thompson, C.H., Kahlig, K.M. and George, A.L. (2011) SCN1A splice variants exhibit divergent sensitivity to commonly used antiepileptic drugs. *Epilepsia*, Vol. 52, No. 5, pp. 1000-1009

Tseng, K.Y., Chambers, R.A. and Lipska, B.K. (2009) The neonatal ventral hippocampal lesion as a heuristic neurodevelopmental model of schizophrenia. *Behav. Brain Res.*, Vol. 204, No. 2, pp. 295-305

Tsien, J.Z., Chen, D.F., Gerber, D., Tom, C., Mercer, E.H., Anderson, D.J., Mayford, M., Kandel, E.R. and Tonegawa, S. (1996) Subregion- and cell type-restricted gene knockout in mouse brain. *Cell*, Vol. 87, No. 7, pp. 1317-1326

Vassilev, L.T. (2004) In vivo activation of the p53 pathway by small-molecule antagonists of MDM2. *Science*, Vol. 303, No. 5659, pp. 844-848

Ventura, A., Kirsch, D.G., McLaughlin, M.E., Tuveson, D.A., Grimm, J., Lintault, L., Newman, J., Reczek, E.E., Weissleder, R. and Jacks, T. (2007) Restoration of p53 function leads to tumour regression in vivo. *Nature*, Vol. 445, No. 7128, pp. 661-665

Weiner, I. and Arad, M. (2009) Using the pharmacology of latent inhibition to model domains of pathology in schizophrenia and their treatment. *Behav. Brain Res.*, Vol. 204, No. 2, pp. 369-386

Yamamoto, A., Lucas, J.J. and Hen, R. (2000) Reversal of neuropathology and motor dysfunction in a conditional model of Huntington's disease. *Cell*, Vol. 101, No. 1, pp. 57-66

Zhu, F., Han, B., Kumar, P., Liu, X., Ma, X., Wei, X., Huang, L., Guo, Y., Han, L., Zheng, C. and Chen, Y. (2010) Update of TTD: Therapeutic Target Database. *Nucleic Acids Res*, Vol. 38, No. Database issue, pp. D787-791

7

Critical Human Hepatocyte-Based *In Vitro* Assays for the Evaluation of Adverse Drug Effects

Albert P. Li
In Vitro ADMET Laboratories LLC and
Advanced Pharmaceutical Sciences Inc., Columbia, MD
USA

1. Introduction

A major challenge in drug development is to accurately estimate human adverse drug effects to allow the selection and advancement of drug candidates with the best safety profile for further development. Due to species differences, safety data obtained with the routine in vivo studies with nonhuman laboratory animals do not always correctly predict human outcome. Human liver-derived systems, especially human hepatocytes, represent physiologically-relevant experimental systems for the evaluation of human adverse drug effects. The assays developed with human-based in vitro experimental systems for the assessment of two major adverse drug effects: drug-drug interactions and drug toxicity can be used routinely during drug development to select and optimize drug candidates to enhance the probability of clinical success.

2. Current challenges in drug development

Efficacy and safety are two co-dependent requirements for successful drug development – clinical failure will result if the drug candidate possesses only one of these two properties. For the past 50 years, drug candidates are evaluated for pharmacological and safety properties using in vivo animal models. It is now known that this paradigm, namely, prediction of human drug properties with animals in vivo, is no longer valid. DiMassi et al (2003)[1] has estimated that for R&D initiated in 2001 with approval 12 years later (based on the average time required for approval), the out-of-pocket cost for a single approved drug is estimated to be U. S. $ 970 million, equivalent to a capitalized cost of U. S. $ 1.9 billion. Frequent clinical trial failure, with lack of efficacy and the occurrence of unexpected adverse drug effects as major reasons, accounts for astronomical time and costs involved in the development of a successful drug. The most recent published estimation of the clinical approval success rate for investigational drugs is 16% [2]. Furthermore, marketed drugs are frequently withdrawn or have their use limited due to adverse effects, with dire consequences to the welfare of the patients and the financial status of the drug manufacturers [3].

3. Overcoming species-species differences

True advancement in the efficiency of drug development can only be made if one accepts that, due to species differences, data from nonhuman laboratory animals do not always predict human drug properties. As in vivo experimentation with humans in vivo during preclinical phases is neither practical nor ethical, surrogates for humans in vivo need to be applied. Experimental models with human tissues and human cells represent practical and relevant surrogates.

A major breakthrough in the acceptance of the reliability of in vitro human-based system in the prediction of human drug properties is the advancement of human-based drug metabolism systems. Human liver fractions (e.g. human liver microsomes), human hepatocytes, and cDNA-derived human drug metabolizing enzymes have been found to provide useful information for the prediction of human metabolism in vivo. These systems are now used routinely for the evaluation of drug metabolism and drug-drug interaction potential of drug candidate in various phases of drug development [4, 5], with the approaches fully endorsed by U. S. FDA [6]. It is interesting to note that the application of in vitro drug metabolism technologies using human-based experimental systems has been attributed to the removal of pharmacokinetics as a major reason for clinical trial failure.

The success in the application of in vitro drug metabolism systems, in combination with data from relevant in vivo animal models, in the prediction of human metabolism suggest that the same approach will also be successful for safety evaluation [7, 8]. Based on the premise that the inability to accurately predict human drug toxicity is due to species-species differences, i. e., there are human-specific drug properties that cannot be revealed by nonhuman animal studies, a safety evaluation strategy is proposed here for the preclinical evaluation of human drug toxicity:

1. Application of **human**-based in vitro systems to provide human-specific toxicity data;
2. Select a relevant animal species to develop **in vivo** parameters;
3. Predict **human in vivo** drug toxicity via a combination of human-specific information obtained in vitro, and in vivo parameters obtained from nonhuman animals in vivo.

Success of this In Vitro-In Vivo Strategy (IVIVS) requires the development of in vitro experimental systems with human-specific properties to cover the key adverse drug effects in humans, and a vigorous set of parameters defining the relevant nonhuman animal species.

4. Human hepatocytes as a key in vitro experimental system for the evaluation of human-specific drug properties

The liver is a key determinant of drug properties. It is a major organ for drug metabolism, and is often a target for drug toxicity [9,10]. Hepatocytes or liver parenchymal cells are the cells in the liver responsible for drug metabolism and are the target cells for hepatotoxic drugs. Isolated hepatocytes therefore represent the most physiologically-relevant experimental system for the evaluation of hepatic drug metabolism and hepatotoxicity [11-13] for the following reasons:

1. Human xenobiotic metabolism: Fresh isolates or cryopreserved fresh isolates of human hepatocytes are known to contain most, if not all, of the in vivo hepatic xenobiotic metabolism capacity [12].

2. Human target cells: The hepatocytes are the cells in the human liver that are damaged by hepatotoxicants, leading ultimately to liver failure [14,15].
3. Endpoints: Myriad of toxicological endpoints allowing measurements of necrosis, apoptosis, nuclear receptor interactions, P450 functions, transporter functions etc. have been developed in hepatocytes for the evaluation of adverse drug properties[15,16].

In the past, the use of human hepatocytes has been severely limited by their availability. This limitation has been overcome in the past decade due to advances in the procurement of human livers for research, and the commercial availability of isolated human hepatocytes. The application of human hepatocytes in drug metabolism studies is greatly aided by the successful cryopreservation of human hepatocytes to retain drug metabolism activities [12, 13, 17]. Recently, the usefulness of cryopreserved human hepatocytes is further extended through the development of technologies to cryopreserve human hepatocytes to retain their ability to be cultured as attached cultures (plateable cryopreserved hepatocytes) which can be used for longer term studies such as enzyme induction studies [12].

Cryopreserved human hepatocytes have several advantages over the use of freshly isolated cells:

1. Experimentation can be readily scheduled;
2. There are little or no deleterious effects of cryopreservation on key hepatocyte properties;
3. Repeat of experimentation can be performed at different times or by different laboratories with cells from the same donor;
4. The hepatocytes can be pre-characterized for properties relevant to a specific study before they are used for experimentation;
5. Hepatocytes from multiple donor can be used in the same study.

5. Critical assays for the evaluation of adverse drug effects

Two adverse drug effects are responsible for clinical failures and drug withdrawal: drug-drug interactions and drug toxicity. Below are the critical assays for these adverse drug effects. In this chapter, the overall scientific concepts behind these assays and the general approaches used in the assays are described.

6. Critical assays for drug-drug interactions

Metabolic drug-drug interaction results from the alteration of the metabolic clearance of one drug by a co-administered drug. There are two major pathways of metabolic drug-drug interactions:

Inhibitory drug-drug interaction: When one drug inhibits the drug metabolism enzyme responsible for the metabolism of a co-administered drug, the result is a decreased metabolic clearance of the affected drug, resulting in a higher than desired systemic burden. For drugs with a narrow therapeutic index, this may lead to serious toxicological concerns. Most fatal drug-drug interactions are due to inhibitory drug-drug interactions.

Inductive drug-drug interactions: Drug-drug interactions can also be a result of the acceleration of the metabolism of a drug by a co-administered drug. Acceleration of metabolism is usually due to the induction of the gene expression, leading to higher rates of protein synthesis and therefore higher cellular content of the induced drug-metabolizing enzyme and a higher rate of metabolism of the substrates of the induced enzyme. Inductive drug-drug interactions can lead to a higher metabolic clearance of the affected drug, leading to a decrease in plasma concentration and loss of efficacy. Inductive drug-drug interactions can also lead to a higher systemic burden of metabolites, which, if toxic, may lead to safety concerns.

Due to the realization that it is physically impossible to evaluate empirically the possible interaction between one drug and all marketed drugs, and that most drug-metabolizing enzyme pathways are well-defined, a mechanism-based approach is used for the evaluation of drug-drug interaction potential of a new drug or drug candidate [18-20], This mechanistic-based approach is endorsed and required by the U. S. FDA (www.fda.Gov/cber /gdlns/interactstud.htm) for new drug applications. The approach consists of the following major studies:

1. Metabolic phenotyping: The major enzymes involved in the biotransformation of the drug candidate are identified. The major emphasis in the past has been on phase 1 oxidation pathways and on P450 isoforms. Elucidation of enzyme pathways involved in the biotransformation of a drug candidate will allow the identification of potential drug-drug interactions with drugs that are known modifiers (inhibitors and inducers) of the pathways.
   a. Metabolite identification: Structural identification of the metabolites allow one to deduce the major pathways of metabolism. Identification of
      i. Experimental systems: Human liver homogenate 9000 x g supernatant (S9); human liver microsomes (HLM); hepatocytes
      ii. General incubation conditions:
      1. S9 or HLM: 0.25 to 1.0 mg protein/mL in 0.1 M phosphate buffer at pH 7.4 containing NADPH or NADPH regenerating system (phase 1 oxidation); uridine 5'-diphospho-glucuronic acid (UDPGA; cofactor for glucuronidation) and 3'-phosphoadenosine 5'- phosphosulfate (PAPS; cofactor for sulfation).
      2. Hepatocytes: 0.5 to 1.0 million cells/mL in Isotonic buffer (e.g. Krebs-Hensleit Buffer) maintained at pH 7.2.
      3. Temperature: 37 deg. C
      4. Compound concentration: Generally 10 uM
      5. Time: Multiple time points up to 30 minutes (HLM); 2 hrs (hepatocytes in suspension); 24 hrs. (hepatocytes in monolayer culture)
      iii. Metabolite identification: HPLC-MS/MS is the most commonly used approach for the initial identification of the metabolites. NMR is used for definitive structural identification.
   b. Major pathway identification: Chemical inhibitors are used to identify of the major oxidative pathways involved in the formation of the metabolites. Inhibition of metabolism of the parent compound, as indicated by metabolic stability or decreased formation of metabolites, would suggest that the participation of the pathway in the metabolism of the compound. Examples of inhibitors for the major pathways are as follows:
      i. P450 inhibition: 1-aminobenzotriazole (S9; HLM; hepatocytes)
      ii. MAO inhibitors: pargyline (S9)
      iii. FMO inhibitiors: 45 deg. C inactivation (S9; HLM).
   c. P450 isoform identification:

i. Experimental system: HLM or cDNA-P450 isoforms
ii. Incubation with HLM in the presence of isoform-selective inhibitors or individual cDNA-P450 isoforms to determine pathway responsible for metabolism. Inhibition of metabolism by an inhibitor of a specific isoform (Table 1) with corroborative data using the identified cDNA-P450 isoform would allow the identification of the isoform for the metabolism of the compound in question.

d. Evaluation of inhibitory potential for drug-metabolizing enzymes: The drug candidate will be evaluated for its ability to inhibit known drug metabolizing enzymes, with emphasis on the P450 isoforms. The incubation conditions are similar to that described above for metabolite identification, using substrates that are selective for the pathways in question (Table 1).
e. Evaluation of induction potential for drug metabolizing enzymes: The drug candidate will be evaluated for its ability to induce known drug metabolizing enzymes. The inducible P450 isoforms: CYP1A, 2B and 3A are the ones required by U. S. FDA. Human hepatocytes are considered the "gold standard" for induction studies, with cryopreserved hepatocytes that can be cultured after thawing and have been characterized to be responsive to prototypical inducers as the preferred system. As of this writing, virtually all known inducers of P450 isoforms in vivo are inducers in human hepatocytes in vitro (Table 1) [12]. Experimental evaluation of enzyme induction involves the treatment of human hepatocytes for several days with the test article followed by evaluation of enzyme activities using P450 isoform-specific substrates [20].

The general experimental conditions are as follows:

i. Experimental system: Primary cultured human hepatocytes
ii. Culturing condition: Matrigel-collagen sandwich (requirement: >80% confluent cultures).
iii. Treatment regiment: Culturing of hepatocytes for 2 days followed by 3 days of treatment
iv. Endpoints: Quantification of CYP1A2, 2B6 and 3A4 gene expression by RT-PCR as well as activities using isoform-specific substrates (Table 1).

7. Higher throughput human hepatocyte-based drug-drug interaction studies

Of the multiple P450 isoforms, CYP3A4 is the most abundant of the isoforms in the human liver. CYP3A4 has been found to be responsible for the metabolism of a large variety of exogenous and endogenous substrates [21, 22]. In drug development, there is a need to evaluate the inhibitory and inductive potential of drug candidates towards CYP3A4 to estimate their drug-drug interaction potential with the myriad drugs that are substrates of this important P450 isoform [23-25]. In our laboratory, we have developed cost- and time-effective higher throughput screening assays for the evaluation of drug-drug interaction potential of drug candidates involving CYP3A4. The assays are as follows:

1. 384-well CYP3A4 inhibition assay [26];
2. 96-well time-dependent CYP3A4 inhibition assay [27];
3. 96-well CYP3A4 induction assay [26].

The throughput of the assays are increased via the use of the following technologies:

a white 96-well plate. After all the solutions are collected from the various time points, 50 uL of Luciferin Detection Reagent is added to each well containing incubated substrate solution followed by quantification of luminescence using a Wallac Victor-3 plate reader. Luminescence signals are converted to pmoles of luciferin based on a standard curve generated from luciferin. Viability of the hepatocytes after treatment is determined after CYP3A4 activity quantification using cellular ATP as an endpoint using a commercially available ATP kit consisting of lysis buffer and ATP detection reagent.

Results are expressed as % remaining activity, which is calculated as a ratio of the activity in the presence of inhibitors to that of the solvent control using the following equation:

% Remaining Activity (%) = [Normalized Activity (Treatment)/Normalized Activity (Solvent Control)] x 100;

whereas activity represents luciferin generated in each well quantified by luminescence normalized by relative activity based on ATP content using the following equations:

Normalized Activity = CYP3A4 Activity/Relative Viability

Relative Viability (%) = ATP Content (Treatment)/ATP Content (Solvent Control)

Enzyme kinetic parameters for TDI are derived as follows: The observed rate of enzyme inactivation (k_{obs}) is determined as the initial slope of the linear regression line of a semi-logarithmic plot of the natural logarithm of remaining activity versus preincubation time. k_{inact} and K_I values are determined based on the double reciprocal Lineweaver-Burk plot (1/k_{obs} versus 1/[I], whereas [I] represents inhibitor concentration), where k_{inact} is estimated as the reciprocal of the Y-intercept and K_I as the negative reciprocal of the x-intercept.

Representative results of the application of this HTS assay to evaluate time-dependent CYP3A4 inhibitory potential of drug substances, using the model time-dependent CYP3A4 inhibitor, 1-aminobenzotriazole, are shown in Fig. 1.

10. 96-well CYP3A4 induction assay with human hepatocytes

Enzyme induction is a major mechanism for drug-drug interactions. Induction of a drug metabolizing enzyme by one drug would lead to the enhanced metabolism of co-administered drugs that are substrates of the induced enzyme.

As freshly isolated hepatocytes possess endogenous activities which may be the result of inducers present in the donor's systemic circulation, the isolated hepatocytes are cultured for 2 to 3 days to allow the P450 enzyme activities to return to a basal level. Testing for induction potential is that initiated by treatment of the cultured hepatocytes for 2 to 3 days to allow full expression of the induced enzyme. Induction is generally evaluated by measuring enzyme activity as activity represents the most relevant endpoint for drug-drug interaction. Both freshly isolated and plateable cryopreserved human hepatocytes can be used for the induction study.

In our laboratory, we have developed a higher-throughput P450 induction assay using 96 well plates[26]. The procedures are as follows:

1. Day 0: Plate human hepatocytes (freshly isolated or plateable cryopreserved human hepatocytes) with 50 uL of cell suspension per well, at a cell density of 1 million cells/mL thereby delivering 50,000 cells per well.

2. Day 1: Change medium to cold (4 to 10 deg. C) medium containing 0.25 mg/mL of Matrigel®.
3. Day 2: Change medium to treatment medium containing test articles at the desired concentrations.
4. Day 3, 4, 5: Continue treatment. Medium change is not necessary unless the test article is known to be unstable under the culturing conditions.
5. Day 6: Measure activity (in situ incubation with LIPA) or extraction of RNA for the evaluation of gene expression.

Representative results of the application of this HTS assay to evaluate CYP3A4 induction potential of drug substances, using model CYP3A4 inducers, are shown in Fig. 1.

11. In vitro evaluation of drug toxicity

The current success in the application of human-based in vitro experimental models in the evaluation of drug metabolism and drug-drug interactions paths the way for a similar approach to evaluate drug toxicity, especially human-specific toxic events that cannot be observed in laboratory animals. In vitro toxicity assays are can be applied in various during phases of drug development:

1. **Early screening of intrinsic toxicity:** Cell-based systems are used for rapid screening of drug candidates, especially structural analogs, to allow the selection of less toxic structures for further development. The screening assay can allow logical evaluation of structures responsible for toxicity (toxicophore) which, hopefully, can be separated from structures for pharmacological activity (pharmacophore). Toxicity screening with in vitro systems require only limited amount of test articles, and is rapid and quantitative. Toxicity is most effective when one has an indication for in vivo toxicity (e.g. hepatotoxicity or nephrotoxicity) for a lead molecule, therefore allowing the selection of the most appropriate in vitro system for screening (e.g. hepatocytes for hepatotoxicity and renal proximal tubule cells for nephrotoxicity).
2. **Mechanistic evaluations:** Mechanistic understanding is critical to drug development. It allows a better understanding of human health risks, defines potential risk factors, and evaluates the relationship between efficacy and adverse effects. Mechanistic studies may be performed after adverse effects are observed in nonhuman animals to aid the prediction of human toxicity as well as the development of approaches for a more acceptable replacement. The defined experimental conditions and the availability of reagents and approaches for multiple endpoints of in vitro experimental systems allow one to define the key pathways involved in a toxicology phenomenon.

The preferred human in vitro systems for the evaluation of drug toxicity are primary cells derived from human organs, used within a period that the cells would retain differentiated functions, thereby serving as surrogates of the similar cells in vivo.

Primary cell culture systems, including stem-cell derived differentiated cells representative of the key cell types in each organ, are currently available and the respective organ-specific toxicity:

- Hepatocytes (hepatotoxicity)
- Renal proximal tubule epithelial cells (nephrotoxicity)
- Vascular endothelial cells (vascular toxicity)
- Neuronal cells, glial cells and astrocytes (neurotoxicity)

- Cardiomyocytes (cardiotoxicity)
- Bone marrow cells (bone marrow toxicity)

12. Overcoming the major deficiencies of in vitro system

An argument routinely raised against the application of in vitro systems in safety evaluation is that toxicity is a complex phenomenon and therefore cannot be adequately modeled by simple in vitro systems such as cell culture assays.

The major deficiencies of in vitro experimental systems can be defined as follows:

1. **Lack of systemic effects.** In vitro experimental systems in general consist of single cell types. Toxic effects are evaluated in the absence of influences from systemic effects that may be critical to drug toxicity. An example is the participation of the immune system in organ toxicity. One hypothesis for idiosyncratic hepatotoxicity, for instance, is the hapten-hypothesis which postulates that liver failure arises from the cytotoxicity of antibodies towards antigens developed between the idiosyncratic drug (or its metabolites) on the plasma membrane of the hepatocytes.
2. **Absence of chronic dosing.** It is generally believe that drug toxicity due to acute cytotoxic events can be studied effectively with in vitro systems. However, toxic effects due to chronic, low-dose treatments may require multiple events that may or may not be obtained with in vitro studies, with cells treated for a relatively short time period (e.g. 24-hours). Long-term treatments (e.g. months to years) of cells in culture is theoretically possible but in practice near impossible. Further, it is extremely difficult to maintain primary cells, the preferred cell system, in a differentiated state for a long time period.

For in vitro systems to be useful, one needs to develop experimental approaches to overcome these deficiencies.

13. In vitro experimental model for multiple organ interactions: Integrated discrete multiple organ co-culture (IdMOC)

One major drawback of in vitro system is that each cell type is studied in isolation. In the human body, multiple organ interactions may be critical to drug toxicity. An example of multiple organ interactions is a drug which is firstly metabolized by one organ (e.g. liver) to form metabolites which may enter the general systemic circulation to cause toxicity in a distant organ (e.g. heart).

The multiple organ interaction is not covered by the TACIT approach[8] using a single cell type, as the initiating events may include effects of a toxicant on a nontarget cell. To overcome this deficiency, we have developed the IdMOC (Independent Discrete Multiple Organ Co-culture) system ([42-44]). The IdMOC allows the co-culturing of cells from different organs as physically separated cultures that are interconnected by an overlying medium, akin to the blood circulation connecting the multiple organs in the human body (Fig. 1). The IdMOC models the multiple organ interaction in the whole organism in vivo, allowing the evaluation of organ-specific effects a drug and its metabolites. The IdMOC represents an improved in vitro experimental system for routine screening of ADMET drug properties.

The IdMOC involves the "wells-in-a-well" concept. The typical IdMOC plate consists of a chamber within which are several wells (Fig. 2). Cells of different origins (e.g. from different organs) are initially cultured, each in its specific medium, in the wells. When the cells are established, the wells are flooded with an overlying medium, thereby connecting all the wells. The multiple cell types now can interact via the overlying medium, akin to the multiple organs in a human body interacting via the systemic circulation.

The IdMOC system can be used for the following:

1. Differential cytotoxicity: Evaluation of the toxicity of a substance on different cell types (e.g. cells from different organs) under virtually identical experimental conditions with multiple cell-type interactions. Aflatoxin B1, a know hepatotoxicant in humans in vivo, is shown to have selectively higher cytotoxicity in hepatocytes in the IdMOC co-culture of hepatocytes, renal proximal tubule cells, and small airway epithelial cells.
2. Differential distribution: Evaluation of the differential accumulation/distribution of a substance among multiple cell types. This application is especially useful for the development of cytotoxic anticancer agent with selective affinity towards cancer cells.
3. Multiple organ metabolism: Evaluate the ultimate metabolic fate of a substance upon metabolism by cells representing multiple organs with metabolic functions (e.g. liver, kidney, lung). This application allows the development of metabolite profiling of drugs which are subjected to both hepatic and extrahepatic metabolism.

Evaluate of organ-specific toxicity is illustrated by the treatment of IdMOC with a known hepatotoxicant, aflatoxin B1, in IdMOC with three human primary cell types: hepatocytes, renal proximal tubule epithelial cells, and pulmonary (small airway) epithelial cells. Aflatoxin B1 was found to be significantly more cytotoxic towards human hepatocytes, presumably due to the higher P450 activities of the cells versus the other two cell types (Fig. 3), as it is known that aflatoxin requires P450 metabolism to toxic metabolites to exert its toxicity.

14. Conclusion

Accurate prediction of human adverse drug effects represents a major challenge for drug development. The high rate of clinical failure of drug candidates that have been carefully selected from preclinical studies illustrates clearly that the routine, "classical" approach of preclinical safety evaluation is inadequate. It is argued here that species-species differences in drug toxicity is a major reason - human-specific toxicity, by definition, cannot be predicted with nonhuman laboratory animals. It is proposed here that human in vivo drug toxicity can be predicted using a combination of human-based in vitro experimental systems and appropriate in vivo laboratory animals - the In Vitro-In Vivo Strategy (IVIVS). The success of IVIVS will depend on the selection of appropriate in vitro models. Human-specific drug metabolism, appropriate target cell populations, and relevant endpoints are three key parameters for the selection of an appropriate in vitro model. Human hepatocytes and human liver fractions represent useful appropriate experimental models to evaluate liver specific events such as hepatic metabolism, drug-drug interactions, and hepatotoxicity. Higher throughput screening assays have been developed to allow early screening of human-specific adverse drug effects. IdMOC allows the co-culturing of multiple cell types modeling in vivo multiple organ interactions and thereby represent a more complete in vitro experimental system for the prediction of in vivo drug properties.

It is to be noted that recent research findings have demonstrated that in addition to drug metabolizing enzyme activities, uptake and efflux transporters also play critical roles in the manifestation of adverse drug effects [10, 45]. Human hepatocyte assays for the evaluation of uptake and efflux transporters have been established and are being applied towards drug development [46-50]. These transporter assays, when applied in conjunction with the assays described in this chapter, should aid the selection of the most appropriate drug candidates for further drug development.

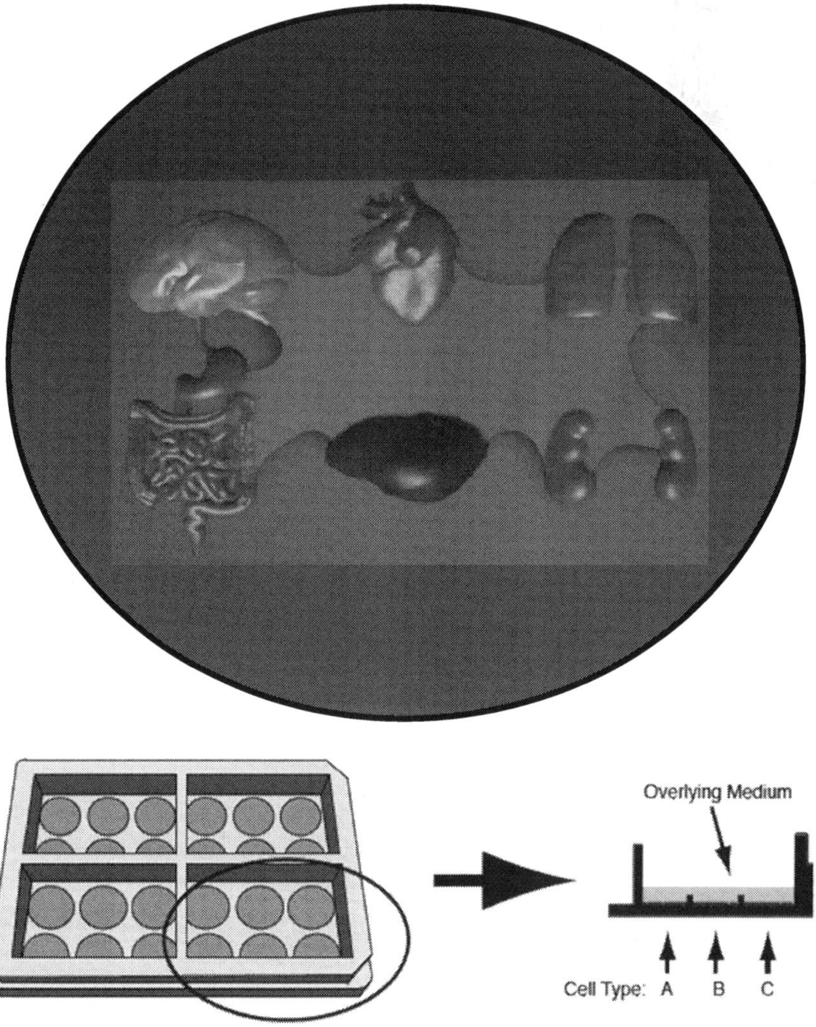

Fig. 2. The Integrated Discrete Multiple Organ Co-culture (IdMOC) experiment system is based on the concept that in the human body consists of multiple organs interacting via the systemic circulation (Top figure). A toxicant may be metabolized by one or more of the organs, and the resulting metabolites may interact with one or more organs via the systemic circulation. This concept is reduced to practice as an IdMOC plate (Lower Figure), with multiple wells within a chamber. Cells from individual organs are cultured physically separated in the wells, with the cells of the multiple organs interconnected via an overlying medium. From Li [43]

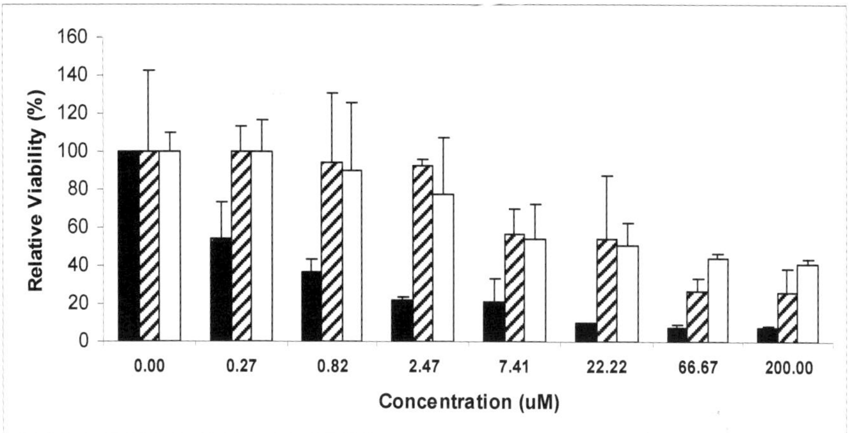

Fig. 3. Application of the Integrated Discrete Multiple Organ Co-culture (IdMOC) experiment system in the evaluation of organ specific toxicity. IdMOC with co-cultures of human hepatocytes (solid bars), renal proximal tubule cells (shaded bars), and small airway epithelial cells (open bars) was used to evaluate the cytotoxicity of the known hepatotoxic agent, aflatoxin B1. While dose-dependent cytotoxicity was observed for all cell types, aflatoxin B1 was significantly more cytotoxic towards human hepatocytes. The results illustrate the application of IdMOC in the evaluation of organ-selective toxicity of drug substances. Other applications of IdMOC include organ-selective drug distribution and integrated multiple organ metabolism.

15. References

[1] DiMasi JA, Hansen RW, Grabowski HG: The price of innovation: new estimates of drug development costs, J Health Econ 2003, 22:151-185

[2] DiMasi JA, Feldman L, Seckler A, Wilson A: Trends in risks associated with new drug development: success rates for investigational drugs, Clin Pharmacol Ther 2010, 87:272-277

[3] Wysowski DK, Swartz L: Adverse drug event surveillance and drug withdrawals in the United States, 1969-2002: the importance of reporting suspected reactions, Arch Intern Med 2005, 165:1363-1369

[4] Li AP, Jurima-Romet M: Overview: pharmacokinetic drug-drug interactions, Adv Pharmacol 1997, 43:1-6

[5] Davit B, Reynolds K, Yuan R, Ajayi F, Conner D, Fadiran E, Gillespie B, Sahajwalla C, Huang SM, Lesko LJ: FDA evaluations using in vitro metabolism to predict and interpret in vivo metabolic drug-drug interactions: impact on labeling, J Clin Pharmacol 1999, 39:899-910

[6] Zhang L, Zhang YD, Zhao P, Huang SM: Predicting drug-drug interactions: an FDA perspective, AAPS J 2009, 11:300-306

[7] MacGregor JT, Collins JM, Sugiyama Y, Tyson CA, Dean J, Smith L, Andersen M, Curren RD, Houston JB, Kadlubar FF, Kedderis GL, Krishnan K, Li AP, Parchment RE,

Thummel K, Tomaszewski JE, Ulrich R, Vickers AE, Wrighton SA: In vitro human tissue models in risk assessment: report of a consensus-building workshop, Toxicol Sci 2001, 59:17-36

[8] Li AP: Human-based in vitro experimental systems for the evaluation of human drug safety, Curr Drug Saf 2007, 2:193-199

[9] Ikeda T: Drug-induced idiosyncratic hepatotoxicity: prevention strategy developed after the troglitazone case, Drug Metab Pharmacokinet 2011, 26:60-70

[10] Assis DN, Navarro VJ: Human drug hepatotoxicity: a contemporary clinical perspective, Expert Opin Drug Metab Toxicol 2009, 5:463-473

[11] Hewitt NJ, Lechon MJ, Houston JB, Hallifax D, Brown HS, Maurel P, Kenna JG, Gustavsson L, Lohmann C, Skonberg C, Guillouzo A, Tuschl G, Li AP, LeCluyse E, Groothuis GM, Hengstler JG: Primary hepatocytes: current understanding of the regulation of metabolic enzymes and transporter proteins, and pharmaceutical practice for the use of hepatocytes in metabolism, enzyme induction, transporter, clearance, and hepatotoxicity studies, Drug Metab Rev 2007, 39:159-234

[12] Li AP: Human hepatocytes: isolation, cryopreservation and applications in drug development, Chem Biol Interact 2007, 168:16-29

[13] Li AP: Human hepatocytes as an effective alternative experimental system for the evaluation of human drug properties: general concepts and assay procedures, ALTEX 2008, 25:33-42

[14] Ulrich RG, Rockett JC, Gibson GG, Pettit SD: Overview of an interlaboratory collaboration on evaluating the effects of model hepatotoxicants on hepatic gene expression, Environ Health Perspect 2004, 112:423-427

[15] Gomez-Lechon MJ, Castell JV, Donato MT: The use of hepatocytes to investigate drug toxicity, Methods Mol Biol 2010, 640:389-415

[16] O'Brien PJ, Chan K, Silber PM: Human and animal hepatocytes in vitro with extrapolation in vivo, Chem Biol Interact 2004, 150:97-114

[17] Loretz LJ, Li AP, Flye MW, Wilson AG: Optimization of cryopreservation procedures for rat and human hepatocytes, Xenobiotica 1989, 19:489-498

[18] Li AP: Preclinical evaluation of drug-drug interactions using human in vitro experimental systems, IDrugs 1998, 1:311-314

[19] Li AP: Primary hepatocyte cultures as an in vitro experimental model for the evaluation of pharmacokinetic drug-drug interactions, Adv Pharmacol 1997, 43:103-130

[20] Li AP: Evaluation of drug metabolism, drug-drug interactions, and in vitro hepatotoxicity with cryopreserved human hepatocytes, Methods Mol Biol 2010, 640:281-294

[21] Li AP, Kaminski DL, Rasmussen A: Substrates of human hepatic cytochrome P450 3A4, Toxicology 1995, 104:1-8

[22] Guengerich FP: Cytochrome P450: what have we learned and what are the future issues?, Drug Metab Rev 2004, 36:159-197

[23] Zhou SF, Xue CC, Yu XQ, Li C, Wang G: Clinically important drug interactions potentially involving mechanism-based inhibition of cytochrome P450 3A4 and the role of therapeutic drug monitoring, Ther Drug Monit 2007, 29:687-710

[24] Flockhart DA, Oesterheld JR: Cytochrome P450-mediated drug interactions, Child Adolesc Psychiatr Clin N Am 2000, 9:43-76

[25] Fujita K: Food-drug interactions via human cytochrome P450 3A (CYP3A), Drug Metabol Drug Interact 2004, 20:195-217

[26] Doshi U, Li AP: Luciferin IPA-Based Higher Throughput Human Hepatocyte Screening Assays for CYP3A4 Inhibition and Induction, J Biomol Screen 2011,

[27] Li AP, Doshi U: Higher Throughput Human Hepatocyte Assays for the Evaluation of Time-Dependent Inhibition of CYP3A4, Drug Metab Lett 2011,

[28] Chauret N, Tremblay N, Lackman RL, Gauthier JY, Silva JM, Marois J, Yergey JA, Nicoll-Griffith DA: Description of a 96-well plate assay to measure cytochrome P4503A inhibition in human liver microsomes using a selective fluorescent probe, Anal Biochem 1999, 276:215-226

[29] Crespi CL, Penman BW: Use of cDNA-expressed human cytochrome P450 enzymes to study potential drug-drug interactions, Adv Pharmacol 1997, 43:171-188

[30] Ogilvie BW, Zhang D, Li W, Rodrigues AD, Gipson AE, Holsapple J, Toren P, Parkinson A: Glucuronidation converts gemfibrozil to a potent, metabolism-dependent inhibitor of CYP2C8: implications for drug-drug interactions, Drug Metab Dispos 2006, 34:191-197

[31] Lu C, Hatsis P, Berg C, Lee FW, Balani SK: Prediction of pharmacokinetic drug-drug interactions using human hepatocyte suspension in plasma and cytochrome P450 phenotypic data. II. In vitro-in vivo correlation with ketoconazole, Drug Metab Dispos 2008, 36:1255-1260

[32] Shitara Y, Li AP, Kato Y, Lu C, Ito K, Itoh T, Sugiyama Y: Function of uptake transporters for taurocholate and estradiol 17beta-D-glucuronide in cryopreserved human hepatocytes, Drug Metab Pharmacokinet 2003, 18:33-41

[33] Maeda K, Kambara M, Tian Y, Hofmann AF, Sugiyama Y: Uptake of ursodeoxycholate and its conjugates by human hepatocytes: role of Na(+)-taurocholate cotransporting polypeptide (NTCP), organic anion transporting polypeptide (OATP) 1B1 (OATP-C), and oatp1B3 (OATP8), Mol Pharm 2006, 3:70-77

[34] Li AP, Lu C, Brent JA, Pham C, Fackett A, Ruegg CE, Silber PM: Cryopreserved human hepatocytes: characterization of drug-metabolizing enzyme activities and applications in higher throughput screening assays for hepatotoxicity, metabolic stability, and drug-drug interaction potential, Chem Biol Interact 1999, 121:17-35

[35] Li AP: Evaluation of luciferin-isopropyl acetal as a CYP3A4 substrate for human hepatocytes: effects of organic solvents, cytochrome P450 (P450) inhibitors, and P450 inducers, Drug Metab Dispos 2009, 37:1598-1603

[36] Zhou ZW, Zhou SF: Application of mechanism-based CYP inhibition for predicting drug-drug interactions, Expert Opin Drug Metab Toxicol 2009, 5:579 605

[37] Wang X, Wang Y, Chunsheng Y, Wang L, Han S: Mechanism-based quantitative structure-phytotoxicity relationships comparative inhibition of substituted phenols on root elongation of Cucumis sativus, Arch Environ Contam Toxicol 2002, 42:29-35

[38] Mori K, Hashimoto H, Takatsu H, Tsuda-Tsukimoto M, Kume T: Cocktail-substrate assay system for mechanism-based inhibition of CYP2C9, CYP2D6, and CYP3A using human liver microsomes at an early stage of drug development, Xenobiotica 2009, 39:415-422

[39] McGinnity DF, Berry AJ, Kenny JR, Grime K, Riley RJ: Evaluation of time-dependent cytochrome P450 inhibition using cultured human hepatocytes, Drug Metab Dispos 2006, 34:1291-1300

[40] Mao J, Mohutsky MA, Harrelson JP, Wrighton SA, Hall SD: Prediction of CYP3A-Mediated Drug-Drug Interactions Using Human Hepatocytes Suspended in Human Plasma, Drug Metab Dispos 2011, 39:591-602

[41] Li AP, Doshi U: Higher Throughput Human Hepatocyte Assays for the Evaluation of Time-Dependent Inhibition of CYP3A4, Drug Metab Lett 2011, 5:183-191

[42] Li AP, Bode C, Sakai Y: A novel in vitro system, the integrated discrete multiple organ cell culture (IdMOC) system, for the evaluation of human drug toxicity: comparative cytotoxicity of tamoxifen towards normal human cells from five major organs and MCF-7 adenocarcinoma breast cancer cells, Chem Biol Interact 2004, 150:129-136

[43] Li AP: In vitro evaluation of human xenobiotic toxicity: scientific concepts and the novel integrated discrete multiple cell co-culture (IdMOC) technology, ALTEX 2008, 25:43-49

[44] Li AP: The use of the Integrated Discrete Multiple Organ Co-culture (IdMOC) system for the evaluation of multiple organ toxicity, Altern Lab Anim 2009, 37:377-385

[45] Morgan RE, Trauner M, van Staden CJ, Lee PH, Ramachandran B, Eschenberg M, Afshari CA, Qualls CW, Jr., Lightfoot-Dunn R, Hamadeh HK: Interference with bile salt export pump function is a susceptibility factor for human liver injury in drug development, Toxicol Sci 2010, 118:485-500

[46] Diao L, Li N, Brayman TG, Hotz KJ, Lai Y: Regulation of MRP2/ABCC2 and BSEP/ABCB11 expression in sandwich cultured human and rat hepatocytes exposed to inflammatory cytokines TNF-{alpha}, IL-6, and IL-1{beta}, J Biol Chem 2010, 285:31185-31192

[47] Maeda K, Sugiyama Y: The use of hepatocytes to investigate drug uptake transporters, Methods Mol Biol 2010, 640:327-353

[48] Rotroff DM, Beam AL, Dix DJ, Farmer A, Freeman KM, Houck KA, Judson RS, LeCluyse EL, Martin MT, Reif DM, Ferguson SS: Xenobiotic-metabolizing enzyme and transporter gene expression in primary cultures of human hepatocytes modulated by ToxCast chemicals, J Toxicol Environ Health B Crit Rev 2010, 13:329-346

[49] Liao M, Raczynski AR, Chen M, Chuang BC, Zhu Q, Shipman R, Morrison J, Lee D, Lee FW, Balani SK, Xia CQ: Inhibition of hepatic organic anion-transporting polypeptide by RNA interference in sandwich-cultured human hepatocytes: an in vitro model to assess transporter-mediated drug-drug interactions, Drug Metab Dispos 2010, 38:1612-1622

[50] Badolo L, Rasmussen LM, Hansen HR, Sveigaard C: Screening of OATP1B1/3 and OCT1 inhibitors in cryopreserved hepatocytes in suspension, Eur J Pharm Sci 2010, 40:282-288

8

The Use of *In Vitro* 3D Cell Models in Drug Development for Respiratory Diseases

Song Huang, Ludovic Wiszniewski and Samuel Constant
Epithelix Sàrl
Switzerland

1. Introduction

In a certain way, drug developers are like the blind men in the well-known tale of "THE BLIND MEN AND THE ELEPHANT", who believe the elephant to be like a water spout, a fan a pillar and a throne since they can only feel a different part but only one part of the elephant's body such as trunk, ear, leg, back. Impossible to test a drug lead on human beings, drug developers also are obliged to forge a whole picture of the "elephant" - how a drug candidate would behave in a whole human body, by using information from the "parts" - models. The task of the drug developers are far more complex and challenging than the blind men, instead of touching only the surface, they have to go deep into the human bodies: organs, tissues, cells, genes, proteins, lipids, hormones ... Furthermore, a living human being is a dynamic and interacting system, in a certain sense, the situation of the drug developers are even worse than the blind men: the blind men touch and feel a real elephant, the information that they get is true; a drug developer, most of the time, works on models, animal models or *in vitro* cell models, which are far from representing a human beings as a whole. As consequences, the information that one gets sometimes could be misleading. For drug developers, the misleading information could have serious consequences in terms of costs and human lives.

This blind men's approach may explain why a drug candidate, even though successfully passed pre-clinical stages, eventually failed at clinical trials. The failure of Torcetrapib, a drug developed by Pfizer, gives an example of just how difficult to develop a drug. Torcetrapib, designed to prevent heart attacks and strokes, is a cholesteryl-ester transfer protein (CETP) inhibitor. Genetic studies of the Japanese populations revealed that people with a deficiency of CETP presented a favorable lipid profile compared with unaffected family members: namely more High Density Lipoproteins (HDL, good) and less Low Density Lipoproteins (LDL, bad) (Inazu et al., 1990; Koizumi et al., 1991). CETP naturally became a target of drug development. Preclinical studies of Torcetrapib on different animal models (mice, rabbits, etc) didn't reveal any severe side effects (Tall et al., 2007). But, medication of Torcetrapib on human beings caused severe hypertension and an increased mortality; apparently there was no obvious beneficial effects on coronary heart disease. The development of Torcetrapib was halted at 2006.

This example illustrates another difficulty in drug development: the genetic heterogeneity of the human populations. The knowledge obtained from one group of people may not be applicable to another group of people. Quite often, this truth has been neglected.

Furthermore, human body is a complex dynamic system, with interconnected networks, equilibrium, feedback, compensation, redundancy, etc..., the cause-effect relationship between the target and the patho-physiological condition is not linear. In the example of CETP, people with the genetic deficiency of CETP, despite of having a favorable lipid profile, also suffer from coronary heart disease (Hirano et al., 1995).

Unfortunately, Torcetrapib is not an exception. According to a statistics, the failure rate at Phase III clinical trials is estimated to be 50% and only 12% of compounds entering into the human phase testing will eventually makes to the market place (Chuang & Stein, 2004).

However, despite of these difficulties, efficient and safe drugs have been successfully developed. The huge increase of the life-span of human populations is the testimony of this success.

The question now is how to improve the success rate of the drug development? In light of the above discussions, we could give a generally recommendations:

1. If possible, use models as close as possible to human patho-physiology and disease conditions.
2. Take into account of the genetic heterogeneity whenever possible during the preclinical studies.
3. Simulate as realistically as possible the dynamic and complex nature of biological responses.

The recent development of 3D human tissue models and the *in silico* models are some attempts to get closer to the human "reality". In this article, authors try to give an overview of the different models for studying the respiratory diseases and for drug development. First of all, in order to develop efficient and safe drugs, it is crucial to understand the nature and the underlying cellular and molecular mechanisms of the pathogenesis of the disease that one would like to treat. In the following sections, we will describe several major respiratory diseases.

2. Respiratory diseases

Respiratory disease is a medical term that encompasses pathological conditions affecting the normal function of the respiratory systems, making the gas exchange impossible. Anatomically, the respiratory system is composed of upper respiratory tract, trachea, bronchi, bronchioles, alveoli, pleura and pleural cavity, and the nerves and muscles of breathing. During the breathing, the respiratory system constantly expose to external insults such as bacteria, virus, particles, gas, etc... making the respiratory system highly vulnerable to various diseases. Indeed, according to the WHO World Health Report 2000, the top five respiratory diseases account for 17.4% of all deaths and 13.3% of all Disability-Adjusted Life Years (DALYs). Lower respiratory tract infections, chronic obstructive pulmonary disease (COPD), tuberculosis and lung cancer are each among the leading 10 causes of death worldwide. There are urgent and unmet needs of better treatments for respiratory diseases.

Respiratory diseases could be classified in various ways. In this article, we will classify them by the cause (etiology) of the disease. As such, the respiratory diseases can be divided into the following categories:

- Inflammatory lung disease
- Obstructive lung diseases
- Respiratory tract infections
- Respiratory tumors

- Pleural cavity diseases
- Pulmonary vascular diseases

We are going to limit our scope to the respiratory tract infections and inflammatory lung diseases. However, it is necessary to point out that one disease may be classified in several categories. For example, asthma is caused by airway inflammation; the consequence is the airway obstruction. Viral infection may also contribute to asthma exacerbation. The interplay of multi-factorial risks makes the drug development even more challenging.

2.1 Respiratory tract infections

Over 200 different viruses have been isolated in patients with respiratory tract infections. The most common virus is the rhinovirus. Other viruses include the coronavirus, parainfluenza virus, adenovirus, enterovirus, and respiratory syncytial virus (RSV) (Mäkelä et al., 1998). Up to 15% of acute pharyngitis cases may be caused by bacteria, commonly Group A streptococcus in Streptococcal pharyngitis ("Strep Throat") (Bisno, 2001). Influenza (the flu) is a more severe systemic illness which typically involves the upper respiratory tract.

During evolution, the viruses as well as bacteria co-evolve and adapt to their host, acquiring so-called tropism, namely the specificity of a given virus or bacterium for a cell type, tissue or species. The well known example is the influenza viruses. Certain strains of influenza A viruses such as H5N1 infect specifically one species: avian, pig, or human, etc... Thanks to this species barrier, the deadly avian H5N1 has not been able to cause "pandemics" within human populations.

Even though there are several determinants of the viral tropism, the main molecular basis of the viral tropism is the specific cell surface receptor(s) for viral entry. A typical and well-studied example is the receptors for influenza viruses (Fig.1. and Fig.2.).

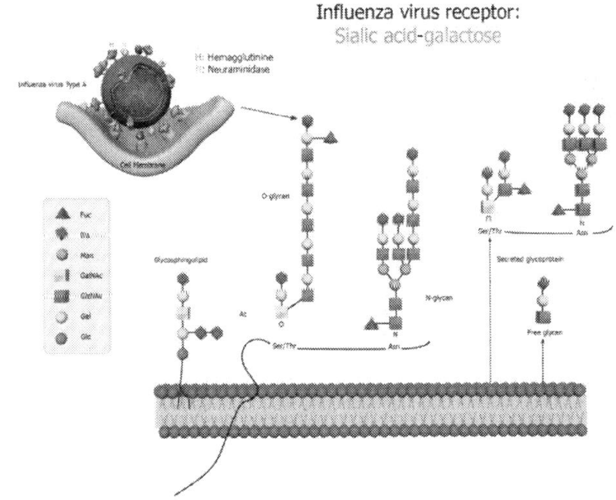

Fig. 1. Schematic representation of the interaction of Influenza virus and its receptors.On the apical surface of the airway epithelial cells, most of the membrane proteins are glycosylated on serine (O-glycan) or asparagine (N-glycan). The glycans are often have a sialic acid (sia) tail linked to galactose (gal), which serves as receptor for Influenza A viruses such as H1N1.

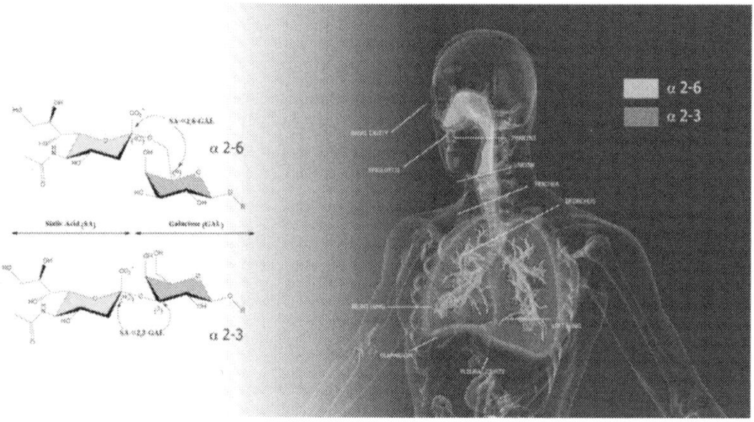

Fig. 2. Two types of linkages which plays an important role in viral tropism. Avian Influenza A viruses prefer α2-3 linkage, human Influenza A viruses, α2-6, porcine Influenza A viruses are adapted to both α2-3 and α2-6. In the human lung, there exists a particular distribution pattern of these two linkages: α2-6 linkage is present mainly on the airway epithelial surface lining the respiratory tracts, from the nose down to the bronchioles. In contrast, α2-3 linkage is located in the alveolar cavity mainly on the type-II cells.

The receptor of influenza A virus is glycosylated-proteins with a terminal sialic acid linked to galactose. There exist two main types of linkages: SA-α2-3-Gal and SA-α2-6-Gal. It has been shown that the avian Influenza A viruses prefer α2-3 linkage, human Influenza A viruses, α2-6, porcine Influenza A viruses are adapted to both α2-3 and α2-6.

What is interesting is the distribution of these two types of linkage in human airway epithelial cells. Using lectin probes specific for each type of linkages, the distribution of these two types of linkages has been studied in the human lungs (Shinya et al., 2006; Van Riel et al., 2006). It has been demonstrated that epithelial cells in the paranasal sinuses, the pharynx, the trachea, the bronchi as well as in the terminal and respiratory bronchioles, mainly express SA-α2-6-Gal. In contrast, SA-α2-3-Gal was found on non-ciliated cuboidal bronchiolar cells at the junction between the respiratory bronchiole and alveolus, and a substantial number of cells lining the alveolar wall also expressed this molecule. Moreover, the SA-α2-3-Gal-positive alveolar cells also reacted to an antibody against surfactant protein A; this suggests that they were alveolar type-II cells (which express surfactant proteinA) (Shinya et al., 2006; Van Riel et al., 2006).

Using similar approach, Varki and Varki confirmed these results. Moreover, they discovered that this distribution pattern seems to be unique of human lungs, it is even absent in the lung of great apes (Varki & Varki 2009).

Since most of the bacteria infect the human respiratory tracts without entering into the cells, the tropism of bacteria is less evident. But, in certain physiological as well as pathological conditions, bacteria preferentially infect certain species or tissues. As example, in patients suffering from cystic fibrosis (the pathology will be discussed below), the respiratory tracts of the patients are chronically colonized by *P. aeruginosa* which can rarely be eradicated. This chronic infection provokes lung inflammation and lung injury, leading to respiratory failure and death (Kerem et al., 1990). The reason of this persistent infection by *P. aeruginosa* is still not clear. But it is reasonable to assume that the respiratory tracts of the CF patients provide a niche particularly favorable to *P. aeruginosa*.

So, given these particular and unique pathogen and host relationship, it is preferable to use human models for drug development for treating viral and bacterial infections of the human respiratory tracts.

2.2 Inflammatory lung diseases

Another category of respiratory diseases is the inflammatory lung diseases such as asthma, cystic fibrosis, emphysema, chronic obstructive pulmonary, characterized by a high neutrophil count. The mechanisms of immune responses in cystic fibrosis, asthma, COPD diseases have been extensively documented. The common feature of these inflammatory airway diseases is the involvement of the respiratory airway epithelia.

Cystic fibrosis (CF) is an autosomal recessive, a multisystem disorder, characterized primarily by defective electrolyte transport in **epithelial cells** and abnormally viscid mucus secretions from glands and mucus epithelia. The impairment of the mucociliary clearance leads to chronic infection and inflammation, ultimately causing cystic bronchiectasis, severe airflow obstruction and death (Boucher, 2004, 2007) (Figure 3).

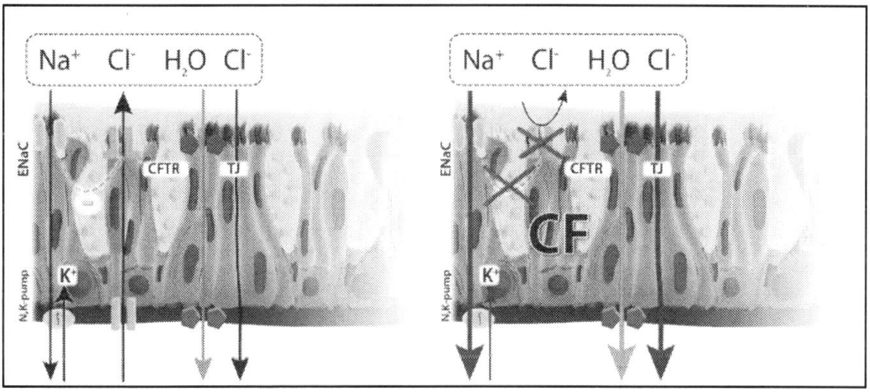

Fig. 3. Schema depicts normal airway epithelial ion transport, dysfunctional transport in CF.Normal airway epithelia (left): CFTR functions as a Cl- and it also regulates Na+ absorption (it inhibits ENaC). The quantity of NaCl on airway surface is optimally regulated to osmotically hydrate the periciliary and mucus layers allowing efficient mucus clearance. CF airway epithelia (right): In the absence of the CFTR protein in the apical membrane consequent to common CF mutations, such as ΔF508 CFTR, the CF epithelium can exhibit unrestrained Na+ absorption and a failure to secrete Cl-. These combined defects reduce the quantity of NaCl on CF airway surfaces, maintain less water osmotically on CF airway surfaces and, hence, lead to depletion of water in the periciliary liquid layer (PCL) and collapse of a thickened mucus layer onto the epithelial surface.

Asthma is an inflammatory disease characterized by allergic reaction to allergens and chemicals. The hallmark of asthma diseases is the antigen-specific IgE production. Even though the effector cells in asthma pathogenesis are immune cells like dendritic cells, helper

T cells (usually CD4+ cells), eosinophils, neutrophils, etc… the airway epithelia play an important role in the induction phase of asthma. Indeed, recent advances suggest that a cytokine named Thymic Stromal Lymphopoietin (TSLP) might play a key role in biasing the Th0 cells to Th2 differentiation pathway (Rochman et al., 2008; Ziegler et al., 2006; Esnault et al., 2008; Shi et al., 2008). What is more, TSLPR-knock-out mice failed to develop lung inflammation upon ovalbumin challenge (Al-Shami et al., 2005). Conversely, the over-expression of TSLP in mice induces spontaneous airway inflammation and atopic dermatis (Zhou et al., 2005; Yoo et al., 2005), suggesting TSLP is an important factor necessary and sufficient for the initiation of allergic airway inflammation. The implication of TSLP in Th2 response is further confirmed by studies of other allergic diseases such as the skin atopic dermatis (Zhou et al., 2005) and intestinal immune homeostasis (Zaph et al., 2007). Interestingly, expression of TSLP is elevated in the bronchial biopsies from the asthmatic patients compared to that of healthy donors (Ying et al., 2005).

Chronic Obstructive Pulmonary Disease (COPD) is now the fifth leading cause of death worldwide (Pauwels & Rabe, 2004) and it will become, as predicted by the World Health Organization (WHO), the third leading cause of death worldwide by 2030 (www.who.int/respiratory/copd/en/index.html). Even though airborne pollutants such as smoke from the burning fuel or coals can cause COPD, the main inducing factor is the cigarette smoke. COPD is a complex syndrome comprised of airway inflammation, mucociliary dysfunction and consequent airway structural destruction. This process is considered non-reversible.

Upon the irritant challenge, the airway epithelial cells synthesize and release pro-inflammatory cytokines and chemokines such as IL-8, MIP-3α, which in turn recruit neutrophils, CD8+ T-lymphocytes, B-Cells, macrophages and dendritic cells to the lumen of the airways. The matrix-metalloproteinases (MMP-6, MMP-9), among other mediators, cause airway injury and remodeling, eventually leading to airway obstruction.

3. The Airway epithelium: Central to the pathogenesis of respiratory diseases

From the above descriptions, it is clear that the airway epithelial cells occupy a central position in the pathogenesis of most respiratory diseases, ranging from infectious diseases, genetic diseases, to most inflammatory diseases. Indeed, it has been long recognized that the airway epithelium is more than just a barrier: it synthesizes and releases a large panel of chemokines, cytokines, lipids, growth factors, proteases, protease inhibitors, for example, IL-8, Il-6, IL-17F, TGFs (Folkerts et al., 1998; Laberge et al., 2004; Suzuki et al., 2007). And the expression of these cytokines and chemokines are induced and modulated by various external insults like viral and bacterial infections, cigarette smokes (Nakamura et al., 2008) and are associated with disease conditions like CF, asthma, and COPD (Fig. 4).

This paradigm provides a theoretic framework for developing more relevant *in vitro* cells models of allergic asthma and COPD, especially the *in vitro* 3D cell models of the human airway epithelium.

4. The experimental models

A survey of the existing models of respiratory diseases may be useful for the readers. Knowing the strengths and limitations of each model will help drug developers to choose the more appropriate tools for their work.

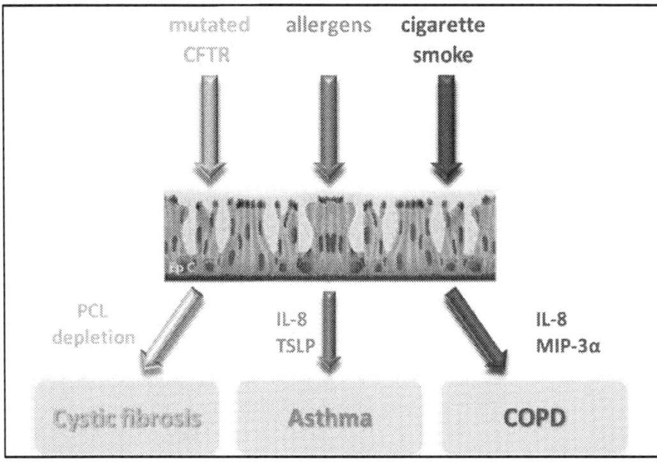

Fig. 4. The Airway epithelium - central to the pathogenesis of respiratory diseases. In addition to its barrier functions, the airway epithelium is also an immune-modulator involved in most of the respiratory diseases.

4.1 Animal models

Animal models are widely used for studying the respiratory diseases and for drug development. Due to the economical and technical reasons, the small rodents like mice and rats are the most popular and widely used animal models. Besides, chicken eggs, rabbits, guinea pig, cats, dogs, sheep, monkeys are also routinely used (Epstein, 2004).

For example, embryonated chicken eggs have been extensively used for growing the influenza viruses and for vaccine production (Potkin & Potkin, 2006; Artenstein, 2009). However, since the dominant linkage in the embryonated chicken eggs is α2-3, some of the field strains grow poorly or not at all in chicken eggs. Furthermore, High mutation rates of RNA viruses like Influenza A allow the generation of viral escape mutants, rendering vaccines and drugs directed against virus encoded targets potentially ineffective (Neumann et al., 2009). A new strategy is to temporarily disable the host cellular factors necessary for viral replication, thus reduce the risk of selecting for resistant viral mutants. Using genome-wide RNAi screen approach, Karlas et al. have identified hundreds of human host factors crucial for influenza A virus (H5N1) replication in A459 cells (Karlas et al., 2010). However, Due to the genetic drift of A549, a cancerous alveolar cell line, it is necessary to confirm these results in primary human pneumocytes. As discussed above, the major concern about pandemic threat of avian influenza A is the possibility of avian flu virus to acquire the ability to infect the upper human airway tracts which are rich in α2-6 linkage.

As animal models, mice and rats are routinely used for studying respiratory diseases. Besides the economical considerations, the biggest advantage of rodent models is the possibility to modify genetically the animals. Indeed, transgenic mice with knock-out CFTR or with delta-F508 mutations have been created (Colledge et al., 1992; Snouwaert et al., 1992; Ratcliff et al., 1993; O'Neal et al., 1993; Hasty et al., 1995). Unfortunately, these transgenic mice don't present lung problems as found in cystic fibrosis patients, highlighting once again the molecular, cellular and physiological differences between animals and human.

As for asthma and COPD animal models, since the rodents don't naturally develop these human diseases, allergic asthma or COPD has to be induced artificially by immunizing and challenging the respiratory tracts with antigen/allergen or proteases/cigarette smokes (for reviews: Epstein, 2008; Churg et al., 2008). Even though some asthmatic symptoms like eosinophil infiltration, mucus hypersecretion, airway hyper responsiveness, and elevated IgE production, can be observed, the lung inflammation is often transient rather than chronic as in human being. Similarly, due to the considerable differences of lung anatomy and susceptibility to injurious agents among species (Bracke et al., 2007), none of the animal COPD models reproduces the exact changes seen in humans (Churg et al., 2008).

Occasionally, naturally occurring animal disease models could also be found and used. For example, Ascaris suum-allergic sheep and flea-allergic dog have been discovered and used for studying asthma diseases and for drug development (Singh et al., 2002; Tang et al., 2003).

One way to get closer to human disease conditions, so-called humanized animal models have also been made to explore the pathogenesis of allergic asthma: the human peripheral blood mononuclear cells were isolated and injected into T and B lymphocyte deficient severe combined immunodeficiency (SCID) mice, creating a human-SCID mouse. Even though it is an innovative approach, due to the complexity of the human immune systems, it is not possible to humanize all the immune cells of the SCID mouse.

In short, animal models, even though useful, indispensable and informative, don't give the true picture of the human respiratory diseases. Sometimes, it is even misleading. Furthermore, none of these animal models can reflect the human genetic heterogeneity which is key for developing safe and efficient drugs.

4.2 Human respiratory disease models

There are several categories of human disease models:

- Cell lines
- Primary cells
- 3D cell models
- Cell co-cultures
- Explants
- *In silico* models

Until now, the most popular human models are cell lines derived from various human tissues.

4.2.1 Epithelial cell lines

The airway epithelia constitute the first line of defense against the external insults. It has a pseudo-layer structure consisted of three main types of cells: ciliated epithelial cells, mucus cells and basal cells. The mucus cells synthesize and secret mucin-rich mucus which trap most of the inhaled particles, virus and bacteria, the later are eliminated from the body by muco-cilliary clearance via the cilia-beating. All the three cell types contribute to the pathogenesis of respiratory diseases, for example, inflammatory reaction, mucus hypersecretion, airway remodeling (Epstein, 2004; Verstraelen et al., 2008).

As airway epithelial cell lines, the most frequently used ones are A549, BEAS-2B, Calu3, 16HBE14o-, etc… The characteristics and uses of these cell lines have been nicely reviewed by Verstraelen et al., 2008.

A549

Origin: This line was initiated in 1972 by D.J. Giard, et al. (Giard, 1972) through explant culture of lung carcinomatous tissue from a 58-year-old Caucasian male. As type II pulmonary epithelial cells (alveolar pneumocyte), it synthesizes lecithin with a high percentage of disaturated fatty acids (surfactants). It is oncogenic when tested in nude mice.
Applications: The cells can be used to screen chemical and biological agents for ability to induce or affect differentiation and/or carcinogenesis. Mechanistic studies, pathway-mapping and target-finding, or ranking of the toxicity potency of chemicals.

BEAS-2B

Origin: BEAS-2B cells were isolated from normal human bronchial epithelium obtained from autopsy of non-cancerous individuals. The cells were infected and immortalized with an adenovirus 12-SV40 virus hybrid Ad12SV40 and cloned. These cells retain the ability to undergo squamous differentiation in response to serum, and stained positively for keratins and SV40 T antigen.
Applications: The cells can be used to test the toxicity of chemicals and biological agents relevant to upper airway epithelia. Suitable for mechanistic studies, pathway-mapping and target-finding.

Calu-3

Unlike most immortal cells, Calu-3 cells form sheets of cells that are welded to each other by tight junctions. These sheets form a fully functional epithelium that can transport large quantities of ions and fluid. In addition, Calu-3 cells have the highest level of natural CFTR expression of any known immortalized cell, even higher than some intestinal cell lines that once held the record. Thus, this cell line is suitable to study cystic fibrosis and drug discovery (Haws et al., 1994).

4.2.2 Immune cells (Effector cells)

Dendritic cells: Although both the skin and lung airway mucosa possess resident dendritic cells, the majority of studies conducted to date have utilized human peripheral blood mononuclear cell-derived dendritic cells (PBMC-DC) due to their relative ease of extraction and the ability to obtain larger quantities of cells (Casati et al., 2005). Several protocols have been established to generate human DC *in vitro*. Starting with blood or bone marrow derived CD34+ hematopoietic progenitor cells (HPC), DC can be generated under various culture conditions with a cocktail of specific cytokines. Despite of the progress made in the field, it is still difficult to obtain sufficient amount of primary DC cell for basic or clinic research. Therefore, the use of cell lines such as THP-1, KG-1, especially the MUTZ-3, proves to be invaluable (Santegoets et al., 2008).
Mast cells, neutrophils, eosinophils, , basophils, are considered as effector cells which are involved in early and late phases of asthma by releasing a plethora of inflammatory mediators. Their roles in broncho-constriction, mucus secretion, and airway remodeling have clearly defined. Many therapeutics are targeting these effector cells and associated key molecules (Casale et al., 2008). These cells can be isolated from the blood or cord blood and cultured *in vitro*. Their behaviors such as migration, free radical production, viability and apoptosis, can be assessed after stimulation by allergen and cytokines (Frieri et al., 2003; Tang et al., 2003; Nilsson et al., 2004).

4.2.3 The drawbacks of cell lines

1. These cells have been transformed by oncogenes one way or other, thus certain signal transduction networks have been deregulated.
2. Genetic aberrations such as chromosomes loss, chromosomes translation, mutations, etc…
3. These cell lines cannot give rise to fully differentiated phenotypes of the original tissues such as cilia formation, mucus secretion, epithelium repair and remodeling.
4. Under the monolayer culture conditions, the cells behave totally different as they do in vivo situations. These differences have been illustrated by comparing the responses of the same cancer cells to drugs (Bissell et al., 2006; Yamada et al., 2006; Griffith & Schartz, 2006).

4.2.4 Fully differentiated 3D human airway epithelial models

To overcome these shortcomings of the cell lines, different techniques have been developed to make 3 dimensional (3D) cultures, by providing a micro-environment or architecture closer to *in vivo* situations. Among these techniques, cellular matrix scaffold, hang-drop culture, perfusion culture chambers, air-liquid interface cultures, etc…
However, in order to simulate the *in vivo* lung conditions, the ALI cultures seem to be more appropriate: the basal-lateral side of the epithelia is immerged in the culture medium and the apical side is exposed to humidified air with 5% CO_2. Furthermore, with the Costar PET Transwell inserts, it is very practical and convenient to use. It is suitable for most of the applications, such as imaging, immune-cytochemistry, toxicity tests, electrophysiological studies (Ussing chamber measurement), assessment of drug permeation and drug formulations, etc…

4.2.4.1 MucilAir

It is a fully differentiated and ready-to-use 3D model of human airway epithelium, constituted with primary human epithelial cells freshly isolated from the nasal or bronchial biopsies. It is commercially available and ready-to-use (Epithelix, www.epithelix.com). MucilAir (Fig. 5.), is not only morphologically and functionally differentiated, but also can also be maintained in a homeostatic state for a long period of time. Using cells from diseased donors, different versions of MucilAir can be made such as asthmatic, allergic, COPD, CF, etc…

4.2.4.2 Applications of MucilAir in drug development

Due to its fully differentiated nature, MucilAir can be used for studying various respiratory diseases. In the following paragraphs, we will give some examples about the applications of MucilAir in drug development.

4.2.4.2.1 Viral infections

MucilAir has been successfully used for studying Pandemic H1N1 2009 influenza virus (Brookes et al., 2010). It is also suitable for other respiratory viruses like Respiratory syncytial virus (RSV) and Human Rhinovirus (HRV) (Fig. 6.). The results are highly reproducible.

4.2.4.2.2 Electro-physiology of the airway epithelia (Ussing chamber measurements)

One of the characteristics of the airway epithelia is the active ion transport which is essential for regulating and maintaining the ion composition and height of the pericilliary liquid layer. The ion channel activities of the airway epithelia can be monitored in a modified Ussing Chamber. In the following figure, the short circuit current mediated by CFTR is absent when stimulated with Isoproterenol which increases the intra-cellular cyclic AMP (see above discussion on CF pathology). Typical recording is shown in Fig. 7.. Related to electrophysiology is the muco-ciliary clearance. It is convenient to use MucilAir for evaluating the drug effects on cilia beating and muco-ciliary clearance.

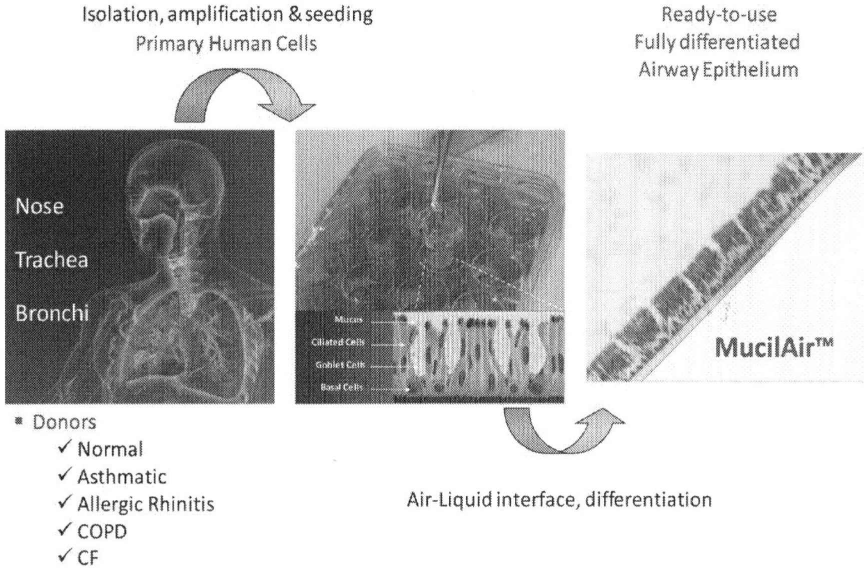

Fig. 5. MucilAir, a fully differentiated 3D in vitro cell model of the human airway epithelia Epithelial cells were freshly isolated from the biopsies (nose, trachea, and bronchi), then seeded onto a semi-porous membrane (Costar Transwell, pore size 0.4 µm). After about 45 days of culture at air-liquid interface, the epithelia were fully differentiated, both morphologically and functionally. Depending on the pathology of the donors, different versions of MucilAir could be made.

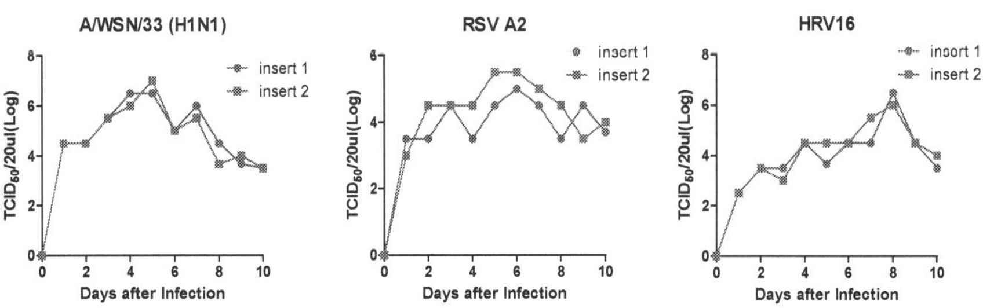

Fig. 6. MucilAir was infected apically: A/WSN/33, H1N1 influenza, 1MOI; RSV A2, 0.1MOI; HRV16, 1MOI. The virions were collected by washing the apical surface with 500 µl culture medium. The titre of the viruses was measured by ELISA.

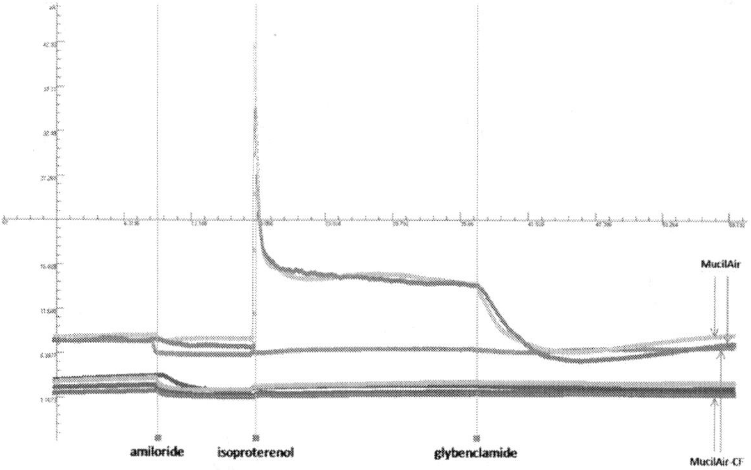

Fig. 7. Measurement of the short-circuit current in modified Ussing chambers. The reconstituted epithelia are placed in modified Ussing chambers and the short-circuit currents are measured after the addition of various blockers and activators of the ionic channels. Addition of Amiloride (blocker of the sodium channels) reduced the current. The addition of Isoproterenol increased the current in normal MucilAir, but in MucilAir-CF. The addition of glybenclamide (an inhibitor of CFTR channel) completely inhibited the currents mediated by CFTR in normal MucilAir.

4.2.4.2.3 Mucociliary clearance analysis

The muco-ciliary clearance is the principal defense mechanism of the respiratory systems. The impairment of this function is the major cause of chronic infection and inflammation, as exemplified in cystic fibrosis disease. For experimental reasons, direct measurements of mucus velocity in human lungs are presently available only for the trachea, with values ranged from 4-6 mm/min. (Hofmann et al., 2002). The only reported value of the mucus velocity in the main bronchi is about 2.4 mm/min (Foster et al., 1982). Interestingly, the same value has been obtained by using an in vitro culture model of the bronchial airway epithelial cells (Masui et al., 1998). However, the velocity of muco-ciliary clearance varies considerable depending on individuals, anatomical location, and disease conditions, etc… Indeed, the values that we obtained from the nasal epithelia are slightly inferior to that of bronchial ones, about 1.8 mm/min (Fig. 8.). Due to the simplicity of *in vitro* methods, it is possible to access the drug effects on muco-ciliary clearance in various disease settings.

4.2.4.2.4 Multi-endpoint test strategy

In addition to its applications in viral infection and cystic fibrosis, MucilAir can also be used for testing the toxicity and efficacy of the drugs candidates. To this end, a multi-endpoint strategy is used (Fig. 9.). The drug candidates can be applied on the apical surface as liquids, solids, gaz, smoke and nanoparticles. The effects of drugs can be monitored by several endpoints: such as the trans-epithelial electric resistance (TEER), cell viability tests (Resazurin, LDH), cilia beating frequency monitoring, muco-ciliary clearance, mucus secretion, release of cytokines/chemokines.

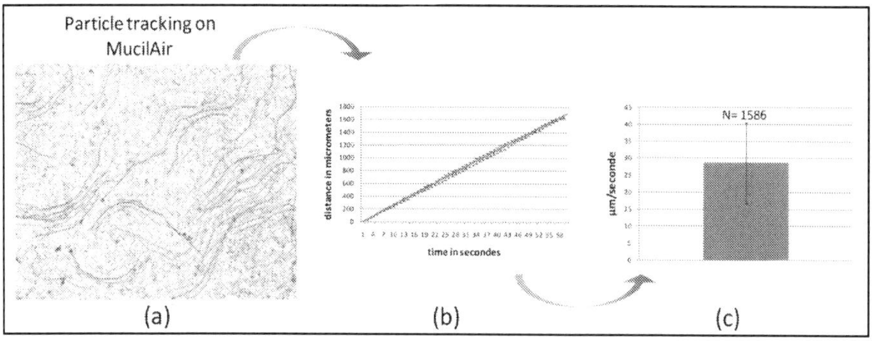

Fig. 8. Due to its fully differentiated nature, muco-ciliary clearance can be easily studied in vitro on MucilAir. Briefly, the mucociliary clearance is monitored using a fully automated setup dedicated to video-microscopy. Microbeads of 5 microns are seeded onto the apical surface of MucilAir-normal or MucilAir-CF cultures. Then, pictures are taken every second during 1 minute in order to reconstitute movies showing the movement of the small particles. The particle movement is then tracked using dedicated software for calculating velocities of beads' movement.

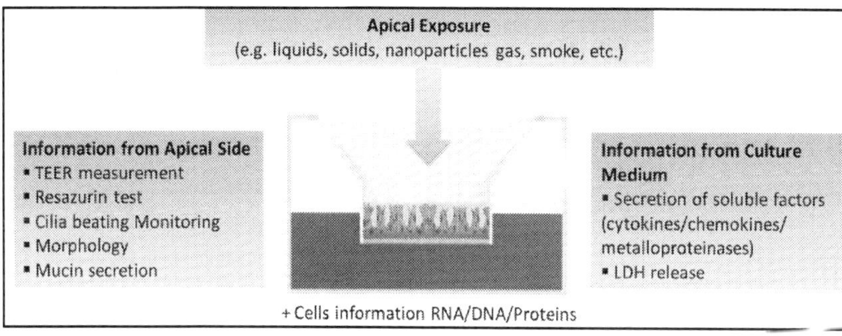

Fig. 9. Multiple end points testing strategy for toxicity testing using MucilAir

4.2.4.2.5 Dextran application

One of the problems that drug developers frequently encounter is the solubility of the compounds: not all the chemicals are soluble or stable in solutions. It is also difficult to test powders or nanoparticles. In order to solve this problem, a procedure which allows testing all kinds of solid substances was developed (PCT/IB2010/053956). The idea is to use inert and neutral substances as carrier. Dextran was successfully used as carrier to deliver the insoluble chemical compounds and nanoparticles onto the apical surfaces of MucilAir. Dextran is a bacterial byproduct; the dextran macromolecule consists of glycan groups linked end to end. It didn't show any harmful effect on MucilAir. The following figure describes the procedure and application of the dextran tablets (Fig. 10.).

4.2.4.2.6 Simulation of chronic airway inflammation

Airway epithelium is more than just a barrier; it is also an immune-modulator. Upon external stimulations, it synthesizes and releases a large panel of chemokines, cytokines, lipids, growth factors, proteases, protease inhibitors. In the following figure (Fig. 11.), the epithelia were repetitively stimulated by Cytomix (TNF-α/LPS). It is remarkable that the airway epithelial cells could recover after repetitive challenge of Cytomix, a relatively physiological stimulus. It was not the cases with some chemical compounds (data not shown).

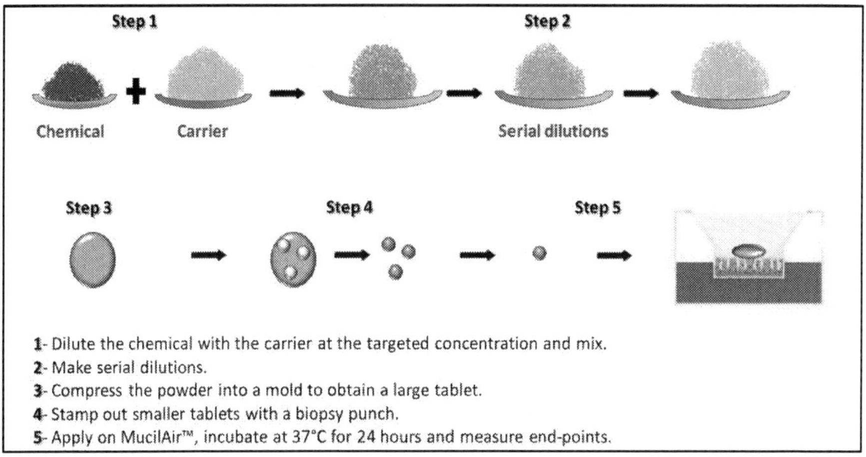

Fig. 10. Preparation and application of the Dextran Tablets

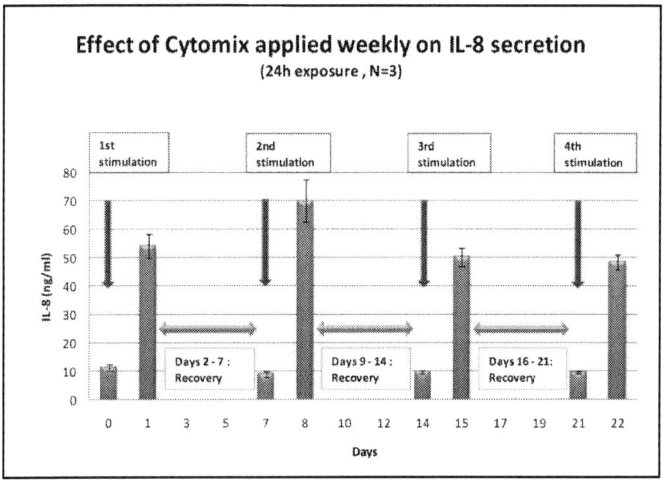

Fig. 11. Inflammatory response of the epithelia. Before the stimulation, the basal level of IL-8 was about 10 ng/ml. After 24 hours of stimulation with pro-inflammatory mediators (Cytomix = TNF-α + LPS), the amount of IL-8 released was increased five-fold. Upon removal of the stimulus, the amount of IL-8 returned to basal level as day 0. The epithelia could respond to the stimulus in a physiological manner again and again.

4.2.4.2.7 Repeated dose and long term toxicity testing using MucilAir

Quite often, it is necessary to perform repeated dose and Long term toxicity/efficacy test of drug candidates. Up to now, this kind of experiments can be performed only on animals. In the following graph, we provide a proof-of-concept for repeated dose tests using an *in vitro* cell model. It is a transposition of the OECD412 guideline for 28 day test on rodents. The TEER was used as endpoint, which is an indicator of the epithelial integrity (Fig. 12.). This is a very sensitive endpoint. The "No Observed Adverse Effect Level"(NOAEL) can be determined (around 10 mM).

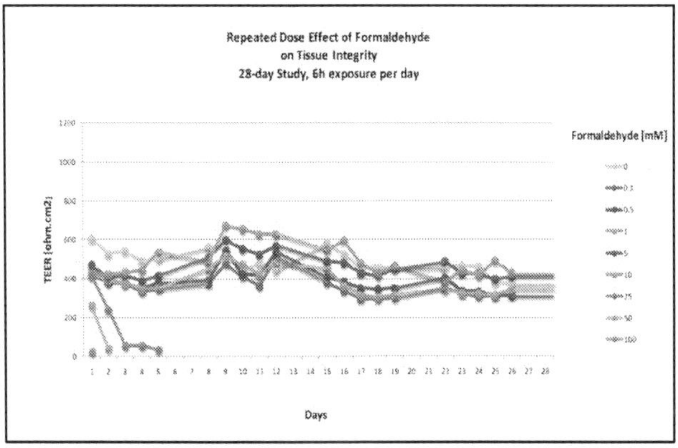

Fig. 12. Repeated dose tests of formaldehyde on MucilAir (28 days repeated dose exposure study). 6 hours per day exposure on MucilAir to Formaldehyde for a period of 28 days. Every day, tissue Integrity (TEER) were measured (N=3) then epithelia were reused for the next exposure.

4.2.4.2.8 Drug permeation

In recent decades, the nasal mucosa has become an established administration site for systemic as well as local drug delivery (Ugwoke et al., 2005). For developing novel drugs intended for this route, reliable methods are needed for assessing the rate and extent of absorption across the nasal epithelium. Desired methods should enable studies of enhancer effects and toxicology. By transposing the Caco-2 protocol (Hubatsch et al., 2007) to MucilAir™, trans-epithelial permeability of drug candidates or xenobiotics can be assessed on MucilAir™. Since epithelium is grown on separable inserts, kinetic studies are facilitated (Fig. 13.). The results obtained are very similar using different batches of MucilAir™ derived from different donors. Apical to basolateral and basolateral to apical permeability studies on height reference compound were performed (Table 1).

4.2.4.2.9 The problem of variability

One of the concerns of using the primary human cells is the variability from donor to donor: researchers don't like variability! Indeed, one of the gold standards of scientific analysis is the reproducibility. If one performs an experiment with a standard operating protocol, one should get the same results. We agree with this principle. But, the genetic heterogeneity of the human population is a reality that drug developers have to face sooner or later: Exposed to the same allergens, only a small percent of people develop asthma. Not all the smokers suffer from COPD. This reality has to be taken into account whenever possible, and as early as possible. Thus, in our opinion, the donor-dependent variation is not a problem; on the contrary, it could be a solution for reducing failure rate at later stages. Using a large collection of frozen primary airway epithelial cells, it is possible to address the issue of the genetic heterogeneity of the human populations. With tools like genomics, proteomics, bio-informatics, etc, it would be possible to pin down cellular and molecular mechanisms underlying the donor to donor variability.

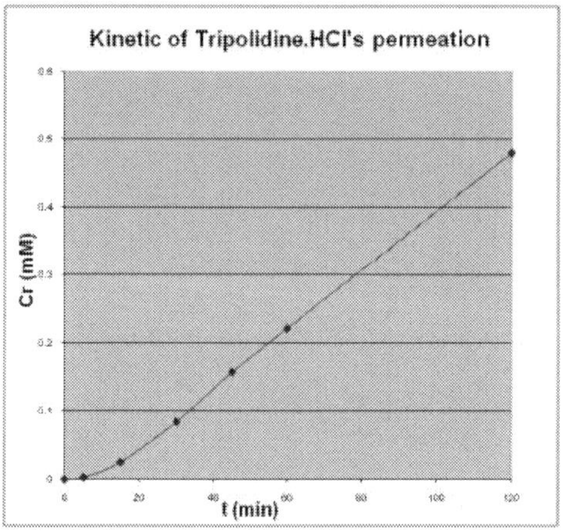

Fig. 13. Time course of the rate of permeability of Tripolidine.HCl from the apical to basolateral side (N=3).

Molecules	Papp (cm/s) A→B	Papp (cm/s) B→A	Asymmetry Ratio
Salicilic Acid	7.7×10^{-5}	1.7×10^{-5}	0.2
Nicotine	2.1×10^{-5}	3.3×10^{-5}	1.6
Propranolol. HCl	1.2×10^{-5}	1.6×10^{-5}	1.3
Ibuprofen	1.1×10^{-5}	1.9×10^{-5}	1.7
Tripolidine. HCl	9.7×10^{-6}	1.2×10^{-5}	1.2
Tetracaïne. HCl	8.0×10^{-6}	1.1×10^{-5}	1.3
Dopamine. HCl	3.0×10^{-6}	2.5×10^{-6}	0.8
Atenolol	2.2×10^{-6}	6.7×10^{-6}	3.0

Table 1. Evaluation of transport of 8 reference compounds across MucilAir (N=3)

4.2.5 Immune competent 3D models

Despite the central rule of the airway epithelia, other cellular components are also implicated and necessary for understanding the pathology of respiratory diseases, especially the immune cells.

Co-culture systems: To study the cross-talks between different types of cells, the simplest way is by co-culturing different cells involved *in vitro*. Such experiments have been carried out using established cell lines: for examples, BEAS-2B are co-cultured with human lung fibroblasts (HFL-1 or WISTAR-38) (Lang et al., 1998), human umbilical vein endothelial cells (ECV304) (Mögel et al., 1998), or eosinophils (Wong et al., 2005), and primary human BECs with alveolar macrophages (Ishii et al., 2005). Using 3D cell models like MucilAir™ and freshly isolated immune cells, more reliable and faithful co-culture systems could be developed for studying the inflammatory respiratory diseases like asthma or COPD diseases and for drug development.

Explants: Another way is to use explants. In other words, part of animal or human lung was excised and cultured *in vitro* for a period of days or weeks. The effects of cytokines or chemical compounds on bronco-constriction have been studied (Wohlsen et al., 2003). Using explants models it is possible to assess immunomodulatory effects (Tan et al., 2009) and understand signaling processes involved in tissue hyperresponsiveness related to asthma (Morin et al., 2005). Precision Cut Lung Slides (PCLS) are now used for studying the effects of sensitizers. PCLS mirrors the complex interplay of different cell types in the living organ and allows physiological processes to be mimicked (Henjakovic et al., 2008). The problem with the lung explants is the rapid degradation of the tissue slices. It is also difficult to obtain health, normal tissues.

Lung on a chip: Ideal is to reconstitute the lung on a chip. Some attempts have been made. For example, Ingber's lab designed and constructed a microfluidics system, so-called Lung on a chip that reproduces both the lung's alveolar-capillary interface and the mechanical effects of breathing on that interface—all on a polymer chip about 2 cm long (Huh et al., 2010). Another example is a so-called **Multi-Compartmental Bioreactor** designed on the basis of allometric scaling laws in order to recreate physiological life conditions of four different human cell types (pancreatic, adipocyte, endothelial and hepatic cells), interconnected each other through media flow (Vozzi et al., 2011). Some physiologically relevant results have been obtained by Vozzi and coworkers, suggesting that interactions, mediated by metabolites present in media flow, have a remarkable effect more than the physical interaction and can lead to a restoration of physiological cell life conditions.

By incorporating the immune cells into these microfluidics systems, it is possible to build an immune-competent human *in vitro* lung model for studying the inflammatory respiratory diseases like asthma and COPD.

4.3 *In silico models*: A systems biological approach - virtual cells, virtual organs, and virtual patients

Despite the spectacular successes of molecular biology, some scientists did feel the drawbacks of the "blind men's approach", and they tried to take a more holistic viewpoint to describe the biological systems (von Bertalanffy, 1968; Noble, 2006). Back to 1960, Noble already developed the first computer model of the heart pacemaker (Noble, 1960). From 2000 onward, so-called systems biology has been gaining popularity and importance. The systems biology tries to put the parts - head, ear, trunk, and legs - together to form a whole elephant: namely to achieve a holistic, quantitative, and predictive understanding through mathematical models that enable an iterative cycle between prediction and experiments (Sauer et al., 2007). Based on systemwide component identification and quantification ("omics" data) at the level of mRNA, proteins, and small molecular weight metabolites, Ishii et al. made a "virtual cell" which includes both the constituting components and the functional state of a metabolic network, providing a proof-of-concept for integrating a heterogeneous data set into a coherent whole (Ishii et al., 2007).

With increasing calculation capacity and better software, it is now possible to simulate more realistically the biological processes at all levels: molecular interaction (ligand-receptor), virtual cells, virtual organs, and even virtual patients (Epstein et al., 2004). The *in silico* approach allows to rapidly integrating new data and novel knowledge, and it can get better and better with time. It is reasonable to hope that in the near future, based on systemwide data collection using relevant human 3D cell/tissue models, we could build a virtual lung for studying the respiratory diseases and for new drug development.

5. Conclusion

Each model has its strengths and weaknesses and there is no perfect respiratory disease model. Depending on the goal or on application, one model could be better than another. Since the drugs are to be used by human beings, it is logic to assess the toxicity and efficacy on cells of human origin, especially on 3D human models. Due to its central role in pathogenesis of respiratory diseases, the 3D *in vitro* cell models of the human airway epithelium deserve more attention in the future. We believe that the 3D cell models like MucilAir are highly relevant and valuable for development of new drugs.

6. Acknowledgments

The authors thank Dr. Kazuhiro Ito from Respivert Ltd. (London) for providing the data on viral infections on MucilAir reported in Fig.6. We also thank the "Ligue Suisse Contre la Vivisection" and the "Fondation E. Naëf pour la recherche *in vitro*" (Geneva) for their continuous support.

7. References

Al-Shami, A. et al. (2005) A role for TSLP in the development of inflammation in an asthma model. *J. Exp. Med.* 202, 829–839

Anderson, M.P., Berger, H.A., Rich, D.P., Gregory, R.J., Smith, A.E. and Welsh, M.J. (1991) Nucleoside triphosphates are required to open the CFTR chloride channel. *Cell*, 67, 775–784.

Artenstein, A.W (2009) "Influenza" In: Vaccines: A Biography Andrew W. Artenstein, ed. pp. 191-205.

Bear, C.E.; Li, C.; Kartner, N.; Bridges, R.J.; Jensen, T.J.; Ramjeesingh, M. and Riordan, J.R. (1992) Purification and functional reconstitution of the cystic fibrosis transmembrane conductance regulator (CFTR). *Cell*, 68, 809–818.

Bisno, A.L. (2001) Acute pharyngitis. *N Engl J Med*: 344:205

Bissell M.J. and LaBarge M.A. (2005) Context, tissue plasticity, and cancer: Are tumor stem cells also regulated by the microenvironment? *Cancer Cell* 7: 17–23

Bracke K.R.; D'hulst A.I.; Maes T; Demedts I.K.; Moerloose K.B.; Kuziel W.A.; Joos G.F.; Brusselle G.G. (2007). Cigarette smoke-induced pulmonary inflammation, but not airway remodelling, is attenuated in chemokine receptor 5-deficient mice. *Clin Exp Allergy* 37: 1467-1479

Casale, T.B. and Stokes, J.R. (2008) Immunomodulators for allergic respiratory disorders. *J Allergy Clin Immunol* 121 (2), 288-296; quiz 297-288

Cheng, S.H.; Rich, D.P.; Marshall, J.; Gregory, R.J.; Welsh, M.J. and Smith, A.E. (1991) Phosphorylation of the R domain by cAMPdependent protein kinase regulates the CFTR chloride channel. *Cell*, 66, 1027-1036

Cheung, M. and Akabas, M.H. (1996) Identification of cystic fibrosis transmembrane conductance regulator channel-lining residues in and flanking the M6 membrane-spanning segment. *Biophys. J.*, 70, 2688-2695

Chuang-Stein, C. (2004). "Seize the opportunities." *Pharmaceutical Statistics*. 3, 157-159

Colledge, W.H.; Ratcliff, R.; Foster, D.; Williamson, R. and Evans, M.J. (1992) Cystic fibrosis mouse with intestinal obstruction. *Lancet*, 340: 680

Esnault, S. et al. (2008) Thymic stromal lymphopoietin (TSLP) as a bridge between infection and atopy. *Int. J. Clin. Exp. Pathol.* 1, 325-330

Epstein, M.M. (2004) Do mouse models of allergic asthma mimic clinical disease? *Int Arch Allergy Immunol* 133 (1), 84-100

Folkerts, G. and Nijkamp, F.P. (1998) Airway epithelium: more than just a barrier! *Trends Pharmacol. Sci.* 19, 334-341

Foster, W. M.; Langenback, E. G. and Bergofsky, E. H. (1982). Lung mucociliary function in man: Interdependence of bronchial and tracheal mucus transport velocities with lung clearance in bronchial asthma and healthy subjects. *Ann. Occup. Hyg.* 26, 227-244.

Friend, S.L. et al. (1994) A thymic stromal cell line supports *in vitro* development of surface IgM+ B cells and produces a novel growth factor affecting B and T lineage cells. *Exp. Hematol.* 22, 321-328

Frieri, M. et al. (2003) Montelukast inhibits interleukin-5 mRNA expression and cysteinyl leukotriene production in ragweed and mite-stimulated peripheral blood mononuclear cells from patients with asthma. *Allergy Asthma Proc* 24 (5), 359-366

Griffith L.G and Swartz M.A. (2006) Capturing complex 3D tissue physiology *in vitro*

Hasty, P. et al. (1995) Severe phenotype in mice with termination mutation in exon 2 of cystic fibrosis gene. *Somat. Cell Mol. Genet.*, 21, 177-187

Haws C.; Finkbeiner W.E.; Widdicombe J.H.; Wine J.J.; (1994) Calu-3: a human airway epithelial cell line that shows cAMP-dependent Cl- secretion., *Am J Physiol.* 266, 493-501

Henjakovic, M. et al. (2008) Ex vivo lung function measurements in precision-cut lung slices (PCLS) from chemical allergen-sensitized mice represent a suitable alternative to in vivo studies. *Toxicol Sci* 106 (2), 444-453

Hirano K.; Yamashita S.; Kuga Y.; Sakai N.; Nozaki S.; Kihara S.; Arai T.; Yanagi K.; Takami S.; Menju M. (1995) Atherosclerotic disease in marked hyperalphalipoproteinemia. Combined reduction of cholesteryl ester transfer protein and hepatic triglyceride lipase. *Arterioscler Thromb Vasc Biol.* ; 15: 1849-1856

Hofmann, W.; Asgharian, B. and Winkler-Heil, R. (2002). Intersubject variability in particle deposition in human lungs. *J. Aerosol Sci.* 33, 219 -235.

Huang S.; Wiszniewski L.; Derouette J.P.; Constant S. (2009), *In vitro* organ culture models of asthma *Drug Discovery Today: Disease Models* Vol. 6, No. 4

Hubatsch, I.; Ragnarsson, E.G.E. and Artursson, P. (2007) Determination of drug permeability and prediction of drug absorption in Caco-2 monolayers. *Nature Protocols* 2: 2111-2119.

Inazu A.; Brown M.L.; Hesler C.B.; Agellon L.B.; Koizumi J.; Takata K.; Maruhama Y.; Mabuchi H.; Tall A.R. (1990) Increased high-density lipoprotein levels caused by a common cholesteryl-ester transfer protein gene mutation. *N Engl J Med.* 323: 1234-1238

Ishii H. et al. (2005) Alveolar macrophage-epithelial cell interaction following exposure to atmospheric particles induces the release of mediators involved in monocyte mobilization and recruitment. *Respir Res* 6: 87

Ishii N. ; Nakahigashi K.; Baba T.; Robert M. et al. (2007) Multiple High-Throughput Analyses Monitor the Response of E. coli to Perturbations. *Science* 316: 593-597

Karlas A., Machuy N.; ShinY.J.; Pleissner K-P; Artarin A.; Heuer; Becker D.; Khalil H.; Ogilvie LA; Hess S.; Maeurer AP; Müller E.; Wolff T.; Rudel T.; Meyer TF (2010) Genome-wide RNAi screen identifies human host factors crucial for influenza virus replication. *Nature* 463: 818-822

Kerem E.; Corey M.; Gold R.; Levison H. (1990) Pulmonary function and clinical course in patients with cystic fibrosis after pulmonary colonization with Pseudomonas aeruginosa. *J Paediatr*; 116: 714d719

Koizumi, J.; Inazu, A.; Yagi, K.; Koizumi, I.; Uno, Y.; Kajinami, K.; Miyamoto, S.; Moulin, P.; Tall, AR.; Mabuchi, H.; et al. (1991) Serum lipoprotein lipid concentration and composition in homozygous and heterozygous patients with cholesteryl ester transfer protein deficiency. *Atherosclerosis.* 90: 189–196

Laberge, S. and El Bassam, S. (2004) Cytokines, structural cells of the lungs and airway inflammation. *Paediatr. Respir. Rev.* 5 (Suppl. A), S41–45

Lang, D.S. et al. (1998) Interactions between human bronchoepithelial cells and lung fibroblasts after ozone exposure *in vitro. Toxicol Lett* 96-97, 13-24

Mäkelä, M.J.; Puhakka, T.; Ruuskanen, O.; Leinonen, M.; Saikku, P.; Kimpimäki, M.; Blomqvist, S.; Hyypiä, T. and Arstila, P. (1998) Viruses and Bacteria in the Etiology of the Common Cold *J Clin Microbiol.* February; 36(2): 539–542

Matsui H.; Grubb B.R.; Tarran R.; Randell S.H.; Gatzy J.T.; normal Ion Composition, in the Pathogenesis of Cystic Fibrosis Airways Disease. *Cell*, Vol. 95, 1005–1015.

Mögel, M.; Krüger, E.; Krug, H.F.; Seidel, A. (1998) A new coculture-system of bronchial epithelial and endothelial cells as a model for studying ozone effects on airway tissue. *Toxicol. Letter* 96-97, 25-32

Morin, C. et al. (2005) Organ-cultured airway explants: a new model of airway hyperresponsiveness. *Exp Lung Res* 31 (7), 719-744

Nakamura, Y. et al. (2008) Cigarette smoke extract induces thymic stromal lymphopoietin expression, leading to T(H)2-type immune responses and airway inflammation. *J. Allergy Clin. Immunol.* 122, 1208–1214

Neumann, G.; Noda, T. & Kawaoka, Y (2009) Emergence and pandemic potential of swine-origin H1N1 influenza virus. *Nature* 459: 931–939

Nilsson, C. et al. (2004) Low numbers of interleukin-12-producing cord blood mononuclear cells and immunoglobulin E sensitization in early childhood. *Clin Exp Allergy* 34 (3), 373-380

Noble D. (1960) "Cardiac action and pacemaker potentials based on the Hodgkin-Huxley equations". *Nature* 188 (4749): 495–497

Noble D. (2006) The music of life: Biology beyond the genome. *Oxford: Oxford University Press*. pp. 176. ISBN 978-0-19-929573-9

O'Neal, W.K.; Hasty, P.; McCray, P.B.; Casey, B.; Rivera-Perez, J.; Welsh, M.J.; Beaudet, A. and Bradley, A. (1993) A severe phenotype in mice with a duplication of exon 3 in the cystic fibrosis locus. *Hum. Mol. Genet.*, 2, 1561–1569

O'Sullivan, BP.; Freedman, SD (2009) Cystic fibrosis. *Lancet*; 373: 1891–904

Pauwels, RA.; Rabe KF (2004) Burden and clinical features of chronic obstructive pulmonary disease (COPD). *Lancet* 364: 613–620

Plotkin, S.L. and Plotkin, S.A. (2008) "A short history of vaccination." *In: Vaccines*, pp. 6-7

Ratcliff, R.; Evans, M.J.; Cuthbert, A.W.; MacVinish, L.J.; Foster, D.; Anderson, J.R. and Colledge, W.H. (1993) Production of a severe cystic fibrosis mutation in mice by gene targeting. *Nature Genet.*, 4, 35–41

Rich, D.P.; Berger, H.A.; Cheng, S.H.; Travis, S.M.; Saxena, M.; Smith, A.E. and Welsh, M.J. (1993) Regulation of the cystic fibrosis transmembrane conductance regulator Cl - channel by negative charge in the R domain. *J. Biol. Chem.*, 268, 20259–20267

Rochman, Y. and Leonard, W.J. (2008) Thymic stromal lymphopoietin: a new cytokine in asthma. *Curr. Opin. Pharmacol.* 8, 249–254

Santegoets, S.J. et al. (2008) Human dendritic cell line models for DC differentiation and clinical DC vaccination studies. *J Leukoc Biol* 84 (6), 1364-1373

Shi, L. et al. (2008) Local blockade of TSLP receptor alleviated allergic disease by regulating airway dendritic cells. *Clin. Immunol.* 129, 202–210

Singh J et al., Identification of potent and novel alpha4beta1 antagonists using *in silico* screening, *J. Med. Chem.* 45 (2002), pp. 2988–2993

Snouwaert, J.N.; Brigman, K.K.; Latour, A.M.; Malouf, N.N.; Boucher, R.C.; Smithies, O. and Koller, B.H. (1992) An animal model for cystic fibrosis made by gene targeting. *Science*, 257, 1083–1088

Suzuki, S. et al. (2007) Expression of interleukin-17F in a mouse model of allergic asthma. *Int. Arch. Allergy Immunol.* 143 (Suppl 1), 89–94

Tall A. R.; Yvan-Charvet, L.; Wang N. (2007) The Failure of Torcetrapib: Was it the Molecule or the Mechanism? *Arterioscler Thromb Vasc Biol* 27 : 257-260.

Tan, L. et al. (2009) Immunomodulatory effect of cytosine-phosphate-guanosine (CpG)-oligonucleotides in nonasthmatic chronic rhinosinusitis: an explant model. *Am J Rhinol Allergy* 23 (2), 123-129

Tang, L. et al. (2003) Expression and characterization of recombinant canine IL-13 receptor alpha2 protein and its biological activity *in vitro*. *Mol Immunol* 39 (12), 719-727

Ugwoke, M.I.; Agu, R.U.; Verbeke, N. and Kinget, R. (2005) Nasal mucoadhesive drug delivery: Background, applications, trends and future perspectives. *Advanced Drug Delivery Reviews* 57, 1640-1665

Van Riel D.; Munster V.J.; De Wit E.; et al. H5N1 attachment to lower respiratory tract. *Science* 2006; 312 : 399

Verstraelen, S. et al. (2008) Cell types involved in allergic asthma and their use in *in vitro* models to assess respiratory sensitization. *Toxicol. In vitro* 22, 1419–1431

Von Bertalanffy L. (1968) General System theory: Foundations, Development, Applications. George Braziller. pp. 295. ISBN 9780807604533.

Welsh M.J. and Smith A. E. (1995) "Cystic Fibrosis." *Scientific American* 273 (6): 52-59.

Wohlsen, A. et al. (2003) The early allergic response in small airways of human precision-cut lung slices. *Eur Respir J* 21 (6), 1024-1032

Wong, C.K. et al. (2005) Role of p38 MAPK and NF-kB for chemokine release in coculture of human eosinophils and bronchial epithelial cells. *Clin Exp Immunol* 139 (1), 90-100

Ying, S. et al. (2005) Thymic stromal lymphopoietin expression is increased in asthmatic airways and correlates with expression of Th2-attracting chemokines and disease severity. *J. Immunol.* 174, 8183–8190

Yoo, J. et al. (2005) Spontaneous atopic dermatitis in mice expressing an inducible thymic stromal lymphopoietin transgene specifically in the skin. *J. Exp. Med.* 202, 541–549

Zaph, C. et al. (2007) Epithelial-cell-intrinsic IKK-beta expression regulates intestinal immune homeostasis. *Nature* 446, 552–556

Ziegler, S.F. and Liu, Y.J. (2006) Thymic stromal lymphopoietin in normal and pathogenic T cell development and function. *Nat. Immunol.* 7, 709–714

Zhou, B. et al. (2005) Thymic stromal lymphopoietin as a key initiator of allergic airway inflammation in mice. *Nat. Immunol.* 6, 1047–1053

Part 3

Tools, Methods, and Biomarkers

9

Chemical Biology: What is Its Role in Drug Discovery?

Lisa Pirrie and Nicholas J. Westwood
School of Chemistry and Biomedical Sciences Research Complex, University of St Andrews and EaStCHEM, St Andrews, Scotland, UK

1. Introduction

For better or worse, there are considerable changes underway in the world of drug discovery. Whilst it is unclear what the future will bring, one possibility is a strategic shift in the *modus operandi* of the large pharmaceutical companies. One consequence of a shift away from high level investment in "in-house" research and development by pharma could be increased industrial interest in early stage research carried out in biotech, government or charity-funded research centres and academia. In many of these institutions, this type of research is often referred to as "chemical biology". But what is chemical biology? In this chapter we take a less-trodden path to addressing this question with the overall aim of shedding some light on areas of chemical biology which are relevant to drug discovery.

Chemical biology is a difficult topic to define in a few sentences since the subject is very wide ranging. Recent attempts have included an excellent review article in ChemBioChem written by some of the experts in the field (Altmann et al., 2009). A book focusing on the new frontiers in chemical biology has also recently been published (Bunnage, 2010). Interestingly, the Editorial in this book identifies "..reducing the high levels of attrition currently seen in "proof-of concept" Phase II clinical trials" as a key future challenge in drug discovery. It goes on to argue that this can only be achieved through "a much deeper knowledge of biological systems in order to identify and validate those biomolecular targets for which there is the highest possible confidence of disease-relevance in humans". The Editor concludes by proposing that chemical biology has great potential to help address the challenges that have been summarised above. So again we ask what is chemical biology?

Several excellent articles cover this issue in the New Frontiers book (Bunnage, 2010), but here we use an alternative method of probing what chemical biology really involves at the grass roots level. Our goal was to reflect on whether chemical biology, as currently practiced, really is and will be of interest to the drug discovery community in the future. Our chosen approach was to provide a review of all the chemical biology papers which were published in 2009 in the RSC journal *Organic and Biomolecular Chemistry*. Due to the number of papers, over 300, coverage of many of these exciting pieces of research is brief. We apologise for this and for any we may have inadvertently overlooked. However, our goal was to bring this body of work together in an organised and accessible form and to try and continue efforts to define what chemical biology involves. The chapter is split into three main sections focusing on: (**1**) advances in the core technologies in chemical biology; (**2**) progress in the established research areas and (**3**) emerging areas in chemical biology. The chapter concludes with a brief discussion of the sub-areas of chemical biology that have been identified and attempts to assess which, if any, are of relevance to the future of drug discovery.

2. The core techniques in chemical biology

The core skills of chemical biology, including synthetic chemistry, molecular biology, protein crystallography and many others, are often viewed as "standard" and we have therefore decided to cover the majority of the developments in these core techniques in section **3** in connection with their applications. However, progress in three areas is highlighted here:

2.1 Analytical techniques in chemical biology

Work continues on the development of novel reagents and methods to address the many analytical challenges presented by chemical biology. For example, the key issue of the detection of post-translational modification (PTM) in proteins has been studied by Stoyanovsky (Sengupta et al., 2009). This work involves the development of a novel method of assessing *S*-nitroso PTMs, that complements the established biotin switch assay (for a schematic representation see Figure 1A). The technique works by trapping the thiyl radical **2**, which is generated when an *S*-nitroso group spits out NO on irradiation with visible light. This method uses 5,5-dimethyl-1-pyrroline-*N*-oxide as the trapping agent to give **3** and the amount of this adduct can be assessed via western blotting methods. Gene silencing requires the selective methylation of the 5-position of cytidines in DNA. This important PTM therefore provides control of gene function. A novel nonenzymatic method for detecting 5-methylcytosine has been reported by reaction of the nucleobase with a photosensitive uridine derivative (Scheme 1B) (Ogino et al., 2009). It was demonstrated that the yield of the photoligation between 5-methylcytosine and photosensitive 5-vinyl-2′-deoxyuridine derivatives was 5-6 fold higher than with cytosine itself, allowing detection of this important PTM.

Progress continues to be made in the synthesis of molecular imprints that are capable of recognising specific proteins in complex mixtures, such as human serum. Micro-contact imprinting was used to prepare an imprint of creatine kinase (Yi-Wen Chen et al., 2009). The use of a fluorescent imprinted polymer for detecting chiral amines has also been reported (Nguyen&Ansell, 2009). Three strategies for the recognition of paracetamol through molecular imprinting of materials have been described (Rosengren-Holmberg et al., 2009). Further exploring aspects of the recognition of biomolecules, a highly sensitive enzyme immunoassay has been developed by raising antibodies to an anthrose-containing trisaccharide derived from *Bacillus anthracis* (Dhenin et al., 2009). Careful characterisation of the epitope recognised by the antibody was reported. An ingenious method of detecting spores from the *Bacillus* phylum of bacteria has also been described (Lusvarghi et al., 2009). In this approach a biotinylated multivalent scaffold was used in conjunction with a spore-binding heptapeptide. A related report describes the ability of resin beads, functionalised with clustered or individual peptides, to bind cells providing a novel cell adhesion assay (Foillard et al., 2009).

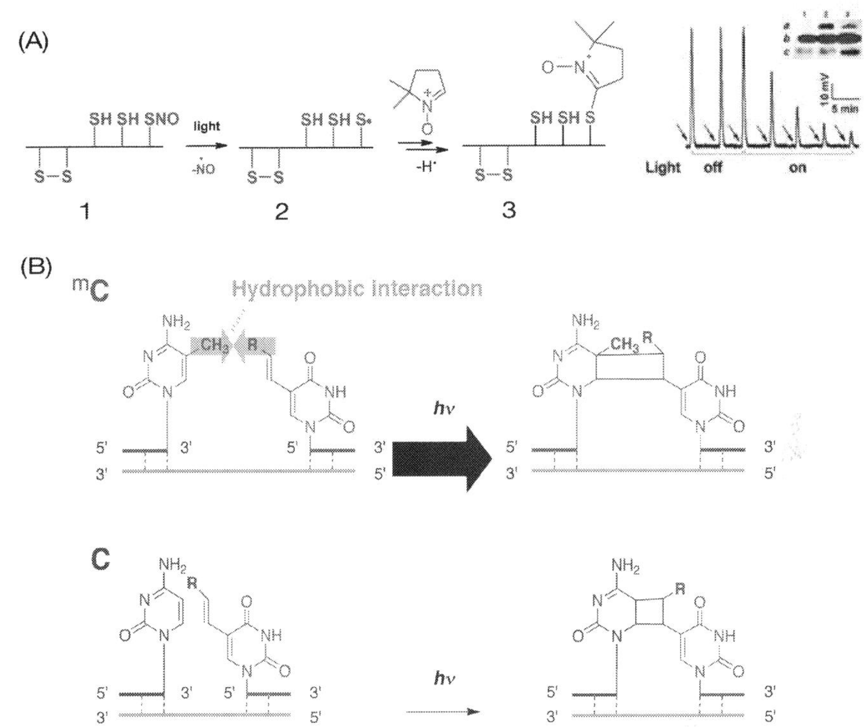

Fig. 1. (A) *S*-(de)nitrosation of thiol-containing protein **1** to give the thiyl radical **2** followed by spin-trapping of this radical by DMPO giving **3**. Chemiluminescence-monitored decomposition of the SNO group upon irradiation and western blotting analysis of the DMPO-tagged proteins (Sengupta et al., 2009). http://dx.doi.org/10.1039/b817981f (B) Strategy for the detection of 5-methylcytosine by photoligation with vinyluridine derivatives. This reaction is enhanced due to an increased hydrophobic interaction between the two reactants (Ogino et al., 2009) http://dx.doi.org/10.1039/b904941j. *Reproduced by permission of The Royal Society of Chemistry.*

The analysis of pH in biological systems is very important. As an aid to this, two novel pH sensors have been reported. One, based on 5(6)-carboxynaphthofluorescein, has been applied to the study of ion channels,(Butterfield et al., 2009) whilst a second study focused on the use of dextran nanoparticles as a means of supporting both a pH indicator dye (FITC) and a reference dye (Schulz et al., 2009). In other work, the analysis of the kinetics of bile acid transport by flow cytommetry has been advanced by the development of novel dansyl-labelled cholic acid derivatives (Rohacova et al., 2009). The assessment of the purity of peptide hormones has also been improved by the use of a dynamic combinatorial chemistry approach to identify a metal-dye combination that delivered a sensor with the required discriminatory power (Zaubitzer et al., 2009). A new assay format for the analysis of the DNA-binding protein NF-κB has been developed (Altevogt et al., 2009).

2.2 Computational techniques

The application of computational methods continues to advance and provide novel insights in chemical biology. Computational methods were used to deduce the mechanism and important residues in the glycoside hydrolysis reaction by endo-β-1,4-xylanase (Soliman et al., 2009; Soliman et al., 2009). By using quantum chemical calculations, a new mechanism for the inhibition of trichodiene synthase by an analogue of farnesyl diphosphate (FPP) containing a cyclopropane ring has been reported (Hong&Tantillo, 2009). The phosphate transfer mechanism of uridine-cytidine kinase 2 has been investigated using computational methods (Smith et al., 2009). The interactions between tryptophan residues of membrane peptides and proteins and the lipid bilayer has been studied using both experimental, NMR titrations, and computational methods (Blaser et al., 2009). Applications of computational chemistry in inhibitor design remain important with, for example, the study of sulfonylhydrazines as potential metalloprotease inhibitors being reported (Rouffet et al., 2009). The results of these studies will be used to guide synthetic efforts towards potent inhibitors. Computational chemistry has also been used to design conjugates of docetaxel with increased solubility for use in a nano-emulsion formulation (Huynh et al., 2009). Other examples of the use of computational methods occur throughout this review.

2.3 The development of imaging methods

The ability to analyse and in some cases image important anions, cations or other chemical entities in live cells is becoming very important in chemical biology. This has triggered considerable activity in the design and synthesis of novel sensors. For example, several novel anion- and cation-sensors have been reported. In the context of anion-sensors, an indole-azadiene conjugate that is a useful fluoride ion sensor has been discovered (Shiraishi et al., 2009). In addition, fluoride ion recognition by urea (Perez-Ruiz et al., 2009) and thiourea-containing (Veale et al., 2009) sensors has been reported. In the thiourea example, a bidirectional PET-based system was shown to be responsive to AcO^- and $H_2PO_4^-$ anions as well as fluoride (Veale et al., 2009). The importance of allosteric effects has been assessed in a tetrapodal imidazolium-derived calix[4]arene receptor that recognises a range of anions (Willans et al., 2009). The use of porphyrin and *N*-confused porphyrin systems to detect anions has also been progressed (Toganoh et al., 2009). The sensing of inorganic phosphate by a *bis*-dipicolylamine ligand has been assessed using calorimetric techniques (Drewry et al., 2009).
Chemosensors for Cu^{2+} in aqueous solution based on an unsymmetrical 4,5-diaminonaphthalimide (Junhai Huang et al., 2009) or calix[4]arenes (Gruber et al., 2009) have been developed. The interesting observation by Jiang that suitably substituted *N*-acylhydrazones are converted to highly fluorescent 1,3,4-oxadiazoles in the presence of Cu^{2+} provided a sensitive method of detecting Cu^{2+} levels (Figure 2A) (Ai-Fang Li et al., 2009). This chemistry has also been applied to the detection of methylmercury ($MeHg^+$) cations in living cells and organisms (Young-Keun Yang et al., 2009). In two separate but related reports a dithiolane-linked thiorhodamine dimer (Weimin Liu et al., 2009) and a tridentate diaza-oxa-containing BODIPY derivative (Lu et al., 2009) have been developed for the detection of Hg^{2+} ions in living cells. A phosphane disulfide derivative has also been shown to be a highly selective and sensitive Hg^{2+} sensor (Ha-Thi et al., 2009). A ruthenium-based metallocrown complex senses the presence of Li^+ ions in both water and in serum providing a fluorescent readout (Rochat et al., 2009). Sensors for other compounds including glucose (Sharrett et al., 2009), spermidine and spermine (Tanima et al., 2009), palmatine and

dehydrocorydaline (Chunju Li et al., 2009), and acetylcholine (Dumartin et al., 2009) have also been described. A novel ditopic receptor based on resocinarene has been reported for the binding of acetylcholine and ammonium cations (Salorinne et al., 2009). An artificial receptor for carbohydrates has been designed and was shown to be selective for disaccharides over monosaccharides in organic solvent (Mazik&Buthe, 2009). A europium-based luminescence assay for the detection of lactate and citrate in biological fluids has been developed by Parker (Figure 2B) (Pal et al., 2009). The results obtained using this approach were compared to those obtained using a commonly used citrate lyase kit and the outcome found to be almost identical. The sensing of biological thiols has also been advanced (Wang et al., 2009). This report describes the synthesis of a merocyanine-based probe that is cleaved by thiols to give two compounds one of which is a chromophore, the other a fluorophore.

Many of the sensors described above rely on the use of established dyes. However, the chemical biology community continues to drive forward the optimisation of existing and the discovery of new fluorophores. The synthesis of a series of novel cyanine dyes, using a combination of solid phase and microwave irradiation, covering the whole colour range has been reported by Bradley (Figure 2C) (Lopalco et al., 2009). The synthesis and characterisation of napthalenediimide cyclophane dyes has also been explored (Gabutti et al., 2009). Novel tetrathiafulvalene-dicyanovinyl donor-acceptor chromophores, (Andersson et al., 2009) and new clickable fluorophores (Kele et al., 2009; Tsou et al., 2009) have also been developed. In one of these systems (Kele et al., 2009), the versatility of the new fluorophore was demonstrated in both cell labelling experiments and applications to the labelling of azide modified surface glycans. The synthesis of novel 7-(dimethylamino)fluorene-based probes and characterisation of their binding to human serum albumin has been described by Park and Hamilton *et al* (Figure 2D) (Park et al., 2009). Competition studies with known human serum albumin binders enabled the binding sites of these probes to be established.

Established imaging techniques involve the use of either radiotracers or lanthanide-based complexes and progress in both of these areas continues at pace. A new synthetic approach to the positron-emitting radiotracer [^{18}F]-2-fluoro-2-deoxy-D-glucose ([^{18}F]-FDG) has been reported (L. J. Brown et al., 2009). The synthesis of [^{18}F]- and [^{13}C]-labeled *N*-benzyl-isatin sulphonamides have also been described. These reagents are of use in the study of apoptosis in living systems (D. Zhou et al., 2009). A novel ^{111}In(III) containing radio-pharmaceutical based on oxytocin has also been shown to have potential applications in the diagnosis of tumours over-expressing oxytocin receptors (Barge et al., 2009). Details of the mechanism of uptake of luminescent lanthanide probes by cells has concluded that the major uptake mechanism is macropinocytosis (New&Parker, 2009). The coupling of Eu(III) complexes to gold nanoparticles (Bonnet et al., 2009), and trinucleotides (DNA only or chimeric RNA/DNA)(Escudier et al., 2009) has also been described. Novel coumarin-based europium complexes have been synthesised and their photophysical properties determined in water (Feau et al., 2009). The preparation of bifunctional chelating agents containing Gd(III) has been achieved using a 4-component Ugi coupling reaction (Tei et al., 2009).

In addition to the further development of existing technologies, a series of novel reports that fall into the imaging category have also appeared. For example, substituted phenothiazine dyes have been shown to aggregate into fluorescent organic nanoparticles (Lin et al., 2009). These particles surprisingly light up the lysosomes of cancer cells but not normal cells. The synthesis and use of novel quadrupolar Bodipy dyes in FLIM experiments in HeLa cells has also been reported (Didier et al., 2009). Imaging of a variant of the protein haloalkane dehalogenase (HD) in cells has also been achieved by the development of a novel fluorogenic affinity label derived from an HD substrate (Watkins et al., 2009). A key feature of the affinity label is that it requires unmasking by an intracellular esterase and the authors envisage applications in pulse-chase experiments and high-content screening amongst other protocols. Fluorescent cholinesterase inhibitors have been used to identify the formation of β-amyloid plaques in brain samples from animals and humans affected with Alzheimer's disease (Elsinghorst et al., 2009).

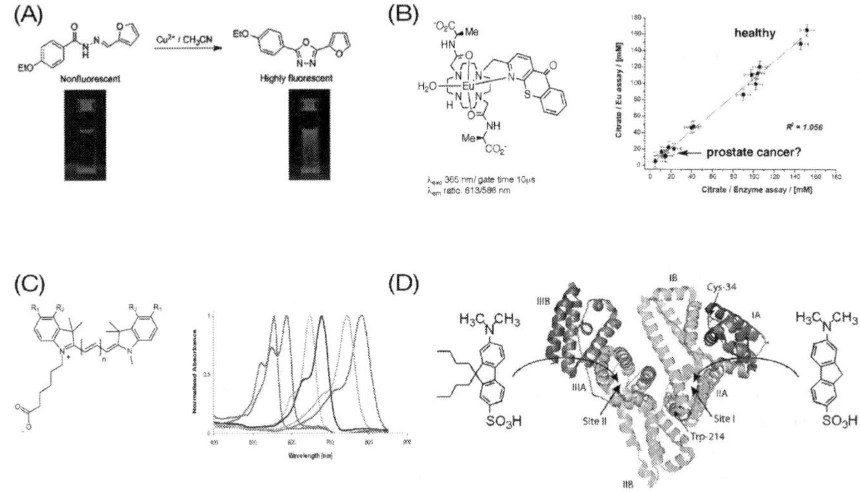

Fig. 2. (A) Conversion of *N*-acylhydrazones which are non-fluorescent to highly fluorescent 1,3,4-oxadiazoles on treatment with Cu^{2+}.(A. F. Li et al., 2009) http://dx.doi.org/10.1039/b811612a (B) Europium(III) complex and a comparison of the results obtained using this new assay to those obtained with a commercially available citrate lyase kit.(Pal et al., 2009) http://dx.doi.org/10.1039/b901251f (C) General structure of the novel cyanine dyes and their corresponding absorption spectra.(Lopalco et al., 2009) http://dx.doi.org/10.1039/b820719b (D) 7-(dimethylamino)fluorene-based probes and their binding sites in human serum albumin.(Park et al., 2009) http://dx.doi.org/10.1039/b911605b *Reproduced by permission of The Royal Society of Chemistry.*

3. Progress in established research areas

3.1 The chemical biology of proteins

This section covers research advances in topics as diverse as amino acid and peptide chemistry, studies on enzyme mechanisms and the use of proteins in synthesis (biocatalysis).

The structure of small peptides and glucopeptides containing the unnatural (1*S*,2*S*)-1-amino-2-hydroxycyclobutane carboxylic acid (C_4Ser) residue has been studied (Fernandez-Tejada et al., 2009). In addition, the synthesis of 2-arylated tyrosine analogues (Bedford et al., 2009) and a diverse series of 5-oxopiperazine-2-carboxylates for use as amino acid isosteres have been reported (Limbach et al., 2009). Penmacric acid, an optically active C-4 substituted pyroglutamic acid has been successfully prepared (Berini et al., 2009). Following optimisation of the conditions required for use of the Dmab amino acid protecting group, the solid phase synthesis of *N*-linked glycopeptides was achieved (Conroy et al., 2009). A new 1,2-dimethylindole-3-sulfonyl group for the protection of the arginine side chain has been reported (Isidro et al., 2009). A novel one-pot hydroformylation/Strecker synthesis of α-aminonitriles has been developed (Subhani et al., 2009). A new route to enone-derived α-amino acids has been described and used to prepare a novel fluorescent α-amino acid for use as a potential biological probe (Fowler et al., 2009). A range of non-proteinogenic phenylalanine analogues were synthesised successfully via a Rh- catalysed cycloaddition reaction (Garcia et al., 2009). The Ru-catalysed synthesis of *N,N*-diallyl and *N,N,O*-triallyl amino acids has been reported without the need for protecting groups (Sundararaju et al., 2009). A novel series of 10-12 membered ring cyclic amino acids containing an enediyne functionality has been reported (Kaiser et al., 2009) The unnatural 4-amino-3-hydroxytetrahydrofuran-2-carboxylic acid has been incorporated into a α,γ-cyclic tetrapeptide that has been shown to self-assemble (Reiriz et al., 2009). A method for the preparation of *N*- or *C*-terminus mercaptoimidazoles from amino acids is described (Crepin et al., 2009). The Ugi multi-component reaction was used in the preparation of azabicyclic derivatives for use as peptide mimics (Basso et al., 2009).

Cyclic peptides, based on the 3_{10} helical Pro138-Gly144 segment of aquaporin-4 were prepared by olefin metathesis (O. Jacobsen et al., 2009). The synthesis of tetravalent peptide conjugates has been reported using a cyclic peptide template and unprotected peptide monomers (Avrutina et al., 2009). A cyclic bile-acid peptide conjugate was synthesised as a mimic of the HNE loop of the measles virus (Bode et al., 2009). This conjugate was shown to bind the same monoclonal antibodies as HNE itself and therefore may be of use as a new measles vaccine. The development of a novel approach to macrocyclic peptoids for use as ionophores has been reported (De Cola et al., 2009). Cyclotides, disulfide rich cyclic peptides, have been isolated for the first time from the *Melicytus* family of plants (Trabi et al., 2009). Using solid phase chemistry, a novel A-chain analogue of human relaxin-3 (INSL7) has been synthesised in which the intramolecular disulfide bond is replaced with a non-reducable carbon-carbon bond (Hossain et al., 2009). A novel class of peptidomimetics, Ψ[CH(CF_3)NH]Gly peptides, have been reported, which utilises a stereogenic trifluoroethylamine group as a peptide bond mimic (Molteni et al., 2009). The Lossen rearrangement has been used to prepare α ureidopeptides (Narendra et al., 2009). The importance of hydrogen bonding for the stability and bioactivity of α-helical anti-HIV inhibitory peptides has been described (Oishi et al., 2009). A procedure for the synthesis of peptides containing *C*-terminal *O*-acyl serine or threonine residues has been established (Yoshiya et al., 2009). A route for the synthesis of non-natural peptide foldamers by the post-assembly reaction of the amino-acid side chains has been developed and used to synthesise a series of novel foldamers (Franz et al., 2009). A method for the solid phase preparation of C-terminal peptide α-ketoacids has been described. This functional group can be reacted further using the α-ketoacid-hydroxylamine ligation reaction to afford peptides (Ju & Bode, 2009). A novel method for the synthesis of peptide alcohols has been developed (A. R. Katritzky et al., 2009). Peptides can also be used as catalysts in organic reactions. A library of histidine-containing octapeptides were screened, as potential catalysts, in the hydrolysis reaction of a pyrene ester (Schmuck et al., 2009). Solid supports have been designed to bind selectively to the phosphate group of peptides which allows any non-phosphorylated peptides to be easily removed by filtration (F. Cass & Tepe, 2009). Activation of spleen tyrosine kinase (Syk) has been achieved by the binding of its SH2 domain to a tetrapeptide motif containing a phosphotyrosine residue (Kuil et al., 2009). Dendrimers conjugated to this tetrapeptide were synthesised and shown to have high binding affinities to the SH2 domain of Syk.

The main methods used for the specific labelling of proteins have been reviewed (Sunbul & Yin, 2009). A detailed and useful discussion of the various types of chemistry and new technologies used to modify proteins chemically was provided. A convenient synthesis of a novel water soluble coumarin-based probe, able to tag biomolecules fluorescently, has been reported (Song et al., 2009). A new system for the specific fluorescent labelling of lysine residues in proteins using a modified microbial *trans*-glutaminase has also been described (Kamiya et al., 2009). Optimisation of the reaction conditions for the low-yielding *S*-nitrosothiol-ascorbate reaction, a reaction frequently exploited to analyse *S*-nitrosocysteinyl residues in proteins, has improved the method (Kirsch et al., 2009). Novel chemiluminescent probes based on dioxetane have been designed and synthesised (Richard et al., 2009). The probes have been used to detect the activities of various proteases. Poly-*N*-(2-hydroxypropyl) methacrylate chains were synthesised and conjugated to the surface of lysozyme (Tao et al., 2009). The number of conjugated chains could be controlled by altering either the pH of the conjugation reaction or the molecular weights of the polymers.

There have been many papers published on deducing specific enzyme mechanisms. The first mechanistic study on a mammalian α-methylacyl-CoA racemase, an enzyme over-expressed in some cancers, has been reported (Darley et al., 2009). The enzymatic reaction mechanism of aristolochene synthase was studied using fluorinated farnesyl analogues by Allemann (Figure 3A) (Miller et al., 2009). Upon incubation of farnesyl analogues **4b** and **4c** with the enzyme, fluorinated germacrene A analogues **6b** and **6c** were obtained, confirming this as an intermediate in the pathway. Since the presence of the fluoro-substituents prevent the formation of the eudesmane cations **7b** and **7c**, a mechanism for the formation of this process could be proposed. Squalene-hopene cyclise (SHC) was used for the cyclisation of a C_{33} polyprenoid (Cheng & Hoshino, 2009). Since the products from this reaction included mono- through to pentacyclic but no hexacyclic compounds, conclusions were drawn about the conformations required for cyclisation to occur. The substrate specificity of UDP-D-galactopyranose mutase from *Klebsiella pneumonia* was probed by Field using substituted analogues of UDP-D-galactose (Figure 3B) (Mann et al., 2009). The enzymatic reaction mechanism of catechol dioxygenase was studied in detail (Brivio et al., 2009) and the Cys69 residue in the photoactive yellow protein has been found to play a key role in its colour regulation (Okamoto et al., 2009). The stereochemistry of the acrylate moiety at the C17 position of chlorophylls C_1 and C_2 was determined and its function elucidated (Mizoguchi et al., 2009). 3,6-Difluorocatechol was used as a probe to study the mechanism for suicide-inactivation of the tyrosinase enzyme, resulting in a new route of inactivation being proposed (Ramsden et al., 2009).

Several groups have worked on the immobilisation and encapsulation of enzymes for use in chemical reactions (Nakashima et al., 2009, Sopaci et al., 2009 & de Hoog et al., 2009). Work has also been carried out on the optimisation of enzymatic reactions. A pH based, colorimetric assay has been designed for the determination of transaminase activity by Truppo and Turner (Truppo et al., 2009). Also reported, are three techniques which can be used to push the reaction towards quantitative conversion (Figure 3C). The stereo- and chemo-selective oxidation of thioanisole to its *S*-sulfoxide has been reported (Ricoux et al.,

2009). This transformation was catalysed by an artificial hemoprotein obtained by inserting Fe(III)-*meso*-tetra-*p*-carboxyphenylporphyrin into xylanase A.

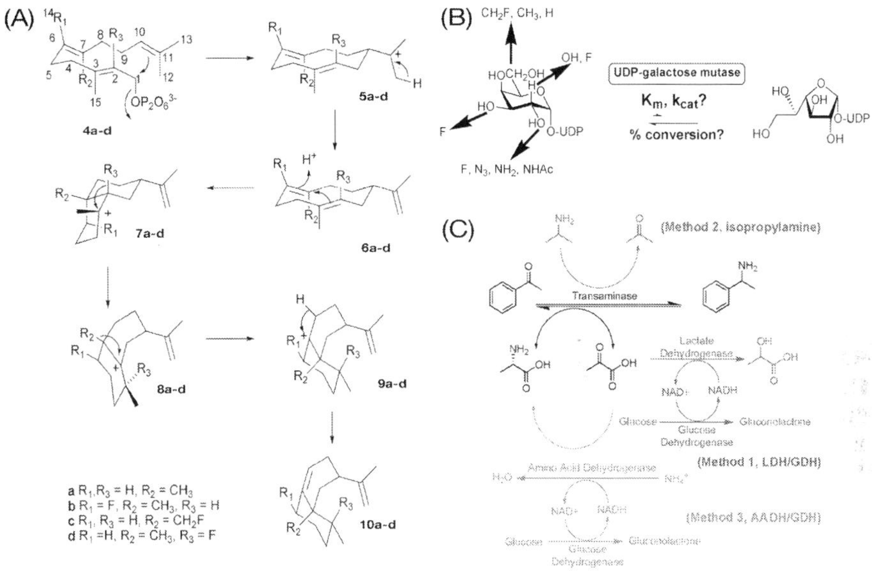

Fig. 3. (A) Aristolochene synthase catalyses the magnesium dependent turnover of FPP (**4a**) into the sesquiterpene (+)-aristolochene (**10a**) (Miller et al., 2009). http://dx.doi.org/10.1039/b817194g (B) Analogues of UDP-D-galactose used to probe the substrate specificity of UDP-D-galactopyranose mutase from *Klebsiella pneumonia* (Mann et al., 2009). http://dx.doi.org/10.1039/b815549f (C) An overview of the transaminase catalysed reaction sequence (Truppo et al., 2009). http://dx.doi.org/10.1039/b817730a *Reproduced by permission of The Royal Society of Chemistry.*

Numerous advances in biocatalysis i.e. the use of enzymes to carry out chemical transformations, have been reported. The substrate specificity of the phospho-mannose isomerise/GDP-mannose pyrophosphorylase bifunctional enzyme was probed by the synthesis of a number of nucleotidediphospho-mannoses and guanidinediphospho-hexoses (Mizanur & Pohl, 2009). The use of FMN-dependant oxidoreductases for the oxidation of α,β-unsaturated carbonyl compounds and thioethers to the corresponding epoxides and sulfoxides has been reported (Mueller et al., 2009). Biocatalysis has been used to prepare many novel compounds including (-)-striatisporolide A (Deska & Backvall, 2009), (*R*)-2-*O*-α-D-glucopyranosyl glycerate (Sawangwan et al., 2009), febrifugine (Wijdeven et al., 2009) and the four different stereoisomers of aszonalenin (W. B. Yin et al., 2009). The solid phase synthesis of peptides using protease catalysis has been described (Haddoub et al., 2009). The chemoenzymatic synthesis of a range of sialyl galactosidases has enabled the substrate selectivity of bacterial sialidases to be explored (Cao et al., 2009). Lipase-catalysed amidation and palladium-catalysed cross coupling of the same substrate were carried out in one pot (Caiazzo et al., 2009). Synthesis and testing of a truncated *N*-glycan hexasaccharide oxazoline, a potential substrate for a glycosylation reaction carried out by endohexosaminidases Endo A and Endo M was also reported (Parsons et al., 2009). The synthesis of enantiopure (*R,R*)-2,3-butanediol from glucose was carried out using *E.coli* and various secondary alcohol dehydrogenases (Yan et al., 2009). An enzyme-mediated synthesis of DNA duplexes containing a large number of locked nucleic acids (LNAs) has been achieved using KOD DNA polymerase (Veedu et al., 2009). A method for the synthesis of polypeptide chains which incorporate an azide-containing sidechain using *in vitro* translation techniques has been developed (Humenik et al., 2009). A novel method for the preparation of peptide thioesters for further reaction using native chemical ligation has been reported (Kang et al., 2009). (5*S*)-Hydroxy-2-hexanone was synthesised in 85% yield with an enantiomeric excess (e.e.) of >99% by the mono-reduction of 2,5-hexanedione using *S.cerevisiae* L13 (Katzberg et al., 2009). A whole cell system, *E.coli* JM 109(pDTG 601), was used to catalyse the dihydroxylation of the aromatic ring of a number of benzoate esters to the corresponding diols, providing useful intermediates for the synthesis of amino cyclitols and pseudo-sugars (Fabris et al., 2009). New ribozymes which catalyse the Diels-Alder reaction of anthracene and maleimide have been designed (Petermeier & Jaschke, 2009).

3.2 Carbohydrates

The chemical biology of carbohydrates is a very active field with the development of new synthetic routes to these challenging molecules dominating the literature in this area. Ducatti has reported the use of polysaccharides from red seaweed in the synthesis of useful carbohydrate building blocks (Ducatti et al., 2009). Others have described the synthesis of tetrafluorinated ribose and fructose (Linclau et al., 2009), 6-deoxy-6-fluorohexoses (Caravano et al., 2009), difluorinated carbasugar phosphates (Anderl et al., 2009), and pyrrolidine homoazasugars (Blanco et al., 2009). The synthesis of unnatural inositol phosphates, 4-*C*-methyl-Ins(1,4,5)P_3 and 4-*C*-methyl-Ins(1,3,4,5)P_4 has been reported (Swarbrick et al., 2009). A novel route for the synthesis of the lipid phosphatidyl inositol 4,5-biphosphate has been reported (Panchal & Gaffney, 2009). The selective chloro-*O*-formylation of sugars using the Vilsmeier reagent (Thota et al., 2009), Rh-catalysed aziridination of glycols (Lorpitthaya et al., 2009), and an appraisal of the utility of the oxoketene cycloaddition methodology in the synthesis of 2,6-dideoxy- and fluorinated 2,6-dideoxysugars have also been described (Audouard et al., 2009). A malonate-containing precursor has been shown to facilitate the synthesis of 2-C-branched carbohydrates (J. Yin & Linker, 2009). The use of the NPPOC photolabile protecting group in the synthesis of glycopyranosides has been explored (Yi et al., 2009) and the synthesis of pseudo-oligosacchasrides using cross-metathesis methods (Ronchi et al., 2009) and pseudodisaccharides based on neamine have also been described (Pang et al., 2009). Several studies on the control of glycosylation reactions have also been reported(Belen Cid et al., 2009; Xiaoning Li et al., 2009; Stalford et al., 2009). Studies towards the synthesis of *C*-glycosyl amino acids have been described using *C*-glycosyl 2-iodopropanes and the chiral auxiliary camphorsultam glyoxylic oxime ester (Bragnier et al., 2009). The synthesis of *C*-glucosyl allothreonine was achieved using this approach. Glucosaminidine ketones have been used as organocatalysts in asymmetric olefin epoxidation reactions (Boutureira et al., 2009).
The structural determination of complex polysaccharides remains a considerable challenge. The relevance of *N*-hexyl-4-amino glycosides in addressing issues of glycan structure and function has been carefully studied (Suzuki et al., 2009). NMR and molecular modelling

techniques have been used to study a bacterial exopolysaccharide with an average molecular weight of 1.3 x 10^6 daltons (Sanchez-Medina et al., 2009). By combining the synthesis and analysis of two oligosaccharides with molecular dynamics simulations, novel insights into the structure of the *S. enteritidis* capsular polysaccharide have been gained (Olsson et al., 2009). *N*-acetyl-α-D-mannosamine 1-phosphate is a repeating unit in the capsular polysaccharide from *Neisseria meningitides* serovar A (Toma et al., 2009). The synthesis and NMR analysis of this compound and its analogues provide further insight into the structure of this complex polysaccharide. A ^{13}C-labelled *N*-acetyl derivative of GAG-heparin has been developed to study GAG-protein interactions in amyloid using solid-state NMR methods (Madine et al., 2009).

The *in vitro* and in cell activity of a series of novel D-glucose derivatives has been reported (van Dijkum et al., 2009). These compounds are proposed to act as chain terminators of cellulose biosynthesis. Two studies on the synthesis and analysis of mannose-functionalised scaffolds have been reported (Andre et al., 2009; Su et al., 2009). In one of these, the nanoparticles ability to bind to concavalin A and sperm surface lectins with high affinity has been reported as a good indicator that these probes will be able to disrupt a range of protein-carbohydrate interactions on the cell surface (Su et al., 2009). A novel approach to the synthesis of oligorotaxanes where the capping group is a carbohydrate has been developed. The conjugates were tested in enzyme linked lectin assays (ELLA) assays for their ability to disrupt carbohydrate-protein interactions (Chwalek et al., 2009).

3.3 The chemical biology of nucleic acids

This section covers a wide range of topics in chemical biology. An attempt has been made to group together related studies although, encouragingly, the boundaries are often blurred.

Driven by a desire to study small molecules that bind to and interact with DNA, researchers have prepared a series of macrocyclic polyamines with an appended anthracene unit (Yu Huang et al., 2009). They have assessed the ability of these molecules to induce site specific photocleavage of DNA. Esters of pyropheophorbides that contain tetraalkyl ammonium groups have been prepared and their intercalating ability assessed (Taima et al., 2009). The reaction of the naturally occurring DNA damaging agent clerocidin with the four DNA bases has been characterised by Richter *et al* (Figure 4A) (Richter et al., 2009). Studies on the individual bases and in the context of DNA provided new insights into the mode of action of this compound mode of action. Molecular modelling was also used to provide further insights into clerocidins direct action on DNA and its ability to react with topoisomerase II. Studies on the protonation state as a function of pH of a dinucleoside monophosphate derivative of the photoadduct that is repaired by the (6-4) photolyase have been carried out (Yamamoto et al., 2009). The selected photoadduct mimics the major UV-induced lesion in DNA. These studies provided an interesting insight into the structure of this compound as well as raising further questions about recognition by and the mechanism of action of the (6-4) photolyase enzyme.

Some of the many challenges inherent in developing RNA intercalators have also been addressed. A hybrid ligand which brings together two weak RNA intercalators has increased binding affinity and enables some specificity to be achieved (Cline & Waters, 2009). In related work, new artificial oligonucleotides have shown selective recognition of short RNA regions over long RNA targets. These probes are particularly useful for the detection of matured miRNAs (Seio et al., 2009). The ability of azacrown-containing Zn(II) complexes to cleave short oligoribonucleotides has been investigated (Laine et al., 2009). Careful analysis of the ability of aminoglycosides to cleave RNA oligonucleotides has progressed the understanding of the mode of action of these drugs (Belousoff et al., 2009). A series of more stable mRNA cap analogues have been synthesised (Rydzik et al., 2009). These compounds were designed to bind tightly to the eukaryotic initiation factor 4E that is responsible for cap binding during initiation of translation and several of the analogues were indeed potent inhibitors of translation. Novel pyrene-labelled uridine derivatives have been used to study RNA bulges, structures that act as molecular handles in RNA (Jeong et al., 2009).

The synthesis of DNA duplexes containing chemically modified nucleotides continues to yield interesting results. The incorporation of "double-headed" monomers containing two nucleobases into oligonucleotides, however, resulted in no detectable pairing of the additional bases (Umemoto et al., 2009). The effect of incorporating a fluorine atom at the 2′ position of 2′-deoxy nucleotides has been investigated (Figure 4B) (Katolik et al., 2009). The resulting oligonucleotide, known as 2′-FANA was considerably more stable to low and high pH than DNA or RNA in the absence of enzymes and an interesting dependence on the stability to cleavage by snake venom phosphodiesterase on the stereochemistry at the 2′-F position was observed. Studies on a new type of internucleotide phosphorodithioate linkage have been reported (Olesiak et al., 2009). A set of four 2′-deoxyborononucloleotides have been prepared and structural studies carried out following their incorporation into dinucleotides (A. R. Martin et al., 2009). 2′-Deoxyuridine-5′-triphosphates, functionalised with various linkers on the 5 position of the uridine moiety, were synthesised and their incorporation into DNA strands using two different polymerases were evaluated (Borsenberger et al., 2009). In addition, 8-aza-2′-deoxyguanosine has been shown to be an excellent mimic of dG. As the anion of this reported nucleotide is highly fluorescent, it has been used in the study of DNA mismatches (Seela et al., 2009). A series of novel 8-aza-7-deazaguanine nucleotide dye conjugates have been reported with the potential to be used in DNA and RNA sequencing or detection (Seela et al., 2009). An anthroquinone-containing nucleotide has also been incorporated into DNA to facilitate the study of duplexes by electrochemical DNA methods (M. F. Jacobsen et al., 2009). Knowledge of the photochemistry of anthracene has enabled the templated synthesis of a bespoke DNA structure (Mukae et al., 2009). A carefully designed system enabled two DNA-conjugated anthracene units to be in sufficiently close proximity that a light-induced dimerisation reaction could occur. The synthesis of α-L-arabino- and α-D-arabino-containing nucleoside analogues and the effects of their incorporation into oligonucleotides has been reported (Gupta et al., 2009). An analysis of the effect of single-base mismatches on excess electron transfer in DNA has been reported using phenothiazine-modified DNA (Ito et al., 2009). The authors were surprised to find that electron transfer was more efficient in duplexes containing a mismatch, possibly because the mismatch site enables electron injection or hopping beyond this site.

Synthetic methods of relevance to DNA and RNA chemistry continue to be developed (Lakshman & Frank, 2009, Kaloudis et al., 2009, Edwards et al., 2009, Ducatti et al., 2009 & Ohkubo et al., 2009).

The chemical biology of DNA quadruplexes continues to develop. The binding of ligands to the human telomeric repeat sequence (h-Tel) and the c-kit promoter has also been explored

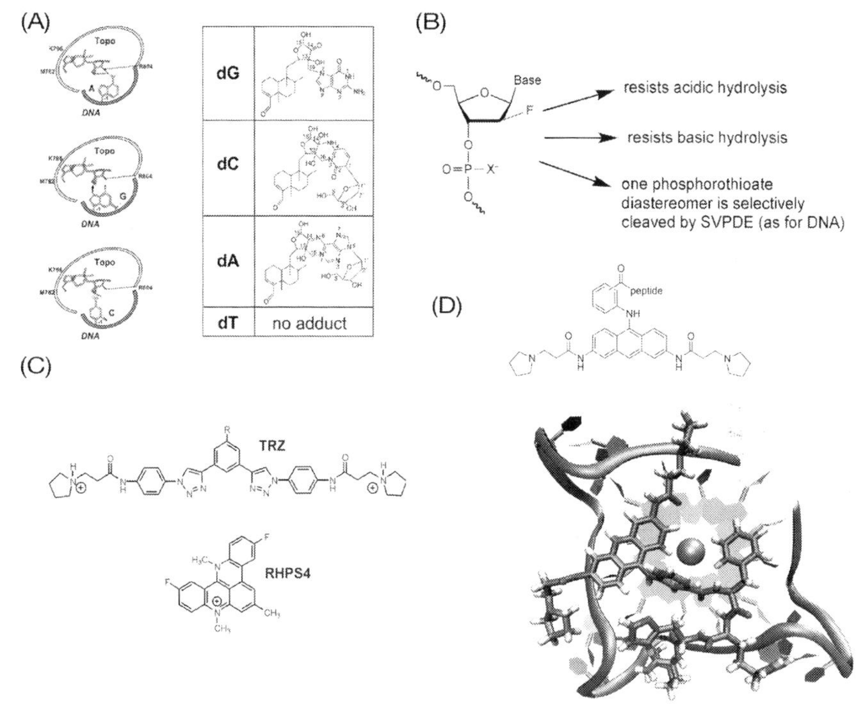

Fig. 4. (A) Schematic representation of clerocidin and dA or dG or dC mutual orientations within the DNA–topoisomerase cleavage complex (enzyme in blue, DNA in red) as suggested by docking experiments and table of the most abundant adducts formed by reaction of clerocidin with DNA deoxyribonucleosides (Richter et al., 2009). http://dx.doi.org/10.1039/b819049f (B) Structure of 2′-FANA and its reported properties (Katolik et al., 2009). http://dx.doi.org/10.1039/b900443b (C) Structures of the small molecule quadruplex binders TRZ and RHPS4 (Garner et al., 2009) http://dx.doi.org/10.1039/b910505k (D) General structure of 9-peptide acridine analogues synthesised and a representative model of a peptide-acridine conjugate docked to the parallel human telomeric quadruplex (Redman et al., 2009) http://dx.doi.org/10.1039/b814682a *Reproduced by permission of The Royal Society of Chemistry.*

by Moses and Searle using a range of techniques (Figure 4C) (Garner et al., 2009). Two different classes of h-Tel ligands were developed and showed selectivity for parallel or anti-parallel conformations respectively. This was rationalised due to the structural plasticity of h-Tel, a property that the c-kit quadruplex does not possess. Research variations in the ability of acridine-peptide conjugates to bind selectively to different DNA quadruplexes as a function of peptide sequence, substitution position on the acridine and the functional group at the C-terminus of the peptide have been investigated by Balasubramanian and Neidle (Figure 4D) (Redman et al., 2009). High degrees of selectivity for the N-ras quadruplex were achieved in some cases. An anti-parallel unimolecular G-quadruplex has been formed by a thrombin binding aptamer in the presence of ammonium ions (Trajkovski et al., 2009). Detailed structural information was gained by the use of solution-state NMR techniques when $15NH_4^+$ cation was used. The platination of human telomeric G-quadruplex has also been explored with the Pt-complexes showing interesting antiproliferative activity (Bertrand et al., 2009). The strength of binding of the Pt- complex to the quadruplexes increased as the aromatic surface area of the terpyridine-based ligand increased. The most strongly bound complex was shown to interact exclusively with the adenine nucleobases in the loop of the quadruplex. A novel potent and selective G-quadruplex ligand based on a trazatruxene core structure has been developed (Ginnari-Satriani et al., 2009). The ligand's anticancer activity has also been assessed.

The exploration of synthetic analogues of DNA has proved a popular area of study with reports on the development of both GNA (glycol nucleic acid) and PNA (peptide nucleic acid) appearing. Novel phosphoramidites that enable the incorporation of hydroxypyridone and pyridopurine homo- and hetero-base pairs into GNA have been prepared. Interestingly, these reagents were used in conjunction with automated GNA solid phase synthesis techniques to compare the metal binding capacity of the resulting GNA to the analogous DNA duplexes (Schlegel et al., 2009). GNA containing fluorescent nucleotides have also been prepared (Hui Zhou et al., 2009). A novel nucleobase known as PPT has been synthesised and incorporated into PNA (Hirano et al., 2009) and interesting studies on novel metal-containing PNAs have been reported (Sosniak et al., 2009). The introduction of a disulfide bond into the main chain of PNA enabled the facile removal of the PNA from its duplex and invasion complexes with DNA (Aiba & Komiyama, 2009). This was achieved following reduction of the disulfide linkage in the complexes leading to the formation of short PNA fragments. The ability of poly(*m*-phenylene) to act as an artificial helical polymer has been studied (Ben et al., 2009).

3.4 The study of bioactive compounds

Researchers interested in the identification, optimisation and study of bioactive compounds remain an important component of the chemical biology community. This is reflected in the number of papers published in this area. In an attempt to provide some structure to this large section of the review it has been split into sub-sections that cover reports on: (1) compound classes that exhibit antibacterial, antiviral, anticancer and other activities; (2) the synthesis, isolation and biosynthesis of natural products; (3) medicinal chemistry which includes studies on approaches to drug delivery and studies on the metabolism of bioactive compounds and (4) chemical genetics.

3.4.1 Bioactives

A large number of bioactive compounds with a range of activities were reported in OBC in 2009. Compounds with antibacterial activity included sulfone-based nucleotide isosteres which were shown to be inhibitors of CMP-sialic acid synthetase, an important enzyme in bacterial polysaccharide biosynthesis (Wong et al., 2009). By using mimics of the substrates and reaction intermediates of 3-deoxy-D-arabino-heptulosonate 7-phosphate (DAH7P) synthase, inhibition of this important bacterial enzyme was achieved (Walker et al., 2009). A synthesis of a library of 2,5-dihydrochorismate analogues has been described by Payne and Abell (Payne et al., 2009). Interestingly, differential activity against 4 different chorismate-utilising enzymes was observed (Scheme 5A). New antimicrobial peptides have also been reported (Mitra et al., 2009). These dipeptide-based amphiphiles exhibited inhibitory activity against a number of gram-positive and gram-negative bacteria. A solid phase synthesis of argifin, a cyclic pentapeptide chitinase inhibitor, was achieved by Eggleston and applied to the synthesis of a number of analogues (Figure 5B) (Dixon et al., 2009). This work highlighted the key peptide residues required to bind to the enzyme. Polyamide-based minor groove binders have been reported by Suckling to show antibacterial activity (Figure 5C) (Breen et al., 2009). The synthesis and biological evaluation of castanospermine and austriline analogues as glucosaminidase inhibitors has been achieved (Pluvinage et al., 2009). Porphyrin-linked nitroimidazole antibiotics have been found to be selective growth inhibitors of *Porphyromonas gingivalis*, a bacterium implicated in periodontal disease (Yap et al., 2009)and a novel triazolyl nucleoside, which acts as a nucleoside triphosphate mimic, was prepared as an ATP-competitive inhibitor of the pantothenate kinase of *B. Anthracis* (Rowan et al., 2009).

The anti-HIV activity of 2′,3′-didehydro-2′,3′-dideoxyuridine (d4U) and 2′,3′-dideoxyuridine (ddU) phosphoramidate derivatives (Mehellou et al., 2009) as well as a series of phosphonate terminated dendrimers have been evaluated (Perez-Anes et al., 2009). A set of hexahydroisobenzofuran nucleosides have been synthesised and tested as potential inhibitors of HIV-1 (Diaz-Rodriguez et al., 2009). One of these compounds had an EC_{50} of 12.3 μM and the activity was rationalised by comparison to the structure of the known HIV drug didanosine. 1,2,3-Triazole acyclonucleotides containing a difluoromethyl phosphonate group have been synthesised and are currently being investigated as potential nucleoside phosphorylase inhibitors (A. Diab et al., 2009). Amongst several possible applications, glycosidase inhibitors, such as a series of novel polyhydroxylated quinolizidines, (Kumari & Vankar, 2009) have been linked to antiviral drug development. Through the synthesis of a series of multivalent iminosugars, as inhibitors of glycosidases, it was demonstrated that the binding affinity and selectivity of glycosidase inhibition could be altered by multivalency (Diot et al., 2009). Ring modified castanospermine analogues have been evaluated as selective β-glucosidase inhibitors (Aguilar-Moncayo et al., 2009).

Potential anti-cancer compounds have been reported including a poly-THF spiroketal-containing compound which is active against both breast and ovarian cancer cell lines (Piccialli et al., 2009). Both enantiomers of (-)-cylindrocyclophane were synthesised and found to have very similar activities against the human colon cancer HCT-116 cells (Yamakoshi et al., 2009). Iron(III)-salen complexes were used to demonstrate that, somewhat surprisingly, the less DNA cleavage activity these compounds showed *in vitro*, the more efficient they were at inducing apoptosis in MCF7 cells (Ansari et al., 2009). Further evidence has been gathered to support the proposal that it is the quinone methide, formed by two electron reduction of prekinamycin, that is responsible for its cytostatic activity (Khdour & Skibo, 2009). A series of substituted thienopyrimidines have been synthesised and shown to be cytotoxic to a number of cancer cell lines (Snegaroff et al., 2009) and substituted *O*-galactosyl aldoximes were prepared as selective galectin-3 inhibitors (Tejler et al., 2009). Pyrrolidine 3,4-diols have been reported as α-L-fucosidase inhibitors (Moreno-Clavijo et al., 2009). A series of new pentacyclic analogues of BRACO-19, a DNA quadruplex binder, have been synthesised and evaluated for their DNA quadruplex binding affinities (Debray et al., 2009). A library of cyclic pentapeptides were synthesised as potential antagonists of CXCR4, a member of the G-protein coupled receptor family, which is implicated in many diseases including cancer (Tanaka et al., 2009). Redox catalysts containing selenium and tellurium have been designed and synthesised since compounds with the ability to alter the redox state in cells have potential anti-cancer activity (Mecklenburg et al., 2009). A number of the compounds prepared possess interesting biological activities.

In other areas, polyfunctionalised quinolizidine alkaloids were synthesised and some analogues were discovered to be potent and selective inhibitors of α-glucosidase with potential anti-diabetes applications (Pandey et al., 2009). Methodology was developed to prepare compounds containing a phenothiazine skeleton (Prasad & Sekar, 2009). This chemistry was illustrated by the synthesis of some anti-histamine agents. A study was carried out to identify selective inhibitors of the human dopamine transporter which did not inhibit the closely related human serotonin and norepinephrine transporters (Riss et al., 2009). Analogues of Salvinorin A have been synthesised and their affinities for the different opioid receptors determined (Simpson et al., 2009). A series of novel proteo-dendrimers, which inhibit apoptosis, have been reported and may be of use in the treatment of apoptosis mediated diseases (Azuma et al., 2009). A detailed study was carried out on Belactosin A, a cyclopropane containing tripeptidic proteasome inhibitor (Yoshida et al., 2009).

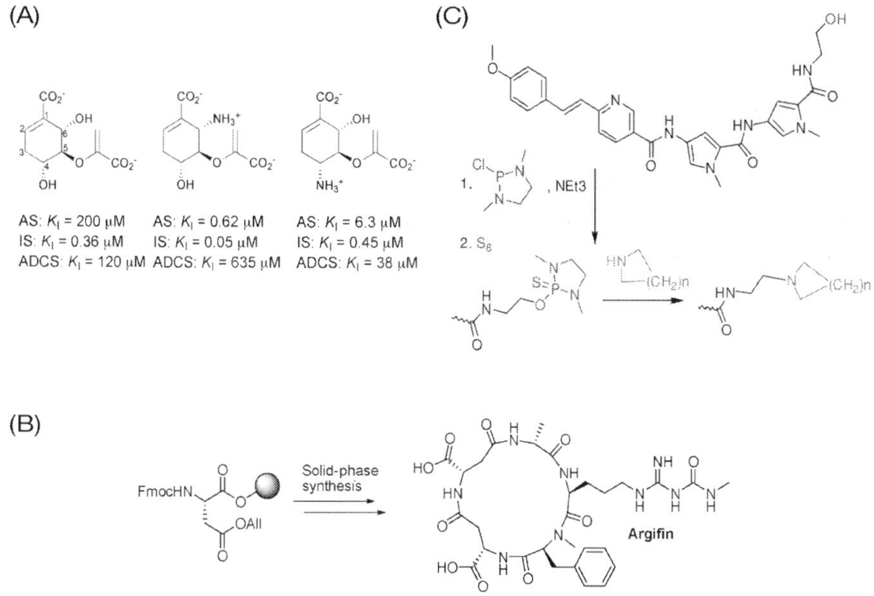

Fig. 5. (A) Inhibition constants for chorismate-utilising enzyme inhibitors (AS = *S. marcescens* anthranilate synthase, IS = *E. coli* isochorismate synthase and ADCS = *E. coli* ADC synthase) (Payne et al., 2009). http://dx.doi.org/10.1039/b901694e (B) General illustration of the solid phase synthesis of analogues of argifin. This approach enabled an assessment of the role of the various amino acids on the activity of the cyclic peptide as a chitinase inhibitor (Dixon et al., 2009). http://dx.doi.org/10.1039/b815077j (C) Synthesis of polyamide minor groove binders (Breen et al., 2009). http://dx.doi.org/10.1039/b814452d *Reproduced by permission of The Royal Society of Chemistry.*

A number of papers have been published on the synthesis of privileged chemical structures which are likely to be of relevance to the discovery of new biologically active molecules. A method for the regioselective synthesis of 1-phenyl pyrazoles, a fragment present in many bioactive compounds, has been reported (Ko et al., 2009). Since isoindolines have been shown to exhibit biological activities including the inhibition of COX-2, a new synthetic strategy for the synthesis of 1-aryl substituted isoindolines has been developed (Clary et al., 2009). An approach for the diversity-oriented synthesis of non-symmetrical malonate analogues has been reported since 2-alkyl and 2-arylmalonates have been shown to posses a wide range of biological activities including the inhibition of HIV-1 and -2 proteases (Ramachary et al., 2009). The synthesis of 3,5-diarylpyrazolines from readily available starting materials has been reported (Mahe et al., 2009). The ring closing metathesis of allyl-seleno compounds has been reported for the synthesis of bicyclic β-lactams containing selenium (Garud et al., 2009). Incorporation of the CF_3 group in a bioactive compound can have a dramatic effect on its properties. For this reason the synthesis of CF_3-substituted heterocyclic boronic acids and esters has been reported and their utility in the synthesis of novel pharmacophores has been demonstrated (Clapham et al., 2009). Using an intramolecular [3+2] azide-alkyne cycloaddition, a number of new heterocyclic core structures were obtained which may possess novel biological activities (R. Li et al., 2009). A novel one-pot cascade reaction of 2H-1,4-benzoxazin-3-(4H)-ones, a scaffold present in the enediyne antitumour antibiotics, has been reported (D. Chen et al., 2009). A series of C-8 arylated adenines have been synthesised using a new direct arylation methodology, which may be used for the synthesis of potential Hsp90 inhibitors (Sahnoun et al., 2009).

3.4.2 Natural products – isolation, synthesis and biosynthesis

The isolation, structural determination and chemical synthesis of natural products continue to be widely studied areas. The first total syntheses of many bioactive natural products was achieved in 2009 (Commeiras et al., 2009, Alvarez-Manzaneda et al., 2009, Alvarez-Manzaneda et al., 2009, Davis et al., 2009 & Ribes et al., 2009). The synthesis of novel aza-analogues of staurosporine, K-252a and rebeccamycin have also been reported (McCort-Tranchepain, 2009). Total syntheses and new approaches to the total synthesis of many other natural products have also been reported (Yi Li et al., 2009, Zhang et al., 2009, Garcia-Egido et al., 2009, Foster et al., 2009, Jiang & Hamada, 2009, Tang et al., 2009, Oh et al., 2009, Shing & Cheng, 2009, Poldy et al., 2009, Luo Yang et al., 2009, Ceccon et al., 2009, Coldham et al., 2009 & Ayats et al., 2009).

The isolation of several new natural products has also been achieved. Two new saponins from *Parthenium hysterophorus* were found to be potent TNF-α inhibitors (Shah et al., 2009). The successful isolation and structure determination of new cyclodepsipeptides has been reported (Zampella et al., 2009). These compounds, named homophymine B-E and A1-E1, were shown to exhibit potent anti-proliferative effects against several human cancer cell lines. Novel dihydro-β-agarofuran sesquiterpenes were isolated and several were shown to be anticancer multi-drug resistant reversal agents (Torres-Romero et al., 2009). Glycosylated analogues of versipelostatin, a GRP78/Bip molecular chaperone down regulator, were isolated (Zhao et al., 2009). It was concluded that the α-L-oleandropyranosyl(1→4)-β-D-digitoxopyranosyl residue of the sugar moiety may be the key feature required for this activity. Five new members of the actinomycin family of antibiotics, Y_1-Y_5, have been isolated (Bitzer et al., 2009). Their structures differ from the Z-type actinomycins and this was shown to affect their biological activities. By examining the structure of (-)-ternatin, an important fat-accumulation inhibitor, by NMR and CD spectroscopy, it was concluded that the β-turn structure is key to the observed inhibitory effect in 3T3-L1 murine adipocytes (Shimokawa et al., 2009). The full relative stereochemistry of 13,19-didesmethyl spirolide C has been assigned by analysis of NMR data and using computational methods (Ciminiello et al., 2009). The preferred conformation of this natural product was also studied and will provide useful information for studies on the mechanism of action of the spirolide class of natural products. The potent bioactivity and unusual structures of the *Garcinia* xanthones led to a study to assign the pharmacophore of this class of natural products (Figure 6A) (Chantarasriwong et al., 2009). Synthesis of various analogues and subsequent biological evaluation led to the conclusion that the ABC ring system with the caged structure of ring C is essential for the observed activity. Studies conducted with cluvenone, a member of this family, demonstrated that these compounds exhibit cytotoxicity in leukemia cells which are multi-drug resistant.

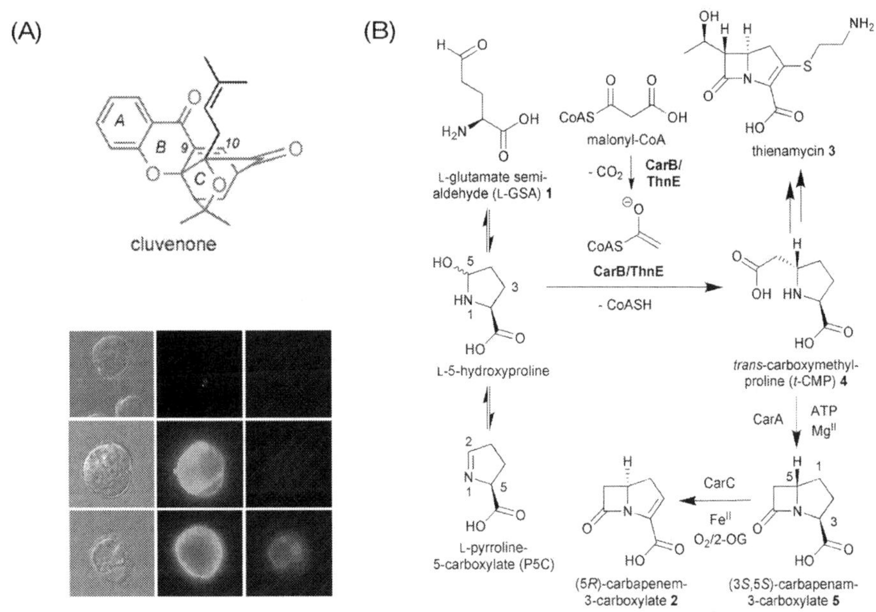

Fig. 6. (A) Structure of cluvenone and the demonstration of induction of apoptosis in HL-60/ADR cells by cluvenone visualised by differential interference contrast microscopy (left column) and fluorescence microscopy (middle and right columns). Control untreated cells are shown in the top row. Treated cells undergoing early and late stage apoptosis are shown in the middle and bottom rows respectively (Chantarasriwong et al., 2009) http://dx.doi.org/10.1039/b913496d (B) Outline of the proposed biosynthesis of the carbapenems. Detailed studies provided novel insights into the chemical transformation catalysed by CarB/ThnE (Ducho et al., 2009). http://dx.doi.org/10.1039/b903312b *Reproduced by permission of The Royal Society of Chemistry.*

Extending our understanding of the biosynthesis of natural products and hijacking these pathways to deliver novel compounds remain important sub-sections of chemical biology. Using labelling experiments it was demonstrated that pyrrolylpolyenes, fungal natural products from *Auxarthron umbrinum* are synthesised from proline, methionine, acetate and pyrrole-2-carboxylate (Clark & Murphy, 2009). The synthesis of key intermediates in several biosynthetic pathways has also been reported and the intermediates used to understand further these pathways. For example, studies on the biosynthesis of Fosfomycin, were carried out by supplementing the growth media with chemically synthesised hypothesised intermediates (McGrath et al., 2009). The synthesis of UDP-Glc-2,3-diNAcA, a key intermediate in the biosynthesis of cell surface polysaccharides, was accomplished and the compound used to study this process (Rejzek et al., 2009). Using synthesised glycosylated seco-iridoid steroisomers, the first steps in monoterpine indole alkaloid biosynthesis were studies (Bernhardt et al., 2009). The stereoselective synthesis of deuterated analogues of L-glutamate was accomplished by Schofield and the analogues used in a study on carbapenem biosynthesis (Figure 6B) (Ducho et al., 2009). A report on the first α-ketoglutarate-dependant dioxygenase with non-heme Fe(II) to catalyse the formation of an endoperoxide bond has appeared (Steffan et al., 2009). This enzyme was shown to convert fumitremorgin B to verruculogen by the insertion of an endoperoxide bond using both oxygen atoms of O_2. Examples of the synthesis of novel natural products by manipulating biosynthetic pathways include the preparation of a new fluorinated analogue of iturin A (Moran et al., 2009). By incubating *Bacillus subtilis* with 3-fluoro-L-tyrosine, this unnatural amino acid is incorporated in the product, replacing D-tyrosine. Since the activity of iturin A is dependent on this tyrosine residue the incorporation of this modified tyrosine may result in a change in its biological activity. Through the overexpression of biosynthetic genes encoding the first steps of the deoxyhexose biosynthetic pathway, TDP-L-olivose was obtained. This carbohydrate was then used as a substrate of spinosyn glycosyl transferase resulting in the synthesis of a novel sugar appended spinosyn analogue (Gaisser et al., 2009). A new chemical biology based approach, known as chemical epigenetics, involves the use of small molecule inhibitors of HDACs and DNA methyltransferases to activate selectively gene clusters that encode biosynthetic enzymes. A novel natural product, nygerone A was produced from the fungus *Aspergillus niger* using this approach (Henrikson et al., 2009).

3.4.3 Medicinal chemistry

Medicinal chemistry is an important and widely studied area of chemical biology. This area encompasses many research topics including drug metabolism, drug/gene delivery as well as detailed SAR studies on biologically active molecules with potential as drugs. The transacylation kinetics of acyl glucoronides (AGs) has been studied in detail (Berry et al., 2009). Since many non-steroidal anti-inflammatory drugs are metabolised as their AGs, this study highlights issues relating to the metabolism and pharmacokinetics of these well-known drugs. The thermal degradation of kynurenines was studied as these compounds may be important in cataract formation (Kopylova et al., 2009) and the synthesis of [1,3,5-$^{13}C_3$] gallic acid was completed for use as an internal standard for studies on the bioavailability and metabolism of tea catechins (Marshall et al., 2009).

A new pro-drug approach for the delivery of cytarabine, a potent anti-tumour agent, has been reported by Tanabe and Nishimoto (Figure 7A) (Hirata et al., 2009). This involved conjugating cytarabine with a 2-oxopropyl group which upon treatment with X-rays releases cytarabine by a one-electron reduction process. It was shown that by using this approach, the drug was released preferentially in hypoxic tumour cells leading to increased cytotoxicity. The intestinal peptide, PepT1, is capable of transporting thiodipeptide prodrugs and may be an interesting target for drug delivery applications (Foley et al., 2009; Foley et al., 2009). Amino acid-quinoline antibiotic conjugates are used as prodrugs for the delivery of the quinoline antibiotics. A new route for the synthesis of these conjugates has been reported (A. R. Katritzky et al., 2009). A "bio-oxidisable" pro-drug strategy has been reported for the delivery of new acetylcholinesterase inhibitors (Bohn et al., 2009) and a series of polyamine conjugated naphthalimides have been prepared to exploit the polyamine transporter for drug delivery (Tian et al., 2009). A novel method for the delivery of cytotoxic peptides into cells has been reported (Foillard et al., 2009). The method relies on the use of an RGA-containing scaffold which is anchored to the required peptide. It has also been demonstrated that a fluorescent peptide could be transported using this method allowing monitoring of its activity in cells. Modifying the structure of compounds to enable them to cross the blood-brain barrier remains a challenging area within medicinal chemistry. Recent work illustrated the ability of the 1,4-dihydroquinoline derivatives to cross the blood-brain barrier (Foucout et al., 2009). Rats were injected with radio-labelled 1,4-dihydroquinoline [^{11}C] and the level of radioactivity in their brains was studied. It was concluded that the [^{11}C] carrier was able to penetrate into the central nervous system (CNS). This concept was exemplified by conjugation of the carrier to GABA, a well-known neurotransmitter which is poor at crossing the blood-brain barrier. After injection in mice their locomotor activity was altered significantly, consistent with the expected effect of GABA once it has entered the CNS.

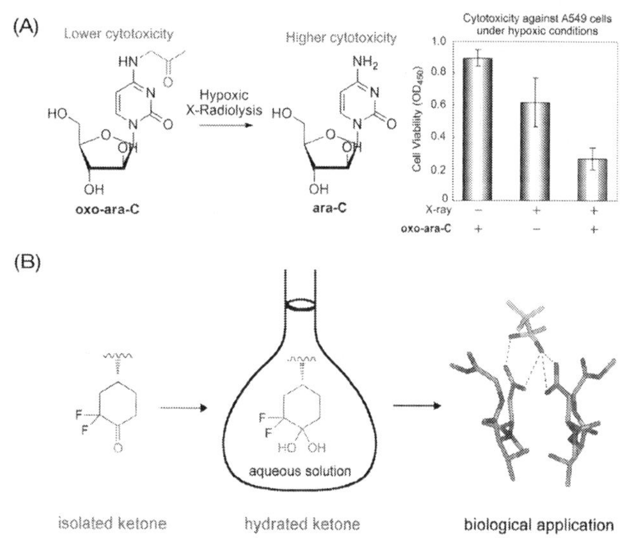

Fig. 7. (A) Cytarabine conjugated with a 2-oxopropyl group which upon treatment with X-rays releases cytarabine. The resulting cytotoxicity against A549 cells is also shown (Hirata et al., 2009) http://dx.doi.org/10.1039/b816194a (B) The structure of alicyclic α,α-difluoroketone hydrates and one of the known binding modes for this structural class of inhibitors in aspartic proteases (Fah et al., 2009). http://dx.doi.org/10.1039/b908489d *Reproduced by permission of The Royal Society of Chemistry.*

Kinases remain an important target in medicinal chemistry and several reports focus on the discovery and/or optimisation of kinase inhibitors. A novel irreversible inhibitor of EGFR tyrosine kinase has been identified (Ban et al., 2009). A series of bisubstrate inhibitors of the Abelson tyrosine kinase, a kinase implicated in CML, has been identified with some of the inhibitors being as potent as the drug Imatinib against this target (Kalesh et al., 2009).

Several examples of research on parasite-derived diseases have been published. SAR studies on the use of a melamine core structure have been reported (Baliani et al., 2009). This structural component exploits the plasma membrane transporters in trypanosomes to transport potent compounds anchored to the core selectively into the parasite. Many compounds demonstrated very promising activity *in vitro*. Diversity-oriented synthesis was used in the synthesis of fused pyrimidine analogues (Gibson et al., 2009). The compounds were tested against pteridine reductases from protozoan parasites and several were found to be active. SAR studies revealed the key structural components required for inhibition. A study by Diederich on the inhibition of plasmepsins, an important target for the treatment of drug resistant forms of malaria, has identified novel alicyclic α,α-difluoroketone hydrates as micromolar inhibitors of isoforms II and IV (Figure 7B) (Fah et al., 2009). Novel SF_5-containing analogues of mefloquine, an anti-malarial, were synthesised and shown to possess both increased selectivity and potency against various malaria-causing parasites (Wipf et al., 2009). A series of inhibitors of protein farnesyltransferase, an important target in both anti-cancer and anti-parasitic fields were also synthesised (Kerherve et al., 2009). Click chemistry was used efficiently in the synthesis of 3-(1,2,3-triazol-1-yl)- and 3(-1,2,3-triazol-4-yl)-substituted pyrazolo[3,4-d] pyrimidin-4-amines (Klein et al., 2009). Two of these compounds were shown to exhibit activity against *Plasmodium falciparum* PfPK7 kinase. These compounds may prove to be interesting lead compounds for the treatment of the most virulent form of malaria.

Known drugs continue to provide a source of inspiration. For example, pyridine and pyrimidine analogues of acetaminophen have been prepared as novel cyclooxygenase inhibitors (Nam et al., 2009). The anthracycline antibiotics are clinically used cancer chemotherapeutics but drug resistance has become an issue and they are known to be cardiotoxic. With this in mind, a new series of glycosylated anthracycline mimics have been synthesised to overcome these problems (Shi et al., 2009). Synthesis of a range of Nefopam analogues was accomplished in a three-step process (Ramachary et al., 2009). Phospha-oseltamivir conjugates were synthesised and used to study influenza neuraminidases (Carbain et al., 2009). Since the 1,4-benzodiazepine moiety is present in well-known drugs such as Valium and Xanax, a study on the synthesis of novel 1,4-benzodiazepin-3-ones was carried out (Pettersson & Bergman, 2009). Novel Milnacipran derivatives were synthesised as potential anti-depressants (Vervisch et al., 2009).

New photosensitizer agents for use in photodynamic therapy (PDT), have also been reported including a novel series of hydrophilic conjugated porphyrin dimers (Balaz et al., 2009). This series has shown very promising results, including good uptake by cells, strong absorption in the necessary range, good photostability and excellent efficiency of generation of singlet oxygen (Kuimova et al., 2009). Importantly, the conjugates are more effective at killing human ovarian adenocarcinoma cells, under both one- and two-photon activation, than the clinically used photosensitisor Visudyne® (Dahlstedt et al., 2009). New glucosylated zinc (II) phthalocyanines have been reported as potential photosensitisor agents (J-Y. Liu et al., 2009). The anti-microbial activity of a 2-aminoimidazole-triazole conjugate, a known biofilm dispersal agent, in combination with a photodynamic inactivation (PDI) agent has been demonstrated (Rogers et al., 2009). This combination of PDI and a biofilm dispersal agent was shown to have a synergistic effect and could be used to control colonisation of drug resistant bacteria.

The design of transfection aids to enable gene therapy is currently a well-studied topic. Elongation of long chain saturated fatty acids (greater than C18) led to increased transfection of cationic lipids, leading to novel compounds with promising transfection abilities (Liberska et al., 2009). Click chemistry was used for the synthesis of β-cyclodextrans as potential systems for gene delivery (Mendez-Ardoy et al., 2009) and the synthesis of poly-6-cationic amphiphilic cyclodextrins has been reported for the same purpose (Byrne et al., 2009). Biotinylated disulfide containing polyethyleneimine was conjugated to avidin to give a novel gene vector which was shown to have high transfection efficacy in HepG2 cells (Zeng et al., 2009). Research has also been ongoing on the use of dendrimers for gene delivery. New carbosilane dendrimers which are capable of acting as dual carriers for therapeutic and imaging agents have been described (Ortega et al., 2009). Small dendritic structures, that are unable to transfect on their own, have been shown to increase the levels of transfection when used in combination with Lipofectamine 2000™, a cationic vector (Hardy et al., 2009).

An analogue of the trisaccharide repeating unit of *Streptococcus pneumonia* capsular polysaccharide was prepared and shown to exhibit similar biological activities to the natural carbohydrate but with increased stability to hydrolysis making it a promising compound for vaccine development (Legnani et al., 2009).

3.4.4 Chemical genetics

The development and use of chemical tools to study biological processes is often referred to as chemical genetics. Papers covering several aspects of the chemical genetic approach appeared in OBC in 2009. Here we focus initially on the synthesis of novel compound collections for use in chemical genetics. The high-throughput synthesis of an azide library for use in "click" reactions was reported (Srinivasan et al., 2009). A small library of novel spiroacetal-containing nucleosides was synthesised which may possess novel bioactivities (Choi & Brimble, 2009). 24- and 48-well silicon carbide plates were evaluated for their use in library synthesis by microwave irridation (Stencel et al., 2009). Libraries of biaryls, 1,4-dihydropyridines and *N*-aryl functionalised β-amino esters were successfully prepared in 48-well plates using this approach. A route to 3,5-isoxazole sulfonamides and sulfonate esters has been developed which will allow access to a diverse library of substituted isoxazole analogues in the future (Lee et al., 2009). A review describing various methods of generating dynamic combinatorial libraries was published which also discussed the utility of these libraries (Herrmann, 2009).

Work carried out in our own lab, in collaboration with researchers at the University of Vermont, is focused on the discovery of novel tools to advance understanding of the important process of host cell invasion by the parasite *Toxoplasma gondii*. We reported the identification of a novel inhibitor of this process, Conoidin A (Haraldsen et al., 2009). Attempts to identify the protein target(s) of Conoidin A led us to evaluate the *T.gondii* protein peroxiredoxin II (TgPrxII) as a possible target. Whilst the use of a TgPrxII knock-out parasites suggested that this was not the relevant target, studies with the purified protein confirmed that Conoidin A was a novel inhibitor of this enzyme. Further studies on the mode of inhibition of TgPrxII by Conoidin A and some novel analogues have also been reported by us recently (G. Liu et al., 2010). Our collaborative team has also focused on the use of the yeast-3-hybrid system for the identification of potential protein targets of small molecules (Walton et al., 2009). In the first report in this series we have described the synthesis and preliminary characterisation of a chemical inducer of dimerisation (CID) based on a *T.gondii* invasion inhibitor. In another approach to protein target identification an affinity matrix derived from the dimeric membrane phospholipid, cardiolipin, was synthesised (Johns et al., 2009). The resulting matrix was used to identify possible protein targets. The synthesis and biological assessment of a set of four stereoisomers of coranatine, a natural phytotoxin, has advanced understanding of the interesting process of stomatal opening in plant guard cells (Okada et al., 2009). In another study involving plant biology, a new family of stringolactone analogues were synthesised and found to promote germination in *Orobanche* seeds (Bhattacharya et al., 2009). 4α-Bromo-5α-cholestan-3β-ol and nor-5α-cholestan-3β-ol derivatives were synthesised and used to study the *in vivo* metabolism of cholesterol through feeding experiments (R. Martin et al., 2009). A series of (25*R*)-cholesten-26-oic acids were synthesised and evaluated as ligands for the hormonal receptor DAF-12.(R. Martin et al., 2009). The synthesis and biological characterisation of novel SAM mimetics has also been reported by Nelson (Joce et al., 2009). The ability of these ligands to promote the binding of the *E.coli* methionine repressor (MetJ) to its operator DNA was explored leading to a deeper understanding of this process (Scheme 8A). The synthesis of mannosyl glycolipids containing perfluoroalkyl membrane anchors has also been reported by Webb and Flitsch (Noble et al., 2009). When studies were carried out in vesicles, the lipids either dispersed or formed artificial rafts in the absence or presence of choleseterol respectively (Scheme 8B). More detailed studies using these new tools led the authors to question current thinking about the preorganisation of glycolipids in lipid rafts.

4. Emerging areas

We finish this review with two sections that, we believe, reflect the ability of chemical biology to impact in new areas that fall outside the traditional areas discussed in the preceding section. It is this continuing desire for researchers in the chemical biology community to ask new and interesting questions that makes the field so vibrant and exciting. The final paper in the chemical genetics section highlights one very interesting and relatively new area - the chemical biology of natural and artificial membranes. The final section describes innovations that have been reported as research in chemical biology merges into biotechnology.

4.1 The chemical biology of membranes

The synthesis of various artificial membranes and ion channels has been described. A novel family of phosphate-linked cyclic oligosaccharides for use as synthetic ionophores has been reported (Licen et al., 2009). Solid phase chemistry was used to prepare novel linear tetra- and penta-ester ion channels (Fyles & Luong, 2009). In a follow-up paper the authors describe the ion transport activity of the synthesised channels (Fyles & Luong, 2009). A report on the synthesis of a new ion channel containing redox active ferrocine has also appeared (Tsikolia et al., 2009). This channel was shown to be capable of transporting both Na^+ and K^+ ions. Amphiphilic zinc porphyrins have been incorporated into liposomal bilayer membranes (Murakami et al., 2009).

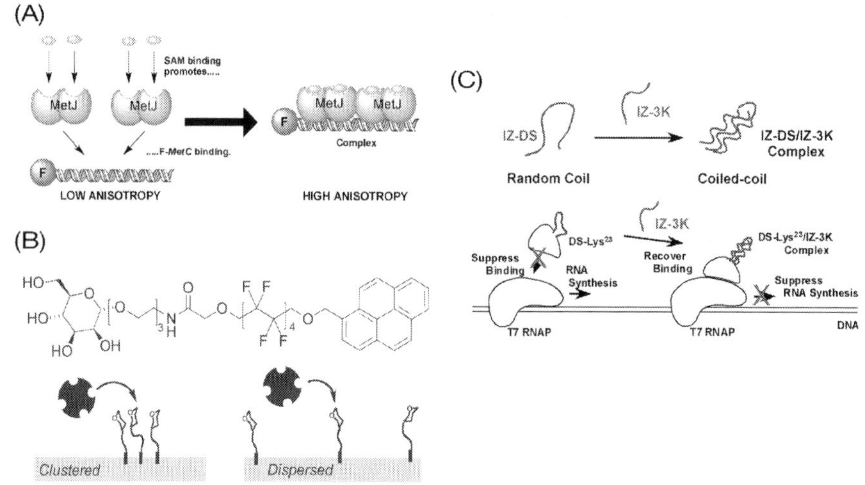

Fig. 8. (A) Cartoon illustrating the fluorescence anisotropy assay. Binding of SAM molecules promotes formation of a SAM-*F-metC*-protein complex, with two MetJ dimers bound to the 18 base-pair DNA duplex (Joce et al., 2009) http://dx.doi.org/10.1039/b816495a (B) Binding of multivalent lectins to mannosylated lipids that are in artificial "lipid rafts" or dispersed over the bilayer surface could change the lateral distribution of these lipids but increasing the distance between the surface and the mannosyl group may facilitate chelation of the multivalent lectin (Noble et al., 2009) http://dx.doi.org/10.1039/b910976e (C) Schematic illustration of the ligand-induced switch that turns off DNA synthesis (Mizuno et al., 2009). http://dx.doi.org/10.1039/b901118h *Reproduced by permission of The Royal Society of Chemistry.*

4.2 From chemical biology to biotechnology

The synthetic accessibility of DNA continues to inspire novel applications in biotechnology. For example, a 2D-DNA nanoarray has been constructed in which different metal complexes are positioned at regular intervals (Ghosh et al., 2009). Nucleobases and nucleoside end capped structures have been incorporated into novel compounds of relevance to the synthesis of molecular tectons for new types of porous solids (Schindler et al., 2009). Novel tectons have also been accessed using click chemistry (Plietzsch et al., 2009). In this case self-complementary DNA chains were incorporated in the tectons. The combination of novel acridinium esters with methyl red has provided a new high sensitivity ligand binding assay format that has been applied to the study of nucleic acid hybridisation (R. C. Brown et al., 2009). A novel detection system has been used to identify a single nucleotide difference on the leukemia-related *bcr/abl* gene (Furukawa et al., 2009). The system takes advantage of a new fluorogenic naphthorhodamine ligand that is reduced when it finds itself in close proximity to a DNA strand ending in triphenylphosphine. This reduction-trigger leads to the reduced ligand fluorescing at 650 nm. A DNase 1 resistant molecular beacon has been synthesised using a benzene-phosphate backbone at its stem (Ueno et al., 2009).

Changes in pH have been used as a trigger to control a gold nanoparticle–peptide interaction (Wagner et al., 2009). Only when the peptide adopts a helical conformation was the nanoparticle able to bind. The synthesis of novel bionanomaterials has been advanced through the use of repeating units of an amyloidogenic peptide derived from the Alzheimer Aβ sequence (van Dijk et al., 2009). The heteromeric self-assembly of gp27-gp5, proteins from the bacteriophage T4, has been used to generate novel bionanomaterials in which the position of fluorescent probes is controlled (Koshiyama et al., 2009). The incorporation of a negatively charged polyelectrolyte within the capsid of the cowpea chlorotic mottle virus has been reported (Minten et al., 2009). The resulting monodisperse 18 nm particles had novel redox properties. The switching of a random coil module, engineered into a protein (T7) lysozyme, to a coiled-coil on addition of a peptide ligand has been used to investigate the effect of the induced structural change on binding of T7 lysozyme to T7 RNAP (Figure 8C) (Mizuno et al., 2009). This system was characterised by studying the effect of the peptide on RNA synthesis. Genetic engineering of the heme binding pocket in human serum albumin has led to the identification of a crucial triad of amino acids at the entrance to the pocket (Komatsu et al., 2009). With the goal of understanding better the role that adhesion and aggregation of cells plays in tissue organisation and growth, detailed studies using large unilamellar vesicles as models for cells have been carried out (Feng & Otto, 2009). An interesting report on novel methods of fingerprint protection has been published (Plater et al., 2009) and decaging methodology has been applied to TRPV1 agonists and antagonists (Van Ryssen et al., 2009).

5. Conclusion

The purpose of this chapter has been to explore at the grass roots level the types of research that currently fall under the chemical biology umbrella and to assess which of these are of potential relevance to the drug discovery process. It is clear that chemical biology is a broad church but it remains important that a clear definition is developed of what research in this field involves. An excellent way to help the greater scientific community comprehend the benefits that chemical biology provides and the challenges it faces, is to consult the established experts in the field. A recent review (Altmann et al., 2009) and a series of excellent books (Schreiber & Kapoor, 2007; Begley, 2009; Bunnage, 2010) have achieved this. Here we take a complementary approach by reviewing the papers that were published in chemical biology in OBC in 2009. We have structured our review to emphasise: i) that chemical biology is built on a core set of research techniques and reagents and that the continued development of these skills and tools is essential; ii) that there remain 4 main areas that the term chemical biology encompasses but the boundaries between these areas are increasingly blurred as the field advances and iii) that new areas are emerging within chemical biology.

Figure 9 shows a breakdown of the 339 papers we reviewed as a function of the category we placed the research in. We believe that several important trends arise from this analysis:

1. The category termed bioactives appears of most direct relevance to drug discovery. It describes research towards novel anti-bacterials, -virals, -parisitics and anticancer agents. It also includes examples of the development of pro-drugs, metabolism studies, advances in photodynamic therapy and transfection reagents for gene therapy.
2. Developments in the synthesis of privileged chemical structures and studies on natural products remain common and, with chemical genetics, have a clear link to drug discovery.
3. The discovery of novel reagents and techniques in analytic aspects of chemical biology, including imaging, are a major focus of the community and this area is developing rapidly. These studies are rapidly enhancing our ability to probe the environment inside cells and this will impact on cell biology studies aimed at defining the function of bioactives.

4. There is considerable interest in the synthesis and analysis of chemical structures that fall outside conventional chemical space including purity assessment of biologics, synthesis and analysis of cyclic peptides and peptoids, carbohydrates and the study of modified DNA, GNA and PNA.
5. The chemical biology community continues to push forward our understanding of how biological systems function through fundamental studies on proteins (eg. enzyme function), carbohydrates and DNA/RNA (eg. DNA quadruplexes). Advances in the analysis of post-translational modifications and the labelling of proteins will also be of importance in this area.
6. What is certain is that the chemical biology community will not stand still and the recent interest in both membrane (chemical) biology as well as the increasing focus on biotechnological applications (particularly of DNA-based or DNA-inspired systems) reflects this. Information on understudied areas of biology and on new technologies may turn out to be of great relevance to drug discovery.

Whilst we, as academic researchers, are probably not the best people to judge which flavour of chemical biology will have the greatest impact on drug discovery, we hope this chapter helps people as they think about its future and the role that chemical biology has to play in it.

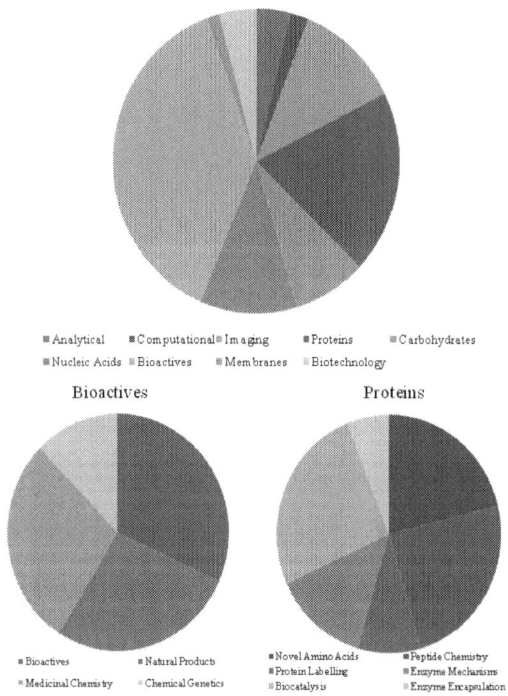

Fig. 9. Numbers of chemical biology papers published in the RSC journal *Organic and Biomolecular Chemistry* in 2009 as a function of category paper was assigned to. A key detailing the various categories is provided above. A breakdown of the two major categories of protein research and bioactives is also given.

6. Acknowledgments

We would like to thank the Royal Society (NJW fellowship), SULSA (LP PhD funding) and CRUK (LP PhD funding) for financial support. We would also like to thank the Royal Society of Chemistry for their permission to use figures taken directly from their journal.

7. References

Aguilar-Moncayo, M., Gloster, T. M., et al. (2009). *Organic & Biomolecular Chemistry* Vol. 7, No. 13, 2738-2747.

Aiba, Y.&Komiyama, M. (2009). *Organic & Biomolecular Chemistry* Vol. 7, No. 24, 5078-5083.

Altevogt, D., Hrenn, A., et al. (2009). *Organic & Biomolecular Chemistry* Vol. 7, No. 19, 3934-3939.

Altmann, K.-H., Buchner, J., et al. (2009). *ChemBioChem* Vol. 10, No. 1, 16-29.

Alvarez-Manzaneda, E., Chahboun, R., et al. (2009). *Organic & Biomolecular Chemistry* Vol. 7, No. 24, 5146-5155.

Amel Diab, S., Hienzch, A., et al. (2009). *Organic & Biomolecular Chemistry* Vol. 7, No. 21, 4481-4490.

Anderl, T., Audouard, C., et al. (2009). *Organic & Biomolecular Chemistry* Vol. 7, No. 24, 5200-5206.

Andersson, A. S., Diederich, F., et al. (2009). *Organic & Biomolecular Chemistry* Vol. 7, No. 17, 3474-3480.

Andre, S., Velasco-Torrijos, T., et al. (2009). *Organic & Biomolecular Chemistry* Vol. 7, No. 22, 4715-4725.

Ansari, K. I., Grant, J. D., et al. (2009). *Organic & Biomolecular Chemistry* Vol. 7, No. 5, 926-932.

Audouard, C., Bettaney, K., et al. (2009). *Organic & Biomolecular Chemistry* Vol. 7, No. 8, 1573-1582.

Avrutina, O., Empting, M., et al. (2009). *Organic & Biomolecular Chemistry* Vol. 7, No. 20, 4177-4185.

Ayats, C., Soley, R., et al. (2009). *Organic & Biomolecular Chemistry* Vol. 7, No. 5, 860-862.

Azuma, H., Yoshida, Y., et al. (2009). *Organic & Biomolecular Chemistry* Vol. 7, No. 8, 1700-1704.

Balaz, M., Collins, H. A., et al. (2009). *Organic & Biomolecular Chemistry* Vol. 7, No. 5, 874-888.

Baliani, A., Peal, V., et al. (2009). *Organic & Biomolecular Chemistry* Vol. 7, No. 6, 1154-1166.

Ban, H. S., Usui, T., et al. (2009). *Organic & Biomolecular Chemistry* Vol. 7, No. 21, 4415-4427.

Barge, A., Cappelletti, E., et al. (2009). *Organic & Biomolecular Chemistry* Vol. 7, No. 18, 3810-3816.

Basso, A., Banfi, L., et al. (2009). *Organic & Biomolecular Chemistry* Vol. 7, No. 2, 253-258.

Bedford, R. B., Haddow, M. F., et al. (2009). *Organic & Biomolecular Chemistry* Vol. 7, No. 15, 3119-3127.

Begley, T. P. (2009). *Wiley Encyclopedia of Chemical Biology*, Wiley.

Belen Cid, M., Alfonso, F., et al. (2009). *Organic & Biomolecular Chemistry* Vol. 7, No. 7, 1471-1481.

Belousoff, M. J., Graham, B., et al. (2009). *Organic & Biomolecular Chemistry* Vol. 7, No. 1, 30-33.

Ben, T., Furusho, Y., et al. (2009). *Organic & Biomolecular Chemistry* Vol. 7, No. 12, 2509-2512.

Berini, C., Pelloux-Leon, N., et al. (2009). *Organic & Biomolecular Chemistry* Vol. 7, No. 21, 4512-4516.

Bernhardt, P., Yerkes, N., et al. (2009). *Organic & Biomolecular Chemistry* Vol. 7, No. 20, 4166-4168.

Berry, N. G., Iddon, L., et al. (2009). *Organic & Biomolecular Chemistry* Vol. 7, No. 12, 2525-2533.

Bertrand, H., Bombard, S., et al. (2009). *Organic & Biomolecular Chemistry* Vol. 7, No. 14, 2864-2871.

Bhattacharya, C., Bonfante, P., et al. (2009). *Organic & Biomolecular Chemistry* Vol. 7, No. 17, 3413-3420.

Bitzer, J., Streibel, M., et al. (2009). *Organic & Biomolecular Chemistry* Vol. 7, No. 3, 444-450.

Blanco, O., Pato, C., et al. (2009). *Organic & Biomolecular Chemistry* Vol. 7, No. 11, 2310-2321.

Blaser, G., Sanderson, J. M., et al. (2009). *Organic & Biomolecular Chemistry* Vol. 7, No. 24, 5119-5128.

Bode, C. A., Bechet, T., et al. (2009). *Organic & Biomolecular Chemistry* Vol. 7, No. 17, 3391-3399.

Bohn, P., Le Fur, N., et al. (2009). *Organic & Biomolecular Chemistry* Vol. 7, No. 12, 2612-2618.

Bonnet, C. S., Massue, J., et al. (2009). *Organic & Biomolecular Chemistry* Vol. 7, No. 15, 3074-3078.

Borsenberger, V., Kukwikila, M., et al. (2009). *Organic & Biomolecular Chemistry* Vol. 7, No. 18, 3826-3835.

Boutureira, O., McGouran, J. F., et al. (2009). *Organic & Biomolecular Chemistry* Vol. 7, No. 20, 4285-4288.

Bragnier, N., Guillot, R., et al. (2009). *Organic & Biomolecular Chemistry* Vol. 7, No. 19, 3918-3921.

Breen, D., Kennedy, A. R., et al. (2009). *Organic & Biomolecular Chemistry* Vol. 7, No. 1, 178-186.

Brivio, M., Schlosrich, J., et al. (2009). *Organic & Biomolecular Chemistry* Vol. 7, No. 7, 1368-1373.

Brown, L. J., Ma, N., et al. (2009). *Organic & Biomolecular Chemistry* Vol. 7, No. 3, 564-575.

Brown, R. C., Li, Z., et al. (2009). *Organic & Biomolecular Chemistry* Vol. 7, No. 2, 386-394.

Bunnage, M. E. (2010). *New Frontiers in Chemical Biology*, RSC Publishing.

Butterfield, S. M., Hennig, A., et al. (2009). *Organic & Biomolecular Chemistry* Vol. 7, No. 9, 1784-1792.

Byrne, C., Sallas, F., et al. (2009). *Organic & Biomolecular Chemistry* Vol. 7, No. 18, 3763-3771.

Caiazzo, A., Garcia, P. M. L., et al. (2009). *Organic & Biomolecular Chemistry* Vol. 7, No. 14, 2926-2932.

Cao, H., Li, Y., et al. (2009). *Organic & Biomolecular Chemistry* Vol. 7, No. 24, 5137-5145.

Caravano, A., Field, R. A., et al. (2009). *Organic & Biomolecular Chemistry* Vol. 7, No. 5, 996-1008.

Carbain, B., Martin, S. R., et al. (2009). *Organic & Biomolecular Chemistry* Vol. 7, No. 12, 2570-2575.

Ceccon, J., Danoun, G., et al. (2009). *Organic & Biomolecular Chemistry* Vol. 7, No. 10, 2029-2031.

Chantarasriwong, O., Cho, W. C., et al. (2009). *Organic & Biomolecular Chemistry* Vol. 7, No. 23, 4886-4894.

Chen, D., Shen, G., et al. (2009). *Organic & Biomolecular Chemistry* Vol. 7, No. 19, 4067-4073.

Chen, Y.-W., Rick, J., et al. (2009). *Organic & Biomolecular Chemistry* Vol. 7, No. 3, 488-494.

Cheng, J.&Hoshino, T. (2009). *Organic & Biomolecular Chemistry* Vol. 7, No. 8, 1689-1699.

Choi, K. W.&Brimble, M. A. (2009). *Organic & Biomolecular Chemistry* Vol. 7, No. 7, 1424-1436.

Chwalek, M., Auzely, R., et al. (2009). *Organic & Biomolecular Chemistry* Vol. 7, No. 8, 1680-1688.
Ciminiello, P., Catalanotti, B., et al. (2009). *Organic & Biomolecular Chemistry* Vol. 7, No. 18, 3674-3681.
Clapham, K. M., Batsanov, A. S., et al. (2009). *Organic & Biomolecular Chemistry* Vol. 7, No. 10, 2155-2161.
Clark, B. R.&Murphy, C. D. (2009). *Organic & Biomolecular Chemistry* Vol. 7, No. 1, 111-116.
Clary, K. N., Parvez, M., et al. (2009). *Organic & Biomolecular Chemistry* Vol. 7, No. 6, 1226-1230.
Cline, L. L.&Waters, M. L. (2009). *Organic & Biomolecular Chemistry* Vol. 7, No. 22, 4622-4630.
Coldham, I., Jana, S., et al. (2009). *Organic & Biomolecular Chemistry* Vol. 7, No. 8, 1674-1679.
Commeiras, L., Thibonnet, J., et al. (2009). *Organic & Biomolecular Chemistry* Vol. 7, No. 3, 425-427.
Conroy, T., Jolliffe, K. A., et al. (2009). *Organic & Biomolecular Chemistry* Vol. 7, No. 11, 2255-2258.
Crepin, A., Wattier, N., et al. (2009). *Organic & Biomolecular Chemistry* Vol. 7, No. 1, 128-134.
Dahlstedt, E., Collins, H. A., et al. (2009). *Organic & Biomolecular Chemistry* Vol. 7, No. 5, 897-904.
Darley, D. J., Butler, D. S., et al. (2009). *Organic & Biomolecular Chemistry* Vol. 7, No. 3, 543-552.
Davis, F. A., Song, M., et al. (2009). *Organic & Biomolecular Chemistry* Vol. 7, No. 24, 5067-5073.
De Cola, C., Licen, S., et al. (2009). *Organic & Biomolecular Chemistry* Vol. 7, No. 14, 2851-2854.
de Hoog, H. M., Nallani, M., et al. (2009). *Organic & Biomolecular Chemistry* Vol. 7, No. 22, 4604-4610.
Debray, J., Zeghida, W., et al. (2009). *Organic & Biomolecular Chemistry* Vol. 7, No. 24, 5219-5228.
Deska, J.&Backvall, J.-E. (2009). *Organic & Biomolecular Chemistry* Vol. 7, No. 17, 3379-3381.
Dhenin, S. G. Y., Moreau, V., et al. (2009). *Organic & Biomolecular Chemistry* Vol. 7, No. 24, 5184-5199.
Diaz-Rodriguez, A., Sanghvi, Y. S., et al. (2009). *Organic & Biomolecular Chemistry* Vol. 7, No. 7, 1415-1423.
Didier, P., Ulrich, G., et al. (2009). *Organic & Biomolecular Chemistry* Vol. 7, No. 18, 3639-3642.
Diot, J., Garcia-Moreno, M. I., et al. (2009). *Organic & Biomolecular Chemistry* Vol. 7, No. 2, 357-363.
Dixon, M. J., Nathubhai, A., et al. (2009). *Organic & Biomolecular Chemistry* Vol. 7, No. 2, 259-268.
Drewry, J. A., Fletcher, S., et al. (2009). *Organic & Biomolecular Chemistry* Vol. 7, No. 24, 5074-5077.
Ducatti, D. R. B., Massi, A., et al. (2009). *Organic & Biomolecular Chemistry* Vol. 7, No. 9, 1980-1986.
Ducatti, D. R. B., Massi, A., et al. (2009). *Organic & Biomolecular Chemistry* Vol. 7, No. 3, 576-588.
Ducho, C., Hamed, R. B., et al. (2009). *Organic & Biomolecular Chemistry* Vol. 7, No. 13, 2770-2779.
Dumartin, M.-L., Givelet, C., et al. (2009). *Organic & Biomolecular Chemistry* Vol. 7, No. 13, 2725-2728.

Edwards, W. F., Young, D. D., et al. (2009). *Organic & Biomolecular Chemistry* Vol. 7, No. 12, 2506-2508.
Elsinghorst, P. W., Hartig, W., et al. (2009). *Organic & Biomolecular Chemistry* Vol. 7, No. 19, 3940-3946.
Escudier, J.-M., Dupouy, C., et al. (2009). *Organic & Biomolecular Chemistry* Vol. 7, No. 16, 3251-3257.
Fabris, F., Collins, J., et al. (2009). *Organic & Biomolecular Chemistry* Vol. 7, No. 12, 2619-2627.
Fah, C., Hardegger, L. A., et al. (2009). *Organic & Biomolecular Chemistry* Vol. 7, No. 19, 3947-3957.
Feau, C., Klein, E., et al. (2009). *Organic & Biomolecular Chemistry* Vol. 7, No. 24, 5259-5270.
Feng, G.&Otto, S. (2009). *Organic & Biomolecular Chemistry* Vol. 7, No. 20, 4289-4295.
Fernandez-Tejada, A., Corzana, F., et al. (2009). *Organic & Biomolecular Chemistry* Vol. 7, No. 14, 2885-2893.
Foillard, S., Dumy, P., et al. (2009). *Organic & Biomolecular Chemistry* Vol. 7, No. 20, 4159-4162.
Foillard, S., Sancey, L., et al. (2009). *Organic & Biomolecular Chemistry* Vol. 7, No. 2, 221-224.
Foley, D., Bailey, P., et al. (2009). *Organic & Biomolecular Chemistry* Vol. 7, No. 6, 1064-1067.
Foley, D., Pieri, M., et al. (2009). *Organic & Biomolecular Chemistry* Vol. 7, No. 18, 3652-3656.
Foster, R. S., Huang, J., et al. (2009). *Organic & Biomolecular Chemistry* Vol. 7, No. 19, 4052-4056.
Foucout, L., Gourand, F., et al. (2009). *Organic & Biomolecular Chemistry* Vol. 7, No. 18, 3666-3673.
Fowler, L. S., Ellis, D., et al. (2009). *Organic & Biomolecular Chemistry* Vol. 7, No. 20, 4309-4316.
Franz, N., Menin, L., et al. (2009). *Organic & Biomolecular Chemistry* Vol. 7, No. 24, 5207-5218.
Frawley Cass, S. M.&Tepe, J. J. (2009). *Organic & Biomolecular Chemistry* Vol. 7, No. 16, 3291-3299.
Furukawa, K., Abe, H., et al. (2009). *Organic & Biomolecular Chemistry* Vol. 7, No. 4, 671-677.
Fyles, T. M.&Luong, H. (2009). *Organic & Biomolecular Chemistry* Vol. 7, No. 4, 725-732.
Fyles, T. M.&Luong, H. (2009). *Organic & Biomolecular Chemistry* Vol. 7, No. 4, 733-738.
Gabutti, S., Schaffner, S., et al. (2009). *Organic & Biomolecular Chemistry* Vol. 7, No. 16, 3222-3229.
Gaisser, S., Carletti, I., et al. (2009). *Organic & Biomolecular Chemistry* Vol. 7, No. 8, 1705-1708.
Garcia-Egido, E., Paz, J., et al. (2009). *Organic & Biomolecular Chemistry* Vol. 7, No. 19, 3991-3999.
Garcia, L., Pla-Quintana, A., et al. (2009). *Organic & Biomolecular Chemistry* Vol. 7, No. 23, 5020-5027.
Garner, T. P., Williams, H. E. L., et al. (2009). *Organic & Biomolecular Chemistry* Vol. 7, No. 20, 4194-4200.
Garud, D. R., Garud, D. D., et al. (2009). *Organic & Biomolecular Chemistry* Vol. 7, No. 12, 2591-2598.
Ghosh, S., Pignot-Paintrand, I., et al. (2009). *Organic & Biomolecular Chemistry* Vol. 7, No. 13, 2729-2737.
Gibson, C. L., Huggan, J. K., et al. (2009). *Organic & Biomolecular Chemistry* Vol. 7, No. 9, 1829-1842.
Ginnari-Satriani, L., Casagrande, V., et al. (2009). *Organic & Biomolecular Chemistry* Vol. 7, No. 12, 2513-2516.

Gruber, T., Fischer, C., et al. (2009). *Organic & Biomolecular Chemistry* Vol. 7, No. 23, 4904-4917.
Gupta, P., Maity, J., et al. (2009). *Organic & Biomolecular Chemistry* Vol. 7, No. 11, 2389-2401.
Ha-Thi, M.-H., Penhoat, M., et al. (2009). *Organic & Biomolecular Chemistry* Vol. 7, No. 8, 1665-1673.
Haddoub, R., Dauner, M., et al. (2009). *Organic & Biomolecular Chemistry* Vol. 7, No. 4, 665-670.
Haraldsen, J. D., Liu, G., et al. (2009). *Organic & Biomolecular Chemistry* Vol. 7, No. 15, 3040-3048.
Hardy, J. G., Love, C. S., et al. (2009). *Organic & Biomolecular Chemistry* Vol. 7, No. 4, 789-793.
Henrikson, J. C., Hoover, A. R., et al. (2009). *Organic & Biomolecular Chemistry* Vol. 7, No. 3, 435-438.
Herrmann, A. (2009). *Organic & Biomolecular Chemistry* Vol. 7, No. 16, 3195-3204.
Hirano, T., Kuroda, K., et al. (2009). *Organic & Biomolecular Chemistry* Vol. 7, No. 14, 2905-2911.
Hirata, N., Fujisawa, Y., et al. (2009). *Organic & Biomolecular Chemistry* Vol. 7, No. 4, 651-654.
Hong, Y. J.&Tantillo, D. J. (2009). *Organic & Biomolecular Chemistry* Vol. 7, No. 19, 4101-4109.
Hossain, M. A., Rosengren, K. J., et al. (2009). *Organic & Biomolecular Chemistry* Vol. 7, No. 8, 1547-1553.
Huang, J., Xu, Y., et al. (2009). *Organic & Biomolecular Chemistry* Vol. 7, No. 7, 1299-1303.
Huang, Y., Zhang, Y., et al. (2009). *Organic & Biomolecular Chemistry* Vol. 7, No. 11, 2278-2285.
Humenik, M., Huang, Y., et al. (2009). *Organic & Biomolecular Chemistry* Vol. 7, No. 20, 4218-4224.
Huynh, L., Leroux, J.-C., et al. (2009). *Organic & Biomolecular Chemistry* Vol. 7, No. 17, 3437-3446.
Isidro, A., Latassa, D., et al. (2009). *Organic & Biomolecular Chemistry* Vol. 7, No. 12, 2565-2569.
Ito, T., Kondo, A., et al. (2009). *Organic & Biomolecular Chemistry* Vol. 7, No. 10, 2077-2081.
Jacobsen, M. F., Ferapontova, E. E., et al. (2009). *Organic & Biomolecular Chemistry* Vol. 7, No. 5, 905-908.
Jacobsen, O., Klaveness, J., et al. (2009). *Organic & Biomolecular Chemistry* Vol. 7, No. 8, 1599-1611.
Jeong, H. S., Kang, S., et al. (2009) *Organic & Biomolecular Chemistry* Vol. 7, No. 5, 921-925.
Jiang, H.&Hamada, Y. (2009). *Organic & Biomolecular Chemistry* Vol. 7, No. 20, 4173-4176.
Joce, C., Caryl, J., et al. (2009). *Organic & Biomolecular Chemistry* Vol. 7, No. 4, 635-638.
Johns, M. K., Yin, M.-X., et al. (2009). *Organic & Biomolecular Chemistry* Vol. 7, No. 18, 3691-3697.
Ju, L.&Bode, J. W. (2009). *Organic & Biomolecular Chemistry* Vol. 7, No. 11, 2259-2264.
Kaiser, J., van Esseveldt, B. C. J., et al. (2009). *Organic & Biomolecular Chemistry* Vol. 7, No. 4, 695-705.
Kalesh, K. A., Liu, K., et al. (2009). *Organic & Biomolecular Chemistry* Vol. 7, No. 24, 5129-5136.
Kaloudis, P., Paris, C., et al. (2009). *Organic & Biomolecular Chemistry* Vol. 7, No. 23, 4965-4972.
Kamiya, N., Abe, H., et al. (2009). *Organic & Biomolecular Chemistry* Vol. 7, No. 17, 3407-3412.
Kang, J., Reynolds, N. L., et al. (2009). *Organic & Biomolecular Chemistry* Vol. 7, No. 23, 4918-4923.

Katolik, A., Viladoms, J., et al. (2009). *Organic & Biomolecular Chemistry* Vol. 7, No. 9, 1904-1910.
Katritzky, A. R., Abo-Dya, N. E., et al. (2009). *Organic & Biomolecular Chemistry* Vol. 7, No. 21, 4444-4447.
Katritzky, A. R., Munawar, M. A., et al. (2009). *Organic & Biomolecular Chemistry* Vol. 7, No. 11, 2359-2362.
Katzberg, M., Wechler, K., et al. (2009). *Organic & Biomolecular Chemistry* Vol. 7, No. 2, 304-314.
Kele, P., Li, X., et al. (2009). *Organic & Biomolecular Chemistry* Vol. 7, No. 17, 3486-3490.
Kerherve, J., Botuha, C., et al. (2009). *Organic & Biomolecular Chemistry* Vol. 7, No. 10, 2214-2222.
Khdour, O.&Skibo, E. B. (2009). *Organic & Biomolecular Chemistry* Vol. 7, No. 10, 2140-2154.
Kirsch, M., Buscher, A.-M., et al. (2009). *Organic & Biomolecular Chemistry* Vol. 7, No. 9, 1954-1962.
Klein, M., Diner, P., et al. (2009). *Organic & Biomolecular Chemistry* Vol. 7, No. 17, 3421-3429.
Ko, Y. O., Chun, Y. S., et al. (2009). *Organic & Biomolecular Chemistry* Vol. 7, No. 6, 1132-1136.
Komatsu, T., Nakagawa, A., et al. (2009). *Organic & Biomolecular Chemistry* Vol. 7, No. 18, 3836-3841.
Kopylova, L. V., Snytnikova, O. A., et al. (2009). *Organic & Biomolecular Chemistry* Vol. 7, No. 14, 2958-2966.
Koshiyama, T., Ueno, T., et al. (2009). *Organic & Biomolecular Chemistry* Vol. 7, No. 12, 2649-2654.
Kuil, J., Branderhorst, H. M., et al. (2009). *Organic & Biomolecular Chemistry* Vol. 7, No. 19, 4088-4094.
Kuimova, M. K., Collins, H. A., et al. (2009). *Organic & Biomolecular Chemistry* Vol. 7, No. 5, 889-896.
Kumari, N.&Vankar, Y. D. (2009). *Organic & Biomolecular Chemistry* Vol. 7, No. 10, 2104-2109.
Laine, M., Ketomaki, K., et al. (2009). *Organic & Biomolecular Chemistry* Vol. 7, No. 13, 2780-2787.
Lakshman, M. K.&Frank, J. (2009). *Organic & Biomolecular Chemistry* Vol. 7, No. 14, 2933-2940.
Lee, C. C., Fitzmaurice, R. J., et al. (2009). *Organic & Biomolecular Chemistry* Vol. 7, No. 21, 4349-4351.
Legnani, L., Fallarini, S., et al. (2009). *Organic & Biomolecular Chemistry* Vol. 7, No. 21, 4428-4436.
Li, A.-F., He, H., et al. (2009). *Organic & Biomolecular Chemistry* Vol. 7, No. 1, 193-200.
Li, C., Li, J., et al. (2009). *Organic & Biomolecular Chemistry* Vol. 7, No. 13, 2699-2703.
Li, R., Jansen, D. J., et al. (2009). *Organic & Biomolecular Chemistry* Vol. 7, No. 9, 1921-1930.
Li, X., Huang, L., et al. (2009). *Organic & Biomolecular Chemistry* Vol. 7, No. 1, 117-127.
Li, Y., Nawrat, C. C., et al. (2009). *Organic & Biomolecular Chemistry* Vol. 7, No. 4, 639-640.
Liberska, A., Unciti-Broceta, A., et al. (2009). *Organic & Biomolecular Chemistry* Vol. 7, No. 1, 61-68.
Licen, S., Coppola, C., et al. (2009). *Organic & Biomolecular Chemistry* Vol. 7, No. 6, 1060-1063.
Limbach, M., Lygin, A. V., et al. (2009). *Organic & Biomolecular Chemistry* Vol. 7, No. 16, 3338-3342.
Lin, H.-H., Su, S.-Y., et al. (2009). *Organic & Biomolecular Chemistry* Vol. 7, No. 10, 2036-2039.
Linclau, B., Boydell, A. J., et al. (2009). *Organic & Biomolecular Chemistry* Vol. 7, No. 4, 803-814.

Liu, G., Botting, C., et al. (2010). *Chemmedchem* Vol. 5, No. 1, 41-45.

Liu, J.-Y., Lo, P.-C., et al. (2009). *Organic & Biomolecular Chemistry* Vol. 7, No. 8, 1583-1591.

Liu, W., Xu, L., et al. (2009). *Organic & Biomolecular Chemistry* Vol. 7, No. 4, 660-664.

Lopalco, M., Koini, E. N., et al. (2009). *Organic & Biomolecular Chemistry* Vol. 7, No. 5, 856-859.

Lorpitthaya, R., Sophy, K. B., et al. (2009). *Organic & Biomolecular Chemistry* Vol. 7, No. 7, 1284-1287.

Lu, H., Xiong, L., et al. (2009). *Organic & Biomolecular Chemistry* Vol. 7, No. 12, 2554-2558.

Lusvarghi, S., Kim, J. M., et al. (2009). *Organic & Biomolecular Chemistry* Vol. 7, No. 9, 1815-1820.

Madine, J., Clayton, J. C., et al. (2009). *Organic & Biomolecular Chemistry* Vol. 7, No. 11, 2414-2420.

Mahe, O., Frath, D., et al. (2009). *Organic & Biomolecular Chemistry* Vol. 7, No. 18, 3648-3651.

Mann, M. C., Fairhurst, S. A., et al. (2009). *Organic & Biomolecular Chemistry* Vol. 7, No. 5, 1009-1016.

Marshall, L. J., Cable, K. M., et al. (2009). *Organic & Biomolecular Chemistry* Vol. 7, No. 4, 785-788.

Martin, A. R., Mohanan, K., et al. (2009). *Organic & Biomolecular Chemistry* Vol. 7, No. 21, 4369-4377.

Martin, R., Saini, R., et al. (2009). *Organic & Biomolecular Chemistry* Vol. 7, No. 11, 2303-2309.

Martin, R., Schmidt, A. W., et al. (2009). *Organic & Biomolecular Chemistry* Vol. 7, No. 5, 909-920.

Mazik, M.&Buthe, A. C. (2009). *Organic & Biomolecular Chemistry* Vol. 7, No. 10, 2063-2071.

McCort-Tranchepain, I. (2009). *Organic & Biomolecular Chemistry* Vol. 7, No. 4, 706-716.

McGrath, J. W., Hammerschmidt, F., et al. (2009). *Organic & Biomolecular Chemistry* Vol. 7, No. 9, 1944-1953.

Mecklenburg, S., Shaaban, S., et al. (2009). *Organic & Biomolecular Chemistry* Vol. 7, No. 22, 4753-4762.

Mehellou, Y., Balzarini, J., et al. (2009). *Organic & Biomolecular Chemistry* Vol. 7, No. 12, 2548-2553.

Mendez-Ardoy, A., Gomez-Garcia, M., et al. (2009). *Organic & Biomolecular Chemistry* Vol. 7, No. 13, 2681-2684.

Miller, D. J., Yu, F., et al. (2009). *Organic & Biomolecular Chemistry* Vol. 7, No. 5, 962-975.

Minten, I. J., Ma, Y., et al. (2009). *Organic & Biomolecular Chemistry* Vol. 7, No. 22, 4685-4688.

Mitra, R. N., Shome, A., et al. (2009). *Organic & Biomolecular Chemistry* Vol. 7, No. 1, 94-102.

Mizanur, R. M.&Pohl, N. L. B. (2009). *Organic & Biomolecular Chemistry* Vol. 7, No. 10, 2135-2139.

Mizoguchi, T., Nagai, C., et al. (2009). *Organic & Biomolecular Chemistry* Vol. 7, No. 10, 2120-2126.

Mizuno, T., Suzuki, K., et al. (2009). *Organic & Biomolecular Chemistry* Vol. 7, No. 15, 3102-3111.

Molteni, M., Bellucci, M. C., et al. (2009). *Organic & Biomolecular Chemistry* Vol. 7, No. 11, 2286-2296.

Moran, S., Rai, D. K., et al. (2009). *Organic & Biomolecular Chemistry* Vol. 7, No. 4, 644-646.

Moreno-Clavijo, E., Carmona, A. T., et al. (2009). *Organic & Biomolecular Chemistry* Vol. 7, No. 6, 1192-1202.

Mueller, N. J., Stueckler, C., et al. (2009). *Organic & Biomolecular Chemistry* Vol. 7, No. 6, 1115-1119.

Mukae, M., Ihara, T., et al. (2009). *Organic & Biomolecular Chemistry* Vol. 7, No. 7, 1349-1354.

Murakami, R., Minami, A., et al. (2009). *Organic & Biomolecular Chemistry* Vol. 7, No. 7, 1437-1444.

Nakashima, K., Kamiya, N., et al. (2009). *Organic & Biomolecular Chemistry* Vol. 7, No. 11, 2353-2358.

Nam, T.-g., Nara, S. J., et al. (2009). *Organic & Biomolecular Chemistry* Vol. 7, No. 24, 5103-5112.

Narendra, N., Chennakrishnareddy, G., et al. (2009). *Organic & Biomolecular Chemistry* Vol. 7, No. 17, 3520-3526.

New, E. J.&Parker, D. (2009). *Organic & Biomolecular Chemistry* Vol. 7, No. 5, 851-855.

Nguyen, T. H.&Ansell, R. J. (2009). *Organic & Biomolecular Chemistry* Vol. 7, No. 6, 1211-1220.

Noble, G. T., Flitsch, S. L., et al. (2009). *Organic & Biomolecular Chemistry* Vol. 7, No. 24, 5245-5254.

Ogino, M., Taya, Y., et al. (2009). *Organic & Biomolecular Chemistry* Vol. 7, No. 15, 3163-3167.

Oh, H.-S., Xuan, R., et al. (2009). *Organic & Biomolecular Chemistry* Vol. 7, No. 21, 4458-4463.

Ohkubo, A., Kasuya, R., et al. (2009). *Organic & Biomolecular Chemistry* Vol. 7, No. 4, 687-694.

Oishi, S., Kamitani, H., et al. (2009). *Organic & Biomolecular Chemistry* Vol. 7, No. 14, 2872-2877.

Okada, M., Ito, S., et al. (2009). *Organic & Biomolecular Chemistry* Vol. 7, No. 15, 3065-3073.

Okamoto, K., Hamada, N., et al. (2009). *Organic & Biomolecular Chemistry* Vol. 7, No. 18, 3782-3791.

Olesiak, M., Stec, W. J., et al. (2009). *Organic & Biomolecular Chemistry* Vol. 7, No. 10, 2162-2169.

Olsson, J. D. M., Landstrom, J., et al. (2009). *Organic & Biomolecular Chemistry* Vol. 7, No. 8, 1612-1618.

Ortega, P., Samaniego, R., et al. (2009). *Organic & Biomolecular Chemistry* Vol. 7, No. 15, 3079-3085.

Pal, R., Parker, D., et al. (2009). *Organic & Biomolecular Chemistry* Vol. 7, No. 8, 1525-1528.

Panchal, N.&Gaffney, P. R. J. (2009). *Organic & Biomolecular Chemistry* Vol. 7, No. 23, 4832-4841.

Pandey, G., Grahacharya, D., et al. (2009). *Organic & Biomolecular Chemistry* Vol. 7, No. 16, 3300-3307.

Pang, L.-J., Wang, D., et al. (2009). *Organic & Biomolecular Chemistry* Vol. 7, No. 20, 4252-4266.

Park, K. K., Park, J. W., et al. (2009). *Organic & Biomolecular Chemistry* Vol. 7, No. 20, 4225-4232.

Parsons, T. B., Moir, J. W. B., et al. (2009). *Organic & Biomolecular Chemistry* Vol. 7, No. 15, 3128-3140.

Payne, R. J., Bulloch, E. M. M., et al. (2009). *Organic & Biomolecular Chemistry* Vol. 7, No. 11, 2421-2429.

Perez-Anes, A., Spataro, G., et al. (2009). *Organic & Biomolecular Chemistry* Vol. 7, No. 17, 3491-3498.

Perez-Ruiz, R., Diaz, Y., et al. (2009). *Organic & Biomolecular Chemistry* Vol. 7, No. 17, 3499-3504.

Petermeier, M.&Jaschke, A. (2009). *Organic & Biomolecular Chemistry* Vol. 7, No. 2, 288-292.

Pettersson, B.&Bergman, J. (2009). *Organic & Biomolecular Chemistry* Vol. 7, No. 6, 1184-1191.

Piccialli, V., Oliviero, G., et al. (2009). *Organic & Biomolecular Chemistry* Vol. 7, No. 15, 3036-3039.

Plater, M. J., Barnes, P., et al. (2009). *Organic & Biomolecular Chemistry* Vol. 7, No. 8, 1633-1641.

Plietzsch, O., Schilling, C. I., et al. (2009). *Organic & Biomolecular Chemistry* Vol. 7, No. 22, 4734-4743.
Pluvinage, B., Ghinet, M. G., et al. (2009). *Organic & Biomolecular Chemistry* Vol. 7, No. 20, 4169-4172.
Poldy, J., Peakall, R., et al. (2009). *Organic & Biomolecular Chemistry* Vol. 7, No. 20, 4296-4300.
Prasad, D. J. C.&Sekar, G. (2009). *Organic & Biomolecular Chemistry* Vol. 7, No. 24, 5091-5097.
Ramachary, D. B., Narayana, V. V., et al. (2009). *Organic & Biomolecular Chemistry* Vol. 7, No. 17, 3372-3378.
Ramachary, D. B., Venkaiah, C., et al. (2009). *Organic & Biomolecular Chemistry* Vol. 7, No. 10, 2053-2062.
Ramsden, C. A., Stratford, M. R. L., et al. (2009). *Organic & Biomolecular Chemistry* Vol. 7, No. 17, 3388-3390.
Redman, J. E., Granadino-Roldan, J. M., et al. (2009). *Organic & Biomolecular Chemistry* Vol. 7, No. 1, 76-84.
Reiriz, C., Amorin, M., et al. (2009). *Organic & Biomolecular Chemistry* Vol. 7, No. 21, 4358-4361.
Rejzek, M., Kannathasan, V. S., et al. (2009). *Organic & Biomolecular Chemistry* Vol. 7, No. 6, 1203-1210.
Ribes, C., Falomir, E., et al. (2009). *Organic & Biomolecular Chemistry* Vol. 7, No. 7, 1355-1360.
Richard, J.-A., Jean, L., et al. (2009). *Organic & Biomolecular Chemistry* Vol. 7, No. 14, 2941-2957.
Richter, S. N., Menegazzo, I., et al. (2009). *Organic & Biomolecular Chemistry* Vol. 7, No. 5, 976-985.
Ricoux, R., Allard, M., et al. (2009). *Organic & Biomolecular Chemistry* Vol. 7, No. 16, 3208-3211.
Riss, P. J., Hummerich, R., et al. (2009). *Organic & Biomolecular Chemistry* Vol. 7, No. 13, 2688-2698.
Rochat, S., Grote, Z., et al. (2009). *Organic & Biomolecular Chemistry* Vol. 7, No. 6, 1147-1153.
Rogers, S. A., Krayer, M., et al. (2009). *Organic & Biomolecular Chemistry* Vol. 7, No. 3, 603-606.
Rohacova, J., Marin, M. L., et al. (2009). *Organic & Biomolecular Chemistry* Vol. 7, No. 23, 4973-4980.
Ronchi, P., Vignando, S., et al. (2009). *Organic & Biomolecular Chemistry* Vol. 7, No. 12, 2635-2644.
Rosengren-Holmberg, J. P., Karlsson, J. G., et al. (2009). *Organic & Biomolecular Chemistry* Vol. 7, No. 15, 3148-3155.
Rouffet, M., Denhez, C., et al. (2009). *Organic & Biomolecular Chemistry* Vol. 7, No. 18, 3817-3825.
Rowan, A. S., Nicely, N. I., et al. (2009). *Organic & Biomolecular Chemistry* Vol. 7, No. 19, 4029-4036.
Rydzik, A. M., Lukaszewicz, M., et al. (2009). *Organic & Biomolecular Chemistry* Vol. 7, No. 22, 4763-4776.
Sahnoun, S., Messaoudi, S., et al. (2009). *Organic & Biomolecular Chemistry* Vol. 7, No. 20, 4271-4278.
Salorinne, K., Tero, T.-R., et al. (2009). *Organic & Biomolecular Chemistry* Vol. 7, No. 20, 4211-4217.
Sanchez-Medina, I., Frank, M., et al. (2009). *Organic & Biomolecular Chemistry* Vol. 7, No. 2, 280-287.

Sawangwan, T., Goedl, C., et al. (2009). *Organic & Biomolecular Chemistry* Vol. 7, No. 20, 4267-4270.
Schindler, D., Ei, et al. (2009). *Organic & Biomolecular Chemistry* Vol. 7, No. 17, 3549-3560.
Schlegel, M. K., Zhang, L., et al. (2009). *Organic & Biomolecular Chemistry* Vol. 7, No. 3, 476-482.
Schmuck, C., Michels, U., et al. (2009). *Organic & Biomolecular Chemistry* Vol. 7, No. 21, 4362-4368.
Schreiber, S. L.&Kapoor, T. M. (2007). *Chemical Biology: From Small Molecules to Systems Biology and Drug Design* Wiley.
Schulz, A., Hornig, S., et al. (2009). *Organic & Biomolecular Chemistry* Vol. 7, No. 9, 1884-1889.
Seela, F., Jiang, D., et al. (2009). *Organic & Biomolecular Chemistry* Vol. 7, No. 17, 3463-3473.
Seela, F., Xiong, H., et al. (2009). *Organic & Biomolecular Chemistry* Vol. 7, No. 7, 1374-1387.
Seio, K., Takaku, Y., et al. (2009). *Organic & Biomolecular Chemistry* Vol. 7, No. 11, 2440-2451.
Sengupta, R., Billiar, T. R., et al. (2009). *Organic & Biomolecular Chemistry* Vol. 7, No. 2, 232-234.
Shah, B. A., Chib, R., et al. (2009). *Organic & Biomolecular Chemistry* Vol. 7, No. 16, 3230-3235.
Sharrett, Z., Gamsey, S., et al. (2009). *Organic & Biomolecular Chemistry* Vol. 7, No. 7, 1461-1470.
Shi, W., Coleman, R. S., et al. (2009). *Organic & Biomolecular Chemistry* Vol. 7, No. 18, 3709-3722.
Shimokawa, K., Miwa, R., et al. (2009). *Organic & Biomolecular Chemistry* Vol. 7, No. 4, 777-784.
Shing, T. K. M.&Cheng, H. M. (2009). *Organic & Biomolecular Chemistry* Vol. 7, No. 24, 5098-5102.
Shiraishi, Y., Maehara, H., et al. (2009). *Organic & Biomolecular Chemistry* Vol. 7, No. 10, 2072-2076.
Simpson, D. S., Lovell, K. M., et al. (2009). *Organic & Biomolecular Chemistry* Vol. 7, No. 18, 3748-3756.
Smith, A. J. T., Li, Y., et al. (2009). *Organic & Biomolecular Chemistry* Vol. 7, No. 13, 2716-2724.
Snegaroff, K., Lassagne, F., et al. (2009). *Organic & Biomolecular Chemistry* Vol. 7, No. 22, 4782-4788.
Soliman, M. E. S., Pernia, J. J. R., et al. (2009). *Organic & Biomolecular Chemistry* Vol. 7, No. 24, 5236-5244.
Soliman, M. E. S., Ruggiero, G. D., et al. (2009). *Organic & Biomolecular Chemistry* Vol. 7, No. 3, 460-468.
Song, H. Y., Ngai, M. H., et al. (2009). *Organic & Biomolecular Chemistry* Vol. 7, No. 17, 3400-3406.
Sopaci, S. B., Simsek, I., et al. (2009). *Organic & Biomolecular Chemistry* Vol. 7, No. 8, 1658-1664.
Sosniak, A. M., Gasser, G., et al. (2009). *Organic & Biomolecular Chemistry* Vol. 7, No. 23, 4992-5000.
Srinivasan, R., Tan, L. P., et al. (2009). *Organic & Biomolecular Chemistry* Vol. 7, No. 9, 1821-1828.
Stalford, S. A., Kilner, C. A., et al. (2009). *Organic & Biomolecular Chemistry* Vol. 7, No. 23, 4842-4852.
Steffan, N., Grundmann, A., et al. (2009). *Organic & Biomolecular Chemistry* Vol. 7, No. 19, 4082-4087.
Stencel, L. M., Kormos, C. M., et al. (2009). *Organic & Biomolecular Chemistry* Vol. 7, No. 11, 2452-2457.

Su, R., Li, L., et al. (2009). *Organic & Biomolecular Chemistry* Vol. 7, No. 10, 2040-2045.
Subhani, M. A., Muller, K.-S., et al. (2009). *Organic & Biomolecular Chemistry* Vol. 7, No. 19, 4000-4008.
Sunbul, M.&Yin, J. (2009). *Organic & Biomolecular Chemistry* Vol. 7, No. 17, 3361-3371.
Sundararaju, B., Achard, M., et al. (2009). *Organic & Biomolecular Chemistry* Vol. 7, No. 19, 3906-3909.
Suzuki, K., Tobe, A., et al. (2009). *Organic & Biomolecular Chemistry* Vol. 7, No. 22, 4726-4733.
Swarbrick, J. M., Cooper, S., et al. (2009). *Organic & Biomolecular Chemistry* Vol. 7, No. 8, 1709-1715.
Taima, H., Yoshioka, N., et al. (2009). *Organic & Biomolecular Chemistry* Vol. 7, No. 6, 1176-1183.
Tanaka, T., Nomura, W., et al. (2009). *Organic & Biomolecular Chemistry* Vol. 7, No. 18, 3805-3809.
Tang, B., Bray, C. D., et al. (2009). *Organic & Biomolecular Chemistry* Vol. 7, No. 21, 4448-4457.
Tanima, D., Imamura, Y., et al. (2009). *Organic & Biomolecular Chemistry* Vol. 7, No. 22, 4689-4694.
Tao, L., Liu, J., et al. (2009). *Organic & Biomolecular Chemistry* Vol. 7, No. 17, 3481-3485.
Tei, L., Gugliotta, G., et al. (2009). *Organic & Biomolecular Chemistry* Vol. 7, No. 21, 4406-4414.
Tejler, J., Salameh, B., et al. (2009). *Organic & Biomolecular Chemistry* Vol. 7, No. 19, 3982-3990.
Thota, N., Mukherjee, D., et al. (2009). *Organic & Biomolecular Chemistry* Vol. 7, No. 7, 1280-1283.
Tian, Z.-y., Xie, S.-q., et al. (2009). *Organic & Biomolecular Chemistry* Vol. 7, No. 22, 4651-4660.
Toganoh, M., Miyachi, H., et al. (2009). *Organic & Biomolecular Chemistry* Vol. 7, No. 15, 3027-3030.
Toma, L., Legnani, L., et al. (2009). *Organic & Biomolecular Chemistry* Vol. 7, No. 18, 3734-3740.
Torres-Romero, D., Munoz-Martinez, F., et al. (2009). *Organic & Biomolecular Chemistry* Vol. 7, No. 24, 5166-5172.
Trabi, M., Mylne, J. S., et al. (2009). *Organic & Biomolecular Chemistry* Vol. 7, No. 11, 2378-2388.
Trajkovski, M., Sket, P., et al. (2009). *Organic & Biomolecular Chemistry* Vol. 7, No. 22, 4677-4684.
Truppo, M. D., Rozzell, J. D., et al. (2009). *Organic & Biomolecular Chemistry* Vol. 7, No. 2, 395-398.
Tsikolia, M., Hall, A. C., et al. (2009). *Organic & Biomolecular Chemistry* Vol. 7, No. 18, 3862-3870.
Tsou, L. K., Zhang, M. M., et al. (2009). *Organic & Biomolecular Chemistry* Vol. 7, No. 24, 5055-5058.
Ueno, Y., Kawamura, A., et al. (2009). *Organic & Biomolecular Chemistry* Vol. 7, No. 13, 2761-2769.
Umemoto, T., Wengel, J., et al. (2009). *Organic & Biomolecular Chemistry* Vol. 7, No. 9, 1793-1797.
van Dijk, M., Dechesne, A. C., et al. (2009). *Organic & Biomolecular Chemistry* Vol. 7, No. 21, 4517-4525.
van Dijkum, E., Danac, R., et al. (2009). *Organic & Biomolecular Chemistry* Vol. 7, No. 6, 1097-1105.
Van Ryssen, M. P., Avlonitis, N., et al. (2009). *Organic & Biomolecular Chemistry* Vol. 7, No. 22, 4695-4707.
Veale, E. B., Tocci, G. M., et al. (2009). *Organic & Biomolecular Chemistry* Vol. 7, No. 17, 3447-3454.

Veedu, R. N., Vester, B., et al. (2009). *Organic & Biomolecular Chemistry* Vol. 7, No. 7, 1404-1409.
Vervisch, K., D'Hooghe, M., et al. (2009). *Organic & Biomolecular Chemistry* Vol. 7, No. 16, 3271-3279.
Wagner, S. C., Roskamp, M., et al. (2009). *Organic & Biomolecular Chemistry* Vol. 7, No. 1, 46-51.
Walker, S. R., Cumming, H., et al. (2009). *Organic & Biomolecular Chemistry* Vol. 7, No. 15, 3031-3035.
Walton, J. G. A., Patterson, S., et al. (2009). *Organic & Biomolecular Chemistry* Vol. 7, No. 15, 3049-3060.
Wang, S.-P., Deng, W.-J., et al. (2009). *Organic & Biomolecular Chemistry* Vol. 7, No. 19, 4017-4020.
Watkins, R. W., Lavis, L. D., et al. (2009). *Organic & Biomolecular Chemistry* Vol. 7, No. 19, 3969-3975.
Wijdeven, M. A., van den Berg, R. J. F., et al. (2009). *Organic & Biomolecular Chemistry* Vol. 7, No. 14, 2976-2980.
Willans, C. E., Anderson, K. M., et al. (2009). *Organic & Biomolecular Chemistry* Vol. 7, No. 13, 2756-2760.
Wipf, P., Mo, T., et al. (2009). *Organic & Biomolecular Chemistry* Vol. 7, No. 20, 4163-4165.
Wong, J. H., Sahni, U., et al. (2009). *Organic & Biomolecular Chemistry* Vol. 7, No. 1, 27-29.
Yamakoshi, H., Ikarashi, F., et al. (2009). *Organic & Biomolecular Chemistry* Vol. 7, No. 18, 3772-3781.
Yamamoto, J., Tanaka, Y., et al. (2009). *Organic & Biomolecular Chemistry* Vol. 7, No. 1, 161-166.
Yan, Y., Lee, C.-C., et al. (2009). *Organic & Biomolecular Chemistry* Vol. 7, No. 19, 3914-3917.
Yang, L., Wang, D.-X., et al. (2009). *Organic & Biomolecular Chemistry* Vol. 7, No. 12, 2628-2634.
Yang, Y.-K., Ko, S.-K., et al. (2009). *Organic & Biomolecular Chemistry* Vol. 7, No. 22, 4590-4593.
Yap, B. C. M., Simpkins, G. L., et al. (2009). *Organic & Biomolecular Chemistry* Vol. 7, No. 14, 2855-2863.
Yi, H., Maisonneuve, S., et al. (2009). *Organic & Biomolecular Chemistry* Vol. 7, No. 18, 3847-3854.
Yin, J.&Linker, T. (2009). *Organic & Biomolecular Chemistry* Vol. 7, No. 23, 4829-4831.
Yin, W.-B., Cheng, J., et al. (2009). *Organic & Biomolecular Chemistry* Vol. 7, No. 10, 2202-2207.
Yoshida, K., Yamaguchi, K., et al. (2009). *Organic & Biomolecular Chemistry* Vol. 7, No. 9, 1868-1877.
Yoshiya, T., Kawashima, H., et al. (2009). *Organic & Biomolecular Chemistry* Vol. 7, No. 14, 2894-2904.
Zampella, A., Sepe, V., et al. (2009). *Organic & Biomolecular Chemistry* Vol. 7, No. 19, 4037-4044.
Zaubitzer, F., Riis-Johannessen, T., et al. (2009). *Organic & Biomolecular Chemistry* Vol. 7, No. 22, 4598-4603.
Zeng, X., Sun, Y.-X., et al. (2009). *Organic & Biomolecular Chemistry* Vol. 7, No. 20, 4201-4210.
Zhang, F., Simpkins, N. S., et al. (2009). *Organic & Biomolecular Chemistry* Vol. 7, No. 9, 1963-1979.
Zhao, P., Ueda, J.-y., et al. (2009). *Organic & Biomolecular Chemistry* Vol. 7, No. 7, 1454-1460.
Zhou, D., Chu, W., et al. (2009). *Organic & Biomolecular Chemistry* Vol. 7, No. 7, 1337-1348.
Zhou, H., Ma, X., et al. (2009). *Organic & Biomolecular Chemistry* Vol. 7, No. 11, 2297-2302.

10

Towards Understanding Drugs on the Molecular Level to Design Drugs of Desired Profiles

Jolanta Natalia Latosińska and Magdalena Latosińska
Faculty of Physics, Adam Mickiewicz University in Poznań, Poland

1. Introduction

The process of drug development proceeds through several stages including discovery, product characterisation, formulation, delivery and packaging development, pharmacokinetics and drug disposition, preclinical toxicology testing and IND (Investigational New Drug) application; bioanalytical testing and clinical trials. In general this process is time-consuming and expensive. According to statistical data, from among 50 thousand to 5 million of compounds subjected to screening only 6 become prospective drugs and the whole process from discovery to implementation takes from 12 to 24 years and costs even up to 800 million USD [1]. The number of new approved drugs partially reflects the progress in research and development. Despite enormous financial outlays, there has been a steady decrease in the number of drugs introduced each year into therapy. While in the 1960s about 70-100 new drugs was introduced in the market, in the 1970s, 60-70, in the 1980s 50, in the 1990s 40 while in 2000th only 20. On the one hand, this is a result of increased demands on safety (average number of clinical trials per new drug increased from 30 in the 1970s through 40 in the 1980s, to 70 in the 1990s), which prolonged the development process from 8 years in the 1960s, 12 in 1970s, 14 in 1980s, 15 in 1990s and 21 currently. On the other hand, the so-called "easy" to discover drugs have already been discovered. Currently 75% of expenditures is absorbed by the research ended in failure and as much as 90% of candidates for drug never reach the market.

Therefore, much effort is directed towards development of new theoretical and experimental tools that would increase the effectiveness of the above process, in particular in its first stages leading to a decision whether a given compound is a prospective drug or not. The necessary and reliable data needed to take such a decision are provided first of all by the methods of analytical characterisation of compounds (identification, physical and chemical properties, structure), methods permitting optimisation of the leading structure (structure-activity relation) and pre-clinical study (toxicity). These early stages of pharmacological studies sometimes (but not always) reveal the whole mechanism of action of a future drug.

Recent research work towards drug development has been conducted in two independent directions. On the one hand, completely new drugs or pro-drugs (drug precursors that become drugs only as a result of metabolic transformations *in vivo*) are searched for, while on the other hand, drugs of second and third generation are proposed that are the improved versions of the so-called first generation ones (e.g. more selective, less toxic, etc.). The search for new areas of applications of the already known drugs is conducted independently. It should be realised that paradoxically the physico-chemical properties or the mechanism of activity of many even commonly used drugs are often unknown. In any case, whenever a completely new or well-known compound becomes a candidate promising to be therapeutically relevant, it must be characterised by determination of its structure, stability, solubility, preferred conditions for maintaining function, toxicity, bioactivity and bioavailability. The physico-chemical methods supported by computer modelling at a high level of theory should always be the first step in drug characterisation.

It is well known that magnetic resonance techniques: Nuclear magnetic resonance (NMR) discovered by Bloch et al. [2] and Purcell et al. [3] in 1946, and Nuclear quadrupole resonance (NQR) originated by Dehmelt and Krüger in 1949 [4] for many years have played invaluable role in the process of drug identification, especially when two or more alternative products could be synthesized or when geometrical isomers should be differentiated. Despite their usefulness, the potential of these methods in drug development at least at first sight seems rather limited in comparison to High-throughput screening (HTS), X-ray diffraction (XRD) or Fourier transform infrared spectroscopy (FTIR). Advances of technology over the last decade have brought modern spectroscopic techniques that are sensitive tools for such purposes, especially in combination with high quality, fast computational quantum chemistry methods like Density Functional Theory (DFT). Apart from revealing structural details (geometrical isomers, enantiomers), the standard key areas for physico-chemical NMR/NQR studies are thermal stability of drugs and structural phase transitions.

A unique and quite a new area of their use is the study of spatial packing. Most of drugs are used in the crystalline form in which the arrangement of molecules forced by weak interactions determines their physico-chemical properties (from melting point, solubility to polymorphism) and thus affects the performance of the drug. What is more, weak, noncovalent and reversible molecular interactions such as hydrogen bondings, *van der Waals* forces, π-π interactions or metal coordination have been only recently found to be crucial for understanding biological activity of drugs and biological processes. As in the absence of conformational effects the environmental effect of the crystal influences the electron density of a single molecule in a very similar way as the enzyme of a drug molecule in the complex drug-enzyme [5], the knowledge of crystal packing provides guidance on the site or method of binding. Thus the problems related to understanding the mechanism of formation and interplay of weak interactions in crystals have evoked recently enormous interest. Additional factor prompting the interest in investigation drugs on molecular level are recent advances in genomics and proteomics that have permitted understanding of internal mechanisms of human diseases. The latter cover the knowledge of the genes alteration caused by disease, its influence on the proteins encoded by them, the interaction of these proteins with each other in living cells, the resulting changes in the specific tissues and finally the affect on the entire body. The achievements in this field delimit new directions in drug discovery and development of drugs addressing the needs of individual patient. Thus new drugs in the near future will be discovered and developed exclusively on the basis of a combination of two factors - the understanding of the mechanisms of diseases and mechanisms of drugs, both at the molecular level.

This chapter highlights the importance of combination of experimental and theoretical methods in investigation aimed at understanding drugs on the molecular level which is fundamental for development of drugs of desirable profiles.

2. Directions in drug design

Throughout the history of medicine the process of new drug discovery has been based on natural sources (berries, herbs, leaves, roots, animal parts or minerals) and drugs have been discovered by serendipity (sheer luck) or in a trial-and-error process [6]. While until the mid-1980s new drugs were discovered mainly by chance, over the next decade, till mid-1990s, the knowledge of structure was the basis for research, then the starting point was to identify a target and a relationship between structure and function. At the beginning of the 21st century a future direction in drug design has been indicated by the knowledge of the human genome, which contains about 23 thousand genes encoding proteins. Although there was some success in treating melanoma, HIV or Parkinson disease, the methods involving gene therapy, whose aims are personalization of drugs, correction of genetic defects or replacement of defective genes are still only a promising methods.

In the last century the demand for effective drugs has increased and a rational drug design has begun to replace old methods. With the progress in the field of chemistry, biology, biochemistry, pharmacology, physics and increase in computational power, drug discovery has become an interdisciplinary area and entered a new phase called Computer-Aided Drug Design (CADD) or Computer-Assisted Molecular Design (CAMD) [7]. The modern methods of rational drug design are capable of designing a biologically active compound, drug (ligand) directly interacting with the distinct so-called molecular target (enzyme, transporter, ion channel or receptor) or components of a microorganism (bacterium, virus, parasite).

In general, CCAD method allows the search for ligands which are predicted to interact strongly with a target or alternatively - the search for a target that will interact strongly with a given ligand. In fact molecules of drugs interact in a very specific way with the targets in organisms and the result of this interaction may include beneficial or adverse effects as well as the excitation of both or biotransformation of the drug [8]. Thus the effective drug design is even more complicated as there are three kinds of targets important in drug discovery process: therapeutic/biological targets (those which drugs specifically bind to and those which elicit therapeutic effects), ADME (absorption, distribution, metabolism, and excretion) associated proteins (responsible for metabolism, important for the efficacy and bioactivity study) and adverse drug reaction (ADR)/toxicity targets (major cause for the failure of drugs).

The CADD approaches can be divided into three categories:

1. **the ligand perspective** - the structure of a ligand or the structure-activity relationship (SAR) are known for a selected ligand and a series of pharmacophores (it requires the assumption that both the protein and ligand have limited degrees of flexibility), which allows identification of the target [9,10]
2. **the target perspective** - the 3D structure of the target is known, which allows identification of the amino acid sequences and their conformations responsible for the binding with ligand [11,12].
3. **the ligand-target interaction perspective** - the interaction between drug and target is known from XDR and NMR structural data [13,14].

The most popular CADD techniques are receptor-based and ligand-based approaches, the former is often called direct while the latter - indirect. Receptor-based drug design requires the knowledge of a 3D structure of the biological target and identification of the protein-binding site or supramolecular host, but the ligand is unknown. Ligand-based drug design uses a known set of ligands with the receptor site unknown. Both approaches are based on the lock and key fit of receptor and drug and finally use docking, thus are actually very similar. In the receptor-based approach to drug design the structure of a target or a binding site is known from 3D XRD or NMR studies, while a ligand fitting the binding pocket of the target is searched for in the database, which permits elimination of the need for synthesis of new lead compounds. Alternatively the ligand is constructed in such a way as to fit the binding pocket (*de novo design*). The most spectacular achievements of this kind of approach was design of the HIV RT inhibitors based on the known HIV reverse transcriptase structure [15], development of dorzolamide - a carbonic anhydrase inhibitor, an anti-glaucoma agent by Merck [16] or investigation of mechanism of activation of temozolomide and its inhibitor-target interaction with DNA [17]. If a 3D structure it is not available, the homology model of the target can be created on the basis of its amino acid sequence and known structure of proteins resembling the target [18,19]. The method makes use of the fact that sequences of related proteins are similar and thus the protein structures of naturally occurring homologous proteins are also similar

Indirect drug design is based exclusively on the knowledge of the way different ligands bind to an unknown biological target. The structural (in fact stereochemical) and physicochemical features of a set of different ligands (active and inactive) allow the creation of a hypothetical receptor site - 3D-pharmacophore - determining the minimum set of requirements that must be met for the ligand to bind to the target. In fact these requirements describe a few specific interactions responsible for the ligand-target binding i.e. define a simplified model of the receptor site. The 3D-pharmacophore used in conformationally flexible search for ligands provides the best lock-key arrangement with a hypothetical receptor site. There are many different methods of construction of a 3D-pharmacophore, however the main types are: quantitative structure-activity relationship (QSAR), quantitative structure-property relationships (QSPR), molecular shape analysis (MSA), receptor surface models (RSM), comparative molecular field analysis (CoMFA), comparative molecular similarity index analysis (CoMSIA), pharmacophore mapping (PM) etc. The most commonly used are QSAR-based techniques, in which a correlation between the structure and biological activity or physico-chemical properties of a ligand is derived.

In analogy to the direct and indirect approaches in CADD, QSAR techniques can be divided to receptor-dependent (RD) and receptor-independent (RI) ones [20].

In RD-QSAR, models are derived directly from the 3D structures of the multiple ligand-receptor complex. This group of five methods includes: static ligand representation (3D), multiple ligand representation (4D), ligand-based virtual or pseudo receptor models (5D), multiple solvation scenarios (6D) and real receptor or target-based receptor model data (7D) [21]. Using the structure of the ligand-receptor complex in which both ligand and receptor are flexible the induced-fit process is performed using molecular dynamics (MD) simulation. The descriptors are the energies of the interaction responsible for the binding between the analogue molecules and the receptor [22]. An example of a successful application of the RD-4D-QSAR approach is the study of 4-hydroxy-5,6-dihydropyrone inhibitors of HIV-1 protease [23], which permitted prediction of the "bioactive" conformations of the docked analogues into the active site of HIV-1 protease close to those found by XRD. Moreover, the requirements of specific interactions (hydrophobic, steric and hydrogen bonding) between the enzyme active site and the binding site of analogues of 4-hydroxy-5,6-dihydropyrone inhibitor with HIV-1 protease, indicate directions of development of new lead HIV-1 protease inhibitors [23].

In RI-QSAR, the geometry of the receptor is not available, or it is neglected because it is not credible or its binding with ligand is not recognised. This group of methods include the "classical" (zero-dimensional), one-dimensional (1D), two-dimensional (2D), three-dimensional (3D), and four dimensional (4D) QSAR approaches [24]. The calculated descriptors are atom and molecular counts, molecular weight, sum of atomic properties (0D-QSAR); fragment counts (1D-QSAR); topological descriptors (2D-QSAR); geometrical, atomic coordinates, or energy grid descriptors (3D-QSAR); and a combination of atomic coordinates and sampling of conformations (RI-4D-QSAR) [24]. Commercial drugs developed with the aid of classical QSAR include: Norfloxacin (broad-spectrum antibacterial agent) Kyorin 1983; Metconazole (Wheat Fungicide), Kureha 1994; Lomerizine (Antimigrane, Antiglaucoma) Organon Japan-Upjohn 1999; Flobufen (Long-acting Antiinflammatory) Kuchar et al., Virbac 2000 [25]. 3D QSAR approaches CoMFA [26] and its extension CoMSIA [26] are popular thanks to their ability to generate highly predictive and easy interpretable models even for flexible molecules, despite the fact that only one conformation of each compound is considered. The CoMFA approach uses in its standard implementation only Lennard-Jones and Coulomb potentials, while in the extended version also the hydrophobic and hydrogen-bond fields are taken into account [27]. The field type used in CoMSIA is similar. Instead of field descriptors based on potentials, the use is made of the so-called similarity index describing steric, electrostatic, and hydrophobic similarity or dissimilarity of molecules. Additionally in CoMSIA, Gaussian-type functionals eliminating singularities at the atomic positions are applied [28-30]. Successful application of CoMFA is illustrated by the studies of inhibitors: trypsin, thrombin, factor Xa [30] or thermolysin [31]. Currently, one of the most advanced QSAR-related techniques is the 4D-QSAR approach [32] which eliminates the restriction to a single conformation and allows averaging of the conventional 3D-QSAR descriptors thanks to the assumed conformational flexibility. It allows consideration of the effects of multiple conformations, alignments, and substructure groups i.e. extension of 'QSAR degrees of freedom' in comparison to those used in 3D-QSAR analysis. In this kind of approach, the so-called grid cell occupancy descriptors are used i.e. the occupancy frequencies of the different atom types (any type, nonpolar, polar-positive charge, polar-negative charge, hydrogen bond acceptor, hydrogen bond donor and aromatic) in the cubic grid cells [33,34]. An example of successful application of the RI-4D-QSAR approach is the study of 5′-arylthiourea thymidine analogues, showing inhibitory activity against thymidine monophosphate kinase from *M. tuberculsosis* (TMPKmt) [35]. Recently, different RI- and RD-4D-QSAR approaches were successfully applied to a variety of enzyme inhibitors of different drug targets, such as HIV-1 protease [36,37], HIV-1 integrase [38], p38-mitogen-activated protein kinase (p38-MAPK) [39], 14-α-lanosterol demethylase (CYP51) [40], enoyl-ACP reductase from *M. tuberculosis* (InhA) [41] etc.

Construction of a model requires determination of the structural elements of the target that would be necessary for the ligand to get recognised and to form a stable active complex. Depending on the availability of experimental data, one or a combination of the above mentioned methods is used. The optimum situation for CADD application is when both a group of ligands of defined activity and the spatial structure of the target are known. The search stage called molecular docking in which a ligand is matched to the receptor site and the quality of the fit (most often expressed in energy) is evaluated, is actually very similar irrespective of whether a direct or indirect approach is used. In both cases it is based on algorithms which simulate the docking process of ligands to the target [42]. The receptor binding pocket or its homology model can be used with auto-docking to find the most appropriate ligands or alternatively 3D-pharmacophore can be used in conformationally flexible (steric interactions) search for ligands that fit to the spatial distribution of the receptor. In order for the ligand-target interaction to occur, a few conditions must be met, such as a sufficient concentration of the drug which depends on the quantity of drug administered, its capacity to reach the target and its affinity and specificity for the target. Only specificity and affinity can be modelled, because they are directly related to the structural and electronic complementarities of the drug and target. The structural complementarity is strictly mechanistic and can be described as hollow/bump or key/lock adjustment. It is facilitated by the flexibility of drug and target i.e. their susceptibility to conformational changes which ensure the mutual compatibility of these two molecules. The electronic complementarity can be described as attraction/repulsion depending on the mutual relation between electron densities of the drug and target. In general it facilitates the approach of the drug to its target and in a consequence its binding. The most desirable combination is both a structural complementarity and an electronic complementarity between drug and target, as it ensures the best affinity. The interaction established between drug and target stabilizing the complex is rarely covalent and typically of low energy (electrostatic, van der Waals, hydrogen bonding). Therefore docking is accomplished by either geometric matching of the ligand and its receptor (faster) or by minimising the energy of interaction (slower, more accurate). Geometric matching is often replaced by the matching based on charge distribution, bond vectors, conformational flexibility, hydrophobic properties or molecular fragments.

Thus the knowledge of the 3D structure and/or the physico-chemical properties (electronic, steric, hydrophobic features etc.) of the drug and its biological target as well as the knowledge of their fluctuations related to their molecular motions, polymorphic transitions or shifts in tautomeric equilibrium of drug, is fundamental to understanding molecular recognition and intermolecular interactions participating in drug-target binding.

Many experimental and theoretical, very sophisticated techniques, provide complementary types of data, which after quick selection are considered to be required or not for the full description or prediction of drug - target interaction. With the development of experimental (e.g. XRD, NMR, NQR) and theoretical methods (e.g. ab initio, DFT at different levels) not only the number of recognised 3D structures of ligands and targets has dramatically increased, but also the amount of information on structural dynamics and electronic properties of drugs. The increased availability of these data is crucial for rational drug design, which in general has to involve many different pathways to achieve one common goal that is a drug more efficient and selective to its therapeutic target which exhibits efficacy in vivo and shows low toxicity. Achievement of this goal does not seem possible without understanding drugs on the molecular level.

3. Understanding of drugs on the molecular level

From the chemical point of view, the most important components of drugs i.e. Active Pharmaceutical Ingredients (API), a substance of a drug which is biologically active, and excipients, inactive substances used as a carrier for the API, are composed of small, organic, low-weight molecules (molecular mass below 100 Da, only rarely 500 Da) mainly obtained through chemical synthesis. However, the interest in drugs available through biological processes (biopolymer-based) steadily increases. It is difficult even to estimate the total number of currently known drugs and targets, as it is continuously in change, the data are scattered over multiple resources and available in a non-uniform manner. Comprehensive Medicinal Chemistry (CMC) lists 8,659 [43], PharmaPendium covers over 4,000 [44], Thomson REUTERS Forecast [45] tracks approximately 3,500 in clinical-stage and marketed drugs (700 strategic drugs). One of the largest databases - the Therapeutic Target Database [46] contains information about 11,978 drugs (including 1,514 approved, 1,282 in clinical trial, 9,182 experimental drugs and 3,645 multi-target agents) covering 140 therapeutic classes and 1,973 targets (including 358 successful, 254 clinical trial, 44 discontinued and 1,317 research targets) covering 61 protein biochemical class. Another database, BindingDB, contains 316,172 small drug-like molecules and 721,721 measured binding affinities for 6,179 protein considered to be drug-targets [47]. The DrugBank database [48] - a unique resource that combines chemical, pharmacological and pharmaceutical data with drug target (i.e. sequence, structure, and pathway) contains 6,816 drug entries including 1,437 FDA-approved small molecule drugs, 134 FDA-approved biotech (protein/peptide) drugs, 83 nutraceuticals and 5,194 experimental drugs.

According to World Health Organization (WHO) reports [49] the number of essential drugs has nearly doubled, from 186 in 1977 (1st edition) to 364 in 2011 (17th edition). It should be remembered that the list of essential drugs is extremely selective and includes only "*those drugs that satisfy the health care needs of the majority of the population; they should therefore be available at all times in adequate amounts and in appropriate dosage forms, at a price the community can afford*" [50]. The US Food and Drug Administration (FDA) agency lists about 800 approved API and there are over 100,000 drug products created from those API collected in Green Book, while 14,309 (primarily small-molecule drugs) are collected in US FDA's Orange Book [51] and about 6,000 biological drugs are listed by the Centre for Biologics Evaluation and Research (CBER) [52]. However, when duplicate APIs, salt forms, supplements, vitamins, imaging agents etc. are removed, the list of unique drugs can be shortened to 1,357, of which 1,204 are 'small-molecule drugs' and 166 are 'biological' drugs. FDA list contains also 11,066 inactive ingredients i.e. excipients.

The widely used classification system for API substances is the Anatomical Therapeutic Chemical (ATC) system [53] introduced in 1976 and controlled by Collaborating Centre for Drug Statistics Methodology (WHOCC). ATC categorizes API at different levels: anatomy, therapeutic properties and chemical properties according to therapeutic aspects. The modern, very recently introduced, system of classification [54] assumes that all current drugs with a known mode-of-action act through 324 distinct molecular drug targets and classifies them according to known targets (biochemical structures like: enzymes, substrates, metabolites and proteins, receptors, ion channels, transport proteins, DNA/RNA and the ribosome, targets of monoclonal antibodies; various physicochemical mechanisms and unknown mechanism of action). Current therapy is based on the above mentioned molecular targets [55,56] of which 270 are encoded by the human genome (45% - G-protein coupled receptors, 28% - enzymes, 11% - hormones, 5% - ion channels and 2% - nuclear receptors). Because each of 10 genes which contribute to multifactorial diseases are typically linked to other 5 - 10 gene products in physiological circuits suitable for pharmaceutical intervention, it is expected that in fact there are at least 10-20 times more targets [57]. Their identification is a priority as it determines the discovery of innovative drugs.

Many API's are intended to be used in solid dosage formulations, which is generally preferred for oral route of administration due to greater stability, smaller volume, accurate and flexible dosage and easy manufacturing. In fact oral small-molecule API's target as many as 227 molecular targets [56]. The modern system of classification of APIs according to known targets in fact classifies them according to their mechanisms of action i.e. the API effect at the molecular level. Understanding the API effect at the molecular level requires the knowledge of fundamental data including spatial 3D structure and physico-chemical properties of API. A combination of the experimental (XRD, NMR, NQR spectroscopic techniques) and theoretical data (ab initio, DFT calculations) in a synergistic manner not only provides the data on structure or properties but also allows prediction of the way in which the specific molecular changes will alter the features of API. This, in turn, indicates the directions of design of new API by taking into account such factors as predisposition to participate in certain intermolecular and intramolecular interactions, tendency to polymorphic or tautomeric transitions, required stability (thermal or photo or radiation stability) or solubility. All these factors are closely related to biological effect therapeutic or toxic thus provide the basis for understanding drugs at a more fundamental level. The examples discussed in the next section will cover some, but not all these aspects.

3.1 Spatial 3D structure

In 1868 Brown and Fraser [58] discovered that biological activity of compounds is related to their chemical structure. Until the mid 1990s, the 3D structure was in fact the main a basis of drug design, but even nowadays it is still a key factor. As previously mentioned, the knowledge of the spatial 3D structure of API itself or its biological target is the core of CADD techniques. 3D structure of API or target can be determined either experimentally, using direct or indirect methods, or can be predicted theoretically.

3.1.1 Experimental structure

XRD

The most important sources of information on the drug structures are direct crystallographic methods, i.e. the methods which derive diffraction phases directly from experimentally measured diffraction amplitudes. The first atomic-resolution crystal structure solved by Bragg in 1914 [59] was that of NaCl - a substance playing a crucial role in maintaining the fluid and electrolyte balance. The standard single crystal XRD, actually providing a resolution of 0.5-3.0 Å, is a main source of information about the molecular conformation and packing in the crystalline structure. For small molecules, the crystal structures are usually well resolved. However, high quality single crystals of sufficient size of many pharmaceuticals have proved impossible to grow, while polycrystalline powders can be readily made. For such substances, the powder X-ray diffraction (PXRD) or small-angle X-ray scattering (SAXS) are used to obtain the relevant structural information, which is in fact less detailed. Despite this, PXRD pattern, considered as a characteristic fingerprint of a crystalline phase, is used to identify and characterise crystal forms including polymorphs (1800 of such a patterns are stored at CSD).

A significant disadvantage of XRD from the point of view of APIs studies is not only the necessity of obtaining crystals, but the difficulty in determining the positions of light atoms such hydrogen (only one electron) resulting in imprecise description of weak intermolecular interactions. Although, various parameters describing the covalent geometry (i.e., bond lengths, bond angles, planes, and chirality) are determined to a very high accuracy [60], the degree of uncertainty of the parameters characterising the weak, nonbonding interactions is still high. The application of neutron diffraction (ND), which due to the interaction of radiation with atomic nuclei gives highly accurate positions of tiny atoms (hydrogen), partially solves this problem. The widely used approach for this purpose is the Hansen-Coppens formalism [61] in which individual atomic densities are described in terms of a spherical core and valence densities. Expansion of the atom-centred spherical-harmonic functions is the main idea of this so-called multipole approach. Another solution is modelling with the use of independent atoms [62], or partial optimisation using quantum chemistry methods ab initio or DFT [63]. However, irrespective of the method, the final result becomes in fact not purely experimental. The most accurate API structures, with respect to both molecular geometry and motional description, still come from low-temperature ND [64]. Despite the above mentioned inconveniences, XRD is the starting point for gathering information about APIs.

XRD is also the oldest and major source of 3D structures of targets as well as drug-target complexes [65,66]. In 1965 Johnson and Philips [65] solved the structure of lysozyme (with 2 Å resolution), a 14,7 kDa enzyme which can be found in tears, saliva and egg white. A milestone in the development of CADD was the invention of X-ray structural analysis techniques that would allow examination of structures of very large molecules - proteins, enzymes. The largest known and resolved by XRD protein is human Titin, which consists of 34,350 amino acids, with the molecular weight of the 'canonical' isoform of the protein being approximately 3,816,188.13 Da [67]. However, its use is still marred with a number of restrictions, the method can be applied to good crystals, so its use is restricted to solids (difficult to obtain for targets), it gives no possibility to examine small parts in the large molecule in details, it is unable to reveal many conformations (molecular motions are neglected) or to determine the secondary structures, which is crucial for the target or drug-target complex. A common but rarely mentioned problem of X-ray crystallography and electron crystallography is radiation damage of the samples studied.

The other worth mentioning techniques, complementary to XRD, are the Small-angle X-ray scattering (SAXS) [68], atomic forces microscopy (ATF) [69] or cryo-electron microscopy [70], which allow studies under physiological conditions and are used for studies of micro or nanoscale particles. However, actually their resolution is still lower than that of XRD. One more technique complementary to XRD is the high-resolution electron microscopy (HREM), which can be successfully applied for crystal structure analysis when the grain size is too small or periodicity is imperfect. Its main advantage over XRD is more convenient observation of light atoms in the presence of much heavier atoms. HREM is able to produce a microscopic image and a corresponding diffraction pattern in the atomic scale, however, for crystalline samples the resolution is too low to reveal individual atoms [70].

There are many other techniques that are useful in the study of crystals, but their description is outside the scope of this paper.

NMR

Some of the limitations of XRD can be easily overcome by other techniques like NMR, which reveals a 3D structure of a molecule not only in crystal but also in its natural - biological environment. Solid state NMR (SS NMR) is one of the most important tools for structural investigation of solid APIs for which it delivers data complementary to XRD (precise bond lengths and angles within a molecule, intermolecular bond lengths and angles). It can be said that it adds the time-dependence to the XRD parameter-set, which allows studies of the kinetics of reactions, molecular motions, conformational changes etc. Depending on the type of experiment, different NMR parameters: isotropic chemical shifts, coupling constants, rate constants, chemical shift tensors, spin diffusion and dipolar interactions etc., provide different information about the chemical environment of the selected nuclei in a molecule. In general, the principles are the same for solution and SS NMR. However, low sensitivity and severe line broadening originating from chemical shift anisotropy (CSA) and dipolar interactions are serious inconveniences for SS NMR. Three techniques: cross polarisation (CP), magic angle spinning (MAS) and high-power^{1}H decoupling are applied to overcome the problems encountered in the solid state NMR. For small compounds like APIs each chemically inequivalent site and functional group can be distinguished on the basis of chemical shift. In fact, unique SS NMR spectroscopy capabilities allow differentiation of isomorphic solids, which are difficult to distinguish by XRD. When the spectra are complicated, the spin-spin splittings or *J*-couplings are used to elucidate and verify a possible structure but this can prove insufficient [71]. Moreover, in large molecules such as e.g. targets, the number of chemical shifts can be extremely large (even several thousand) and can suffer from incidental overlaps. The use of sophisticated techniques like multidimentional 2D-4D NMR is then required [72-76]. The most popular are 2D homonuclear NMR experiments: correlation spectroscopy (COSY) [71] and total correlation spectroscopy (TOCSY) [72], which correlate different spins via scalar spin–spin couplings or nuclear Overhauser effect spectroscopy (NOESY) [73], which describes dipole–dipole coupling between pairs of nuclei or Incredible Natural Abundance Double Quantum Transfer Experiment (INADEQUATE) [77], which correlates different carbon nuclei. Each of them produces two-dimensional spectra mapping chemical shifts and reflecting adjacent atoms (COSY) or all atoms if they are connected by a continuous chain of protons (e.g. side chains of amino acids) (TOCSY). Apart from this, the method is also able to reveal the spatial proximity between the atoms (NOESY). As the intensity of a NOESY peak is reciprocally proportional to the 6th power distance, thus it reveals the distance. Because the intensity-distance relationship is approximate thus NOESY derived distance is not exact. The other disadvantages of NOESY are separations no farther than 5 Å and the ambiguous assignment of peaks that are close in space but do not belong to the sequential residues. For such a purpose the technique of labelling of proteins (with ^{13}C, ^{15}N or ^{2}D) is used. Instead of NOESY one or more of the six HSQC-type experiments (HNCO, HNCACO, HNCA, HNCOCA, HNCACB and CBCACONH) can be used, which are capable to resolve overlap in the carbon dimension. The most widely used is the HCCH-TOCSY method (i.e. TOCSY resolved in an additional carbon dimension). Apart from distances, NMR provides estimation of the torsion angles (on the basis of *J*-coupling constants - Karplus equation or chemical shifts). The introduction of isotope labelling and multidimentional experiments extended the area of NMR applications to targets. However, fast relaxation and broader and weaker peaks, which can easily disappear are important limitations. Recently, two techniques dedicated to large target studies have been introduced: residual dipolar couplings (RDC) [78,79], which can be used in particular for the reveal the orientation of the N-H as well as the whole structure refinement, transverse relaxation optimised spectroscopy (TROSY) [80,81] and cross-correlated relaxation-enhanced polarisation transfer (CRINEPT) [82]. These modern techniques allow studies of targets larger than 150kDa. It should be emphasised that the structural information provided by NMR is indirect because no simple relationship between the experimental data and Cartesian coordinates is available. While XRD delivers the approximated coordinates of atoms in target, the NMR gives the estimations of distances between the pairs of target atoms. Therefore, the final conformation of a target is obtained, by solving a geometry-distance problem. Because the actual conformation depends on the properties of the environment, thus the use of NMR to study its influence is possible, for example the influence of different solvents. The resolution of NMR, 2-5 Å, is much lower than XRD since the information got from the same material is much more complex. For the same reason, NMR allows determination of the 3D structure of smaller molecules than XRD. The most spectacular NMR result is the determination of the protein in complex with the 900 kDa chaperone GroES-GroEL [83]. Unique advantages of NMR are the capability of solving secondary structures [84-86] and mapping the binding sites of the substrate [87,88]. At the current state-of-the art methodologies, XDR is still much more efficient than NMR, even in solving a structure of a target. While NMR is expensive - requires isotope labelling, sophisticated spectrometers and time consuming - a determination a high-resolution structure of proteins <40 kDa may take even a year, XDR routinely solves it in weeks to months. Despite these limitations, the role of NMR is continually expanding, as evidenced by the fact that NMR has evolved into one of the two major techniques for elucidation of structure and dynamics of targets and target-drug complexes.

Taking into account advantages and disadvantages of both methods the optimum method for solving structure of API is XRD, while a combination of XRD and NMR studies provides 3D structures of targets or drug-target complexes.

Against the background of the above mentioned methods, NQR, which gives quadrupole coupling constants (e^2qQ/h) and asymmetry parameters (η) from experimental frequencies, seems to have very limited capabilities. Moreover its use involves a number of restrictions; it can be applied only to high purity solids (crystalline or polycrystalline), only for selected isotopes and practically its applications are limited to API. In fact, however, this underappreciated technique has some unique advantages and is an effective tool for preliminary study of crystal structure in the absence of X-Ray data. It allows measurements of distances but only NH or OH bond lengths, gives the number of inequivalent molecules in the elementary cell, permits differentiation of isomers, enantiomers, polymorphs etc.

Successful application of NQR to analysis of structural aspects is illustrated by the studies of the most widely used cytotoxic agent most effective in the treatment of epithelial malignancies such as lung, head and neck, ovarian, bladder and testicular cancer, i.e.cisplatin cis -diamminedichloroplatinum (II). Although cisplatinum and its complexes are widely used as anti-cancer drugs, neither its isomer - transplatin *trans* - diamminedichloroplatinum (I) - nor its complexes have therapeutic properties. Possible explanations of different biological activity of the *cis* and *trans* isomers are that *cis* compounds make platinum-DNA adducts inhibiting DNA replication or transcription to a greater extent than those formed by transplatin, and alternatively, that DNA adducts formed by *trans* compounds may be repaired more efficiently [89]. Thus, differentiation between the *cis* and trans isomers is essential. Isomers distinction for any platinum compounds showing *trans* - *cis* isomerism with ^{35}Cl-NQR is easy as the difference in the resonance frequencies is high enough and reaches 2.13 MHz: 16.18 MHz for *cis*-platinum and 18.31MHz for *trans*-platinum [90]. Another interesting example of NQR capabilities is the study of serine, which occurs in the active sites of many enzymes like chymotrypsin, trypsin and plays an important catalytic function. The enzyme serine racemase converts L-serine into the less common D-isomer (a co-agonist of the N-methyl-D-aspartate receptor in glutamate neurotransmission) and can be used to develop treatments for neurodegenerative diseases (schizophrenia). The sophisticated high sensitivity SQUID technique allows studies of chirality i.e. distinction of L-serine and D-serine and its racemate DL-serine [91] on the basis of small differences in the frequencies (0.018 and 0.023 MHz), quadrupole coupling constants (0.004 MHz) and asymmetry parameters (0.066 MHz). One more illustrative example are NQR studies of diuretic drugs: the highly active and thus widely used one - hydrochlorothiazide (HCTZ) and the weak one and thus used only to alter the mode of furosemide activity - chlorothiazide (CTZ). Both are used in the treatment of hypertension, congestive heart failure, symptomatic oedema and prevention of kidney stones. The difference is only in one bond (in CTZ either the bond N(2)-C(3) or C(3)-N(4) is double, while in HCTZ one hydrogen atom occurs at N(2) and N(4), and the two bonds N(2)-C(3) and C(3)-N(4) are single). This structural difference results in a significant (1.26 MHz) difference in frequencies, which makes the distinction of both compounds very easy [92].

As far as large structures are concerned, a striking example of NQR application was a direct observation of Zn^{2+} in Carbonic Anhydrase (CA), the first enzyme whose activity was recognised to be related to the presence of Zn^{2+}, which was postulated as the activator of bound H_2O. CA, which commonly occurs in all mammalian tissues, plants, algae, and bacteria, is perhaps one of the best recognised metalloprotein. The ^{67}Zn QCC values, being sensitive to changes in the structure and bonding associated with water or hydroxide have been found independent of pH over the range of 5 to 8.5 [93], whereas, according to the hitherto commonly assumed model, Zn^{2+} should be coordinated by H_2O, and as a result, at these pH values the ^{67}Zn NQR spectrum should be three to five times broader than that at pH 8.5. This observation was in contradiction to the widely accepted mechanism and led to acceptance of an alternative one proposed by Merz, Hoffmann, and Dewar [94]. The above example demonstrates the significance of zinc NQR spectroscopy in delineating the structure and mechanism of activity of this class of metalloproteins.

These examples show that NQR has a potential to provide vital structural information about the drug, target and the drug-target interaction.

3.1.2 Predicted structure

Prediction of the structure of single molecules, the so-called geometry optimisation, is available within different approaches starting from molecular mechanics up to very sophisticated levels of the quantum chemical theory. But a single molecule structure is far from that in crystal, especially for flexible molecules. Although it is known that molecules in crystals are bonded via intermolecular interactions, which are weak and numerous, but they act at long ranges and have little directionality, which makes crystals difficult to model [95]. Thus crystal structure prediction (CSP), which includes the prediction of the crystal structures of solids from first principles, is a much more complicated task. Reliable methods for the prediction of crystal structure only on the basis of molecular structure have been searched for since the 1950s [95]. Until recently, crystal structure could not have been predicted computationally from first principles because of the nature of forces acting between the molecules in crystals. Reliable CSP requires assumption of clearly defined criteria of the quality of structure reproduction. One possibility is a comparison of the predicted structure with those experimentally determined. A good test of CSP quality is the validity of reproducing structures that differ only slightly as those of different polymorphs. Indeed, many unsuccessful attempts to predict the structures of polymorphs of sulphonamide have been undertaken. It was believed that the reason for the failure was the kinetic nature of crystallization. But it turned out that successful CSP for small drug molecules is possible [96,97]. Only recently, the structures of three known polymorphs of

sulphanilamide have been correctly predicted from ab initio [98]. The prediction of target or target-drug structure is still an issue for the future.
Much faster is the CSP validation based on experimental parameters. For example NQR, which is a very sensitive technique, provides parameters directly describing the local environment of a nucleus in the molecule. However CPS, based only on these data is impossible, but in combination with DFT it can be used for example to evaluate the degree of structural refinement. A valuable example is triclosan (5-chloro-2-(2′,4′-dichlorophenoxy)-phenol, TCS) active pharmaceutical ingredient (API) of a known potent wide spectrum of antibacterial, antimicrobial and antifungal agents used in many drugs as well as antiseptic or disinfectant formulations. The crystalline structure of TCS, which crystallizes in the space group $P3_1$ with one molecule in the asymmetric unit has been solved by XRD and refined to a final *R*-factor of 2.81% at room temperature [99] and 3.74% at 90 K [100]. The conformation adopted by diphenyl ether of TCS in solid is temperature independent, typical of diphenyl ethers but the opposite to that adopted when it is bound to different inhibitors. The importance of this finding is the suggestion of the presence of two enantiomers of triclosan, which would nicely explain a wide spectrum of its activity. The smooth changes in NQR frequency with temperature increasing from 77 K to 300 K [101] and similar parameters of the unit cells at RT and at 90 K (a=12.5225 Å, b=12.5225 Å and c=6.6809 Å [100] versus a=12.6410 Å, b=12.6410 Å and c=6.7163 Å [99]) confirmed no phase transformation from RT to 90 K during the data collection. The differences in RT and 90K structures seem relatively small but the NQR spectrum of triclosan was much better reproduced at the B3LYP/6-311++G(d,p) level of theory assuming the room temperature structure than 90K one. The scattering of NQR frequencies was found to be a good indicator of the quality of the crystallographic structure resolution [99].

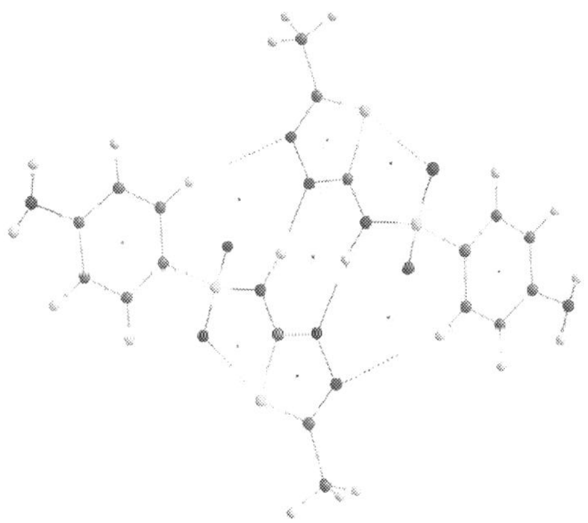

Fig. 1. Predicted structure of sulfamethizole.

NQR combined with DFT can be also used for structure prediction. An interesting example is the structure of sulfamethizole, known to be able to crystallize in different polymorphic forms [102,103] of which none, even the most stable one, was solved. In a single molecule of sulfamethizole there are four nonequivalent nitrogen positions, but within the NQR experimental resolution five nitrogen positions have been detected [104]. This indicated either two nonequivalent molecules in the unit cell or two polymorphic crystal forms of sulfamethizole. The lines at the-NH- and -NH_2 nitrogen positions do not show any splitting within the experimental resolution. A possible explanation of the ^{14}N NQR spectra is that the sulfamethizole molecules form slightly asymmetric hydrogen bonded pairs, similar to the symmetric pairs formed by the acetazolamide molecules. The NQR parameters obtained by B3LYP/6-311++G(d,p) assuming putative dimeric structure, Fig.1., were in a very good agreement with the experimental data [104].

Studies of isostructurality and annular 50:50 prototropic tautomerism of pentabromobenzimidazoles make another example of the successful prediction of crystalline structure performed by NQR and DFT/QTAIM combined [105]. On the basis of three known XRD structures of 4,5,6,7-tetraiodo-1H-benzimidazole, 4,6-dibromo-5,7-diiodo-1H-benzimidazole and 4,6-dichloro-5,7-diiodo-1H-benzimidazole the crystalline structures of a set of pentabromo-benzimidazoles have been proposed and the most stable polymorphic form (alpha) has been predicted.

3.2 Intermolecular interactions pattern

Intermolecular interaction pattern can be analysed using structural data, but more detailed information can be derived from the electron density distribution, which can be determined either experimentally or theoretically. The electron density distribution is a purely physical property of molecules and an observable, thus it can be approached experimentally directly (as maps) or indirectly (as parameters).

For single molecules electron density distribution can be derived from gas electron diffraction (GES) while for solid formulations of drugs from diffraction methods like XRD or neutron diffraction. Using the intensities (measured directly) and phases of the scattered X-Rays (obtained indirectly for example by intelligent guess i.e. Hautpmann-Karl method, through isomorphic substitution or a comparison of intensities at a range of wavelengths near the K_{α} edge of a heavy atom in the crystal) the electron distribution in the crystal after 3D Fourier transform can be mapped as a contour plot, the so-called Fourier map of electron density. According to Parseval's theorem [106], the rms error in Fourier map is proportional to the rms error in the structure factor thus minimisation of rms error in electron density distributions ensures getting a structural factor that minimises the rms error in the complex plane. Importantly, X-ray is in fact an imaging technique because the Fourier transform of the observed structure yields an electron density map of the molecule.

SS NMR, which is complementary to XRD taking into account structure solving, does not deliver an electron density distribution per se but the variations in chemical shielding (or its isotropic chemical shifts) that reflect the variations in this distribution (lower electron density is reflected by smaller chemical shifts). The reliable and experimental parameters directly describing electron density distribution - quadrupole coupling constants and asymmetry parameters - are delivered by NQR. They reflect the electron distribution in the vicinity of the quadrupolar nucleus, thus provide a very sensitive tool for investigation of short range interactions (in contrast to the long range periodic order seen by the XRD). The disadvantage of NQR is the fact that it is not an imaging technique i.e. it does not deliver Fourier maps.

The electron density distribution can be also obtained theoretically using quantum chemical calculations at different levels of theory (semiempirical, *ab intio* or DFT).

Detailed analysis of topology of the electron density distribution, obtained experimentally or theoretically, can be performed within the Quantum Theory of Atoms in Molecules,

QTAIM formulated by Bader [107]. Within this approach the electron density $\rho(r)$ of a molecule, treated as a scalar field, can be examined by analysis of its gradient vector field and a Laplacian. An atom is defined as a region of real space bounded by surfaces through which there is a zero flux in the gradient vector field of the electron density. The values of $\rho(r)$ at the start and end points of a gradient path, which follows the largest increase in $\rho(r)$, take extremes: maxima or minima, or saddle points in the electron density. Depending on the nature of the extreme they are called the nuclear attractor-, bond-, ring-, and cage-critical points and denoted as NACP, BCP, RCP and CCP, respectively. The type of the critical point can be easily determined with the help of a Hessian matrix composed of nine second-order derivatives of $\rho(r)$. The knowledge of electron density distribution allows evaluation of many one-electron properties (e.g. electric dipole moment, electrostatic potential, electric field, electric field gradient, Laplacian of electron density, molecular orbitals) describing the bonds in molecules and intermolecular interactions pattern in molecular crystals. The electron density $\rho(r)$ at BCP and its Laplacian are the indicators of the character of the bond and allow classification of the bondings according to the following rules:

- $\rho(r) > 0$, $\Delta\rho(r) < 0$; covalent (pure closed-shell)
- $\rho(r) \sim 0$, $\Delta\rho(r) > 0$; ionic (pure shared shell)
- $\rho(r) > 0$, $\Delta\rho(r) > 0$; charge shift (transit closed shell)

A number of books [107,108] and review articles [109-111] have described this technique and given examples of its application. The electron density (and thus properties of a molecule) varies according to the local geometry (binding partners, bond lengths, angles between bonds etc.) or external factors (temperature, pressure, solvent, external electric field etc.). Additionally, the electron density can be also influenced by another molecule to the extent dependent on polarisability. This factor is very important for slightly charged atoms having a great number of electrons, like sulphur or iodine, which permits their participation in intermolecular interactions.

Highlighted below are the examples wherein SS NMR and especially NQR spectroscopy combined with DFT has been used to extract detail information on APIs. In this section, particular instances of application of NQR spectroscopy, which provide unique quality information for CADD i.e. for crystal engineering strategies and structure-property relationships are presented.

3.2.1 Polymorphism

Polymorphism (Greek: *polys -multiple, morfé - shape*) is the ability of a substance to exist in more than one crystalline form (polymorph) depending on the crystallisation conditions. While initially most polymorphs have been discovered by chance [111-115], recently identification of polymorphism is a result of a systematic search or is even required by the FDA standards. According to McCrone suggestion, "*in general, the number of forms known for a given compound is proportional to the time and money spent in research on that compound*" [116]. Approximately 70% of API exhibit polymorphism and rarely the differences between two polymorphs and their properties are subtle (e.g. aspirin - acetylsalycilic acid [117]).

Polymorphs differ in physico-chemical properties (e.g. solubility, dissolution rate, permeability, chemical reactivity, melting point, optical and electrical properties, vapour pressure, crystal shape, compressibility, density, hardness, resistance to degradation), which makes a very important problem from the point of view of pharmaceutical industry. It can cause crucial problems not only with the manufacturing or the quality of the formulation but also with the biodisponibility of the active substance and drug stability (i.e. shelf life of a drug). Thus characterisation of solid-state properties of API as well as excipients is of particular interest. In fact API exhibiting structural polymorphism received regulatory approval for only one single crystal form or a specific polymorph. An example is Cefdinir, broad-spectrum antibiotic, for which a lot of companies (Fujisawa, Biochemie, ACS Dobfar, Orchid, Abbott, Aurobindo, Novartis, Lupin, Rambaxy) patented 11 polymorphs related to 5 crystalline forms [118], atorvastatin calcium - a statin lowering blood cholesterol, for which more than 60 solid forms have been patented [119], piroxicam - a non-steroidal anti-inflammatory drug, synthesized in more than 50 forms [120] and sulfathiazole a local antimicrobial agent for which more than 100 forms have been described [121]. From among multicomponents the one showing the optimum properties from the biological activity point of view is chosen.

For pharmaceutical companies, the phenomenon of polymorphism is rather a disadvantage, however sometimes it is used to extend original patents on existing API ,but this procedure requires checking that one polymorph does not decompose or transform to another (infringement of another patent). A well-known example is the patent litigation between pharmaceutical companies Glaxo and Novopharm concerning two polymorphs of ranitidine hydrochloride - a histamine H_2-receptor antagonist that inhibits stomach acid production [122], the problem of "disappearing polymorphs" of ritonavir [123] - an inhibitor of HIV-protease manufactured by Abbot Laboratories or paxil - anti-depressant manufactured by SmithKline Beecham (GlaxoSmithKline). Therefore, the original companies use a stable polymorph, while the generic companies a meta-stable polymorph. The way of labelling of polymorphs is inconsistent (e.g. I, II, III ...; A, B, C...; α,β,γ...) and has no relation to a polymorph stability; it occasionally happens that identical forms are named differently.

In general, polymorphism results from different crystal packing of rigid molecules (packing polymorphism) e.g. acetazolamide, cloxiquine, the presence of different conformations of a flexible molecule (conformational polymorphism) e.g. sulfanilamide, chlorpropamide, or can be a result of inclusion of water or solvent molecules in the lattice i.e. hydration or solvation, respectively (pseudopolymorphism or solvatomorphism) e.g. chloral hydrate, cefdinir. The packing polymorphism is much rarer than the conformational one. In practice usually the mixed types of polymorphism are encountered. The most frequent case is dimorphism. There is a tight connection between the synthons arrangement (packing polymorphism) or the molecular conformation (conformational polymorphism) and the crystal packing in a an elementary unit. The weak noncovalent interactions (hydrogen-bonds, Van der Waals forces, coulombic interactions, steric repulsions π-π interactions) are responsible for the bonds between molecules or supramolecular synthons in the crystal. In general, the molecular energy and the lattice energy of the crystals are not independent, but in fact they control each other. Changes in the weak interaction pattern are able to induce further changes for example in torsion angles, which can result in stabilization of different molecular conformations close to the most stable equilibrium one. Consequently, various nearly energetically equal molecular conformations can force crystallization in different polymorphs. Therefore, a study of molecular motions is sometimes used for the characterisation of polymorphs. Elucidation of the very origin of polymorphism is often crucial to understanding drugs at the molecular level. Polymorphism is a widespread phenomenon among small molecules of APIs, mostly because of their flexibility, the presence of hydrogen bond donor/acceptor sites or overlapping of p-orbitals in π-conjugated systems.

The differences in crystalline structures between polymorphs result in differences in their properties, of which solubility and dissolution rate are considered to be the most important. The solubility in aqueous media is of particular interest because it may influence bioavailability. Although a typical ratio of solubility of two polymorphs is less than two, it is not a rule. For example the ratio of two polymorphs of acetazolamide (I and II) is 1.11 [124], while for premafloxacin (I and III) or chloramphenicol (A and B) it exceeds 10 [125]. When the differences between the solubility of polymorphs are great, the minimum therapeutic concentration in the blood of the poorer soluble polymorph (according to the Hammond rule [126], the poorer soluble polymorph can be more therapeutically active) can be insufficient for its effective activity. It is a rule that anhydrates/ansolvates of API are better soluble than its hydrated/solvated forms.

There are a number of methods that can be used to characterise polymorphs of a drug substance [127] but the single crystal XRD is currently regarded as bringing definitive qualitative and quantitative evidence of polymorphism. Facility of XRD data acquisition and XRD usefulness as a screening technique make it is more often used than the other physico-chemical methods commonly used for the investigation of polymorphism, like hot-stage microscopy (melting point), solid-state infrared spectroscopy (IR), X-ray powder diffraction (PXRD), differential scanning calorimetry (DSC), thermogravimetric analysis (TGA), differential thermal analysis (DTA), FT-Raman spectroscopy and scanning electron microscopy (SEM). However, XRD analysis is not always possible, for example, when no single crystal of sufficient size, quality or stability can be obtained. The complementary tools of ever-growing value for the solid-state characterisation of API, excipients or drug formulations are the solid-state nuclear magnetic resonance spectroscopy (SS NMR) and a more sophisticated but less popular - nuclear quadrupole resonance (NQR). As compared to the IR, Raman, and XRD techniques, SS NMR or NQR are bulk techniques in which the particle size of the substance studied does not matter. In contrast to XRD, they can be applied even to amorphous samples (in the case of NQR after freezing in liquid nitrogen), although it is not easy because of great line widths. Both techniques are non-invasive and non-selective which means that low molecular weight components in the sample can be detected in a single experiment. In a sense they can be defined as selective because they allow detection of signals from the selected types of nuclei. Both techniques are quantitative, i.e. can be used to measure the content of API in a sample. Compared to other techniques, SS NMR and even more NQR are less sensitive and require more expensive equipment, which is their main drawback. Although in many cases SS NMR or NQR can be very effective, the majority of studies of pharmaceutical polymorphs are still performed in conjunction with other analytical techniques. While NMR has become in recent years very popular in studies of drugs, the use of NQR spectroscopy is rather scarce as from over 250 compounds whose polymorphism has been studied by this method [128] fewer than 20 were API, pharmaceutical formulations or excipients.

In general, the suitability of solid-state NMR or NQR for investigation of polymorphism follows from the fact that each polymorph is crystallographically different, which means that a certain nucleus in each polymorph is in a slightly different local molecular environment. Since the local environment at the nucleus site of interest is different, the SS NMR or NQR spectra differ slightly. In consequence, the isotropic chemical-shift / CSA tensor or NQR frequency/quadrupole coupling constant and asymmetry parameter derived from these spectra also differ for the corresponding sites. Thus the analysis and spectral assignment of the solid-state NMR or NQR spectra of the polymorphs provides easy identification of polymorphic forms based only on the spectra recorded. More sophisticated analysis of the experimental solid-state NMR or NQR data often combined with modelling on the basis of quantum chemistry calculations (DFT or ab initio) can lead to the origin of differences in the structure of particular polymorphs.

For the first time the differences in the SS NMR spectra being a result of polymorphism have been reported by Byrn et al. for benoxaprofen (non-steroidal anti-inflammatory drug), nabilone (antiemetic, an adjunct analgesic for neuropathic pain) and pseudo-polymorphism of cefazolin (first-generation cephalosporin antibiotic broad-spectrum) [129]. The method of choice was then PXRD, but surprisingly the solid-state ^{13}C CP/MAS NMR spectrum of each polymorph was found to be distinctly different. These studies performed on bulk API material initiated more systematic studies of polymorphism by SS NMR. The first NQR studies of API polymorphism have been reported much earlier than those by SS NMR [130,131]. The first studied API was chloral hydrate (trichloroacetaldehyde monohydrate, 2,2,2-trichloro-1,1-ethanediol), one of the oldest synthetic agents, a sedative and hypnotic drug. Significant improvement in sensitivity and resolution meant that both methods have become important complementary tools in the studies of polymorphism. SS NMR has been recently accepted by US and Japan Pharmacopeia as a method for polymorphism determination, NQR studies having been too scarce and not so popular.

3.2.1.1 Packing polymorphism

The packing polymorphism occurs when rigid molecules of the same conformation are packed in different ways in a crystal.

Glycine

An interesting example and the most intensively studied organic polymorph, is glycine, the simplest amino acid, a precursor to proteins, an inhibitory neurotransmitter in the central nervous system, anti-cancer, chronic multiple sclerosis and schizophrenia drug, also widely applied as excipient to drugs. In the solid state, glycine crystallizes in three forms α, β and γ, which can be distinguished by XRD [132-134] or neutron diffraction [135,136]. The α form is stable, the β form is unstable and readily transforms to α [132], while the γ form is stable at room temperature, but irreversibly converts to α upon heating above 438K. The internal arrangement of molecules in layers is the same for α, β, which crystallize in monoclinic, P21/n and $P2_1$, respectively, while γ crystallizes with a trigonal hemihedral symmetry, in hexagonal, $P3_1$. In general, in all three forms the glycine molecules are zwitterions, the hydrogen-bonded double layers of molecules are packed by van der Waals forces and the only difference in the two forms results from the nature of the hydrogen bonding. Polycrystalline samples can be distinguished using X-ray powder diffraction [138] or infrared (IR) spectroscopy [133, 139]. The well-marked differences in the N-H stretching frequency in IR spectra (3164 cm^{-1} for α-glycine, 3191 cm^{-1} for β-glycine, and at 3105 cm^{-1} for γ-glycine) allow fast identification of the polymorphs in a polycrystalline sample [140].

The polymorphs of glycine can be also distinguished using solid ^{13}C NMR or ^{15}N NMR by a direct comparison of the isotropic chemical shifts and/or chemical shift tensor components [139, 141]. However, the differences in these values are relatively small, at most of an order of 1ppm, Table 1. The sources of differences in the components of the chemical shift tensor, especially σ_{yy} at ^{13}C and σ_{zz} at ^{15}N for polymorphs have been revealed by the quantum chemistry methods, DFT [142]. These differences have been explained by changes in the hydrogen bonding arrangement of α-glycine and β-glycine. In addition, polymorphs can be readily identified by the spin-lattice relaxation times $^{1}H\ T_{1\rho}$ and $^{15}N\ T_1$, which are much shorter for α-glycine and β-glycine than for γ form.

SITE	FORM I α					FORM II β					FORM III γ				
	σ_{iso} [ppm]	σ_{xx} [ppm]	σ_{yy} [ppm]	σ_{zz} [ppm]	T_1, $T_{1\rho}$ [s]	σ_{iso} [ppm]	σ_{xx} [ppm]	σ_{yy} [ppm]	σ_{zz} [ppm]	T_1, $T_{1\rho}$ [s]	σ_{iso} [ppm]	σ_{xx} [ppm]	σ_{yy} [ppm]	σ_{zz} [ppm]	T_1, $T_{1\rho}$ [s]
^{13}C	176.5 177.0 176.5	 243.5 244	 178.9 180	 108.7 105	12 , 0.18 (C=O) 11, 0.043 (NCH_2)	175.5 175.4	 243.5	 176.5	 106.0	8, 0.012 (C=O) 2.3, 0.30 (NCH_2)	174.5 174.9 174.6	243.2 243	174.9 173	106.6 108	55, 0.27 (C=O) 22, 0.053 (NCH_2)
^{15}N	32.3 32.5	 40.2	 33.1	 24.3	0.240 0.93	-	-	-	-	-	32.9 32.8	 40.5	 33.6	 26.7	0.150 0.018

Table 1. The isotropic chemical shifts and CSA tensor components, spin-lattice relaxation times T_1, $T_{1\rho}$ - in glycine forms α, β and γ [140, 141].

The use of ^{14}N NQR for differentiation of polymorphs is even much easier than the use of NMR, as the frequencies (ν), quadrupole coupling constants e^2Qq/h and asymmetry parameters (η) for β and γ-glycine, are significantly higher than for α - form, Table 2. The changes in quadrupole coupling constants and asymmetry parameters reflect the differences in the hydrogen bonding length pattern.

FORM I α					FORM II β					FORM III γ				
ν_+ [MHz]	ν_- [MHz]	ν_0 [MHz]	e^2Qq/h [MHz]	η [-]	ν_+ [MHz]	ν_- [MHz]	ν_0 [MHz]	e^2Qq/h [MHz]	η [-]	ν_+ [MHz]	ν_- [MHz]	ν_0 [MHz]	e^2Qq/h [MHz]	η [-]
1.100	0.785	0.315	1.257	0.501	1.133	0.843	0.290	1.317	0.440	1.044	0.822	0.222	1.244	0.357
0.988	0.705	0.283	1.129	0.501			-	-	-			-	-	-

Table 2. ^{14}N NQR frequencies, quadrupole coupling constants and asymmetry parameters - in glycine forms α, β and γ [143,144].

Acetazolamide

An example of packing polymorphism is acetazolamide, the first non-mercurial diuretic drug, used clinically as antiglaucoma, antiepileptic or antiulcer, benign intracranial hypertension, altitude sickness, cystinuria and dural ectasia drug. Acetazolamide crystallizes in two polymorphic forms I and II [145], which differ in the spatial molecular arrangement and hydrogen bonding pattern, but not in the conformation of molecules. Thus the polymorphism of acetazolamide is classified as a packing type or pure combining association type. Interesting results concerning the interaction pattern have been obtained using NMR, NQR and DFT/QTAIM calculations [104]. The marked differences in the ^{14}N NQR frequencies, quadrupole coupling constants and asymmetry parameters at the nitrogen sites in the thiadiazole ring and $-NH_2$ on going from phase I to phase II allow distinction of both polymorphs, Table 3. Surprisingly the changes in the NQR parameters are negligible at -NH site. Moreover, the change in the parameters at the $-NH_2$ nitrogen site is significant.

As the source of this diversity can be either different hybridisation or participation in different hydrogen bonds or other weak intermolecular interactions, a detailed examination of the closest-neighbourhood of each site in acetazolamide molecule was necessary. The XRD data were available but they could not explain the differences. Therefore each form was analysed within DFT/QTAIM, which shed some light on the bonding pattern in both polymorphs, Fig. 2. Table 3 [104].

Form	Nitrogen position	NQR					T [K]	DFT B3LYP/6-311++G(d,p)*	
		ν_+ [MHz]	ν_- [MHz]	ν_0 [MHz]	e^2qQ/h [MHz]	η [-]		e^2Qq/h [MHz]	η [-]
I	$-NH_2$	3.320	2.280	1.040	3.730	0.557	295	4.378	0.578
	-NH-	2.830	1.930	0.900	3.170	0.567		3.400	0.833
	N(4)	3.650	3.040	0.610	4.460	0.274		5.231	0.154
	N(3)	3.520	2.400	1.120	3.950	0.568		4.247	0.719
II	$-NH_2$	3.555	2.515	1.040	4.045	0.514	210	4.321	0.678
	-NH-	2.840	1.940	0.900	3.190	0.565		3.375	0.827
	N(4)	3.660	3.070	0.590	4.490	0.263		5.218	0.166
	N(3)	3.570	2.510	1.060	4.050	0.523		4.263	0.706

* cluster of 14 (form I) and 6 (form II) molecules

Table 3. ^{14}N NQR frequencies, quadrupole coupling constants and asymmetry parameters - in acetazolamide form I at T = 295 K and acetazolamide form II at 210 K.

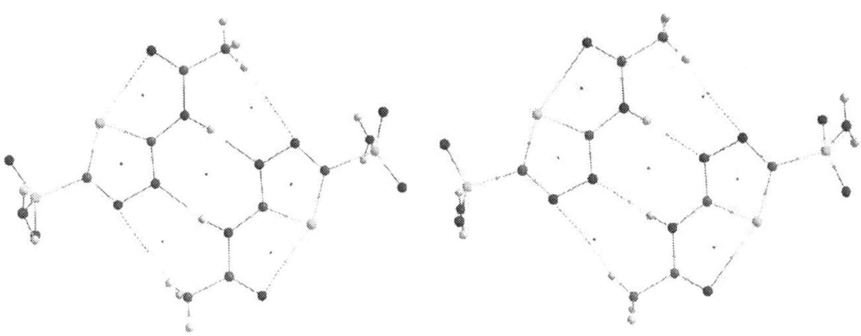

FORM I FORM II

Fig. 2. Polymorphic structures of acetazolamide.

In form I an $-NH_2$ group (proton donor) forms a relatively strong NH…N hydrogen bond of 3.080 Å in length with the nitrogen N(4) from the thiadiazole ring (hydrogen bond acceptor), i.e. that which does not participate in the formation of the molecular pair mentioned earlier. The additional two hydrogen bonds, NH…O, of 2.958 Å and 3.026 Å in lengths, are formed by the oxygen from a sulfone group as a hydrogen bond acceptor and N from $-NH_2$ group as a hydrogen bond donor. In form II, the second of the two atoms in the 1,3,4-thiadiazole ring, N(4) (hydrogen bond acceptor) forms a very weak CH…N hydrogen bond of the length 3.695 Å at 93.2K with the carbon atom from $-CH_3$ (hydrogen bond donor). Besides, two sulfonamide groups are bound by two identical N-H…O hydrogen bonds of the lengths 2.988 Å and energy -20.8 kJ/mol at 93.2 K. Each $-NH_2$ group forms also a bit stronger hydrogen bond NHO with a neighbouring acetyl group, of the length 2.896 Å and with the energy -28.4 kJ/mol at 93.2 K, Table 4..

FORM	BOND	ρ [a.u.]	Δ(ρ) [a.u.]	ε [-]	E [kJ/mol]
I	N(4)...HC	-	-	-	-
RT	N(3)H....N(acetyl)	0.0319	0.084745	0.0727	-29.49
Proton opt.	S1...O(acetyl)	0.0258	0.082293	0.0035	-24.20
II	N(4)...HC	0.0069	0.0211	0.0934	-4.72
93.2 K	N(3)H....N(acetyl)	0.0408	0.1014	0.0682	-44.06
Proton opt.	S1...O(acetyl)	0.0200	0.0630	0.0510	-18.51
I	N(4)...HC	0.0034	0.0115	2.3682	-2.55
RT	N(3)H....N(acetyl)	0.0182	0.0723	0.1108	-15.01
X-Ray	S1...O(acetyl)	0.0259	0.0823	0.0038	-24.22
II	N(4)...HC	0.0042	0.0134	0.1359	-2.96
93.2K	N(3)H....N(acetyl)	0.0325	0.1021	0.0827	-33.12
X-Ray	S1...O(acetyl)	0.0202	0.0622	0.0612	-18.22

Table 4. Topological parameters of ρ(r) for acetazolamide (the electron density at BCP (ρ_{BCP} (r), its Laplacian ΔBCP(ρ), the ellipticity of the bond (ε) and estimated hydrogen bonding energy according to Espinosa (E_E) calculated at the B3LYP/6-311++G(d,p) level of theory).

Thus the largest differences in the symmetry of electron distribution between I and II forms should be observed at the $-NH_2$ site. Indeed, the asymmetry parameter for $-NH_2$ site is higher in I than in form II because in form I the nitrogen atom from $-NH_2$ participates in three different intermolecular interactions, while in form II it participates only in two interactions. For the same reason e^2Qqh^{-1} is smaller at $-NH_2$ site in polymorph I in comparison to that in form II. Differences in bonding schemes of the terminal $-NH_2$ group in the two crystallographic modifications are found to be responsible for a significantly different ^{14}N NQR parameters, which can be used as a measure of the strength of hydrogen bonds [104].

Cloxiquine

An unusual case of packing polymorphism has been noted for cloxiquine (5-Chloro-8-hydroxyquinoline) API of antibacterial, antifungal, antiaging and antituberculosis drugs. In the solid state, cloxiquine crystallizes in two forms I and II differing in the arrangement of rigid molecules. Both forms can be easily distinguished by XRD [145]. In both forms the hydroxyl hydrogens are capable of forming a multicentre i.e. bifurcated O-H...N hydrogen bonds, one intramolecular and the other intermolecular, which simultaneously lead to formation of five-membered hydrogen-bonded chelate rings [N, C(9), C(8), O, H(8)] and to dimerisation of the molecules. Such patterns, usually termed supramolecular synthons [146], are according to XRD data, independent of the polymorphic form, however in the dimeric structure of cloxiquine form I the paired molecules in the units are twisted, while in form II they are not. Due to this subtle difference in the planarity of dimeric structures which consist of the paired molecules linked by bifurcated hydrogen bonds in the units - twisted in form I, and planar in form II [146], accompanied by change in the hydrogen bond lengths, the structure units can be differently packed to yield the two polymorphs. XRD indicated that the supramolecular synthons expand into a column by π-π stacking interactions, along the crystallographic c axis in I and b axis in II [146]. The columns constructed in this way are stabilized in the 3D crystal structure by Van der Waals forces.
The pronounced differences in ^{14}N and ^{14}O NQR spectra (frequency shifts: 0.175, 0.156, 0.020 and 0.107, 0.234, 0127 MHz, respectively) but only slight in ^{35}Cl (frequency shifts by 0.033MHz) allows distinction between forms I and II [148]. The elongation of the hydrogen bond in form I in comparison to form II is reflected by a change in the asymmetry

parameter. DFT/QTAIM formalism was applied to study supramolecular synthon pattern in detail and estimate the strength and character of hydrogen bonds. The intramolecular N-H...O bonds in cloxiquine form II are weak and slightly stronger than the intermolecular N-H...O bonds, but generally weaker than typical and mainly electrostatic ones, while intermolecular N-H...O bonds in cloxiquine form I are moderate and partially covalent in nature. The large differences in strength of the corresponding H-bonds in both cloxiquine forms, suggest the interplay in H-bonds linking adjacent molecules in dimers, Fig. 3. The strong interactions between monomers being components of supramolecular synthon of cloxiquine form II, i.e. the two competitive (intra- and intermolecular) O-H...N hydrogen bonds, the former slightly stronger than the latter, and an additional intermolecular hydrogen bond C-H..O, which in contrast to form I links atoms in the same dimer and thus is more than twice stronger, are responsible for drastic differences in polarity of supramolecular synthons and result in the planarity of form II. Moreover, the strength of stacking π···π interactions is found to be strongly dependent on planarity thus they are much weaker in form I than in form II of cloxiquine. The NQR parameters have been correlated with both the molecular density of the packing and the distance between stacking layers, as a consequence of different hydrogen bonding strength and different π···π overlaps [148]. Both forms differ in water solubility and dissolution rate (form II is 1.47 times better soluble than form I) [146].

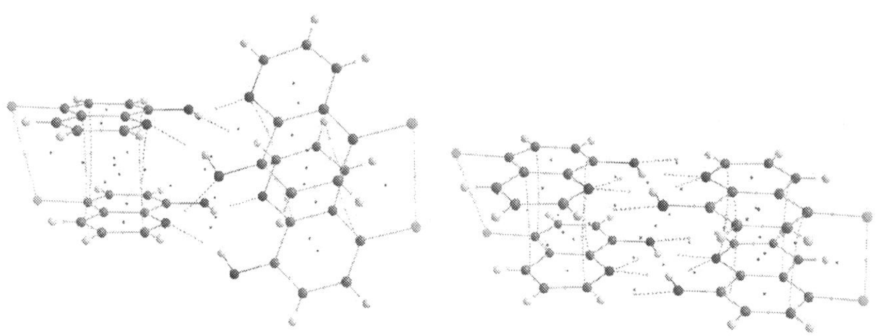

FORM I FORM II

Fig. 3. Polymorphic structures of cloxiquine.

3.2.1.2 Conformational polymorphism

Conformational polymorphism occurs when flexible molecules with different conformations are packed in different ways in the same crystal unit.

The group of sulfonamides, of well-known antibacterial activity, make a good illustration of conformational polymorphism. These compounds have been more or less systematically studied since their discovery in the late 1930s. Till 1948 more than 5,000 derivatives have been synthesised, among which several drug classes have been identified (e.g. antibacetrial, hypoglycemics, carbonic anhydrase inhibitors, saluretics, and tubular transport inhibitors). The antibacterial effectiveness of sulfonamides, classified as the sulfa drugs, is determined by a highly polar sulfonyl group, which is responsible for the similarity of sulfonamides to the p-aminobenzoate ion. Their intermolecular interactions patterns have some common features i.e. amido protons show a greater preference for hydrogen bonding to amidine nitrogens and cocrystal guests, whereas the amino protons show a greater preference for hydrogen bonding to sulfonyl oxygens [149]. The dominant hydrogen-bond pattern is a chain with an eight atom repeat unit. Molecules of sulfonamides are extraordinarily versatile due to conformational (amine and amide) and hydrogen-bonding capabilities. Thus sulfonamides reveal the ability to crystallize in multiple solid-state structures i.e. exhibit polymorphism. In fact many polymorphs and hundreds of solvates have been discovered for this class of compounds [102].

Sulfanilamide

The most intensively studied compound from this class is sulphanilamide (4-aminobenzenesulfonamide) - a sulfonamide antibiotic used in treatment of streptococcal infections. In the solid state, it crystallizes in four forms α, β, γ, [149-151] and δ [152-154] fully investigated by XRD. The different d-spacing of three strongest XRD diffraction lines (4.91, 6.57, 3.57; 6.12, 4.49, 4.23; and 3.90, 3.78, 33.6 for α, β, γ, respectively) allows easy distinction of each polymorph. The form stable at room temperature is β- sulfanilamide. The remaining forms gradually revert to this form on storage. On slow heating, β-sulfanilamide slowly transforms to α and then to γ. The forms β and γ are considered to be enantiotropically related. The origins of polymorphism of sulfanilamide were found to be connected with the versatile hydrogen-bonding capabilities [154]. The differences in the chemical shifts at ^{13}C and at ^{15}N permitting the distinction between individual polymorphs Table 5, [156] are of the same order as in glycine. However, the chemical shifts at N(1) site were almost the same for the three polymorphs. The spin-lattice relaxation times ^{1}H T_1 and ^{1}H $T_{1\rho}$ allow distinction of **β**-sulfanilamide from the other polymorphs, while ^{15}N $T_{1\rho}$ allows distinction of all three polymorphs and what is more, point to substantial differences in mobility around N(1) and N(2) sites. This result has pointed to different molecular mobility in the solid-state at each site in each polymorph.

ISOT.	SITE	FORM I α				FORM II β				FORM III γ			
		σ_{iso} [ppm]	ζ [ppm]	η [-]	T_1, $T_{1\rho}$	σ_{iso} [ppm]	ζ [ppm]	η [-]	T_1, $T_{1\rho}$	σ_{iso} [ppm]	ζ [ppm]	η [-]	T_1, $T_{1\rho}$
^{13}C	C(1)	153.7	-	-	-	153.4	-	-	-	151.0	-	-	-
	C(4)	128				127.1				127.1			
	C(2),C(6)	113.1, 115.3				112.3,117.1				112.7, 115.1			
	C(3),C(5)	128.3				129.5				129.6			
	C(1)	166.5,157.6	-	-	-	165.5, 156.0	-	-	-	165.5, 156.0	-	-	-
	C(4)	134.5				135.6				137.1			
	C(2),C(6)	118.8, 124.0				118.3,123.1				120.0, 122.5			
	C(3),C(5)	134.5				133.3				135.0			
^{15}N	N(1)	-312.2	±46	1	0.64ms	-312.1	43	0.8	0.64 ms	-312.1	±45	1	1.5 ms
	N(2)	-288.8	70	0.4	6.5ms	-284.1	71.2	0.4	10ms	-280.6	67.3	0.3	4.2ms
^{1}H	--	-	-		94 s	-	-	-	8 s	-	-	-	82 s
					7.2 s				7.1 s				3.0 s

Table 5. The isotropic chemical shifts and CSA tensor components - in sulfanilamide forms α, β and γ [156].

The pronounced differences in ^{14}N NQR spectra, Table 6, [157] make the differentiation of α and β polymorphs of sulfanilamide much easier than with the use of SS NMR. The shifts in frequencies (ν) and differences in quadrupole coupling constant e^2Qq/h and asymmetry parameter (η) with reference to those of α form (0.555, 0.522, 0.410 and 0.693 MHz) are evident.

FORM I α			FORM II β			T [K]
ν [MHz]	e^2Qq/h [MHz]	η [-]	ν [MHz]	e^2Qq/h [MHz]	η [-]	
3.460 2.527 0.933	3.990	0.47	2.905 2.005 0.900	3.270	0.55	210
3.115 2.603 0.512	3.810	0.27	2.705 1.910 0.790	3.080	0.51	255

Table 6. ^{14}N NQR frequencies, quadrupole coupling constants and asymmetry parameters - in sulfanilamide form I at T = 295 K and form II at 210 K [156].

Thus NQR seems an even more suitable technique for identification of polymorphs and studies of changes in the intermolecular pattern due to polymorphic transitions.

While the number of drugs studied by solid state NMR is large, ^{14}N NQR was successfully applied for the studies of a group of sulfonamides exhibiting confomational polymorphism including sulfapyridine (4-amino-*N*-pyridinylbenzene sulfonamide), sulfadiazine (4-amino-*N*-pyrimidin-2-yl-benzenesulfonamide), sulfamerazine (4-amino-*N*-(4-methylpyrimidin-2-yl)benzenesulfonamide), sulfamethazine (4-amino-*N*-(4,6-dimethylpyrimidin-2-yl)benzene-sulfonamide), sulfathiazole (4-amino-*N*-(1,3-thiazol-2-yl)benzenesulfonamide)[157]. Interesting results have been also obtained for non-steroidal anti-inflammatory drug piroxicam ((8*E*)-8-[hydroxy-(pyridin-2-ylamino)methylidene]-9-methyl-10,10-dioxo-10λ^6-thia-9-azabicyclo[4.4.0]deca-1,3,5-trien-7-one) [158]. ^{35}Cl NQR was successfully applied in the study of chloral hydrate (trichloroacetaldehyde monohydrate, 2,2,2-trichloro-1,1-ethanediol), one of the oldest synthetic agents of sedative and hypnotic effects [130], non-steroidal anti-inflammatory diclofenac (2-[2-(2,6-dichlorophenyl) aminophenyl] acetic acid) [159], anti-diabetic chloropropamide (1-(4-chlorophenyl)sulfonyl-3-propyl-urea) [159], diuretic furosemide (4-chloro-2-furfurylamino-5-sulfamoyl-benzoic acid) [160]. Differentiation of the polymorphic forms of these compounds is not difficult because of a distinct shift in the ^{14}N-NQR or ^{35}Cl NQR frequency (0.65, 0.425, 0.58 and 0.18MHz for sulfamerazine, 0.23, 0.48, 0.42, 0.30, 0.10 and 0.08MHz for sulfathiazole, and 0.142MHz for furosemide; 0.287MHz for chloral hydrate, 0.176MHz for diclofenac, 0.306 MHz for chloropropamide) while, at the accuracy of determination of the order of 0.001 MHz (^{14}N NQR) and 0.010 MHz (^{35}Cl NQR) even for broad lines.

Apart from typical NQR parameters, polymorphs are often readily identified (similarly as in NMR study) on the basis of changes in the NQR linewidth (1.5kHz for sulfapyridine, 10kHz for chloropropamide) or in the spin-lattice (sulfapyridine 70-fold, chloropropamide 2-fold) or spin-spin (chloropropamide 10%) relaxation times. However, sometimes the estimation of the amount of polymorphs in a mixture on the basis of these parameters can be misleading [156].

It is known that in some cases SS NMR was helpful in explaining contradictions concerning polymorphism following from IR, XRD and DSC studies [118]. A briliant example indicating the usefulness of SS NMR is cefinidir, a broad-spectrum antibiotic, proven effective for common bacterial infections of the ear, sinus, throat, and skin. The use of XRPD and IR was not sufficient and Abbott's 'new polymorph' discovered using these techniques in 2003 was proved to be not a polymorph, but a pyridinium salt. [118]. Up to now no examples of such spectacular NQR applications had been given, but it does not mean that the potential of this method will not be exploited for this purpose in future.

Solid-state NMR or NQR can be powerful methods for comparing physical forms of the drug substance after pharmaceutical processing or manufacturing. Variation in the chemical shift or NQR frequency from polymorph to polymorph allows identification of differences in the atomic environment. In addition, NMR and NQR are quantitative analytical techniques, i.e. the intensity of their respective signals is directly proportional to the number of nuclei in the sample [158,160,161]. Thus it is possible to estimate the quantitative polymorphous composition or a relative proportion of polymorphs in a sample and the result is reliable. NMR is an important spectroscopic tool for the study of solid-state drug formulations. NQR method has such a potential. Both methods can be used for analysis of pure API or mixtures of polymorphs in pure drug substance and in dosage formulations. A detailed analysis of this aspect of NMR or NQR applications is beyond the scope of this chapter.

3.2.2 Tautomerism

Tautomerism (Greek: *tautos-identical; isomerism - Laar, 1985* [162]) can be defined as a reversible structural isomerism involving the sequential processes of bond cleavage, skeletal bond migration and bond reformation. Tautomerisation plays an important role in mutations or enzymatic reactions. Thus the inspection of the most stable tautomeric forms allows further discussion of the functional implications of tautomerism for recognition and binding to DNA, proteins or enzymes. Many purines and pyrimidines occur in tautomeric forms whose relative stabilities depend on the environment. Any alteration or modification in the base pairing scheme of DNA due to the existence of different tautomeric forms also may result in perturbation to the replication process or spontaneous mutations, i.e. to a reduced stability of DNA. The presence of an abnormal tautomer can be even more deleterious to the stability of DNA. On the other hand, these unique capabilities of modifying DNA may be relevant for the process of designing of DNA binding drugs of distinct antitumor efficacy. The fact that often the less abundant tautomer is the most reactive one (Hammond rule [126]) further reinforces the relevance of investigation of intermolecular interactions in the solid state. The preference for different tautomeric forms is a clear indication of the importance of intermolecular interactions, in particular H-bonding, in determination of the structure of the condensed phase.

Polyhalobenzimidazoles

An example are the studies of annular tautomerism of polyhalobenzimidazoles, Fig.4, [105]. NQDR and DFT results have suggested the presence of prototropic annular tautomerism 50:50, which is in a good agreement with the XRD and ^{1}H-NMR data. According to the XRD data, all halogenobenzimidazole crystals are isostructural and have the same space group $I4_1/a$. The intermolecular hydrogen bonds N1-H···N3′ and N1′···H-N3 which link each molecule with two neighbouring ones, occur between the molecules related by the fourfold screw symmetry axis along the c direction of the tetragonal cell, Fig. 4. According to QTAIM analysis, the N-H···N bonds formed by both nitrogen atoms (N1 and N3) differ insignificantly in strength (by less than 0.4 kJ/mol), which is in a good agreement with the differences in their lengths.

Comparison of the HB strength and electron density at the hydrogen bond critical points in a group of polyhalogenobenzimidazoles suggests that hydrogen bonds are of similar strength. The differences in e^2Qqh^{-1} and η observed for both nitrogen sites suggests that hydrogen bonds are asymmetric and should be described by a proton double minimum potential, which is confirmed by the QTAIM analysis. As the compounds crystallise in the centrosymmetric group, the polar chains of the molecules arranged in one direction are accompanied by antiparallel chains arranged in the opposite direction and this spatial ordering is very close to that observed in the α form of 1H-benzimidazole. This suggests that a packing polymorphism similar to that in 1H-benzimidazole can be expected in polyhalogenobenzimidazoles. Additionally QTAIM calculations have revealed weak intermolecular interactions in polyhalogenobenzimidazole structures i.e. N···X (X = H, Cl, Br or I) and two kinds of Y···Z (Y, Z=Cl, Br or I) contacts, which are much weaker than hydrogen bonds. The local potential energy density at BCPs indicated the following ordering of the intermolecular interactions according to increasing bond strength (E) : N1-H···N3 ~ N1-H···N3 < N1···X < X···Y (X, Y from the same ring) < X···Y (X, Y from the different rings). The pattern of intermolecular contacts has been found responsible for the specific crystal arrangement and the annular prototropism [105].

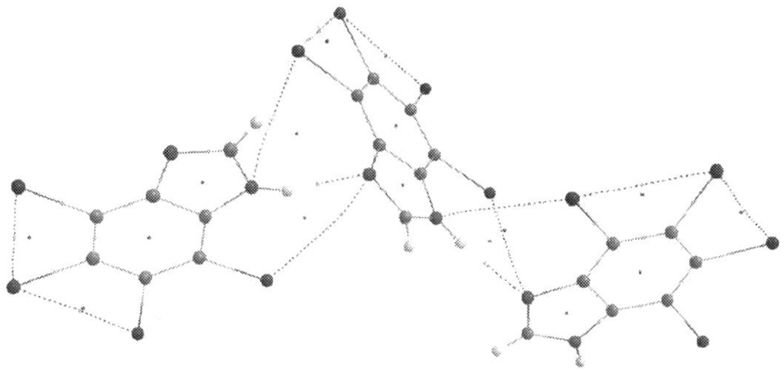

Fig. 4. The intermolecular hydrogen bonds pattern in polyhalogenobenzimidazoles.

2-thiocytosine and cytosine

The solid-state tautomerism studies are well illustrated by those performed for canonical natural nucleic acid base cytosine, and its analogue 2-thiocytosine. The replacement of cytosine by 2-thiocytosine may perturb base-pairing process of DNA or it can produce spontaneous mutations i.e. reduced stability of DNA. The compound of 2-thiocytosine is a potential anti-leukaemic and anticancer agent [163,164]. Numerous derivatives including 1-(β-D-arabinofuranosyl)-2-thiocytosine and its analogues and complexes with trimethyl platinum have been synthesized and their enzymatic reactivity and antitumor activity have been studied [165]. The cytotoxic activity of some of them has been found even higher than that of cisplatin and was manifested even against cisplatin resistant cell lines [165]. The arrangement of molecules in the crystals of 2-TC is essentially the same as that found for cytosine, but more complicated due to the existence of two inequivalent molecules in the elementary cell, Fig. 5, [166].

In the 2-thiocytosine crystalline structure, supramolecular synthons (dimers) are linked to the neighbouring supramolecular synthons by intermolecular interactions of the same pattern i.e. weaker H-bonds: N(1)-H(1)...N(3') and N(4')-H(4')...S(2) of 3.114 and 3.408 Å. Neighbouring ribbons are linked together by much longer, thus considered weak, N-H...S bonds of the lengths 3.466 and 3.551 Å [166]. The application of QTAIM allows detection and distinction of many weaker interactions in the crystalline structure of 2-thiocytosine [167], which was not possible in a standard X-Ray study [166]. Indeed in the crystalline structure of 2-thiocytosine, the QTAIM analysis has revealed the presence of four varieties of intermolecular interactions not involving hydrogen atoms (N…N, N…C and N…S), apart from the hydrogen-bonds (N-H…N, N-H…S, C-H…S and C-H…C).

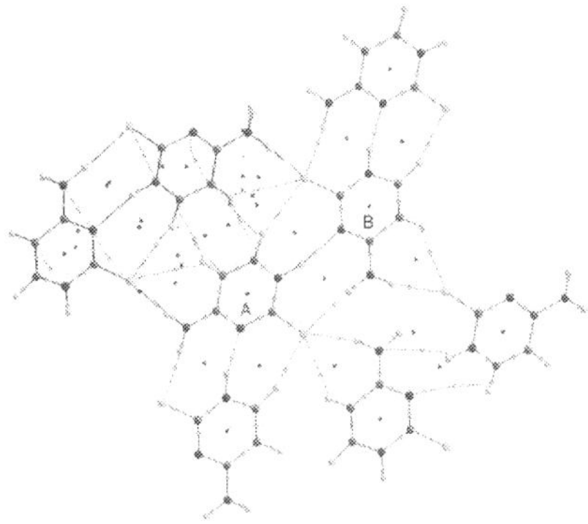

2-THIOCYTOSINE

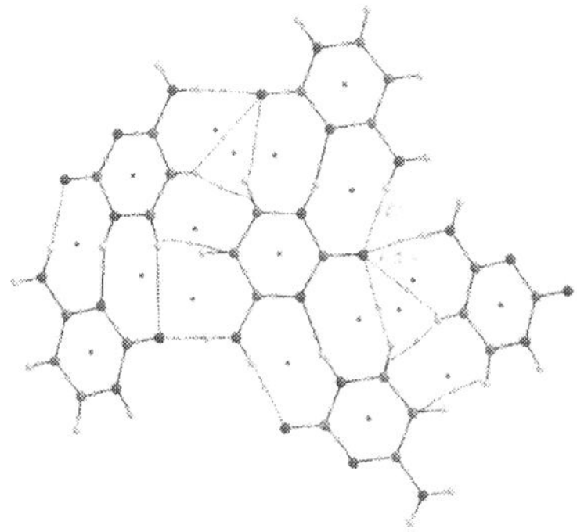

CYTOSINE

Fig. 5. Arrangement of molecules in the crystals of 2-thiocytosine and cytosine.

In general, the hierarchy of structures in crystals of 2-thiocytosine molecules-dimers-ribbons-stacks is reflected by the progressively weaker bonds. The N(1')-H(1')…N(3) interaction is found to be the strongest (-23.18 kJ/mol), followed by N(4)-H(4)...S(2') (-17.13 kJ/mol). The third H-bond linking adjacent molecules into a dimer C(6)-H(6)…S(2'') of 3.532 Å (-9.43 kJ/mol) is much weaker and thus not revealed by X-ray [165]. The hydrogen bonds linking adjacent supramolecular synthons are: N(1)-H(1)...N(3') of 3.114 Å and -16.10 kJ/mol, N(4')-H(4')...S(2) of 3.408 Å and -13.95kJ/mol. The H-bonds linking neighbouring ribbons are: N(4)-H(4)...S(2′) of 3.466 Å (-3.17 kJ/mol) and 3.551 Å (-8.01 kJ/mol) and C(5)-H(5)...S(2′) bond of length 4.037 Å (-2.85 kJ/mol), two C(5)-H(5)...C(6′) and C(5′)-H(5′)...C(6) of 3.688 Å (-3.99 kJ/mol) and 3.943 Å (-1.91 kJ/mol), respectively. Additionally between layered dimers a few π-π interactions involving non-H atoms, purely van der Waals in nature, were detected: N(1)…N(3″), N(1)…C(5″) and N(3)…S(2″) of the lengths 4.094, 3.411 and 3.516 Å and roughly estimated energies -1.14, -4.06 and -4.01 kJ/mol [167]. It is worth noting that N(4) from the NH_2 group, in contrast to N(1) and N(3), does not participate in this stacking π-π interactions. The differences between the isosurface representations of Laplacian at nitrogen sites in both inequivalent molecules are small, however they suggest that -NH- site exhibits more symmetrical electron density distribution in molecule A than B, while -N= and -NH_2 sites exhibit more symmetrical distribution in molecule B than A, which is in a good agreement with experimentally obtained results [167].

3.2.3 Stability

The term 'stability' of drugs refers to their chemical and physical integrity and can be influenced by many factors (temperature, light, air, humidity and pressure), as well as the package components. In the pharmaceutical context the influence of temperature and /or irradiation is of particular interest. These factors can lead to the transition to undesirable meta-stable polymorph or degradation products, which means reduction of bioavailability, loss of activity or even toxicity.

3.2.3.1 Thermal stability

Solid state NMR and NQR are particularly well suited for fast monitoring of temperature effect on the thermal stability of API. Temperature studies of chemical shifts on different isotopes, or ^{1}H NMR second moment or ^{35}Cl or ^{14}N NQR frequencies or different spin-lattice relaxation times (r.g. T_1(^{1}H NMR), T_1(^{35}Cl NQR) or T_1(^{14}N NQR)) provide the information on the compounds stability, including the phase transitions (changes in the crystallographic structure and ordering). For many vitamins and drugs, the temperature dependencies of second moment of ^{1}H NMR or spin-lattice relaxation time have been studied along with molecular motions - hindered rotations, reorientations, proton transfer, but the pharmaceutical context has been neglected. Similarly, for a few APIs including urotropine (HMT), an antiseptic used for the prophylaxis of urinary tract infections, or chloral hydrate - a local anaesthetic, the temperature dependencies of NQR frequency and phase transition have been studied more or less systematically [168-170], but not in the pharmaceutical context.

The thermal stability aspect most important and interesting from the pharmaceutical point of view is the phase transitions of APIs, especially the uncontrolled ones. The unstable polymorphs often convert into more stable ones by phase transitions. Uncontrolled polymorph transitions of API may happen during the final crystallisation, storage in the parent solution, drying, wet granulation, micronization, tablet pressing, or even in shelf life (storing). In general two types of polymorphous transitions are distinguished the enantiotropic and the monotropic ones. The enantiotropic transition occurs at a specific temperature at which the originally more stable polymorph transforms into another finally stable polymorph. Transitions of this type are often reversible and well-defined. The second type of polymorphous transitions, the monotropic one does not occur at a specific temperature in solid state. The polymorph transition passes over the liquid phase, which means crystallisation from a different solvent. Most of polymorphous transitions of APIs are monotropic and not enantiotropic which is a negative phenomenon.

Interesting results have been obtained for hydrochlorothiazide (HCTZ), a diuretic drug applied to beat high blood pressure and heart failure. Among the DTA, NMR, NQR and XRD methods [171,172] the most sensitive to its phase transitions was NQR [172]. The anomalies in the temperature dependence of the ^{35}Cl NQR frequency for HCTZ, the change in the linewidth (being a result of an increase in the spin-lattice relaxation time), small but notable changes in the slope and the jump in frequency observed at 253 K, not exceeding 0.05 MHz, together with the lack of hysteresis (which distinguishes the first- and second-order transitions) indicated a second-order transition. This transition was not revealed by the temperature dependencies of the ^{1}H second moment or ^{1}H spin-lattice relaxation time (NMR), which were able to detect only trans-gauche jumps of $-NH_2$. Moreover, the phase transition clearly visible in NQR was only weakly indicated by the thermal dependence of heat capacity (DTA measurements) [171]. This phase transition was interpreted as a change in the structural ordering connected with the reorientation of the $-NH_2$ group in a specific temperature in solid state i.e. the enantiotropic one. Indeed, in a short time after detection of the conformation phase transition, the polymorphs of HCTZ, Fig. 6, have been crystallised and their structure by XRD have been resolved [173]. Thus the NQR studies contributed to the evidencing of polymorph transforms and understanding of the nature of phase transition.

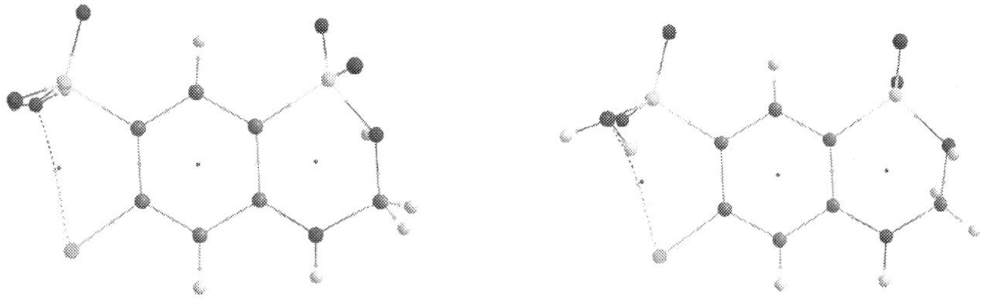

FORM I FORM II

Fig. 6. Polymorphic structures of hydrochlorothiazide.

Another interesting case is chloropropamide for which NQR was able to detect not only the A to C phase transition, but also different molecular dynamics manifested as a difference in the slope of the temperature dependencies of NQR frequencies for A and C polymorphs [159]. Temperature dependencies of NQR frequencies can also bring information on the stability of a compound studied. For instance, a smooth temperature dependence of NQR frequency for triclosan suggests that its ring maintains almost the same conformation in the temperature range studied (no ring rotation), which has been confirmed by XRD results [98]. One more interesting example illustrating the potential of molecular dynamic NQR studies are the results obtained for antipsychotic and antihistaminic drug - phenothiazine [174]. ^{14}N NQR frequencies measured in both the low- and high-temperature phases indicated the presence of large thermal librations of the phenothiazine molecules in both crystallographic phases as well as an order-disorder phase transition associated with reorientations of the quite rigid phenothiazine molecules [175] around the orthorhombic axis. The quadrupole coupling constant have not been affected by the phase transition, while the asymmetry parameter reflected this phase transition even more evidently than the ^{14}N NQR frequencies. Thus the NQR studies contributed to the understanding of the microscopic mechanism of the phase transition.

3.2.3.2 Photostability

In the solid state, the temperatures required for different types of degradation differ, thus the mechanisms of thermal and photochemical degradation are expected to be different. Because light irradiation of drugs is known to have a very strong, often negative effect on their activity, the integral part of research on API are photostability studies. Photostability of API depends on the factors connected with the irradiation features (wavelength, intensity and time of exposure) as well as on a variety of physico-chemical features characterising the API substance itself (formulation type: solution, powder, crystal; presence of specific molecular fragments). Although a large number of drugs have the form of solid formulations, most studies on photostability have been performed in artificial conditions, i.e. in dilute solutions in specific organic solvents in which such processes can be easily observed. However, it should be mentioned that in such conditions the drug's photostability may be totally different than in solid. Even the addition of excipients may affect the photostability of drug formulation.

The main phenomenon responsible for deterioration of the useful properties of a drug, that is the loss of its activity or increased toxicity, is photodegradation. Photodegradation of a drug is significant under irradiation with light of wavelength longer than 330 nm. However, even in such favourable conditions, photoreaction can be easily unnoticed when it is very slow, especially in solid state. The typical approach to study photodegradation is based on a combination of different techniques. The widely applied procedure includes studies of photodegradation products using different techniques including chromatographic techniques gas/liquid chromatography (GLC), thin layer/chromatography (TLC) or high pressure liquid chromatography (HPLC), electron paramagnetic resonance (EPR), differential thermal analysis (DTA), nuclear magnetic resonance (NMR), and *Fourier transform infrared* reflection absorption spectroscopy (FT-IR RAS). Although the above mentioned methods are very sensitive but they require the use of solvents which may cause further degradation of drug during the analysis. The alternative for the identification of photodegradation products are solid state methods, which allow credible identification of the compounds in solid, guaranteeing elimination of the above mentioned solvent side effects.

An interesting example illustrating the studies of photostability is nifedipine, mainly used for treatment of hypertension, coronary heart/artery diseases and arrhythmias, or as cardiovascular organ-protective agent [176]. Nifedipine is known as one of the most photolabile APIs, extremely sensitive to UV-VIS radiation up to 450 nm and to the ionising radiation. The loss of therapeutic properties by NIF due to photodegradation is well documented [177]. The photodegradation of NIF in solution has been widely studied [178] whereas only a few authors have studied it in solid [179]. The photostability and the photostabilization of NIF in different solid formulations including powders and tablets have received considerable attention [180]. A typical approach to study these phenomena is based on a combination of different techniques. The products of photodegradation are studied using different techniques including EPR, DTA, NMR, FT-IR-RAS but the isolation of the products is performed by chromatographic techniques: gas/liquid chromatography (GLC), thin layer/chromatography (TLC) or high pressure liquid chromatography (HPLC).

Unfortunately, solid ^{13}C NMR is not always able to detect the photoproducts. A striking example is nifedipine whose degradation effect manifested as shifts of signals assigned to C(4), C(3) and C(5) as well as C(2') sites was observed only in solution [181]. Instead, a combination of ^{14}N NQDR and DFT methods proved to be effective because the nitrogen sites in nifedipine and its photoproduct differ significantly, (-NH- versus -N= and $-NO_2$ versus -NO). ^{14}N NQDR seems the best experimental method of choice for non-destructive detection of NIF to NO-NIF photoconversion in solid [182]. It is worth noting that the electron density distribution at the -N=, -NH, $-NO_2$, -NO sites can be accurately and fully experimentally evaluated using this technique. Thus ^{14}N NQDR should be of particular importance for the studies of photodegradation of solid drugs, especially nitro-compounds. Additionally within QTAIM formalism it has been possible to predict the sites in nifedipine most affected by irradiation -NH, $-NO_2$ and -CH.

It is known that NQR is suitable for determination of the degree of ^{35}Cl release from a given pharmaceutical under the effect of UV irradiation, which is manifested as a decrease in the signal intensity or even as its disappearance (e.g. for furosemide), but when the radicals formed undergo fast recombination the relevant changes in the NQR spectra are undetectable (e.g. thiazides).

4. Conclusions

According to James Black, a Nobel laureate in Physiology or Medicine 1988, '*The most fruitful basis for the discovery of a new drug is to start with an old drug.*' [183]. Actually among 700,000 crystal structures from monatomic metals to proteins and viruses systematically collected from the late 1960s and early 1970s are available in five comprehensive and fully retrospective world depositories: Cambridge Structural Database (CSD), Worldwide Protein Data Bank (wPDB), Nucleic acid database (NDB), Metals and intermetalics database (CRYSTMET) and Inorganic Crystal Structure Database (ICSD) only about 10% are structures of APIs and targets. The largest database, CSD, nowadays contains over 500,000 structures ("small molecules" - less than 1000 atoms) of which 99% were determined by XRD [61,62]. The number of drug-like structures in CSD exceeds 60,000. The largest protein archive, wPDB, contains 73,699 experimentally-determined structures of proteins, nucleic acids, and complex assemblies, of which 87% were determined by XRD, 12% by NMR, less than 1% by electron microscopy and hybrid methods.

Thus among the large number of known, classified drugs and targets only a small fraction has been investigated using SS NMR and even a smaller one - using NQR. In fact the application of both methods in drug development studies has definitely a short history. Despite this, significant improvements in the past few years, resulting in a remarkable enhancement of the speed and the efficacy of this approach permit expecting a great increase in its role in the near future. SS NMR and NQR in combination with computational methods like ab initio or DFT will play a crucial role in modern crystallography and medicinal chemistry. An important advantage of SS NMR or NQR spectroscopy over XRD, is that SS NMR and NQR spectroscopies are sensitive to local or short-range order (<5 Å), while XRD detects comparatively long-range order (>100 Å). Thus SS NMR and especially NQR provides unique insight into intermolecular interactions that are not easily obtained by other methods. A combination of experimental and theoretical techniques has certainly much to offer for the studies of drugs or potential drugs in early phases of drug research. Their capabilities in particular when applied to the known drugs, have been well documented in literature [92,99,101,104,105,148,156-161,184-189].

Although in some fields the NMR or NQR are not competitive to IR, UV or XRD the examples of combined studies given above show that both techniques have a potential to elicit structural and physico-chemical information about a molecule of dug, target or the interaction drug-target.

5. References

[1] DiMasi J.A.; Hansen R. W.; Grabowski H. G. (2003). The price of innovation: new estimates of drug development costs, Journal of Health Economics, 22, pp. 151-185, ISSN: 0167-6296

[2] Bloch F.; Hansen W.W., Packard M. (1946). The nuclear induction experiment, *Physical Review*, 70, pp. 474-485.

[3] Purcell E.M.; Torrey H.C.; Pound R.V. (1946). Resonance absorption by nuclear magnetic moments in a solid, *Physical Review* 69 pp. 37-38.

[4] Dehmelt H.; Krueger H. (1950). Kernquadrupolfrequenzen in festem Dichloraethylen, *Naturwissenschaften*, 37, pp. 111-112, ISSN 0028-1042.

[5] Mladenovic, M.; Arnone, M.; Fink, R. F.; Engels, B. (2009). Environmental effects on charge densities of biologically active molecules: do molecule crystal environments indeed approximate protein surroundings?, *Journal of Physical Chemistry B*, 113, pp. 5072-5082, ISSN 1089-5647.

[6] Sneader W. (1990). Chronology of drug introductions. In: *Comprehensive Medicinal Chemistry*, Hansch (Ed.), Pergamon Press, vol.1. pp. 7-80, ISBN: 978-0080325309.

[7] Waterbeemd H.; Carter R.E.; Grassy G.; Kubinyi H.; Martin Y.C.; Tute M.S.;Willet P. (1998). Glossary of terms used in computational drug design, Tech. Rep. 2:17 Albany Molecular Research Inc. pp. 1-15

[8] Kapetanovic I.M., (2008). Computer-aided drug discovery and development (CADDD): In silico-chemico-biological approach, *Chemico-Biological Interactions*, 171, pp. 165-176, ISSN 0009-2797.

[9] Saunders J.; Freedman S.B. (1989). The design of full agonists for the cortical muscarinic receptor, *Trends in Pharmacological Sciences* (December 1989); Suppl: pp. 70-75, ISSN: 0165-6147.

[10] Sim E.; Dimoglo A.; Shvets N.; Ahsen V. (2002). Electronic-topological study of the structure-activity relationships in a series of piperidine morphinomimetics, *Current Medicinal Chemistry*, 9, pp. 1537-1545, ISSN: 0929-8673.

[11] Fritz T.A.; Tondi D.; Finer-Moore J.S,.; Costi M.P.; Stroud R.M. (2001). Predicting and harnessing protein flexibility in the design of species-specific inhibitors of thymidylate synthase, *Chemistry & Biology*, 8, pp. 981-995. ISSN: 1099-4831.

[12] Wheatley M. (1998). Understanding neurotransmitter receptors: molecular biology-based strategies, Essays in Biochemistry, 33, pp.15-27. ISSN:0071-1365.

[13] Haugh J.M.; Wells A.; Lauffenburger D.A. (2000). Mathematical modeling of epidermal growth factor receptor signaling through the phospholipase C pathway: mechanistic insights and predictions for molecular interventions, *Biotechnology and Bioengineering*, 70, pp. 225-238. ISSN: 0006-3592.

[14] Wender P.A.; Hinkle K.W.; Koehler M.F.; Lippa B. (1999). The rational design of potential chemotherapeutic agents: synthesis of bryostatin analogues, *Medicinal Research Reviews*, 19, pp. 388-407, ISSN: 0198-6325.

[15] Tantillo C.; Ding J.; Jacobo-Molina A.; Nanni R.G.; Boyer P.L.; Hughes S.H.; Pauwels R.; Andries K.; Janssen P.A.; Arnold E. (1994). Locations of anti-AIDS drug binding sites and resistance mutations in the three-dimensional structure of HIV-1 reverse transcriptase. Implications for mechanisms of drug inhibition and resistance, *Journal of Molecular Biology*, 243, pp. 369-387, ISSN: 0022-2836.

[16] Kubinyi H. (1999). Chance favors the prepared mind--from serendipity to rational drug design. *Journal of Receptors and Signal Transduction Research,* 19, pp. 15–39. ISSN: 1079-9893.

[17] Denny B.J.; Wheelhouse R.T.; Stevens M.F.; Tsang L.L.; Slack J.A. (1994). NMR and molecular modeling investigation of the mechanism of activation of the antitumor

drug temozolomide and its interaction with DNA, *Biochemistry*, 9, pp. 9045-9051, ISSN: 0006-2960.

[18] Teeter M.M.; Froimowitz M.; Stec B.; DuRand C.J.; (1994). Homology modeling of the dopamine D2 receptor and its testing by docking of agonists and tricyclic antagonists. *The Journal of Medicinal Chemistry*, 37, pp. 2874-2888, ISSN: 0022-2623.

[19] Hazaia E.; Bikád A. (2008). Homology modeling of breast cancer resistance protein (ABCG2), *Journal of Structural Biology*, 162, pp. 63-74 , ISSN: 1047-8477.

[20] Esposito, E.X.; Hopfinger, A.J.; Madura, J.D. (2004). Chemoinformatics: concepts, methods, and tools for drug discovery. In *Chemoinformatics: Concepts, Methods, and Tools for Drug Discovery*; Bajorath, J. (Ed.), Humana Press: Totowa, NJ, USA, vol. 275, pp. 131–213, ISBN: 978-1588292612.

[21] Polanski J. (2009). Receptor dependent multidimensional QSAR for modeling drug--receptor interactions, *Current Medicinal Chemistry*, 16, pp. 3243-57, ISSN: 1568-0118.

[22] Santos-Filho, O.A.; Hopfinger, A.J.; Cherkasov, A.; de Alencastro, R.B. (2009). The receptor-dependent QSAR paradigm: an overview of the current state of the art. *Med. Chem. (Shāriqah (United Arab Emirates)), 5*, 359–366, ISSN:1573-4064.

[23] Santos-Filho, O.A.; Hopfinger, A.J. (2006). Structure-based QSAR analysis of a set of 4-hydroxy-5,6-dihydropyrones as inhibitors of HIV-1 protease: an application of the receptor-dependent (RD) 4D-QSAR formalism, *The Journal of Chemical Information and Modeling*, 46, pp. 345–354, ISSN: 1549-9596.

[24] Terfloth, L. *Chemoinformatics: A Textbook* ; Gasteiger, J., Engel, T., Eds.; Wiley-VCH: Weinheim, Germany, 2003; pp. 401–437. ISBN 3-527-30681-1

[25] Fujita, T, (1995). QSAR and Drug Design: New Developments and Applications, Elsevier Science Pub Co. pp. 508, ISBN-13: 978-0444886156.

[26] Cramer III, R. D.; Patterson, D. E.; Bunce, J. D.(1988). Comparative Molecular Field Analysis (CoMFA) 1.Effect of Shape on Binding of Steroids to Carrier Proteins, *Journal of the American Chemical Society*, 110, 5959, ISSN: 0002-7863.

[27] Thibaut, U. (1993). *Applications of CoMFA and related 3D QSAR approaches*. In Kubinyi, H. (Ed.), 3D QSAR in drug design, ESCOM, Leiden, The Netherlands, , pp. 661–696, ISBN 978-0-7923-4791-0.

[28] Klebe, G. (1998). Comparative Molecular Similarity Indices: CoMSIA.*3D QSAR in Drug Design*, Kubinyi, H.; Folkers, G.; Martin, Y. C. (Eds.), Kluwer Academic Publishers, Great Britain, 3, 87-104, ISBN: 0852954409.

[29] Klebe, G.; Abraham, U.; Mietzner, (1994). T. Molecular Similarity Indices in a Comparative Analysis (CoMSIA) of Drug Molecules to Correlate and Predict Their Biological Activity, *Journal of Medicinal Chemistry, 37*, pp. 4130-4146, ISSN: 0022-2623.

[30] Bohm, M.; Sturzebecher, J.; Klebe, G. (1999). Three-Dimensional Quantitative Structure-Activity Relationship Analyses Using Comparative Molecular Field Analysis and Comparative Molecular Similarity Indices Analysis To Elucidate Selectivity Differences of Inhibitors Binding to Trypsin, Thrombin, and Factor Xa. *Journal of Medicinal Chemistry, 42*, pp. 458-477, , ISSN: 0022-2623.

[31] DePriest S.A.; Mayer D. .; Naylor Ch.B. .; Marshall G.R. (1993). 3D-QSAR of angiotensin-converting enzyme and thermolysin inhibitors: a comparison of

CoMFA models based on deduced and experimentally determined active site geometries, *Journal of the American Chemical Society*,115, pp 5372–5384, ISSN: 0002-7863.

[32] Hopfinger, A.; Reaka, A.; Venkatarangan, P.; Duca, J.; Wang, S. (1999). Construction of a virtual nigh throughput screen by 4D-QSAR analysis: Application to a combinatorial library of glucoseinhibitors of glycogen phosphorylase b, *Journal of Chemical Information and Computer Sciences*, 39, pp. 1151–1160, ISSN: 0095-2338.

[33] Albuquerque, M.; Brito, M.; Cunha, E.; Alencastro, R.; Antunes, O.; Castro, H.; Rodrigues, C. (2007).Multidimensional-QSAR: Beyond the third-dimension in drug design. *Current Methods in Medicinal Chemistry and Biological Physics*, Carlton A. Taft , Carlos H. T. P. Silva (Eds), *1*, 91–100. ISBN: 81-308-0141-8.

[34] Albuquerque, M.G.; Hopfinger, A.J.; Barreiro, E.J.; de Alencastro, R.B. (1998). Four-dimensional quantitative structure-activity relationship analysis of a series of interphenylene 7-oxabicycloheptane oxazole thromboxane A2 receptor antagonists. *Journal of Chemical Information and Computer Sciences, 38, pp.* 925–938, ISSN: 0095-2338.

[35] Van Daele, I.; Munier-Lehmann, H.; Froeyen, M.; Balzarini, J.; Van Calenbergh, S. (2007). Rational design of 5'-thiourea-substituted alpha-thymidine analogues as thymidine monophosphate kinase inhibitors capable of inhibiting mycobacterial growth. *Journal of Medicinal Chemistry*, 50, pp. 5281–5292, ISSN: 0022-2623.

[36] Oprea T.I; Waller C.L; Marshall G.R. (1994). Three-dimensional quantitative structure-activity relationship of human immunodeficiency virus (I) protease inhibitors. 2. Predictive power using limited exploration of alternate binding modes. *Journal of Medicinal Chemistry*, 37, pp. 2206-2215. ISSN: 0022-2623.

[37] Senese, C.L.; Duca, J.; Pan, D.; Hopfinger, A.J.; Tseng, Y.J. (2004). 4D-fingerprints, universal QSAR and QSPR descriptors. *Journal of Chemical Information and Computer Sciences*, 44, pp. 1526–1539, ISSN: 0095-2338.

[38] Iyer, M.; Hopfinger, A.J. (2007). Treating chemical diversity in QSAR analysis: modeling diverse HIV-1 integrase inhibitors using 4D fingerprints. *The Journal of Chemical Information and Modeling*, 47, pp. 1945–1960, *ISSN*:1549-960X.

[39] Romeiro, N.C.; Albuquerque, M.G.; de Alencastro, R.B.; Ravi, M.; Hopfinger, A.J. (2005). Construction of 4D-QSAR models for use in the design of novel p38-MAPK inhibitors. *The Journal of Computer-Aided Molecular Design, 19,* pp. 385–400, ISSN: 0920-654X.

[40] Liu, J.; Pan, D.; Tseng, Y.; Hopfinger, A.J. (2003). 4D-QSAR analysis of a series of antifungal p450 inhibitors and 3D-pharmacophore comparisons as a function of alignment. *Journal of Chemical Information and Computer Sciences*, 43, pp. 2170–2179, ISSN: 0095-2338

[41] Pasqualoto, K.F.M.; Ferreira, E.I.; Santos-Filho, O.A.; Hopfinger, A.J. (2004). Rational design of new antituberculosis agents: receptor-independent four-dimensional quantitative structure-activity relationship analysis of a set of isoniazid derivatives. *Journal of Medicinal Chemistry*, 47, pp. 3755–3764 ISSN: 0022-2623.

[42] Krumrine, J.; Raubacher, F.; Brooijmans, N.; Kuntz, I. (2005) Principles and Methods of Docking and Ligand Design, in Structural Bioinformatics, Volume 44 (Eds P. E.

Bourne; H. Weissig), John Wiley & Sons, Inc., Hoboken, NJ, USA, ISBN: 9780471202004.

[43] Comprehensive Medicinal Chemistry, J.T. Triggle, (Ed.) ISBN: 978-0-08-044513-7

[44] PharmaPendium, https://www.pharmapendium.com/

[45] ThomsonReuters forecast, http://thomsonreuters.com/content/science/pdf/tr-forecast-cqa-en.pdf

[46] Chen X., Ji Z.L., Chen Y.Z. (2002), TTD: Therapeutic Target Database, *Nucleic Acids Research,* 30, pp. 412–5. , ISSN: 0305-1048.

[47] Liu,T., Lin,Y., Wen,X., Jorrisen, R.N. Gilson,M.K. (2007). BindingDB: a web-accessible database of experimentally determined protein-ligand binding affinities, *Nucleic Acids Research,* 35, pp. D198-D201, ISSN: 0305-1048.

[48] Wishart D.S., Knox C., Guo A.C., Cheng D., Shrivastava S., Tzur D., Gautam B., Hassanali M. (2008). DrugBank: a knowledgebase for drugs, drug actions and drug targets, *Nucleic Acids Research,* 36, pp. D901–6, ISSN: 0305-1048.

[49] World Health Organization (WHO). March 2011.
http://whqlibdoc.who.int/hq/2011/a95053_eng.pdf.

[50] The Use of Essential Drugs, Ninth Report of the WHO Expert Committee, Technical Report Series, No. 895, 2000. online:
http://www.searo.who.int/en/Section1257/Section2263/info-kit/who-model-drug_list.pdf

[51] FDA: Orange Book: Approved Drug Products with Therapeutic Equivalence Evaluations, *http://www.accessdata.fda.gov/scripts/cder/ob/default.cfm*

[52] FDA: Center for Biologics Evaluation and Research,
http://www.fda.gov/AboutFDA/CentersOffices/CBER/ucm122880.htm

[53] Anatomical Therapeutic Chemical (ATC) system,
http://www.whocc.no/atc/structure_and_principles/

[54] Imming, P.; Sinning, C.; Meyer, A. (2006). Drugs, their targets and the nature and number of drug targets, *Nature Reviews Drug Discovery,* 5, 821–834, ISSN : 1474-1776.

[55] Overington J.P.; Al-Lazikani B.; Hopkins A.L. (2006). How many drug targets are there?, *Nature Reviews Drug Discovery,* 5, pp. 993-996, ISSN : 1474-1776.

[56] Drews J. (2000). Drug discovery: a historical perspective, *Science,* 287, pp. 1960-1964, ISSN: 0036-8075.

[57] Zheng C.J.; Han L.Y.; Yap C.W.; Ji Z.L.; Cao Z.W..; Chen Y.Z. (2006). Therapeutic targets: progress of their exploration and investigation of their characteristics, *Pharmacological Reviews,* 58, pp. 259–79, ISSN: 0031-6997.

[58] Crum-Brown A.; Fraser T.R. (1868-1869). On the connection between chemical constitution and physiological action. Pt 1. On the physiological action of the salts of the ammonium bases, derived from Strychnia, Brucia, Thebia, Codeia, Morphia, and Nicotia. *Transactions of the Royal Society of Edinburgh,* 25, pp. 151-203, ISSN: 0263-5933.

[59] Bragg W.L. (1913). The Structure of Some Crystals as Indicated by their Diffraction of X-rays, *Proceedings of the Royal Society of London,* A89, pp. 248-277, ISSN: 0080–4630.

[60] Engh R. A.; Huber R. (1991). Accurate bond and angle parameters for X-ray protein structure refinement, *Acta Crystallographica,* A47, pp. 392-400, ISSN: 0365-110X.

[61] Hansen N.K.; Coppens P. (1978). Testing aspherical atom refinement on small molecules data sets, *Acta Crystallographica,* A34, 909–921, ISSN: 0365-110X.

[62] Allen F.H. (1986). A systematic pairwise comparison of geometric parameters obtained by X-ray and neutron diffraction, *Acta Crystallographica,* B42, pp. 515-522, ISSN: 0108-7681.

[63] Parr R.G.; Weitao Y. (1994). Density-Functional Theory of Atoms and Molecules, Oxford University Press, pp. 333. ISBN 0195092767.

[64] Allen, F.H. (2002). The Cambridge Structural Database: a quarter of a million crystal structures and rising, *Acta Crystallographica, B58,* pp. 380-388, ISSN: 0108-7681.

[65] Groom, C. R.; Allen, F. H. (2011), The Cambridge Structural Database: experimental three-dimensional information on small molecules is a vital resource for interdisciplinary research and learning. *Wiley Interdisciplinary Reviews: Computational Molecular Science,* 1: pp. 368–376, ISSN: 1759-0884.

[66] Johnson L.N.; Phillips D.C. (1965). Structure of some crystalline lysozyme-inhibitor complexes determined by X-ray analysis at 6 Angstrom resolution, *Nature,* 206, pp. 761-3, ISSN: 0028-0836.

[67] Zou, P.; Pinotsis, N.; Lange, S.; Song, Y.H.; Popov, A.; Mavridis, I.; Mayans, O.M.; Gautel, M., Wilmanns, M. (2006). Palindromic assembly of the giant muscle protein titin in the sarcomeric Z-disk, *Nature* 439, pp. 229-233, ISSN: 0028-0836.

[68] Svergun D.I.; Koch M.H.J. (2003). Small-angle scattering studies of biological macromolecules in solution, *Reports on Progress in Physics,* 66, pp. 1735–82, ISSN: 0034-4885.

[69] Czajkowsky D.M.; Shao Z. (1998). Submolecular resolution of single macromolecules with atomic force microscopy, *FEBS Letters,* 430, pp. 51-54, ISSN 0014-5793.

[70] Fan H.-f. (2010). Direct methods beyond small-molecule crystallography, *Physica Status Solidi A,* 207, pp. 2621-2638, ISSN: 1862-6300.

[71] Harris R. K., Joyce S. A., Pickard C. J., Cadars S. , Emsley L. (2005). Assigning Carbon-13 NMR Spectra to Crystal Structures by the INADEQUATE Pulse Sequence and First Principle Computation: A Case Study of Two Forms of Testosterone, *Physical Chemistry Chemical Physics,* 8, pp. 137 - 143, ISSN 1463-9076.

[72] Aue W.P.; Bartholdi E.; Ernst R.R. (1976). Two-dimensional spectroscopy. Application to nuclear magnetic resonance, *The Journal of Chemical Physics,* 64, pp. 2229-46, ISSN 0021-9606.

[73] Wüthrich, K., Wider, G., Wagner, G. and Braun, W. (1982). Sequential resonance assignments as a basis for determination of spatial protein structures by high resolution proton nuclear magnetic resonance, *Journal of Molecular Biology, 155, pp. 311–319,* ISSN: 0022-2836.

[74] Kumar A., Ernst, R.R. ; Wüthrich, K. (1980). A two-dimensional nuclear Overhauser enhancement (2D NOE) experiment for the eclucidation of complete proton-proteon cross-relaxation networks in biological macromolecules, *Biochemical and Biophysical Research Communications,* 95, pp. 1–6, ISSN 0006-291X.

[75] Ernst R.R.; Bodenhausen G.; Wokaun A. (1987). *Principles of nuclear magnetic resonance in one and two dimensions,* Clarendon Press (1987), Oxford University Press, Oxford, pp. 610, ISBN: 9780198556299

[76] Keeler, J.(2010). *Understanding NMR Spectroscopy* (2nd ed.). Chichester Wiley. pp. 184–187, ISBN: 9780470746080.

[77] Bax A.; Freeman R.; Kempsell S.P. (1980).Natural-abundance 13C-13C coupling observed via double-quantum coherence, *Journal of the American Chemical Society,* 102, 4849–4851, ISSN: 0002-7863.

[78] Lipsitz R.S.; Tjandra N. (2004). Residual dipolar couplings in nmr structure analysis, *Annual Review of Biophysics and Biomolecular Structure,* 33, pp.387–413, ISSN: 1056-8700.

[79] Pervushin, K.; Riek, R.; Wider, G. ; Wüthrich, K. (1997). Attenuated T2 relaxation by mutual cancellation of dipole–dipole coupling and chemical shift anisotropy indicates an avenue to NMR structures of very large biological macromolecules in solution. *Proceedings of the National Academy of Sciences,* 94, pp. 12366–12371, ISSN: 0027-8424.

[80] Riek, R. (2001). Enhancement of the steady-state magnetization in TROSY experiments, *Journal of Biomolecular NMR,* 21, 99-105, ISSN: 0925-2738.

[81] Riek, R.; Pervushin, K.; Wüthrich, K. (2000). TROSY and CRINEPT: NMR with large molecular and supramolecular structures in solution, *Trends in Biochemical Sciences,* 25, pp. 462-468, ISSN: 0968-0004.

[82] Riek, R.; Wider, G.; Pervushin, K.; Wuthrich, K (1999). Polarisation transfer by cross-correlated relaxation in solution NMR with very large molecules *Proceedings of the National Academy of Sciences,* 96, pp. 4918–4923, ISSN: 0027-8424.

[83] Fiaux J.; Bertelsen E.B.; Horwich A.L; Wüthrich K (2002). "NMR analysis of a 900K GroEL GroES complex". *Nature,* 418, pp. 207–11, ISSN: 0028-0836.

[84] Wishart D.S.; Sykes B.D.; Richards F.M. (1992) The chemical shift index: a fast and simple method for the assignment of protein secondary structure through NMR spectroscopy, *Biochemistry,* 31, 1647-1651, ISSN: 0001527X

[85] Wishart D.S.; Sykes B.D. (1994). The 13C chemical-shift index: a simple method for the identification of protein secondary structure using 13C chemical-shift data. *Journal of Biomolecular NMR,* 4, 171-180, ISSN: 0925-2738.

[86] Cornilescu G., Delaglio F.; Bax A. (1999). SimShiftDB; local conformational restraints derived from chemical shift similarity searches on a large synthetic database, *Journal of Biomolecular NMR,* 13, pp. 289-302, ISSN: 0925-2738.

[87] Van Horn W.D.; Kim H.J.; Ellis Ch.D.; Hadziselimovic A.; Sulistijo E.S.; Karra,M.D.; Tian Ch.; Sönnichsen F.D.; Sanders Ch.R., (2009). Solution Nuclear Magnetic Resonance Structure of Membrane-Integral Diacylglycerol Kinase, *Science,* 324, pp. 1726-1729, ISSN 0036-8075.

[88] Hu H.-Y.; Horton J.K.; Gryk M.R.; Prasad R.; Naron J.M.; Sun D.-A.; Hech S.M.; Wilson S.H.; Mullen G.P. (2004). Identification of Small Molecule Synthetic Inhibitors of DNA Polymerase β by NMR Chemical Shift Mapping, *The Journal of Biological Chemistry,* 279, pp. 39736–39744, ISSN 0021-9258.

[89] Johnson N.P.; Lapetoule P.; Razaka H.; Villani G., (1986). Biological and biochemical effects of DNA damage caused by platinum compounds, In D.C.McBrien and T.Slatter, (Eds), Biochemical Mechanisms of Platinum Antitumor Drugs. IRL Press, Oxford, pp. 1-28.

[90] Patterson H.H., Tewksbury J.C., Martin M., Krogh-Jespersen M.B.,.Lomenzo J.A, Hooper H.O., Viswanath A.K. (1981). Luminescence, absorption, MCD, and NQR study of the cis and trans isomers of dichlorodiammineplatinum(II), *Inorganic Chemistry*, 20, 2297-2301, ISSN 0020-1669.

[91] Werner-Zwanziger U.; Zigeweid M.; Black B.; Pines A. (1994). Nitrogen-14 SQUID NQR of L-Ala-L-His and of Serine, *Zeitschrift für Naturforschung,* A49A, pp.1188-1192, ISSN 0932-0784.

[92] Latosińska J.N., Structure-activity study of thiazides by magnetic resonance methods (NQR, NMR, EPR) and DFT calculations, *Journal of Molecular Graphics and Modelling*, 23, 329-37 (2005), ISSN: 1093-3263.

[93] Lipton A.S.; Heck R.W.; Ellis P. D. (2004). Solid-state NMR spectroscopy of human carbonic anhydrase: implications for the enzymatic mechanism, *Journal of the American Chemical Society*, 126, 4735-39, ISSN: 0002-7863.

[94] Merz K. M.; Hoffmann R.; Dewar M. J. S. (1989). The model of action of carbonic anhydrase, *Journal of the American Chemical Society*, 111, 5636-49, ISSN: 0002-7863.

[95] Desiraju G. R. (2002). Cryptic crystallography, *Nature Materials,* 1, pp. 77–79 ISSN: 1476-1122.

[96] Day, G. M.; Cooper, T. G.; Cruz-Cabeza, A. J.; Hejczyk, K. E.; Ammon, H. L.; Boerrigter, S. X. M.; Tan, J. S.; Della Valle, R. G.; Venuti, E.; Jose, J.; Gadre, S. R.; Desiraju, G. R.; Thakur, T. S.; van Eijck, B. P.; Facelli, J. C.; Bazterra, V. E.; Ferraro, M. B.; Hofmann, D. W. M.; Neumann, M. A.; Leusen, F. J. J.; Kendrick, J.; Price, S. L.; Misquitta, A. J.; Karamertzanis, P. G.; Welch, G. W. A.; Scheraga, H. A.; Arnautova, Y. A.; Schmidt, M. U., van de Streek, J.; Wolf, A. K. ; Schweizer, B. (2009). Significant progress in predicting the crystal structures of small organic molecules - a report on the fourth blind test". *Acta Crystallographica,* B65, pp. 107-125, ISSN: 0108-7681.

[97] Neumann, M.A.; Leusen F. J.J., Kendrick J. (2008). A Major Advance in Crystal Structure Prediction, *Angewandte Chemie International Edition,* 47,pp. 2427–2430, ISSN 0570-0833.

[98] Chan S.; John K.; Leusen F.J.J, (2011). Moleculel VI, a Benchmark Crystal-Structure-Prediction Sulfonimide: Are Its Polymorphs Predictable? *Angewandte Chemie International Edition*, 50, pp. 2979–2981, ISSN 0570-0833.

[99] Latosińska J.N; Latosińska M.; Tomczak M.A.; Seliger J.; Zagar V.; Maurin, J.K. (2011). Conformations and intermolecular interactions pattern in solid chloroxylenol and triclosan (API of anti-infective agents and drugs). A ^{35}Cl NQR, ^{1}H-^{14}N NQDR, X-Ray and DFT/QTAIM study *Magnetic Resonance in Chemistry, in press,* ISSN: 0749-1581.

[100] Ramos A. I.; Braga S. S.; Almeida Paz F. A., (2009). Triclosan, *Acta Crystallographica,* C65, 404-5, ISSN: 0108-2701.

[101] Latosińska J.N.; Tomczak M.A.; Kasprzak J. (2009). *Chemical Physics Letters,* 469, pp.201-206, ISSN: 0009-2614.

[102] Yang S. S.; Guillory J. K. (1972). Polymorphism in sulfonamides, *The Journal of Pharmaceutical Sciences*, 61, pp. 26-40, ISSN: 0022-3549.

[103] Kato Y., Watanabe H., Maeyama N., Kido K. (1979). Pulverization method for sulfamethizole and its physicochemical properties, *Chemical & Pharmaceutical Bulletin*, 1979, 27, pp. 366-373, ISSN: 0009-2363.

[104] Seliger J., Žagar V., Latosińska J.N., Phys.Chem.Chem.Phys. 2010.

[105] Latosińska J.N.; Latosińska M.; Seliger J.; Žagar V.; Maurin J.; Orzeszko A.; Kazimierczuk Z. (2010). Structural Study of Polyhalogenated Benzimidazoles (Protein Kinase CK2 Inhibitors) by Nuclear Quadrupole Double Resonance, X-RAY and Density Functional Theory, *The Journal of Physical Chemistry A*, 114, pp. 563-575, ISSN: 1089-5639.

[106] Goodman J.W., (1996). Introduction to Fourier Optics, 2nd ed.,McGraw-Hill, New York, , ISBN:9780070242548.

[107] Bader R.F.W.; (1990). Atoms in Molecules: A Quantum Theory; Oxford University Press: Oxford, U.K.

[108] Popelier P.L.A. (2000). Atoms in Molecules: An Introduction; Harlow. Prentice Hall: London, pp. 164, ISBN: 9780582367982.

[109] Bader, R.F.W. (1999).Can There Be More Than A Single Definition Of An Atom In A Molecule", *Canadian Journal of Chemistry*, 77, 86 - 93

[110] Gatti C. (2005). Chemical bonding in crystals: New directions, *Zeitschrift für Kristallographie*, 220, 399–457, ISSN 0044-2968.

[111] Bader R.F.W. (1998). A Bond Path - A Universal Indicator of Bonded Interactions, *Journal of Physical Chemistry A*, 102, pp. 7314 - 7323 ISSN: 1089-5639.

[112] Tutton A.E.H., (1922). Crystallography and Practical Crystal Measurement, pp. 796, ISBN: 1148686746.

[113] Cholerton T.J., Hunt J.H., Klinkert G., Martin- Smith M. (1984). Spectroscopic Studies on Ranitidine-its Structure and the Influence of Temperature and pH, *Journal of the Chemical Society, Perkin Transactions 1*, 2, pp. 1761-1766, ISSN: 1472-7781.

[114] Chemburkar, S. R.; Bauer, J.; Deming, K.; Spiwek, H.; Patel, K.; Morris, J., Henry, R., et al. (2000). Dealing with the impact of ritonavir polymorphs on the late stages of bulk drug process development. *Organic Process Research Development*, 4, pp. 413-417, ISSN: 1083-6160.

[115] Lommerse, J.P.M.; Motherwell, W.D.S.; Ammon, H. L.; Dunitz, J. D., Gavezzotti; A., Hofmann, D.W.M.; Leusen, F.J.J.; Mooij, W.T.M.; Price, S. L.; Schweizer, B.; Schmidt, M. U.; van Eijck, B. P.; Verwer, P.; Williams, D. E. (2000). A Test of Crystal Structure Prediction of Small Organic Molecules. *Acta Crystallographica*, B56 pp. 697-714, ISSN: 0108-7681.

[116] McCrone WC (1965) In polymorphism in physics and chemistry of the organic solid state. Interscience, New York, p 726.

[117] Bond A.,D.; Boese R.;Desiraju G.R. (2007). On the polymorphism of aspirin, *Angewandte Chemie-International Edition*, 46, pp. 615-617, ISSN:0570-0833.

[118] W. Cabri, P. Ghetti, G. Pozzi, M. Alpegiani, (2007). Polymorphisms and patent, market, and legal battles: Cefdinir case study, *Organic Process Research Development*, 11, pp. 64-72, ISSN: 1083-6160.

[119] Hájková M.; Kratochvíl B.; Rádl S. (2008), Atorvastatin - the World's Best Selling Drug, *Chemické Listy,* 102, pp. 3-14, ISSN 1213-7103.

[120] Childs S.L.; Hardcastle K. I. (2007). Cocrystals of Piroxicam with Carboxylic Acid, *Crystal Growth & Design, 7,* pp. 1291-1304, ISSN 1213-7103.Bingham A.L.; Hughes D.S.; Hursthouse M.B.; Lancaster R.W.; Tavener S. (2001). Threlfall

[121] T.L.: Over one hundred solvates of sulfathiazole, *Chemical Communications,* pp. 603-604, ISSN: 1359-7345.

[122] Bernstein J. (2002). Polymorphism in Molecular Crystals. Oxford University Press: New York, New York, pp.298.

[123] Bauer J. ; Sponton S. ; Henry R. ; Quick J. ; Dziki W. ; Porter W. ; Morfia J. (2001). Ritonavir: An Extraordinary Example of Conformational Polymorphism. *Pharmaceutical Research,* 18, pp. 859-866, ISSN: 0724-8741.

[124] Urakami K.; Shono Y.; Higashi A.; Umemoto K.; Godo M. (2002). A novel method for estimation of transition temperature for polymorphic pairs in pharmaceuticals using heat of solution and solubility data, *Chemical and Pharmaceutical Bulletin,* 50, pp. 263—267, ISSN: 0009-2363.

[125] Pudipeddi M.; Serajuddin A.T.M.: Trends in Solubility of Polymorphs, *The Journal of Pharmaceutical Sciences,* 94, pp. 929-939, ISSN: 0022-3549.

[126] Hammond G.S. (1955), A Correlation of Reaction Rates, *The Journal of the American Chemical Society,* 77, pp.334-338, ISSN: 0002-7863.

[127] Haleblian J.K., (1975).Characterisation of Habits and Crystalline Modification of Solids and their Pharmaceutical Applications, *The Journal of Pharmaceutical Sciences,* 64, 1269, ISSN: 0022-3549.

[128] Chihara H., Nakamura N., NQR Spectroscopy Data in Landolt-Börnststein New Series III, ed. O. Madelung (Spinger, Berlin, 1982-1997), ISBN: 9783540560500.

[129] Byrn S.R., Gray G., Pfeiffer R.R., Frye J., (1985) Analysis of solid-state carbon-13 NMR spectra of polymorphs (benoxaprofen and nabilone) and pseudopolymorphs (cefazolin), *The Journal of Pharmaceutical Sciences,* 74, pp. 565–568, ISSN: 0022-3549.

[130] Biedenkapp D.; Weiss A. (1967). Nuclear quadrupole resonance study of 35Cl in chloral hydrate, $CCl_3CH(OH)_2$, and chloral deuterate, $CCl_3CH(OD)_2$., *Zeitschrift für Naturforschung A,* 22, pp. 1124-1126, ISSN: 0932-0784.

[131] Allen H C Jr (1953). Pure Quadrupole Spectra of Molecular Crystals, *The Journal of Physical Chemistry,* 57, pp.501-504, ISSN: 1089-5639.

[132] Marsh R.E. (1958). A refinement of the crystal structure of glycine. *Acta Crystallographica* 11, pp.654–663, ISSN: 0365-110X.

[133] Iitaka Y. (1960). The crystal structure of β-glycine. *Acta Crystallographica* 13, pp.35- 45, ISSN: 0365-110X.

[134] Iitaka Y. (1958). The crystal structure of γ -glycine. *Acta Crystallographica* 11, pp.225–226, ISSN: 0365-110X.

[135] Jonsson P.G.; Kvick A. (1972). Precision neutron diffraction structure determination of protein and nucleic acid components. III. The crystal and molecular structure of the amino acid α-glycine. *Acta Crystallographica,* B28, pp. 1827–1833, ISSN: 0108-7681.

[136] Power L.F.; Turner K.E.; Moore F.H. (1976). The crystal and molecular structure of α-glycine by neutron diffraction–a comparison. *Acta Crystallographica* B32, pp. 11–16, ISSN: 0108-7681.

[137] Kvick A, Canning WM, Koetzle TF, Williams GJB. 1980. An experimental study of the influence of temperature on a hydrogen-bonded system: the crystal structure of α-glycine at 83 K and 298 K by neutron diffraction. *Acta Crystallographica* B36, pp. 115–120, ISSN: 0108-7681.

[138] Chongprasert S.; Knopp S.; Nail S. (2005). Characterisation of frozen solutions of glycine. *The Journal of Pharmaceutical Sciences,* 90, pp. 1720 –1728, ISSN: 0022-3549.

[139] Kimura H.; Nakamura K.; Eguchi A.; Sugisawa H.; Deguchi K.; Ebisawa K.; Suzuki E.; Shoji A. (1998). Structural study of α-amino-acid crystals by 1H CRAMPS NMR spectroscopy. *Journal of Molecular Structure,* 447 pp.247–255, ISSN: 0022-2860.

[140] Taylor, R.E. (2004). 13C CP/MAS: Application to Glycine, *Concepts in Magnetic Resonance Part A* 22A, pp. 79–89, ISSN: 1552-5023.

[141] Potrzebowski M.J.; Tekely P.; Dusausoy Y. (1998). Comment to 13C-NMR studies of α and γ polymorphs of glycine, *Solid State NMR,* 11, pp. 253–257, ISSN: 0926-2040.

[142] Malkin V.G., Malkina O.L., Salahub D.R. (1995). Influence of intermolecular interactions on the 13C NMR shielding tensor in solid α-glycine, *The Journal of the American Chemical Society,* 117, pp. 3294–3295, ISSN: 0002-7863.

[143] Edmonds D. T.; Summers C. P. (1976). Quadrupole resonance of 14N and 2D in glycine, a model compound, *Chemical Physics Letters,* 41, pp. 482-485, ISSN: 0009-2614.

[144] Rabbani S. R.; Edmonds D. T.; Gosling P.; Palmer M. H. (1987). Measurement of the 14N quadrupole coupling constants in glycine, diglycine, triglycine, and tetraglycine and a comparison with calculation, Journal of Magnetic Resonance 72, pp. 230-237, ISSN: 1090-7807.

[145] Griesser U. J.; Burger A.; Mereiter K. (1997). The polymorphic drug substances of the European pharmacopoeia. Part 9: Crystal structure and thermodynamic properties of Acetazolamide crystal forms, *The Journal of Pharmaceutical Sciences,* 86, 352-358, ISSN: 0022-3549.

[146] Zhenbo M. (2009), A Novel Polymorph of 5-Chloro-8-Hydroxyquinoline with Improved Water Solubility and Faster Dissolution Rate, *The Journal of Chemical Crystallography,* 39, pp. 913–918, ISSN: 1074-1542.

[147] Desiraju, G. R. (2005). Supramolecular Synthons in Crystal Engineering. A New Organic Synthesis, *Angewandtc Chemie International Edition,* 34, pp. 2311- 2327, ISSN 0570-0833.

[148] Latosińska J.N; Latosińska M.; Tomczak M.A.; Seliger J.; Zagar V. (2011). Supramolecular synthon pattern in solid clioquinol and cloxiquine (APIs of antibacterial, antifungal, antiaging and antituberculosis drugs) studied by ^{35}Cl NQR, ^{1}H- ^{17}O and ^{1}H- ^{14}N NQDR and DFT/QTAIM, *Journal of Molecular Modelling,* 17, 1781-1800, ISSN: 0002-7863.

[149] Adsmond D.A.; Grant D.J.W. (2001). Hydrogen bonding in sulfonamides, *The Journal of Pharmaceutical Sciences,* 90, pp. 2058-2077, ISSN: 0022-3549.

[150] O'Connor B.H.; Maslen E.N. (1965). The crystal structure of α-sulphanilamide, *Acta Crystallographica*, 18, 363-366, ISSN: 0108-7681.

[151] Alléaume M.; Decap J. (1965). Affinement tridimensionnel du sulfanilamide β, *Acta Crystallographica*, 18, 731-736, ISSN: 0108-7681.

[152] Alléaume M.; Decap J. (1965). Affinement tridimensionnel du sulfanilamide γ, *Acta Crystallographica*, 19, 934-938, ISSN: 0108-7681.

[153] Sekiguchi K, Tsuda Y, Kanke M. (1975). Dissolution behavior of solid drugs. VI. Determination of transition temperatures of various physical forms of physical forms of sulfanilamide by initial dissolution, *Chemical & Pharmaceutical Bulletin*, 23, pp. 1353-1362, ISSN: 0009-2363.

[154] Lin H.O.; Baenziger N.C.; Guillory J.K. (1974). Physical properties of four polymorphic forms of sulfanilamide I: Densities, refractive indexes, and X-ray diffraction measurement, *The Journal of Pharmaceutical Sciences*, 63, pp. 145-146 ISSN: 0022-3549.

[155] Gelbrich T; Bingham A.L.; Threlfall T.L.; Hursthouse M.B. (2008). δ-Sulfanilamide, *Acta Crystallographica* C64, o205-o207, ISSN: 1600-5759.

[156] Portieri A., Harris R.K., Fletton R.A., Lancaster R.W., Threlfall T.L. (2004). Effects of polymorphic differences for sulfanilamide, as seen through ^{13}C and ^{15}N solid-state NMR, together with shielding calculations, *Magnetic Resonance in Chemistry*, 42, pp. 313-320, ISSN: 0749-1581.

[157] Blinc R., Seliger J., Zidans A., Zagar V., Milia F., Roberts H., (2006). ^{14}N nuclear quadrupole resonance of some sulfa drugs, *Solid State NMR*, 30, pp.61-68, ISSN: 0926-2040.

[158] Lavrič, Z., Pirnat, J., Lužnik, J., Seliger, J., Žagar, V., Trontelj, Z. and Srčič, S. (2010), Application of ^{14}N NQR to the study of piroxicam polymorphism, *Journal of Pharmaceutical Sciences*, 99, pp. 4857–4865, ISSN: 0022-3549.

[159] Perez S.C., Cerioni L., Wolfenson A.E., Faudone S., Cuffini S.L., (2005). Utilization of pure nuclear quadrupole resonance spectroscopy for the study of pharmaceutical crystal forms, *International Journal of Pharmaceutics*, 298, 143-152, ISSN: 0378-5173.

[160] Balchin E., Malcolme-Lawes D.J., Poplett I.J.F., Smith M.J.A.S., Pearce G.E.S., Wren S.A.C., (2005). Potential of Nuclear Quadrupole Resonance Pharmaceutical Analysis, *Analytical Chemistry*, 77, 3925-3930, ISSN: 0003-2700.

[161] Reutzel-Edens, S.M. (2008). NMR Crystallography and the Elucidation of Structure-Property Relationships in Crystalline Solids, *NATO Science for Peace and Security Series B: Physics and Biophysics*, 2008, 351-374, ISBN: 9781402068225.

[162] Laar P.C., Ber. Dtsch. Chem. Ges. 18, 648 (1885).

[163] Roosaf R.A.; DeLamater E.D. (1960). A Cytological Evaluation of Combined Therapy in the 6C3HED Lymphosarcoma, I. -SH-containing Analogs in Combination with Nitrogen Mustard and Mapharsen *Cancer Reserach* 20, pp.1543-1554, ISSN: 1538-7445.

[164] Timson J.; Price D.J. (1972) Chromosomes Today vol. 3, Eds. Darlington C D. and Lewis K.R, Hafner P.F. John Wiley, New York p. 118, ISBN 978-1-4020-0091-1.

[165] Vetter C.; Wagner Ch.; Kaluđerović G.N.; Paschke B.R.; Steinborn D. (2009). Synthesis, Characterisation, and Cytotoxicity of Trimethylplatinum(IV) Complexes with

2-Thiocytosine and 1-Methyl-2-thiocytosine Ligands, *Inorganica Chimica Acta,* 362, pp. 189-195, ISSN: 0020-1693.

[166] McClure R.J., Craven B.M. (1973). New investigations of cytosine and its monohydrate, *Acta Crystallographica* B 29, pp.1234-1238, ISSN: 0108-7681.

[167] Latosińska J.N.; Latosińska M.; Seliger J.; Žagar V.; Burchardt, D.V. (2011). A comparative study of hydrogen bonding pattern and prototropism in solid 2-thiocytosine (potential anti-leukemic agent) and cytosine studied by 1H-14N NQDR and QTAIM/DFT, *Journal of Molecular Modeling,* in press.

[168] Alexander S., Tzalmona A. (1965). Relaxation by Slow Motional Processes. Effect of Molecular Rotations in Pure Quadrupole Resonance, *Physical Review,* 138, A845-855, ISSN: 1943-2879.

[169] Kasprzak J., Pietrzak J., Pietrzak A. (1989). The temperature dependence of ^{35}Cl NQR spectrum and study of spin-lattice relaxation times in chloral hydrate, *Journal of Molecular Structure,* 192, pp. 379-382, ISSN: 0022-2860.

[170] Hashimoto M., Weiss A. (1980). A chlorine NQR study on the phase transformation of chloral hydrate. *Journal of Molecular Structure,* 58, pp. 243-252, ISSN: 0022-2860.

[171] Latosińska J.N., Latosińska M., Utrecht R., Mielcarek S., Pietrzak J., (2004) Molecular dynamics of solid benzothiadiazine derivatives (thiazides). A study by NMR, DTA and DFT methods, *Journal of Molecular Structure,* 694, 211-217, ISSN: 0022-2860.

[172] Latosińska J.N., Kasprzak J., Utrecht R., (2002), Molecular Dynamics of Thiazides Studied by ^{35}Cl-NQR Spectroscopy, Appl.Magn. Reson. 23, 193 ISSN 0937-9347.

[173] Florence A.; Johnston A.; Fernandes P.; Shankland K.; Stevens H.N.E.; Osmundsen E.; Mullen A.B. (2005). Powder study of hydrochlorothiazide form II, *Acta Crystallographica,* E61, o2798-o2800, ISSN: 1600-5368.

[174] Zagar V.; Seliger J. (1994).^{14}N nuclear quadrupole resonance study of the structural phase transition in phenothiazine, *Journal of Physics Condensed Matter,* 6, 6027-6038, ISSN: 0953-8984.

[175] McDowell J.H., *(1976).* The crystal and molecular structure of phenothiazine, *Acta Crystallographica,* B32, pp. 5-10, ISSN: 0108-7681.

[176] Pontremoli R., Leoncini G., Parodi A., (2005). Use of nifedipine in the treatment of hypertension, *Expert Review of Cardiovascular Therapy,* 3, pp. 43-50, ISSN: 1477-9072.

[177] Al-Turk W.A.; Majeed I.A.; Murray W.J.; Newton D.W.; Othman S. (1988). Some factors affecting the photodecomposition of nifedipine, *International Journal of Pharmaceutics,* 41, pp. 227-230, ISSN: 0378-5173.

[178] Matsuda, Y.; Teraoka, R.; Sugimoto, I. (1989). Comparative evaluation of photostability of solid-state nifedipine underordinary and intensive light irradiation conditions. *International Journal of Pharmaceutics* 54, pp. 211–221, ISSN: 0378-5173.

[179] Teraoka R.; Otsuka M.; Matsuda Y., (1999). Evaluation of photostability of solid-state dimethyl 1,4-dihydro-2, 6-dimethyl-4-(2-nitro-phenyl)-3,5-pyridinedicarboxylate by using Fourier-transformed reflection-absorption infrared spectroscopy, *International Journal of Pharmaceutics,* 184, pp. 35–43, ISSN: 0378-5173.

[180] Sadana, G.S., Ghogare, A.B., 1991. Quantitative proton magnetic resonance spectroscopic determination of nifedipine and its photodecomposition products

from pharmaceutical preparations. *Journal of Pharmaceutical Sciences,* 80, pp. 895–898 , ISSN: 0022-3549.

[181] Zielinska M., Wawer I., Pisklak D.M., Tkaczyk M., unpublished results.

[182] Latosińska J.N.; Latosińska M.; Seliger J.; Žagar V., *Journal of Pharmaceutical Sciences,* submitted.

[183] Raju T.N.K. (2000). The Nobel chronicles. *Lancet,* 355, p. 1022, ISSN: 0140-6736.

[184] Wawer I, Bernd D., Holzgrabe U., NMR Spectroscopy in Pharmaceutical Analysis, Elsevier LTD, Oxford, ISBN: 9780444531735.

[185] Harris R.K. (2007), Applications of Solid-State NMR to Pharmaceutical Polymorphism and Related Matters. *Journal of Pharmacy and Pharmacology,* 59, pp. 225 - 239, ISSN: 0022-3573.

[186] Holzgrabe U., Deubner R., Schollmayer C. Waibel B. (2005). Quantitative NMR spectroscopy—Applications in drug analysis, *Journal of Pharmaceutical and Biomedical Analysis,*38, pp. 806-812, ISSN: 0731-7085.

[187] Latosińska J.N., (2007). Applications of nuclear quadrupole resonance spectroscopy in drug development, *Expert Opinion on Drug Discovery,* 2, 225-248 ISSN: 1746-0441.

[188] Latosińska J.N., (2005). Structure-activity study of thiazides by magnetic resonance methods (NQR, NMR, EPR) and DFT calculation, *Journal of Molecular Graphics and Modelling,* 23, pp. 329-337, ISSN: 1093-3263.

[189] Latosińska J.N., (2005). Nuclear quadrupole resonance spectroscopy in studies of biologically active molecular systems-a review. *Journal of Pharmaceutical and Biomedical Analysis,* 38, 557-587, ISSN: 0731-7085.

11

De-Risking Drug Discovery Programmes Early with ADMET

Katya Tsaioun[1] and Steven A. Kates[2]
[1]*Apredica, a Cyprotex Company, Watertown, MA*
[2]*Ischemix LLC, Maynard, MA*
USA

1. Introduction

Drug attrition that occurs in late clinical development or during post-marketing is a serious economic problem in the pharmaceutical industry (1). The cost for drug approvals is approaching $1 billion USD, and the cost of advancing a compound to Phase 1 trials can reach up to $100 million USD according to the Tufts Center for the Study of Drug Development, Tufts University School of Medicine (2). The study also estimates a $37,000 USD direct out-of-pocket cost for each day a drug is in the development stage and opportunity costs of $1.1 million USD in lost revenue (2). Given these huge expenditures, substantial savings can accrue from early recognition of problems that would demonstrate a compound's potential to succeed in development (3).

The costs associated with withdrawing a drug from the market are even greater. For example, terfenadine is both a potent hERG cardial channel ligand and is metabolized by the liver enzyme Cyp3A4. Terfenadine was frequently co-administered with Cyp3A4 inhibitors ketoconazole or erythromycin (4). The consequent overload resulted in increases in plasma terfenadine to levels that caused cardiac toxicity (5) resulting in the drug to be withdrawn from the market (6) at an estimated cost of $6 billion USD. Another example is the broad-spectrum antibiotic trovafloxacin, which was introduced in 1997 and soon became Pfizer's top seller. The drug was metabolically activated *in vivo* and formed a highly reactive metabolite causing severe drug-induced hepatotoxicity (7). Trovafloxacin was black labeled in 1998 (8) costing Pfizer $8.5 billion USD in lawsuits (9). With the new ability to measure hERG and other important ADMET (Absorption, Distribution, Metabolism, Excretion and Toxicity) parameters early in the discovery and development process, such liabilities are now recognized earlier allowing for safer analogs to be advanced to more expensive formal preclinical and clinical stages.

The purpose of preclinical ADMET also referred to as early DMPK (drug metabolism and pharmacokinetics) is to reduce the risk similar to above and avoid spending scarce resources on weak lead candidates and programs. This allows drug-development resources to be focused on fewer, but more-likely-to-succeed drug candidates. In 1993, 40 % of drugs failed in clinical trials because of pharmacokinetic (PK) and bioavailability problems (10). Since then, major technological advances have occurred in molecular biology and screening to allow major aspects of ADMET to be assessed earlier during the lead-optimization stage. By the late 1990s the pharmaceutical industry recognized the value of early ADMET assessment and began routinely employing it with noticeable results. ADME and DMPK problems decreased from 40% to 11% (4). Presently, a lack of efficacy and human toxicity are the primary reasons for failure (11).

The terms "drugability" and "druglikeness" were first described by Dr. Christopher Lipinski, who proposed "Lipinski's Rule of 5" due to the frequent appearance of a number "5" in the rules (12). The Rule of 5 has come to be a compass for the drug discovery industry (13). It stipulates that small-molecule drug candidates should possess:

- a molecular weight less than 500 g/mol
- a partition coefficient (logP - a measure of hydrophobicity) less than 5
- no more than 5 hydrogen bond donors
- no more than 10 hydrogen bond acceptors

A compound with fewer than three of these properties is unlikely to become a successful orally bioavailable drug. There are exceptions to Lipinski's Rule of 5 that have become marketed drugs, such as those taken up by active transport mechanisms, natural compounds, oligonucleotides and proteins.

The drug discovery industry is experiencing dramatic structural change and is no longer just the domain of traditional large pharmaceutical companies. Now venture-capital-funded startups, governments, venture philanthropy and other non-profit and academic organizations are important participants in the search for new drug targets, pathways, and molecules. These organizations frequently form partnerships, sharing resources, capabilities, risks and rewards of drug discovery. Thus, it is becoming increasingly important to ensure that investors, donors, and taxpayers' money is efficiently used so that new safe drugs for unmet medical needs may be delivered to the public. ADMET profiling has been proven to remove poor drug candidates from development and accelerate the discovery process.

Although lack of efficacy and unexpected toxicity are the major causes of drug failure in clinical trials, a prime determinant is the ability of a drug to penetrate biological barriers such as cell membranes, intestinal walls, or the blood brain barrier (BBB). For drugs that target the Central Nervous System (CNS) such as stroke, *in vitro* efficacy combined with the inability to penetrate the BBB typically result in poor *in vivo* efficacy in patients. The delivery of systemically administered drugs to the brain of mammals is limited by the BBB as it effectively isolates the brain from the blood because of the presence of tight junctions connecting the endothelial cells of the brain vessels. In addition, specific metabolizing enzymes and efflux pumps such as P-glycoprotein (P-gp) and the multi-drug-resistance protein (MRP), located within the endothelial cells of the BBB, actively pump exogenous molecules out of the brain (14, 15). This is one of the reasons for CNS drugs having a notoriously high failure rate (16). In recent years, 9% of compounds that entered Phase 1 survived to launch and only 3-5% of CNS drugs were commercialized (16). Greater than 50% of this attrition resulted from failure to demonstrate efficacy in Phase 2 studies. Over the last decade, Phase 2 failures have increased by 15%. Compounds with demonstrated efficacy against a target *in vitro* and in animal models frequently proved to be ineffective in humans. Many of these failures occur due to the inability to reach the CNS targets such as in stroke due to lack of BBB permeability. For drugs targeted to reduce damage from a stroke, the delivery method, BBB permeability, and drug metabolism and clearance can provide life or death to a patient if the drug is not delivered to the target tissue in its active form in a matter of hours from the event.

Due to the extraordinary cost of drug development, it is highly desirable to have effective, cost-efficient and high-throughput tools to measure BBB permeability before proceeding to expensive and time consuming animal BBB permeability studies or human clinical trials. With *in vitro* tools available, promising drug candidates with ineffective BBB penetration may be improved by removing structural components that mediate interaction(s) with efflux proteins, and/or lowering binding to brain tissue at earlier stages of development to increase intrinsic permeability (17).

The development of drugs targeting CNS requires precise knowledge of the drug's brain penetration. Ideally, this information would be obtained as early as possible to focus resources on compounds most likely to reach the target organ. The physical transport and metabolic composition of the BBB is highly complex. Numerous *in vitro* models have been designed to study kinetic parameters in the CNS, including non-cerebral peripheral endothelial cell lines, immortalized rat brain endothelial cells, primary cultured bovine, porcine or rat brain capillary endothelial cells and co-cultures of primary brain capillary cells with astrocytes (18, 19, 20). *In vitro* BBB models must be carefully assessed for their capacity to reflect accurately the passage of drugs into the CNS *in vivo*.

Alternatively, several *in vivo* techniques have been used to estimate BBB passage of drugs directly in laboratory animals. *In vivo* transport across the BBB was first studied in the 1960s using the early indicator diffusion method (IDM) of Crone (21). Other *in vivo* techniques were later proposed including brain uptake index (BUI) measurement (22), *in situ* brain perfusion method (23, 24), autoradiography and intracerebral microdialysis (25). Unfortunately these methods have limitations including sophisticated equipment, technical expertise, mathematical modeling, species differences, invasiveness, and low throughput and render them unsuitable for use during early stages of drug discovery and development. Hence, *in vitro* and *in vivo* models remain mere approximations of the complex BBB and their relevance to human pharmacology must be carefully considered. The most appropriate method to conduct controlled experiments is to cross-compare the BBB passage of a series of compounds evaluated with both *in vitro* and *in vivo* models. This enables cross-correlations of pharmacokinetic data and the assessment of the predictive power of *in vitro* and *in vivo* tests.

2. The evolving science of ADMET

Regulatory authorities have relied upon *in vivo* testing to predict the behavior of new molecules in the human body since the 1950s. Bioavailability, tissue distribution, pharmacokinetics, metabolism, and toxicity are assessed typically in one rodent and one non-rodent species prior to administering a drug to a human to evaluate safety in a clinical trial (Phase 1). Biodistribution is assessed using radioactively labeled compounds later in development because it is expensive both in terms of synthesizing sufficient amounts of radioactively labeled compound and for performing the animal experiments (22).

Pharmacodynamic (PD) effectiveness of test compounds is typically assessed initially through *in vitro* models such as receptor binding, followed by confirmation through *in vivo* efficacy models in mice or rats. The predictive ability depends on the therapeutic area and the animal model. Infectious disease models are considered to have the best predictive ability, whereas CNS and oncology animal models are generally the least predictive of human efficacy. Understanding the PK/PD relationship is crucial in determining the mechanism of action and metabolic stability of the molecule which can explain and support efficacy results. *In vivo* pharmacokinetic (PK) studies in a variety of animal models are routinely used for lead optimization to assess drug metabolism and absorption. There are significant differences in absorption and metabolism among species from animal studies, which may cause conflicting predictions of degradation pathways of new chemical entities (NCEs).

Toxicity and safety studies are performed in models that are relevant to the NCE's mode of action and therapeutic area. *In vivo* toxicity models are required for IND (Investigational New Drug Application) to the US Food and Drug Administration, but have substantial predictive weaknesses. In a retrospective study of 150 compounds from twelve large pharmaceutical companies, the combined animal toxicity study of rodents and non-rodents accurately predicted only 50% of the human hepatotoxicity. This poor level of accuracy in animal toxicity studies caused large numbers of compounds to be removed from development without proceeding into clinical trials with the potential of demonstrating safety in human subjects (26). The other ~50% whose toxicity could not be predicted was attributed to "idiosyncratic human hepatotoxicity that cannot be detected by conventional animal toxicity studies". Although it is widely recognized that mechanisms for toxicity are frequently quite different between species, animal testing remains the "gold standard" for required regulatory and historical data reasons. The US FDA and other regulatory agencies are in the process of evaluating alternatives to animal testing, with the aim of developing models that are truly predictive of human mechanisms of toxicity, and limiting *in vivo* toxicology testing.

3. The ADMET feedback loop

As discussed above, historically ADMET studies were focused on *in vivo* assays. These are time- and resource-intensive, and generally low throughput assays resulting in their implementation later in the development process, when more resources are released to study the few molecules that have advanced to this stage. With the advent of *in vitro* high-throughput screening, molecular biology and miniaturization technologies in the 1990s, early ADMET assays were developed to predict *in vivo* animal and human results, at a level of speed and cost-effectiveness appropriate for the discovery stage. This produced a major advance in the science of ADMET and has created a new paradigm that drug discovery programs follow in advancing compounds from hit to lead, from lead to advanced lead, and on to nominated clinical candidates. Now, early in the discovery phase, using human enzymes and human-origin cells, drug discovery programs are able to obtain highly actionable information about the drug-likeness of new molecules, the potential to reach target organ, and early indications of known human mechanisms of toxicities. ADMET assessment of varying complexity is currently routinely performed on compounds that have shown *in vitro* efficacy and in conjunction with or just prior to demonstrating early proof of principle *in vivo*.

The application of early ADMET is unique to each drug discovery program. The development path from discovery to IND is not straightforward and is dependent on the therapeutic area, route of administration, chemical series, and other parameters. Correspondingly, the importance of the various ADMET assays is based upon the specifics of the drug discovery program. ADMET assays can also be categorized into those that are routine and those reserved for more advanced profiling. This division is also a function of cost effectiveness and the need for the specific information. For instance, data regarding induction of human liver enzymes and transporters are not relevant during the hit-to-lead phase and is normally obtained for fewer more advanced candidates.

In some cases the FDA requests data from *in vitro* ADMET assays. For example, *in vitro* drug-drug interaction (DDI) studies may now be conducted under the guidance from FDA dated September 2006. The guidance document precisely outlines methods to conduct CYP-450 inhibition and induction and P-gp interaction studies (27). This package is now typically included in an IND submission.

How should a discovery team employ early ADMET? The answer is not simple and formulaic – it is a process. It is useful to start from the ultimate goal and work backwards towards discovery. The drug discovery and development team should first define the target product profile (TPP), which includes indication, intended patient population, route of administration, acceptable toxicities, and ultimately will define the drug label. The TPP invariably will evolve during the life of the project, but having major parameters of TPP established initially maintains a collaboration and focus between disciplines such as biology and chemistry, discovery and development, pre-clinical and clinical groups. Once the TPP is identified, then major design elements of the Phase 2 and 3 clinical trials can be outlined leading to questions about the tolerability, toxicity and safety of the molecule. These parameters will then define the GLP toxicity studies in animals, which will guide the team to the discovery and preclinical development data to be addressed in an early ADMET program.

How is this information implemented in the discovery phase? If a compound has high target receptor binding and biological activity in cells and in relevant *in vivo* animal models, what are the chances of it becoming a successful drug? A molecule needs to cross many barriers to reach its biological target. In order to obtain this goal, a molecule must be in solution and thus the first step is typically to assess the solubility of a compound. A solubility screen provides information about the NCE's solubility in fluids compatible with administration to humans. Chemical and metabolic stability is a further extension of the intrinsic properties of a molecule. Chemical stability in buffers, simulated gastric and intestinal fluids, and metabolic stability in plasma, hepatocytes or liver microsomes of different species can be measured to predict the rate of decay of a compound in the different environments encountered in the human body.

The second step is to define the absorption properties and the bioavailability of a molecule. Measurement of permeability across Caco-2 cell monolayers is a good predictor of human oral bioavailability. For CNS drugs, assessment of BBB penetration would be performed at this stage and is usually a key component of lead optimization campaigns. Passive BBB permeability may be assessed using BBB-PAMPA assays whereas potential for active uptake or efflux may be determined using *in vivo* models or cell lines naturally expressing endogenous human intestinal or BBB transporters (such as CaCO-2 cell line) or cell lines overexpressing specific transporters (such as MDCK-MDR1).

Measurement of binding to plasma proteins indicates the degree of availability of the free compound in the blood circulation. This is critical as only unbound drugs are able to reach the target and exert their pharmacologic effects. Metabolism and drug-drug interaction issues are discovered by screening for inhibition of cytochrome P450 liver enzymes (CYP450). All these assays allow chemists and biologists to obtain actionable information and provide a link between structure-activity (SAR) and structure-properties (SPR) relationships that drive decisions on selection of chemical series and molecules.

The next step is the involvement of drug-drug interactions and is required for advanced lead optimization. The effect of drug transporters on permeability and the effect of drugs on transporter activity can be measured in Caco-2, MDCK-MDR1 or other models. P-gp interactions are particularly important for CNS drugs due to high expression of these efflux transporters in the human BBB. Early knowledge about these interactions is instrumental to the medicinal chemistry strategy and helps drive lead optimization.

The effect of a compound on CYP-450 metabolism can be identified by determining the 50% inhibitory concentration (IC_{50}) for each CYP-450. These relationships between the NCE and metabolizing enzymes need to be evaluated in the context of the human effective dose and maximum effective plasma concentrations. These human data are not normally available at early stages of discovery, but could be extrapolated from animal PK/PD results for compounds in more advanced stages of development. It is important to understand these transporter and CYP-450 relationships for the following.

1. The compound may affect the effective plasma concentrations of other concomitantly administered drugs if metabolized by the same CYPs (i.e., terfenadine).
2. If the parent drug is a CYP inducer, it may increase the clearance rate of concomitantly administered drugs which are metabolized by these CYPs. This may result in a decrease in these drugs' effective plasma concentrations, thus decreasing their pharmacologic effect.
3. Metabolites formed *via* CYP metabolism may be responsible for undesirable side effects such as organ toxicity.
4. The metabolite of a compound may actually be responsible for compound's efficacy, and not the parent compound. The metabolite may even have a better efficacy, safety, and pharmacokinetics profile than its parent. As a result, metabolism can be exploited to produce a better drug which will impact the medicinal chemistry strategy.
5. The identification of drug-metabolizing enzymes involved in the major metabolic pathways of a compound assists to predict the probable drug-drug interactions in humans. This information also may be used to design human clinical trials to detect unnecessary drug-drug interaction.

ADMET is a tool that supports overall program goals. Similar to the Rule of 5 that requires only 3 of the 4 conditions to be met, seldom will negative results from a single ADMET assay terminate a compound's development or the overall program. The results are more likely to alter the medicinal chemistry direction.

After assessing compounds in a few simple mechanistic systems such as plasma and liver microsomal stability screens in relevant species, lead optimization phase is started that includes assays which identify potential liabilities. Finally, at the stage of advanced lead optimization and development, more-complex systems are used to more thoroughly understand a compound's metabolic fate and absorption mechanism to drive efficient development. As ADMET roadblocks are discovered, the cycle is repeated until a clear path is found (Figure 1).

4. Impact of ADMET

Early ADMET provides the data necessary for selecting preclinical candidates by providing crucial information to medicinal chemists and accelerates the timelines for IND and subsequently NDA submission which translates to lengthier commercialization under patent protection and greater profits. For investors, this is a major parameter. For philanthropic organizations and from standpoint of public policy, it means increasing the time of clinical benefit to the public. Data compiled by the Tufts Center for Drug Discovery have identified that for a typical, moderately successful proprietary drug ($350 million USD annual sales) each day's delay equates to $1.1 million USD in lost patent protected revenues that provide the return on investment needed to fund drug discovery (3). Further, shorter discovery and development timelines provide faster liquidity events for venture capital and angel investors. As drug discovery requires a longer commercialization than any other form of product development, its slowness to produce returns is a major impediment for obtaining investment. Accelerating drug discovery and development should attract more investment in drug discovery research.

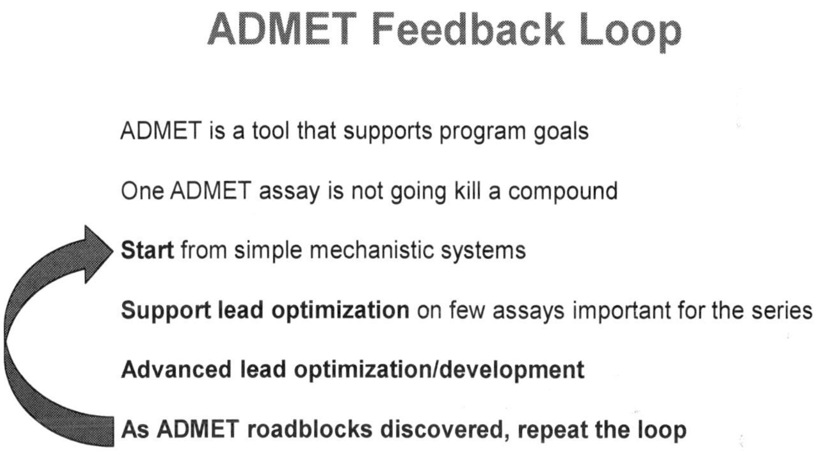

Fig. 1. ADMET Feedback Loop.

ADMET technologies remain an active area of research. There are many challenges in accurately measuring BBB penetration which may be one of the reasons for poor human efficacy of CNS drug candidates. Another challenge is detection of all mechanisms of human idiosyncratic toxicity. These mechanisms cause the most expensive, harmful, and disheartening form of drug attrition - post-commercialization toxicity. Many idiosyncratic drug reactions are due to formation of short-lived reactive metabolites that bind covalently to cell proteins (28). The extent to which a compound will generate these metabolites can now be detected before a compound is administered to humans signifying progress. Other mechanisms of human toxicity can be observed early in discovery and are briefly described in the following section.

5. New ADMET tools

Penetrating the BBB is a challenge particular to CNS drug discovery. Another obstacle caused by BBB permeability is that many drugs not intended as CNS therapeutics cause neurotoxicity. Artificial membrane permeability assays (PAMPA and BBB-PAMPA) offer a cost-effective and high-throughput method of screening for passively absorbed compounds but do not predict active transport in or out of the brain.

5.1 *In Vitro* model of human adult Blood-Brain Barrier

Many new drugs designed for CNS may show exceptional therapeutic promise due to their high potency at the target site, but lack general efficacy when administered systemically. In many cases, the problem is due to lack of penetration of the BBB and this has become a major problem that has impeded the discovery and development of active CNS drugs. CEA Technologies previously reported the development of a new co-culture-based model of human BBB able to predict passive and active transport of molecules into the CNS (29). This new model consists of primary cultures of human brain capillary endothelial cells co-cultured with primary human glial cells (18, 29). The advantages of this system include:

i. made of human primary culture cells
ii. avoids species, age and inter-individual differences since the two cell types are removed from the same person
iii. expresses functional efflux transporters such as P-gp, MRP-1, 4,5 and BCRP.

This model has potential for assessment of permeability of drug and specific transport mechanisms, which is not possible in PAMPA or other cell models due to incomplete expression of active transporters.

One important step in development of any *in vitro* model is to cross-correlate *in vitro* and *in vivo* data in order to validate experimental models and to assess the predictive power of the techniques (30). The human BBB model was validated against a "gold standard" *in vivo* model and has shown an excellent *in vitro-in vivo* correlation (29, 31). In this carefully designed *in vivo-in vitro* correlation study the authors reported the evaluation of the BBB permeabilities for a series of compounds studied correlatively *in vitro* using a human BBB model and *in vivo* with quantitative PET imaging (29). Six clinical PET tracers with different molecular size ranges (Figure 2) and degree of BBB penetration were used including [^{18}F]-FDOPA and [^{18}F]-FDG, ligands of amino acid and glucose transporters, respectively. The findings demonstrate that the *in vitro* co-culture model of human BBB has important features of the BBB *in vivo* including low paracellular permeability, well developed tight junctions, functional expression of important known efflux transporters and is suitable for discriminating between CNS and non-CNS compounds. To further demonstrate the relevance of the *in vitro* human system, drug permeation into the human brain was evaluated using PET imaging in parallel to the assessment of drug permeability across the *in vitro* model of the human BBB. *In vivo* plasma - brain exchange parameters used for comparison were determined previously in humans by PET using a kinetic analysis of the radiotracer binding. 2-[^{18}F]Fluoro-A-85380 and [^{11}C]-raclopride show absent or low cerebral uptake with the distribution volume under 0.6. [^{11}C]-Flumazenil, [^{11}C]-befloxatone, [^{18}F]-FDOPA and [^{18}F]-FDG show a cerebral uptake with the distribution volume above 0.6. The *in vitro* human BBB model discriminates compounds similar to *in v*ivo human brain PET imaging analysis. This data illustrates the close relationship between *in vitro* and *in vivo* pharmacokinetic data (r^2 0.90, $p < 0.001$) (Figure 2). Past *in vivo-in vitro* studies often did not have good correlations for substances transported into or out of the brain *via* active transport. Presumably this is due to experiments being performed either with models that did not have adequate expression of active human transporters (such as PAMPA or MDCK cells) or using too high concentrations of compounds *in vitro*, which are known to saturate the transporters. Using the radioactive labeled probes and the small amounts of compounds avoids these issues.

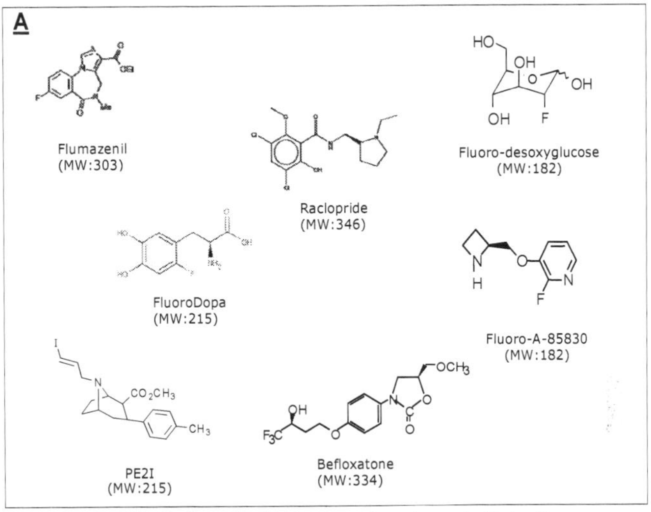

A. Chemical structures of radioligands investigated and used clinically.

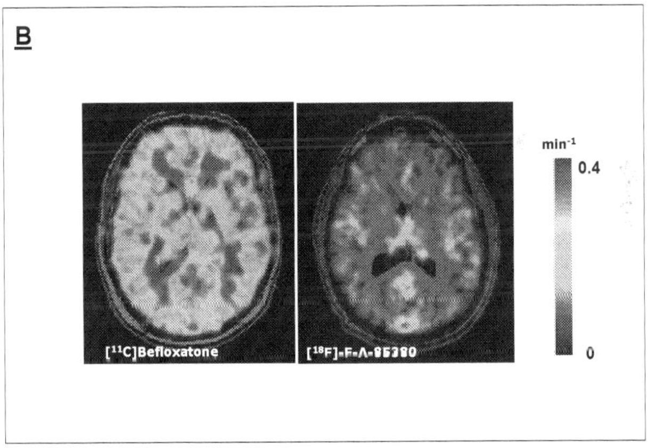

B. Typical imaging data. Co-registered PET-MRI images representing the k1 obtained in human after intravenous injection of [^{11}C]-Befloxatone (left) and [^{18}F]-F-A-85380 (right). The PET images representing the k1 are as follows: PET image obtained at 1 min post injection (mean value between 30 sec and 90 sec) is considered as independent to the receptor binding. This image (in Bq/mL) is corrected from the vascular fraction (Fv in Bq/mL, considered as 4% of the total blood concentration at 1 min) and divided by the arterial plasma input function (AUC0-1 min of the plasma concentration, in Bq*min/mL). The resulting parametric image, expressed in min^{-1}, represent an index of the k1 parameter of the radiotracer.

Fig. 2. *In vitro-in vivo* drug transport correlation.

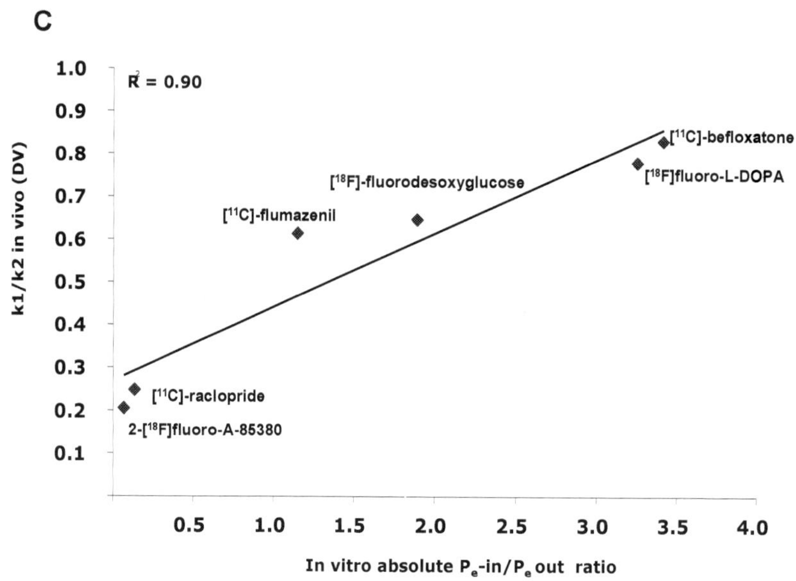

C. *In Vivo* Distribution Volume (DV) as function of the in vitro P_e-out/P_e-in ratio (Q). Regression line was calculated, and correlation was estimated by the two tailed non parametric Spearman test. [11C]PE2I radioligand was not plotted in the figure since the *in vivo* K1/k2 parameter in human is not available.

Fig. 2. *In vitro-in vivo* drug transport correlation (continued).

In conclusion, this *in vitro* human BBB model offers great potential for both being developed into a reproducible screen for passive BBB permeability and determining active transport mechanisms. Due to its high-throughput potential, the model may provide testing large numbers of compounds of pharmaceutical importance for CNS diseases. Validation work is in progress in which activity of transporters that are important in CNS BBB are being assessed in a functional assay and compared between CaC0-2 and hBBB models (31).

5.2 Mechanisms of human toxicity

Idiosyncratic hepatotoxicity or drug-induced liver injury (DILI) occurs in only one out of about 10,000 patients and is usually statistically impossible to discover during clinical trials. In spite of its name which means "rare event with undefined mechanism", some mechanisms have now been defined including mitochondrial toxicity and the formation of reactive metabolites. Another mechanism of human toxicity that is not limited to the liver, but may also affect lung, spleen, and heart tissues is phospholipidosis.

5.2.1 Mitochondrial toxicity

Mitochondrial toxicity is increasing implicated in drug-induced idiosyncratic toxicity. Many of the drugs that have been withdrawn from the market due to organ toxicity have been found to be mitochondrial toxicants (32). Mitochondrial toxicants injure mitochondria by inhibiting respiratory complexes of the electron chain, inhibiting or uncoupling oxidative phosphorylation, inducing mitochondrial oxidative stress, or inhibiting DNA replication, transcription, or translation (33).

Toxicity testing of drug candidates is usually performed in immortalized cell lines that have been adapted for rapid growth in a reduced-oxygen atmosphere. Their metabolism is often anaerobic by glycolysis despite having functional mitochondria and an adequate oxygen supply. Alternatively, normal cells generate ATP for energy consumption aerobically by mitochondrial oxidative phosphorylation. The anaerobic metabolism of transformed cell lines is less sensitive to mitochondrial toxicants causing systematically underreporting in toxicity testing (33, 34). To address this issue, HepG2 and NIH/3T3 cells can be grown in media in which glucose is replaced by galactose (32). The change in sugar results in the metabolism of the cell to possess a respiratory substrate that is both more similar to normal cells and sensitive to mitochondrial toxicants without reducing sensitivity to non-mitochondrial toxicants (Figure 3).

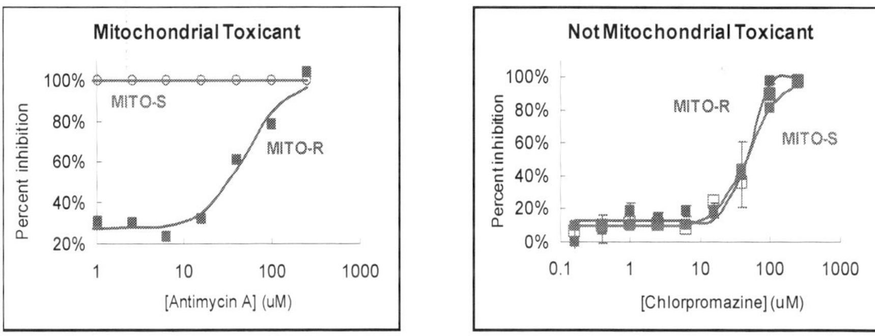

A. Actinomycin A **B. Imipramine**

Fig. 3. Effect of Antimycin A, a compound known to be toxic to mitochondria (A) and Imipramine (B) on parent HepG2 cells (Mito-R - blue) and a HepG2 cell line that has been developed to become sensitive to mitochondrial toxicants (Mito-S - red).

5.2.2 Reactive metabolites formation

Another property of compounds that can cause idiosyncratic toxicity is their ability to form reactive intermediates (35). Formation of short-lived reactive metabolites is known to be the mechanism of toxicity of some compounds such as acetaminophen (36). The formation of reactive metabolites can be identified by incubating test compounds with liver microsomes and adding glutathione to trap the reactive intermediates which are then identified by LC/MS/MS (Figure 4). Conversion of more than 10% of the test agent to reactive intermediates indicates that the compound may be implicated in idiosyncratic toxicity.

5.2.3 Phospholipidosis

Phospholipidosis is a lysosomal storage disorder and can be caused by drugs that are cationic amphiphiles (37). The disorder is considered to be mild and often can self-resolve. However, drugs that cause phospholipidosis can also produce organ damage, and thus this disorder is a concern to the regulatory agencies (37). A cell-based assay for phospholipidosis has been developed (38) which involves accumulation of a fluorescent phospholipid resulting in an increase of fluorescence in the lysosomes of cells that have been treated with drugs that cause phospholipidosis (Figure 5). If phospholipidosis is absent, the phospholipid is degraded and fluorescence does not increase. Increases in fluorescence are normalized to cell numbers since many of these drugs are also cytotoxic (Figure 5).

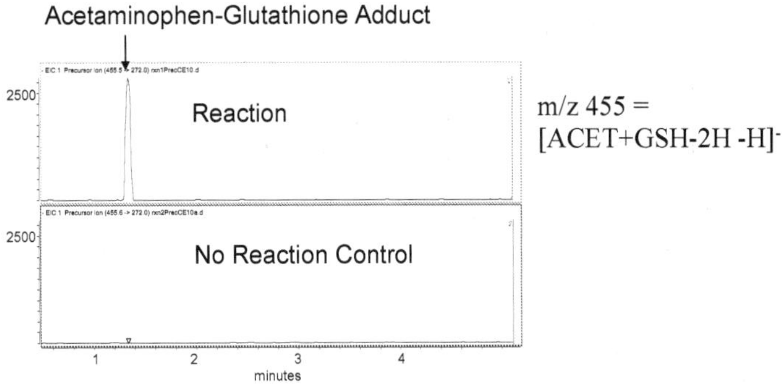

Fig. 4. Formation of Reactive Metabolites of Acetaminophen. Acetaminophen was incubated with microsomes and glutathione in the presence and absence of NADPH. An adduct of glutathione with acetaminophen was formed in the presence of NADPH. When NADPH was absent (No Reaction Control), no adduct was formed.

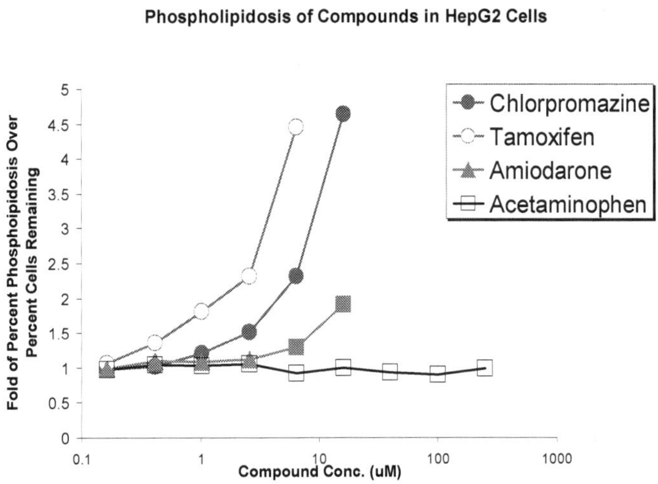

Fig. 5. Drug-induced phospholipidosis (PLD) is determined by measuring the accumulation of a fluorescent phospholipid in cells treated with increasing drug concentrations. Fluorescence is measured and normalized to cell number. Fluorescence is increased in cells treated with compounds that are known to cause PLD (chlorpromazine, tamoxifen, amiodarone), but it is not increased in cells treated with a compound that is known not to cause PLD (acetaminophen).

5.2.4 High-content toxicology: The present and future of predictive toxicology

Drug safety is a major concern for the pharmaceutical industry with greater than 30% of drug candidates failing in clinical trials as a result of toxicity (3, 10). Furthermore, there are numerous examples of drugs which have been withdrawn from the market or given black box warnings as a result of side effects not identified in clinical trials. Developing and commercializing a drug is a large financial commitment and failure at this stage can be catastrophic for a company. To address this problem, there has been a significant drive to incorporate toxicity assessment at much earlier stages in the drug discovery and development process.

It is well recognized that animal models are often not reflective of human toxicity. This is corroborated by a large percentage of drugs fail in the clinic through toxicity despite having progressed through costly preclinical animal studies. Human hepatotoxicity, as well as hypersensitivity and cutaneous reactions, are particularly difficult to identify during regulatory-based animal studies. Only 50% of drugs found to be hepatotoxic in clinical studies showed concordance with animal toxicity results (39, 40). In addition, there are profound ethical issues associated with the widespread use of animals for this purpose. Initiatives such as ECVAM, ICCVAM and NC3Rs are currently addressing this problem by identifying alternatives to animal safety testing. The cosmetics industry is at the forefront and starting in 2013 there is an anticipated total EU ban of the sale of cosmetics tested on animals.

The introduction of more relevant and sophisticated *in vitro* human systems is essential to overcome these issues and will enable higher throughput screening assays to be implemented earlier and more cost effectively. The widespread use of *in vitro* methods has to some extent been hampered by their relatively poor predictive capability as traditionally only single markers of toxicity have been investigated. However, in many cases, drug toxicity is a highly complex process which can manifest itself *via* multiple different mechanisms. Predictions of toxicity can only be improved by investigating a broad panel of markers and their relationship to each other.

6. The power of high content screening

Technologies such as high content screening (HCS) have transformed cell biology and enabled subtle changes in multiple cellular processes to be tracked within the same cell population and well. The technique uses either fluorescently labeled antibodies or dyes to stain specific areas of the cell which have critical roles in cell health or the maintenance of cellular function. The impact of concentration-dependent and time-dependent drug exposure on these cellular processes can be investigated and related to specific toxicological or efficacious responses. The ability to analyze multiple end points simultaneously, yet selectively, is a major advantage and as well as being more sensitive, allows greater predictivity and an improved mechanistic understanding over traditional single endpoint measurements (41).

The power of HCS in toxicity assessment was illustrated in two key papers authored by scientists at Pfizer (41, 42) where a panel of 6 to 8 key toxicity markers were identified and used to predict human hepatotoxicity. The articles highlight the improved predictive power of HCS over existing conventional *in vitro* toxicity assays and over traditional preclinical animal tests. HCS technology is now routinely used for *in vitro* toxicity assessment in large pharmaceutical companies.

7. CellCiphr™ – bridging the gap between *in vitro* and *in vivo*

It is critical to link the *in vitro* HCS information to animal or human pathology and establish a relationship to the *in vivo* data. The patterns observed in the key toxicity markers are often characteristic of specific mechanisms of known pathology.

The CellCiphr™ system utilizes the powerful technique of HCS and combines this with a novel classifier system which is underpinned by a large database of information for drugs with known toxicological profiles. Using this system the toxicological profiles generated by HCS can be compared with known drugs for which animal or clinical data are available. Specific changes in cellular function observed for particular mechanisms of toxicity can then be recognized and used to predict for unknown NCEs.

It is well recognized that toxicological events can be organ specific, time-dependent and concentration-dependent. The CellCiphr™ system investigates three different panels which represent general cytotoxicity (using HepG2 cells) or organ specific toxicity (using primary rat hepatocytes as a model for hepatotoxicity or H9c2 cardiomyocytes as a model for cardiotoxicity). The panels have been validated for the most relevant parameters for each particular cell type. Depending on the panel, these include the following cell health parameters: cell cycle arrest, nuclear size, oxidative stress, stress kinase activation, DNA damage response, DNA fragmentation, mitochondrial potential and mass, mitosis marker, cytoskeletal disruption, apoptosis, steatosis, phospholipidosis, ROS generation, hypertrophy and general cell loss. To assess early and late stage toxic responses, CellCiphr™ investigates exposure at 3 different time points. Dose dependent effects are investigated by exposing the cells to 10 different concentrations of the compound.

Data are represented as AC_{50} (concentration at which average response is 50% of control activity) for each cell health parameter, and the collection of AC_{50} values over the entire cell feature set comprises the response profile. Proprietary visual and quantitative data mining tools including CellCiphr™ Classifiers, correlation analysis and cluster analysis are used to analyze the profiles (Figure 6). Using the CellCiphr™ approach, there are a number of different ways by which the data can be interpreted.

1. Similarity profile plots can identify potential mechanisms of actions by correlating unknown test compound response with known control compounds where the mechanisms of action are already known.
2. The relative toxicity of compounds in a series can be predicted by the CellCiphr™ Classifier and used to rank compounds for prioritization of the most promising candidates.
3. The most potent or earliest cellular response can be extracted from the data which may highlight the optimal endpoint(s) for designing higher throughput systems to investigate SAR within a series.

Detailed mechanistic data can be generated for specific compounds. In the case of nimesulide which has been withdrawn from the market for severe hepatotoxicity, the CellCiphr™ Hepatotoxicity Profiling Panel scored this drug as the most toxic of the nonsteroidal anti-inflammatory drugs (NSAIDS). The toxicity was associated with a specific mechanistic profile characterized by an early oxidative stress response captured as a decreased mitochondrial membrane potential after 1 hour of exposure. This insult drives the development of an apoptotic response at subsequent times points measured in the release of cytochrome C from the mitochondria and activation of the DNA damage response. Finally, prolonged exposure to nimesulide is marked by the accumulation of lipids in lysosomes and other vesicles (Figure 7). The early effect on cell loss may also indicate a necrotic response in addition to apoptosis.

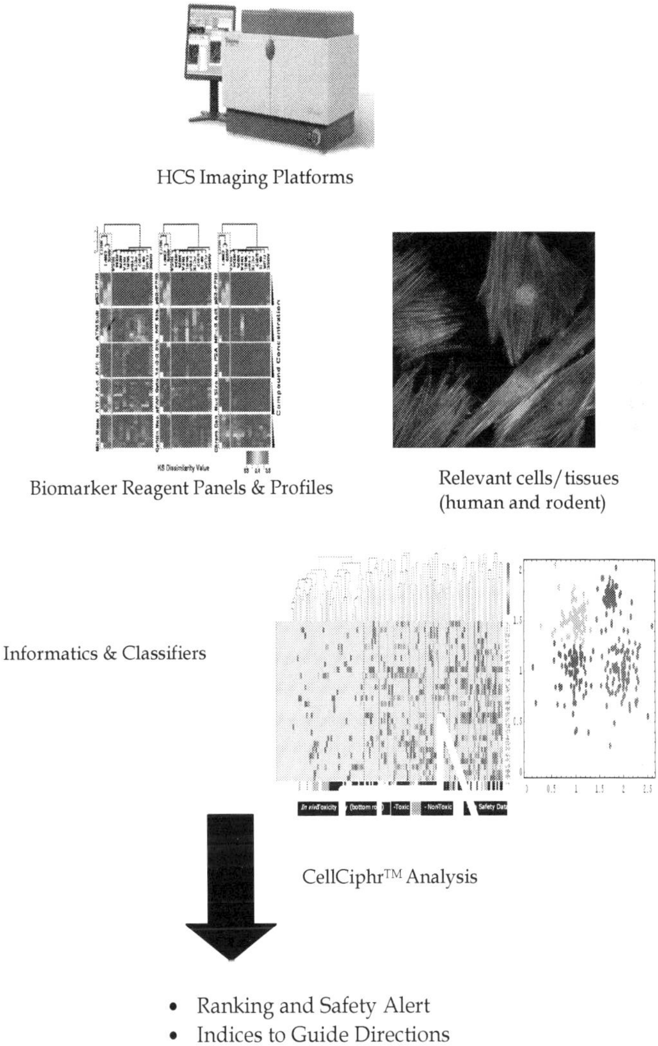

Fig. 6. The CellCiphr™ system uses HCS imaging platforms to identify specific patterns of biomarker response following exposure to multiple concentrations of compound at multiple time points. Proprietary visual and quantitative data mining tools have been developed to analyse the profiles and compare unknown compound response against known in vivo pathology.

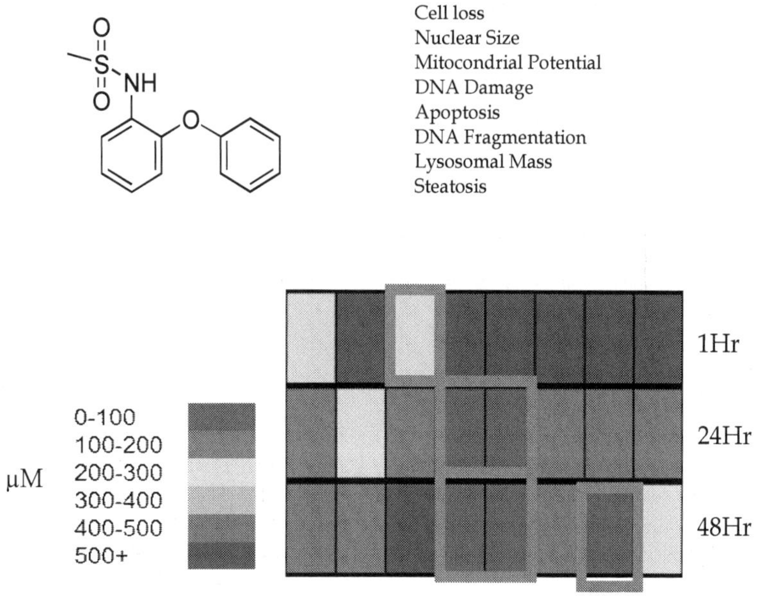

Fig. 7. Nimesulide, which has been withdrawn from the market in several countries over concerns of severe hepatotoxicity, was scored as the most toxic of the NSAIDS by the CellCiphrTM Hepatotoxicity Profiling Panel. The toxicity is associated with a specific mechanistic profile at sub-lethal doses.

7.1 Future strategies

In summary, CellCiphrTM is shown here as an example of a novel approach which identifies time dependent, sub-lethal effects on cell health and function. The system illustrates significant improvements over existing single end point assays and has the ability to predict mechanistic outcomes by correlating with known compound profiles and pathology. By expanding the CellCiphrTM database, improving bioinformatics platform and increasing the number of panels to cover new organ specific cells, it will continue to improve the reliability of the classification.
Toxicological response is influenced by many factors including dose administration (including tissue exposure levels), time of exposure and/or accumulation in specific cells. Many of these factors are influenced by the pharmacokinetics of the drug administered and its effect on absorption, distribution, metabolism and excretion. Considering ADME data in conjunction with multiparametric measurements of *in vitro* toxicology is likely to be an important consideration in the future direction of predictive toxicology. Incorporation of human PK parameters prediction in models such as CellCiphr to ensure that cytotoxicity is relevant to projected tissue exposure is actively being pursued.

8. Genotoxicity

Genotoxicity of drugs is an important concern to the regulatory authorities. The FDA recommends a number of *in vitro* and *in vivo* tests to measure the mutagenic potential of chemical compounds, including the Ames test in *Salmonella typhimurium* (43). GreenScreen GC, a new, high-throughput assay that links the regulation of the human GADD45a gene to the production of Green Fluorescent Protein (GFP) has become available. The assay relies on the DNA damage-induced up-regulation of the RAD54 gene in yeast measured using a promoter-GFP fusion reporter (44). The test is more specific and sensitive for genotoxicity than those currently recommended by the FDA such as the Ames and mouse lymphoma tests.

9. Current challenges and future directions

A large amount of progress in the field of ADMET profiling has occurred in the last 15 years. This progress has decreased the proportion of drug candidates failing in clinical trials for ADME reasons providing optimism in an otherwise declining productivity in drug discovery. The principal barrier now is the toxicity portion of ADMET. The prediction of human-specific toxicology must be improved.

Cell-based assays using established cell lines and co-cultures have been used to determine toxicity to various organs, but many of these cell lines have lost some of the physiological activities present in normal cells. HepG2 cells, for instance, have greatly reduced levels of metabolic enzymes. Primary human hepatocytes can be used but are expensive, suffer from high donor-to-donor variability, and maintain their characteristics for only a short time. Three-dimensional models have been developed for cell-based therapies including micropatterned co-cultures of human liver cells that maintain the phenotypic functions of the human liver for several weeks (45). This development should provide more accurate information about toxicity when used in ADMET screening and could be extended to other organ-specific cells leading to integrated tissue models in the "human on a chip" (46). The potential of stem cells to differentiate into cell lines of many different lineages may be exploited to develop human and animal stem-cell-derived systems for major organ systems (47).

High content screening (HCS) has been used for early cytotoxicity measurement since 2006 and provides great optimism (41). This method has been optimized for hepatocytes and is more predictive of hepatotoxicity than other currently available methods and in the future could be applied to cells of other organs.

Molecular profiling is another alternative and is defined as any combination or individual application of mRNA expression, proteomic, toxicogenomic, or metabolomic measurements that characterize the state of a tissue (48). This approach has been applied in an attempt to develop profiles or signatures of certain toxicities. Molecular profiles, in conjunction with agents that specifically perturb cellular systems, have been used to identify patterns of changes in gene expression and other parameters at sub-toxic drug concentrations that might be predictive of hepatotoxicity including idiosyncratic hepatotoxicity (49). In the future, larger data sets, high-throughput gene disruptions, and more-diverse profiling data will lead to more-detailed knowledge of disease pathways and will facilitate in target selection and the construction of detailed models of cellular systems for use in ADMET screening to identify toxic compounds early in the discovery process. The combination of *in silico, in vitro,* and *in vivo* methods and models into multiple content data bases, data mining, and predictive modeling algorithms, visualization tools, and high-throughput data-analysis solutions can be integrated to predict systems' ADMET properties. Such models are starting to be built and should be widely available within 10 years (50). The use of these tools will lead to a greater understanding of the interactions of drugs with their targets and predict their toxicities.

To conclude, the future should provide a decrease in late-stage development failures and withdrawals of marketed drugs, faster timelines from discovery to market, and reduced development costs through the reduction of late-stage failures.

10. References

[1] Kaitin KI. (2008). Obstacles and opportunities in new drug development. *Clinical Pharmacology & Therapeutics* 83, 210-212.

[2] DiMasi, J.A., Hansen, R.W.& Grabowski, H.G. (2003). The price of innovation: new estimates of drug development costs. *Journal of Health Economics* 22, 151–185.

[3] Kola, I. & Landis, J. (2004). Can the pharmaceutical industry reduce attrition rates? *Nature Reviews Drug Discovery* 3,711-715.

[4] Honig, P.K., Woosley, R.L., Zamani, K., Conner, D.P. & Cantilena, L.R., Jr. (1992). Changes in the pharmacokinetics and electrocardiographic pharmacodynamics of terfenadine with concomitant administration of erythromycin. *Clinical Pharmacology & Therapeutics* 52, 231-238.

[5] Honig, P.K., Wortham, D.C., Zamani, K., Conner, D.P., Mullin, J.C. & Cantilena, L.R. (1993). Terfenadine-ketoconazole interaction. Pharmacokinetic and electrocardiographic consequences. *Journal of the American Medical Association* 269, 1513-1518.

[6] US Food and Drug Administration. (1998). Seldane and generic terfenadine withdrawn from market. FDA Talk Paper T98-10. Available at http://www.fda.gov/bbs/topics/answers/ans00853.html.

[7] Ball, P., Mandell, L., Niki, Y. & Tillotson, G. (1999). Comparative tolerability of the newer fluoroquinolone antibacterials. *Drug Safety* 21, 407-421.

[8] US Food and Drug Administration. Public Health Advisory. Trovan (trovafloxacin/alatroflocacin mesylate). June 9, 1999. Available at http://www.fda.gov/cder/news/trovan.

[9] Stephens, J. (May 7, 2006). "Panel Faults Pfizer in '96 Clinical Trial In Nigeria". *The Washington Post*: p. A01. *Available* at http://www.washingtonpost.com/wp-dyn/content/article/2006/05/06/AR2006050601338.html.

[10] Kubinyi, H. (2003). Drug research: myths, hype and reality. *Nature Reviews Drug Discovery* 2, 665-668.

[11] Schuster, D., Laggner, C. & Langer, T. (2005). Why drugs fail - a study on side effects in new chemical entities. *Current Pharmaceutical Design* 11, 3545-3559.

[12] Lipinski, C.A., Lombardo F., Dominy, B.W. & Feeney, P.J. (1997). Experimental and computational approaches to estimate solubility and permeability in drug discovery and development settings. *Advanced Drug Delivery Reviews* 23, 3–25.

[13] Lipinski, C.A. (2000). Drug-like properties and the causes of poor solubility and poor permeability. *Journal of Pharmacological and Toxicological Methods* 44, 235-249.

[14] Schinkel, A.H., Smit, J.J., van Tellingen, O., Beijnen J.H., Wagenaar, E., van Deemter, L., Mol, C.A., van der Valk, M.A., Robanus-Maandag, E.C., te Riele H.P., Berns, A.J.M., & Borst, P. (1994). Disruption of the mouse mdr1a P-glycoprotein gene leads to a deficiency in the blood-brain barrier and to increased sensitivity to drugs. *Cell* 77(4), 491-502.

[15] Schinkel, R.S. & Minn, A. (1999). Drug metabolizing enzymes in cerebrovascular endothelial cells afford a metabolic protection to the brain. *Cell Mol Biol* 45, 15-23.

[16] Hurko, O. & Ryan, J.L. (2005). Translational research in central nervous system drug discovery. *NeuroRx* 2(4), 671-82.

[17] Liu, X. & Chen, C. (2005). Strategies to optimize brain penetration in drug discovery. *Curr Opin Drug Discov Devel* 8(4), 505-12.

[18] Megard, I., Garrigues, A., Orlowski, S., Jorajuria, S., Clayette, P., Ezan, E., Mabondzo, A. (2002). A co-culture-based model of human blood-brain barrier: application to active transport of indinavir and in vivo-in vitro correlation. *Brain Res* 927(2), 153-67.

[19] Begley, D.J., Lechardeur, D., Chen, Z.D., Rollinson, C., Bardoul, M., Roux, F., Scherman, D., Abbott, N.J. (1996). Functional expression of P-glycoprotein in an immortalised cell line of rat brain endothelial cells, RBE4. *J Neurochem* 67, 988-95.

[20] Deli, M.A., Abraham, C.S., Kataoka, Y., Niwa, M. (2005). Permeability studies on *in vitro* blood-brain barrier models: physiology, pathology and pharmacology. *Cell Mol Neurobiol* 25, 59-120.

[21] Crone, C. (1963). The Permeability of Capillaries in Various Organs as Determined by Use of the 'Indicator Diffusion' Method. *Acta Physiol Scand* 58, 292-305.

[22] Oldendorf, W. H. (1970). Measurement of brain uptake of radiolabeled substances using a tritiated water internal standard. *Brain Res* 24(2), 372-6.

[23] Takasato, Y., Rapoport, S.I. & Smith, Q.R. (1984). An in situ brain perfusion technique to study cerebrovascular transport in the rat. *Am J Physiol* 247(3 Pt 2), H484-93.

[24] Kakee, A., Terasaki, T., Sugiyama, Y. (1996). Brain efflux index as a novel method of analyzing efflux transport at the blood-brain barrier. *J Pharmacol Exp Ther* 277(3), 1550-9.

[25] Elmquist, W.F. & Sawchuk, R.J. (1997). Application of microdialysis in pharmacokinetic studies. *Pharm Res* 14(3), 267-88.

[26] Olson, H., Betton, G., Robinson, D., Thomas, K., Monro, A., Kolaja, G., Lilly, P., Sanders, J., Sipes, G., Bracken, W., Dorato, M., Van Deun, K., Smith, Berger P.B., & Heller, A. (2000). Concordance of the toxicity of pharmaceuticals in humans and in animals. *Regulatory Toxicology and Pharmacology* 32, 56–67.

[27] US Food and Drug Administration Website. Guidance for Industry, Drug Interaction Studies – Study Design, Data Analysis, and Implications for Dosing and Labeling September, 2006 Available at:
http://www.fda.gov/CDER/guidance/6695dft.

[28] Uetrecht, J. (2008). Idiosyncratic drug reactions: past, present, and future. *Chemical Research in Toxicology* 21, 84-92.

[29] Josserand, V., Pélerin, H., de Bruin, B., Jego, B., Kuhnast, B., Hinnen, F., Ducongé, F., Boisgard, R., Beuvon, F., Chassoux, F., Daumas-Duport, C., Ezan, E., Dollé, F., Mabondzo, A., Tavitian, B. (2006). Evaluation of drug penetration into the brain: a double study by in vivo imaging with positron emission tomography and using an in vitro model of the human blood-brain barrier. *J Pharmacol Exp Ther* Jan 316(1), 79-86.

[30] Pardridge, W.M., Triguero, D., Yang, J. & Cancilla, P.A. (1990). Comparison of in vitro and in vivo models of drug transcytosis through the blood-brain barrier. *J Pharmacol Exp Ther* 253(2), 884-91.

[31] Jacewicz, M., Guyot, A.-C., Annand, R., Gilbert, J., Mabondzo, A., Tsaioun, K. Contribution of Transporters to Permeability Across Cell Monolayers. Comparison of Three Models. Apredica, CEA. American Association of Pharmaceutical Scientists, poster presentation, Atlanta, GA, November 2008

[32] Dykens, J.A. & Will, Y. (2007). The significance of mitochondrial testing in drug development. *Drug Discovery Today* 12,777-785.

[33] Rodríguez-Enríquez, S., Juárez, O., Rodríguez-Zavala, J.S., & Moreno-Sánchez, R. (2001). Multisite control of the Crabtree effect in ascites hepatoma cells. *European Journal of Biochemistry* 268, 2512–2519.

[34] Marroquin, L.D., Hynes, J., Dykens, J.A., Jamieson, J.D. & Will, Y. (2007). Circumventing the Crabtree effect: Replacing media glucose with galactose

increases susceptibility of HepG2 cells to mitochondrial toxicants. *Toxicological Sciences* 97, 539-547.

[35] Williams, D.P. & Park, B.K. (2003) Idiosyncratic toxicity: the role of toxicophores and bioactivation. *Drug Discovery Today* 8, 1044-1050.

[36] Liu Z.X. & Kaplowitz, N. (2006). Role of innate immunity in acetaminophen-induced hepatotoxicity. *Expert Opinion on Drug Metabolism & Toxicology* 2, 493-503.

[37] Ademuyiwa, O., Agarwal. R., Chandra, R., and Behari, J.R. (2009). Lead-induced phospholipidosis and cholesterogenesis in rat tissues. *Chemical & Biological Interactions* 179, 314-320.

[38] Natalie, M., Margino, S., Erik, H., Annelieke, P., Geert, V. & Philippe, V. (2009). A 96-well flow cytometric screening assay for detecting in vitro phospholipidosis-induction in the drug discovery phase. *Toxicology In Vitro* 23, 217-226.

[39] Olson, H., Betton, G., Stritar, J. & Robinson, D. (1998). The predictivity of the toxicity of pharmaceuticals in humans from animal data - an interim assessment. *Toxicol Lett* 102–103, 535–538.

[40] Olson, H., Betton, G., Robinson, D., Thomas, K., Monro, A., Kolaja, G., Lilly, P., Sanders, J., Sipes, G., Bracken, W., Doratoi, M., Van Deun, K., Smith, P., Berger, B. & Heller, A. (2000) Concordance of Toxicity of Pharmaceuticals in Humans and Animals. *Regul Toxicol Pharmacol* 32, 56–67.

[41] O'Brien, P.J., Irwin, W., Diaz, D., Howard-Cofield, E., Krejsa, C.M., Slaughter, M.R., Gao, B., Kaludercic, N., Angeline, A., Bernardi, P., Brain, P. & Hougham, C. (2006). High concordance of drug-induced human hepatotoxicity with in vitro cytotoxicity measured in a novel cell-based model using high content screening. *Arch Toxicol* 80, 580-604.

[42] Xu, J.J., Henstock, P.V., Dunn, M.C., Smith, A.R., Chabot, J.R. & de Graaf, D. (2008). Cellular Imaging Predictions of Clinical Drug-Induced Liver Injury. *Toxicol Sci 105(1),* 97-105.

[43] US Food and Drug Administration Guidance for Industry. S2B Genotoxicity: A Standard Battery for Genotoxicity Testing of Pharmaceuticals. Available at: http://www.fda.gov/CDER/guidance/1856fnl.

[44] Hastwell, P.W., Chai, L.-L., Roberts, K.J., Webster T.W., Harvey J.S., Rees R.W., & Walmsley, R.M. (2006). High-specificity and high-sensitivity genotoxicity assessment in a human cell line: Validation of the GreenScreen HC GADD45a-GFP genotoxicity assay. *Mutation Research* 607, 160–175.

[45] Khetani, S.R. & Bhatia, S.N. (2008). Microscale culture of human liver cells for drug development. *Nature Biotechnology* 26, 120-126.

[46] Viravaidya, K. & Shuler, M.L. *(2004).* Incorporation of 3T3-L1 cells to mimic bioaccumulation in a microscale cell culture analog device for toxicity studies. *Biotechnology Progress* 20, 590-597.

[47] Yang, L., Soonpaa, M.H., Adler, E.D., Roepke, T.K., Kattman, S.J., Kennedy, M., Henckaerts, E., Bonham, K., Abbott, G.W., Linden, R.M., Field, L.J. & Keller, G.M. (2008). Human cardiovascular progenitor cells develop from a KDR^{+} embryonic-stem-cell-derived population. *Nature* 453, 524-529.

[48] Stoughton, R.B. & Friend, S.H. (2005). How molecular profiling could revolutionize drug discovery. *Nature Reviews Drug Discovery* 4,345-350.

[49] Kaplowitz, N. (2005). Idiosyncratic drug hepatotoxicity. *Nature Reviews Drug Discovery* 4, 489-499.

[50] Ekins, S., Nikolsky, Y. & Nikolskaya, T. (2005). Techniques: application of systems biology to absorption, distribution, metabolism, excretion and toxicity. *Trends in Pharmacological Sciences* 26, 202-209.

12

Novel Approach to High Throughput Screening for Activators of Transcription Factors

Natalya Smirnova[1], Dmitry Hushpulian[2], Rajiv Ratan[1] and Irina Gazaryan[1]
[1]*Burke Medical Research Institute, Department of Neurology and Neuroscience, Weill Medical College of Cornell University, NY*
[2]*Department of Chemical Enzymology, M. V. Lomonosov Moscow State University, Moscow*
[1]*USA*
[2]*Russia*

1. Introduction

There is growing body of evidence that many diseases require a systemic treatment approach rather than targeting just a single enzyme or receptor. Neurodegenerative diseases affect a wide spectrum of the population and, in most cases, lead to physical and/or mental incapacity, involving memory, cognition, language and personality. Aging contributes to the development of neurodegeneration by shifting the equilibrium between oxygen-dependent and independent mechanisms of energy production towards mitochondria-generated ATP. Mitochondrial capacity degenerates with aging, making cells susceptible to both ischemic and oxidative insults. Although all mechanisms of hypoxic preconditioning are very far from complete understanding, it is clear that cell is equipped with the necessary molecular machinery to respond to the changes in intracellular oxygen content. However, aging significantly compromises this response. Turning on the existent molecular machinery to compensate for hypoxic and oxidative stress may lead to comprehensive and safe therapeutic strategy for age-related neurodegenerative disorders.

To restore homeostatic balance destroyed as a result of acute or chronic injury, one needs to activate intrinsic genetic programs silent or insufficiently active in the damaged cells. Activation of cellular defensive systems requires stabilization of corresponding transcription factors which govern expression of cassettes of genes turning on a particular program such as antioxidant, anti-inflammatory, or anti-hypoxic one. Hence, one of the emerging strategies in drug screening becomes a hunt for activators (or inhibitors) of transcription factors. In some cases there is an enzyme responsible for a rate-limiting conversion of a transcription factor, in some not. The well-known and commonly used approach to screening of activators of transcription factors is the use of luciferase gene cloned under the promoter activated by a specified transcription factor. For example, cell-based screening for activators of hypoxia induced factor 1 (HIF1) is performed using HRE (hypoxia response element)-luciferase (Semenza et al 1996), and for Nrf2 - using ARE (antioxidant response element)-luciferase reporter assay (Moehlenkamp & Johnson 1999). Promega has just begun to offer commercially such type of constructs with any desired promoter for research and drug screening purposes.

Although these reporters are obviously of great help in research, they provide an integrated response and are affected by many steps such as transcription factor stabilization, phosphorylation, translocation to nucleus, interaction with transcription cofactors, etc. As a result, the response of these reporters is not immediate: it is delayed by many hours, the magnitude of activation effect is very modest, and there is always uncertainty in the actual site of their effect along the path leading to activation of a particular promoter.

The important general pathway effectively regulating the cellular response to hypoxia, oxidation and inflammation is specific regulation of protein stability of the corresponding transcription factors or their modulators by ubiquitination and proteasomal degradation. Protein degradation by the proteasome is one of the major regulatory mechanisms in the cell. The proteasome mediates the degradation of most short-lived proteins that control cell cycle, transcription, DNA repair, apoptosis and other cellular processes. Under normal conditions, the stress response transcription factors are expressed constitutively, but on the protein level, these transcriptional factors are unstable: they undergo ubiquitination either directly, or upon specific covalent modification(s) of the targeted amino acids residues (like hypoxia inducible factor, HIF). Considering the protein stability of transcription factors as the most important and limiting step in the stress response we have recently developed a different approach to high throughput screening (HTS) of stabilizers of transcription factors. The approach is based on stable expression of a fusion between luciferase and a transcription factor minimum domain recognized by ubiquitination machinery (Fig.1).

Minimum domain is the portion of a transciption factor that is necessary and sufficient for recognition and ubiquitination steps to occur. The overexpressed luciferase-labeled surrogate of a transcription factor undergoes the same recognition and transformation steps as an endogenous one. The time-course of reporter signal changes can be easily followed: the luminescent readings are extremely sensitive and provide monitoring just minutes after drug administration.

This new approach to HTS was developed in this laboratory and successfully used to discover novel activators of HIF1 and Nrf2 as exemplified below.

2. Development, validation and application of novel reporters for the purposes of HTS

2.1 Neh2-luciferase reporter construction and performance (Smirnova et al 2011)

The key transcription factor that orchestrates antioxidant response is Nrf2 (Moi et al 1994, Motoyashi & Yamamoto 2004, Kaspar et al 2009). Compounds that activate Nrf2 make the cell more resistant to subsequent xenobiotic attack or oxidative stress. This has major implications for human health: (1) Nrf2 activators can be considered as medications for cancer prevention; (2) while an increased level of Nrf2 makes cancerous cells more resistant to chemotherapy; and (3) Nrf2 activators can both prevent and treat neurodegenerative diseases. There is a consensus that oxidative stress either derived from gene mutations or environmental toxins is a mediator of neurodegenerative diseases and thus, Nrf2 has been justified as a pharmacological target for neuroprotective therapies in Parkinson's, Huntington's and other neurodegenerative diseases.

2.1.1 Nrf2 - Keap1 interaction mode

Nrf2 is composed of Nehl-Neh6 domains, among which Neh2 (1-98 aa) is the putative negative regulatory domain that interacts with Keapl, while Neh4 and Neh5 are transactivation domains, and Neh1 is the binding domain for ARE. The functional domains of Keap1 are the Broad complex, Tramtrack and Bric-a-Brac, the intervening region, the double glycine repeats domain, and the C-terminal region (Zhang et al 2006). Two motifs in the Neh2 domain, i.e. ETGE and DLG (Tong et al 2006 a, 2006b), are recognized by the Keap1 homodimer in a hinge-latch mode (see Fig.2 and 3). Keap1 mediates polyubiquitination of the lysines positioned within the central α-helix of the Neh2 domain under homeostatic conditions. Under oxidative/electrophilic stress, most reactive cysteines within Keap1 (Cys 151, Cys273, Cys288) are modified and Keap1 undergoes conformational changes which lead to Nrf2 stabilization (see Fig.3) (Cullinan et al 2004).

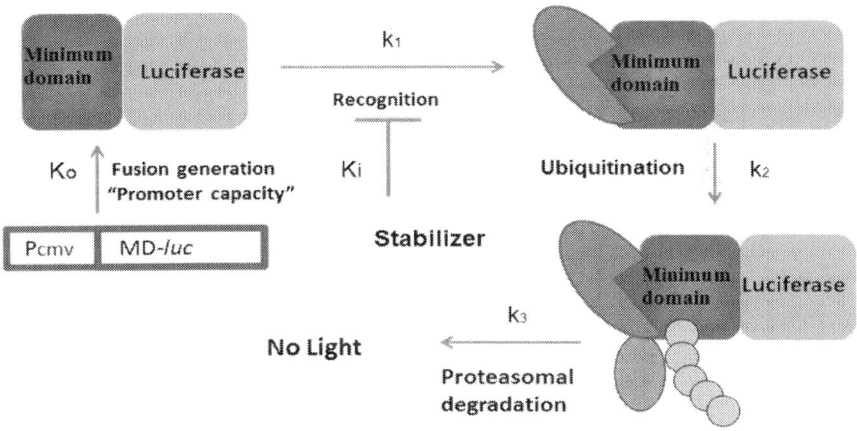

Fig. 1. Schematic presentation of reporter performance based on constitutive expression of luciferase-labeled minimum domain of a transcription factor. The background luminescent signal corresponds to the sum of all forms of labeled surrogate except for its proteolytic fragments: [MD-luc]= $Ko\Sigma(1/k_i)$. Specific stabilizers of a transcription factor must work at the recognition step: each reporter requires validation to demonstrate that this particular step is rate limiting, meaning that [MD-luc]= $Ko\Sigma(1/k_1)$. If this is the case, HTS will select for specific stabilizers of a transcription factor working at the recognition step.

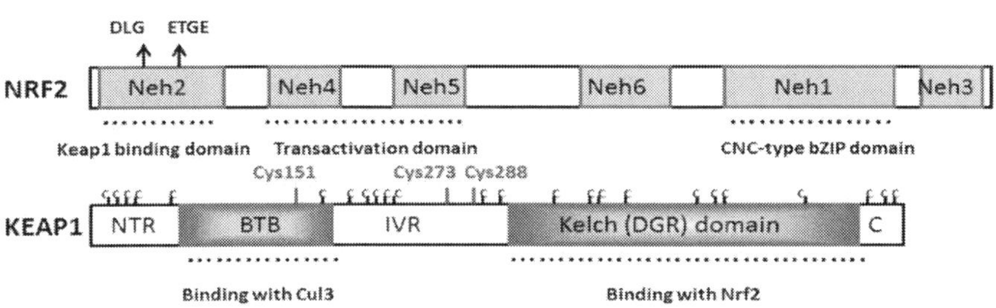

Fig. 2. Schematic presentation of domain structures of Keap 1 and Nrf2.

Nrf2 translocates to the nucleus, interact with Maf protein, and induces expression of the cytoprotective enzymes such as glutathione reductase, thioredoxin reductase, glutathione S-transferase (GST), hemeoxygenase-1 (HO1), catalase, etc. Alkylating agents are supposed to target Cys151 to detach Cul3 ubiquitin-ligase and inhibit ubiquitination (Zhang et al 2004). Keap1 thiols Cys273 and Cys 288 are supposedly responsible for dimer conformation capable of binding Nrf2: changes in Keap1 conformation disrupt dimeric structure and also result in inhibition of ubiquitination. The yet unknown specific stabilizers of Nrf2 should disrupt interaction between DLG domain of Nrf2 and Keap1 and thus prevent ubiquitination of Neh2 lysines and result in Nrf2 stabilization.

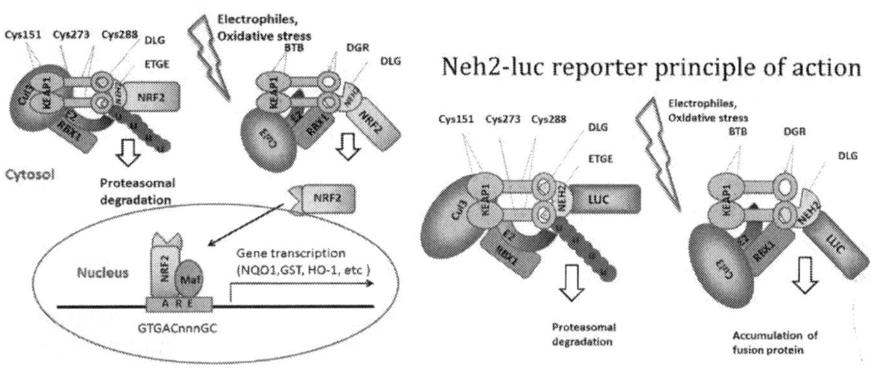

Fig. 3. Schematic presentation of Nrf2 stabilization and transcription activation (left) versus the performance of Neh2-luc reporter (right). Keap1-bound Nrf2 is subject to ubiquitination, and then underegoes proteasomal degradation. Upon oxidative stress, Keap1 thiols are either alkylated (Cys 151) resulting in detachment of Cul3 ubiquitin ligase or modified (Cys273 and Cys288) leading to a conformation change in Keap1 dimer and release of Nrf2 from the complex. In both cases Nrf2 protein is stabilized, and the same mechanism of stabilization applies to the Neh2-luc reporter performance. Luciferase labeling of Neh2 permits easy monitoring of fusion accumulation upon oxidative stress induced by small molecule activators.

2.1.2 Neh2-luciferase reporter validation

The P_{cmv}-driven Neh2-luc reporter supports the constitutive, intracellular synthesis of a novel fusion protein composed of the Neh2 domain and firefly luciferase in human neuroblastoma cell line SH-SY5Y. **Validation studies** (see Smirnova et al 2011) included: (1) Testing of canonical activators of Nrf2, such as 15-deoxy-prostaglandin J2 (15d-PGJ2), sulforaphane and tert-butylhydroquinone (TBHQ), which were shown to produce a significant increase (> 20-fold) in the background luciferase signal within 3-4 h following the treatment of SH-SY5Y human neuroblastoma cells stably expressing the Neh2 reporter; (2) Forced expression of Keap1 in the Neh2- luc reporter cell line led to a 3.5-fold decrease in the background luminescence; (3) Keap1 reduction by siRNA resulted in a steady state increase in Neh2-luc reporter luminescence and an induction of transcription of Nrf2-regulated genes; (4) Immunoblot with antibodies against luciferase confirmed that an increase in luminescence corresponds to the accumulation of the fusion protein upon incubation with commonly used Nrf2 activators. Validation studies demonstrated that Keap1 regulates the stability of the Neh2-reporter in the same manner as for endogenous Nrf2 and that the rate-limiting step in Neh2-luc cell line is controlled by the disruption of the Neh2-Keap1 complex which results in inhibition of ubiquitinylation. The Neh2-luc reporter system is a novel tool to monitor the direct effect of a particular compound on the first step controlling Nrf2 stability, i.e. Nrf2-Keap1 and/or Keap1-Cul3 interaction.

2.1.3 Neh2-luciferase reporter sensitivity

All manual screenings were performed using 96-well plates with 100 µL serum per well dispensed with WellMate multichannel dispenser from Matrix (Thermo Fisher Scientific). Drugs were added after overnight culture incubation, 3hr later serum removed, lysis buffer added, and luminescence measured with either BrightGlo reagent (Promega) or common luciferase reagent made by ourselves. The background luminescence signal calibrated with recombinant luciferase allows us to estimate the steady-state concentration of the Neh2-luciferase fusion protein: the backround is ca. 15-20 rlu, which corresponds to 0.25-0.33 pg luciferase protein and is more than two orders of magnitude lower than that observed for the cell line expressing wild-type luciferase under control of the same promoter. The low steady state luciferase activity (recalculated as 0.6-0.8 nM fusion protein for 30,000 cell/well density and 233 μ^3 single cell volume) suggests that in spite of the forced expression of the Neh2-luciferase fusion protein, it is successfully recognized by the endogenous Keap1-Cul3 complex and almost fully degraded. The reporter exemplifies the action of an "ideal Nrf2 activator" which stabilizes endogenous Nrf2 by competing for Keap1 binding and not by modifying Keap1 chemically. The new reporter is advantageous over the ARE-luc reporter or especially ARE-GFP reporter (Shaw et al 2010) and other methods such as immunoblotting of Nrf2 (or luciferase in our case) or RT-PCR of Nrf2-induced genes because all other methods are at least 5-6 hr delayed as compared to immediate response of the newly constructed reporter. Moreover, ARE-luc reporter background signal is at the single rlu digits and activation for TBHQ is only 3-fold compare to 16-20 fold activation in the case of Neh2-luc reporter (see Smirnova et al 2011).

There are no examples of the literature on the application of the same approach to screening purposes, except for the recently publsihed paper on the reporter construct expressing a fusion between three domains of Nrf2 and beta-galactosidase (Hirotsu et al 2011). The authors validated the construct and showed the advantages of the reporter over the commonly used ARE-luciferase. Nrf2d-LacZ protein consists of Nrf2 N-terminal region (containing Neh2, Neh4, and Neh5) and SV40 nuclear localization signals (NLS)-β-galactosidase, it is specific to Nrf2 activators. However, the Nrf2d-LacZ reporter it is still less sensitive than the one developed in our laboratory. Nrf2d-LacZ reporter provides ca. 5-fold activation over the background signal upon addition of a classic Nrf2 activator, TBHQ, and requires at least 1 hr incubation to get the first time-point (see Fig 3C in Hirotsu et al 2011), compared to 20-fold activation for TBHQ (see above) and the possibility to minotor the reporter effect minutes after drug addition.

2.1.4 Neh2-luciferase reporter optimization for HTS format

For HTS purposes, the assay was optimized to 384-well format: SH-SY5Y-Neh2-luc cells were plated into 384 well, white, flat-bottom plates at 7000 cell/well in 30 µl serum and incubated overnight at 37°C, 5% CO_2. The next day compounds were added to two final concentrations of 10 μM and 20 μM, plates were incubated for 3 hr at 37°C, and luciferase activity was measured using SteadyGlo™ reagent (Promega). Each plate had two internal standards, TBHQ (100%) and DMSO (0%). This format provides Z values above 0.7. The reporter activation (%) was calculated as a ratio $(L-L_{DMSO})/(L_{TBHQ}-L_{DMSO})$. Hits were defined as those greater than 25%. The pilot screen of Spectrum library revealed 224 hits exhibiting Neh2-luc reporter activity equal or higher than 25% of TBHQ; among those, 100 showed activation of at least 75% of that induced by TBHQ. Thus, 5% of biologically active compounds and drugs presented in the Spectrum library are at least 75% as potent as TBHQ in activation of Nrf2. The prevalence of hits does not indicate the low specificity of the reporter, it simply reflects the important role that Nrf2 plays in xenobiotic detoxification of a large number of chemical entities. Ideally, any compound disturbing cellular redox balance should be a hit in Neh2-luc screen.

HTS of Spectrum library of 2,000 biologically active and FDA-approved compounds was performed using a control cell line expressing plain luciferase under the same promoter to evaluate the effect of compounds on luciferase activity. None were found to inhibit/enhance the luciferase activity under the experimental conditions, while 46 compounds were found to be toxic at 3 hr incubation and were excluded from consideration. Cell death was monitored simultaneously with luciferase assays by plating cells, in parallel, in the transparent bottom plates and performing two independent assays of cell viability along with luciferase: MTT reduction and phase contrast observation. In all cases, MTT agreed with our morphological assay. The use of robotics for cell plating results in uniform concentration of cells along the plate, and we have found after validation no need to continue normalization to the cell protein. As one might expect, additional manipulations in the same well result in increasing the errors in following activity measurements as we established during the HTS optimization.

Further HTS screens are performed with two reporters in parallel, e.g. Neh2-luc and HIF1 ODD-luc (see 2.2), in this case each reporter serves as a control for the other. Hits that are equally active in both reporters are excluded from further consideration (could be either metal chelators, redox active compounds, or proteasomal inhibitors). Hits that do not overlap are subject to further studies. In the particular case of HTS for non-alkylating Nrf2 activators, hits are passed through the sructural filters to remove pro-oxidant, alkylating and other reactive motifs recently described by Baell & Holloway 2010.

2.1.5 Challenge to find specific Nrf2 stabilizers: Advantages of real-time monitoring

A major challenge in the development of effective Nrf2 activators is to identify those that lead specifically to Nrf2 stabilization and subsequent promoter activation, without imposing general oxidative/electrophilic stress. Such activators should exhibit higher affinity for Keap1 and work by competing with Nrf2 Neh-2 domain for Keap binding. The novel reporter for the first time provides the possibility of real time monitoring for changes in the stability of Nrf2 in the form of the luciferase labeled Neh2 domain. By following the kinetics of reporter activation one may expect to discriminate the mechanism of action of various Nrf2 activators, i.e. direct activators will exert immediate effects, while those acting indirectly will show lag-periods of different durations. Kinetics of reporter activation were measured by adding varied fixed concentrations of an inhibitor at different time points followed by simultaneous cell lysis and activity measurement in the whole 96-well plate;

this assay format minimizes experimental error originating from the well-known instability of a luciferase reagent.

There are 6 types of experimentally observed kinetics of reporter activation (Fig.4).

Type 1 is characteristic for alkylating agents such as sulforaphane, pyrithione, auranofin, etc. and shows an immediate linear increase in reporter signal in a concentration-dependent manner, and eventually reaches a threshold plateau (determined as a background signal magnitude in the control wild-type luciferase line).

Type 2 shows lag-periods that shorten with rising concentrations and eventually disappear pointing to a switch in the rate-limiting step to the one affected by the added compound: this time-course is typical for proteasomal inhibitors and is observed for both Neh2-luc and HIF ODD-luc reporters (see Fig.1 in Smirnova et al, 2011).

Type 3 shows a prolonged lag-period which duration shortens with rising concentrations to a some limit, but never disappears: such time-course indicates that the drug effects on a step with a limited contribution to the rate-limiting step. It has been seen only for cadmium among the activators studied: the duration of a lag-period was decrerased to 1 hr, and the subsequent increase in cadmium concentration had no effect.

Type 4 shows prolonged lag-period, which duration is concentration independent. This type is characteristic for drugs working either upstream of Nrf2 stabilization step (such as Hsp90 inhibitors showing 3 hr lag-period), or those drugs which must be initially oxidized to be able to modify Keap1 thiols (catechol with 20 min lag-period, or o-phenylene diamine with 40 min lag-period).

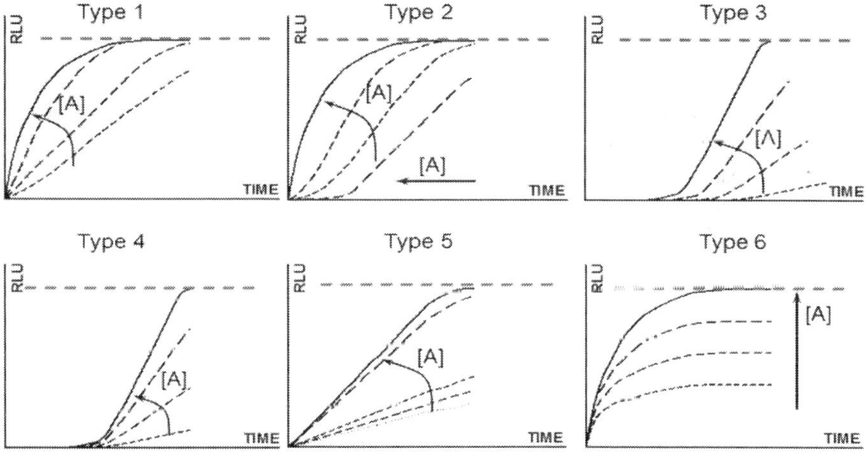

Fig. 4. Schematic representation of various types of reporter activation time-course (see text for explanation). Arrows indicate rising concentrations of Nrf2 activator, [A]; red thresholds show maximum reporter activation determined using a control cell line expressing wild-type luciferase under the same promoter.

Type 5 has been observed for two best hits in Spectrum library, nordihydroguaiaretic acid (NDGA) and fisetin, and shows an immediate switch-type response: there is negligible growth in signal up to a specific concentration (ca. 1.5-2 μM) which brings the system to the maximum rate of signal increase. At this point, we can speculate that Keap1 serves as a redox sensor, possibly via zinc atom bound to some of its thiols. There is evidence for zinc presence *in vitro* for recombinant Keap1, no data available on zinc binding to Keap1 *in vivo*. Future studies are necessary to clarify the target for these two compounds, which were confirmed to be extremely potent Nrf2 stabilizers (Smirnova et al 2011).

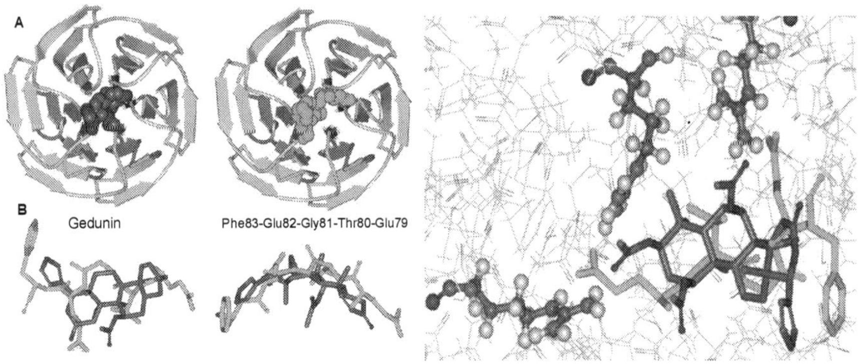

Fig. 5. Gedunin (Left: A & B) and 7-deacetoxy-7oxokhivorin (Right) docking into Keap1 in comparison with the corresponding portion of Neh2 16-mer peptide (green). **Docking experiments** are performed using the CDOCKER algorithm, followed by force field minimization and binding energy calculations using the molecular mechanics algorithm CHARMm (as implemented in Discovery Studio 2.5, Accelrys, San Diego, CA). The crystal structure of the human Keap1 kelch domain with the bound 16-mer peptide of human Neh2 (2FLU.pdb) with polar hydrogen atoms added was used as the starting template structure.

Type 6 is the one that is most promising in terms of specific Nrf2 stabilization: a time-course with a concentration dependent re-equilibration plateau is usually a characteristic of competitive binding. This type of kinetics has been observed for gedunin and some of its derivatives. Gedunin fits perfectly into the same Keap1 binding pocket as Nrf2 closely following the bending of the 83FEGTE79 portion of Nrf2 peptide (Fig. 5 left). Moreover, its oxykhivorin analog with Michael's motif removed and replaced with two acetoxy-groups fits just perfectly, and is a more powerful activator of the Neh2-reporter than gedunin itself (Fig.5 right).

We consider targeting the site of Neh2 binding in Keap1 as the most promising approach for the development of Nrf2 activators not imposing general oxidative stress. Another approach has been recently proposed by Wu et al (2010) who constructed a model of Keap1 including intervening region. Targeting this region one may expect to disturb Keap1 conformation in such a way that Nrf2 is released from the complex. This approach in general is less specific since Nrf2 is not the one client of Keap1.

The authors performed virtual screening using their model and identified a number of structures showing decent docking scores (Fig. 6). Experimental testing of the identified compounds showed that only B10, B31, and B40 are good inducers of Nrf2-dependent genes. The confirmed hits are redox-active molecules and their effect on Keap1-Nrf2 interaction may be not specific.

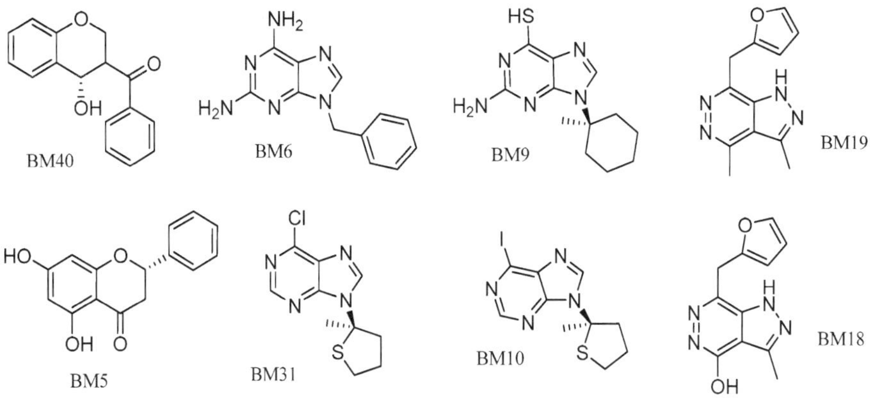

Fig. 6. Virtual hits targeting intervening region of Keap1 (Wu et al 2010).

2.1.6 Criteria for selection of compounds for hit-to-lead program

Depending on a particular goal, an algorithm for drug development efforts will involve a number of steps confirming the nature of the drug action mechanism. For example, if our goal is to develop Nrf2 specific activators that work specifically via disruption of Nrf2-Keap1 interaction by competitively displacing the Neh2-portion of Nrf2, and not by non-specific alkylation of Keap1 thiols, we must perform biological analysis to confirm this. The detailed structure-activity relationship studies (SAR) will employ (a) concentration titration experiments; (b) time-course of reporter activation; (c) *in silico* modeling; the hits obtained from screening the library will be used to help refine the *in silico* model; (d) Keap1 labeling experiments in the presence of selected hits to prove the non-alkylating nature of activation (see Smirnova et al 2011 Fig. S5A & B and protocol therein); (e) hits testing for the ability to upregulate Nrf2-dependent genes (RT-PCR); (f) evaluation of toxicity using primary culture neurons; (g) hits that upregulate Nrf2 may be analyzed by microarray for non-specific activation of Nrf2-independent pathways; (h) hits that are neuroprotective *in vitro* are tested for ADME (**A**bsorption, **D**istribution, **M**etabolism and **E**limination).

We have chosen two of our hits from Spectrum library - NDGA and gedunin for hit-to-lead program which is currently in progress. Both compounds are the key components of well known herbal medicines used for centuries by Native Amrecians (chapparal) and Indians (neem tree), respectively. For both compounds, ADME studies have been already done, and the compounds are neuroprotective in the *in vivo* model of MPTP-induced toxicity.

In vitro ADME studies have always played a critical role in optimizing the pharmacokinetics (PK) properties of lead compounds thereby increasing their success rate (Thompson 2000). The ideal PK properties for an oral drug are favorable bioavailability, clearance and metabolic stability to provide adequate systemic exposure to elicit a pharmacodynamic response with low potential for dose-dependent toxicities. These *in vivo* properties should be assessed as early as practical using *in vitro* ADME prediction tools (Balani et al 2005). In 1991, PK properties were attributed to more failure of drugs (40%) than efficacy or safety in clinical trials. With the application of advanced ADME techniques, the contribution of PK properties resulting in drug failure dropped dramatically to 10% in 2000 (Kola & Landis 2004). Recently, *in vitro* ADME and cytotoxicity screening assays have been incorporated with structure-activity relationship (SAR) studies in the earliest stages of drug discovery. The incorporation of early, high throughput ADME screening in parallel with efficacy screening has significantly reduced cycle time involved in moving compounds from "hit" to "lead" status.

2.2 Cell-based screening using HIF1 ODD-luc reporter system

Major advantage of cell-based screens is that we automatically exclude non-permeable and toxic compounds because they provide either no activation or even lower the background signal. In addition, there is no need to specifically formulate the composition of a reaction medium for an enzymatic reaction because the intracellular medium of cell lines is very close to that existing in the human body. Another advantage is that compared to *in vitro* enzymatic assay we rule out enzyme stability problem. The best example for this is the reaction catalyzed by HIF prolyl hydroxylase (HIF PHD). Below we present a detailed comparison of enzymatic screens versus cell-based screen for HIF1 activators working via inhibition of HIF PHD.

2.2.1 HIF and HIF prolyl hydroxylase: HTS assay development problems

Hypoxia-inducible factor (HIF) is a transcriptional factor that regulates gene expression in mammalian development, physiology and disease pathogenesis (Wang et al 1995). HIF consists of an oxygen-sensitive α-subunit and a continuously expressed β-subunit. HIF-1α is induced and stabilized in hypoxic conditions and functions as a master regulator of oxygen homeostasis. HIF-1α proteolysis is mediated via hydroxylation of two highly conserved Pro residues, which causes its direct interaction with von Hippel-Lindau protein (VHL). HIF-1α hydroxylation is catalyzed by human prolyl-4-hydroxylases (PHDs). Pro564 is located in the so called oxygen degradable domain (ODD) and is considered as the major site for hydroxylation catalyzed by all PHD isoforms. For HIF PDHs, the general reaction mechanism (Solomon et al 2000) includes activation of molecular oxygen to convert α-ketoglutarate into succinate and CO_2 while hydroxylating the prime substrate, HIF-α subunit (Kaelin 2005). The reaction proceeds via the formation of oxoferryl-intermediate as shown in Fig.7.

The proposed mechanism is based on the reported incorporation of ^{18}O into HIF-α substrate and succinate, the available crystal structures for PHD2, and the recent stopped-flow kinetics for taurine/α-ketoglutarate dioxygenase and prolyl-4-hydroxylase from *Parameticum bursaria Chlorella virus 1*(Price et al 2005). The mechanism suggests the initial binding of iron to the active site, then α-ketoglutarate coordination via C-1 carboxylate and ketone oxygen by iron, followed by the binding of HIF peptide (as a substrate) which results in displacing the water molecule from the 6th coordination position. This displacement guarantees oxygen binding and activation. The uncoordinated oxygen of the bound oxygen attacks the ketone carbonyl of α-ketoglutarate to form a bicyclic Fe(IV)-peroxyhemiketal complex, in which decarboxylation occurs concomitantly with formation of an oxo-ferryl (Fe(IV)=O) intermediate. The latter one hydroxylates proline via a substrate radical intermediate as evidenced by the formation of prolyl radical: i.e. oxo-ferryl attacks proline residue to withdraw hydrogen atom, and then introduces the hydroxyl radical. The presence of the water molecule in the 6th position does not prevent oxygen from binding and activation completely: in the absence of the substrate the enzymes of this class are known to catalyze the so called uncoupled reaction, i.e. ketoglutarate decarboxylation in the absence of HIF or HIF peptide. However, the rate of the reaction is rather slow.

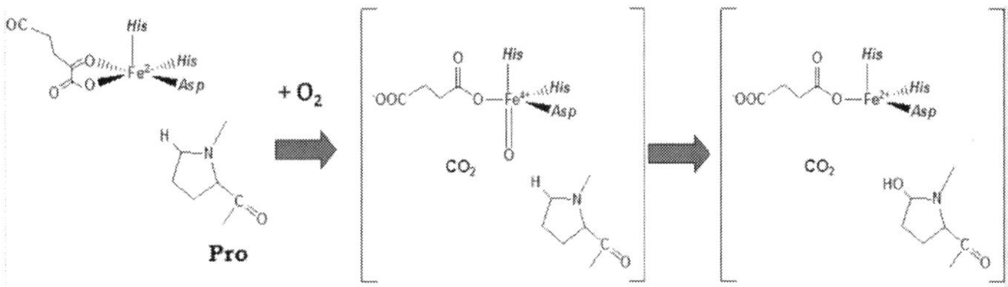

Fig. 7. Schematic presentation of two half-reactions of HIF prolyl hydroxylase catalytic cycle (see detailed explanation below). The reaction substrates are ketoglutarate, oxygen and HIF or HIF peptide, and the reaction products are succinate, cabon dioxide, and hydroxylated HIF or HIF peptide.

PHDs 1-3 (also known as EGLN 2,1, and 3) in human are represented by three isozymes with catalytic domains very homologous to each other (Bruick & McKnight 2001). PHD3 contains the catalytic domain only, contrary to PHD1 and PHD2, which have additional N-terminal domains. The crystal structure of PHD2 catalytic domain was resolved by two independent groups. PHD2 exists as a monomer in solution. The enzyme contains double-stranded β-helix core fold common to the Fe(II)-αKG-dependent dioxygenase family. The active site comprises a relatively deep pocket compared to other αKG oxygenases. Iron is coordinated in an octahedral manner by His-313, His-374 and Asp-313, inhibitor (occupying two sites) and water molecule (Fig.8). The similarity in the structure of catalytic domains of PHDs1-3 and identical αKG binding residues (according to the homology modeling) makes the task of developing specific inhibitors based on αKG analogues doubtful.

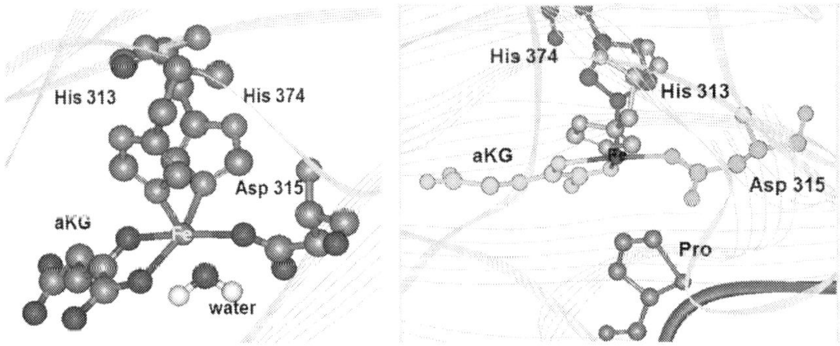

Fig. 8. Displacement of active site water (left) upon binding of HIF peptide (right) initiates oxygen binding and the catalytic cycle of ketoglutarate decarboxylation accompanied by formation of ferryl iron, subtraction of hydrogen from Proline 564, and subsequent hydroxylation of the latter.

There are 3 different ways to assay PHD activity (Hewitson et al 2007):

- The assay of the first half-reaction substrates and products (O_2 and a-ketoglutarate consumption; CO_2 evolution, succinate production); this format should account for the uncoupled reaction, which is non-specific.

- The assay of the second half-reaction oxidized product (mass-spec of hydroxylated peptides); mass-spec analysis is difficult to make suitable for HTS format.
- The so-called "capture assay" monitoring interaction of the hydroxylated product with VHL; requires recombinant HIF, reticulocyte-produced VHL, protein/peptide labelling and corresponding antibodies.

The most reliable way to monitor the formation of hydroxylated product is either by mass-spectrometry, or using the "capture assay". The latter is known in three different formats:

- **End-point** immunochemical assay is based upon the tight interaction between pVHL and the hydroxylated Pro564 of HIF-1α. Iimmobilized HIF-peptide which, after hydroxylation, is recognized by the thioredoxin-labeled VHL-elongin B-elongin C complex (expressed in *E.coli* and purified), which is its turn, is detected by anti-thioredoxin antibodies by the method of double antibodies with the second, peroxidase-labeled, antibodies.
- **Continuous** fluorescence polarization assay: HIF-peptide modified with a fluorescent label upon capture by VHL-elongin B-elongin C shows higher polarization signal (Cho et al 2005).
- **Continuous** homogeneous time-resolved fluorescence resonance energy transfer (TR-FRET) assay: VCB-Eu complex recognizes hydroxylated P564-HIF-1α peptide, preliminary biotinylated, followed by interaction with streptavidin labeled allophycocyanin (Fig.9). This assay, developed by Amgen team, is the best one in terms of sensitivity and applicability for HTS. The assay, in addition to other expensive reagents, utilizes Europium (Dao et al 2009).

All enzymatic assays are based on the use of PHD2 recombinant enzyme produced in either baculovirus or *E.coli* expression system. High throughput screening for PHD inhibitors using an enzyme assay is a challenge both in terms of the enzyme source and the assay format. The enzymatic activity and stability of purified PHD is very low (Tuckerman et al 2004), and enzyme assays suitable for HTS require large quantities of recombinant enzyme supplemented with iron. One of challenges in the search for selective HIF PHD inhibitors or other regulators of HIF stability is to discriminate between non-specific iron chelation in solution and specific iron chelation inside the active center of the PHD enzyme (see 2.2.4). Given the non-physiological conditions under which screening for inhibitors occurs with recombinant PHD2, it is not surprising that the IC_{50} value determined in the enzyme *in vitro* assay did not correlate with the IC_{50} for VEGF activation reported in the same study (Warshakoon et al. 2006d). Another limitation is the use of a 19-mer HIF peptide, whose affinity for the HIF PHDs is orders of magnitude lesser than the full length protein. So far only Amgen team used recombinant HIF protein in HTS of their internal collection, although again they had been varying the concentration of αKG, not HIF, when determining the inhibition constant for their best hit (Tegley *et al.* 2008). A negative consequence of the test tube strategy is the assay format is more likely to yield inhibitors competitive with respect to αKG than those competing with HIF itself.

The screening for PHD2 inhibitors based on enzymatic assays with recombinant PHD2 was performed by Fibrogen, Procter&Gamble, Amgen, and some other groups. The Procter&Gamble team published 4 papers analyzing structure-activity relationship (SAR) for 3 different groups of compounds possessing clear iron binding motifs that dock into the PHD2 active site. The hydroxylation assay was performed by mass-spectrometry. In addition, the ability of some inhibitors to induce VEGF was judged by a VEGF ELISA using

HEK293 cells. The total number of compounds reported was ca.50. The screening for PHD inhibitors based on the αKG mimetic structures yielded a number of different classes of inhibitors with the inhibition constants in the μM range. The best inhibition constant among substituted pyridine derivatives was exhibited by *p*-chloro phenyl-substituted 5-pyridine carboxyamide (15 μM) and those with the pyrazole moiety in the 5th position of the pyridine ring (5-20 μM) (Warshakoon et al, 2006a); the further work resulted in the significantly improved affinity (1-2 μM) of the newly designed inhibitors of pyrazolopyrimidines series (Warshakoon et al, 2006a). Imidazo[1,2-a]pyridine derivatives showed the apparent inhibition constants in the 4-27 μM range (Warshakoon et al, 2006b), and 8-hydroxyquinoline derivates exhibited the apparent inhibition constants in the range of 3-10 μM (Warshakoon et al, 2006c). However, taking into account that the screening for potential inhibitors was performed using a 19-mer peptide, which shows at least 1 order of magnitude worse K_m than HIF-ODD, the range of the apparent inhibitor constants obtained may be insufficient for the inhibition of the enzyme activity *in vivo*.

Very recently, the Amgen team developed a time-resolved fluorescence resonance energy transfer-based assay based on interaction of the hydroxylated HIF peptide with VHL and performed HTS of their "internal compounds collection" to reveal a lead compound of IC50 of ca. 72 nM from a novel hydroxyl-thiazole class, followed by lead optimization. 30 new derivatives have been synthesized and assayed. The inhibition constant was determined from single-point measurements done in triplicate at pH 6.0, which was found to be optimal for the *in vitro* reaction catalyzed by human full-size recombinant PHD2. The best inhibitors have a long hydrophobic tail that screens the entrance to the active site. Flexibility of the tail (benzyl instead of phenyl) enhances affinity by orders of magnitude as the IC50 is improved from dozens nM to single digits. These are the best inhibitors reported in literature thus far.

The conformation of recombinant PHD2 may be different from that of the native enzyme, in addition, PHD2 like all enzymes of this family is highly unstable in the absence of reducing agents such as DTT. The recently reported crystal structure of PHD2 with a 17-mer HIF peptide (Chowdhury *et al.* 2009) shows no active site water displacement, which appears to be a mandatory requirement for the initiation of the catalytic cycle. Given these biases, it is not surprising that all PHD inhibitors developed using the recombinant enzyme explored only the αKG-binding motif inside PHD2 active site and had a carboxyl group interacting with Arg-383 in addition to a clearly defined iron-binding motif (Tegley et al. 2008, Warshakoon et al. 2006a, Warshakoon et al. 2006b, Warshakoon et al. 2006c, Warshakoon et al. 2006d, Ivan et al. 2002). The reaction mixture has to be supplemented with excess of iron, alpha-ketoglutarate, and HIF peptide, making the selection of mild inhibitors impossible. Majority of PHD inhibitors identified in HTS are presented by iron chelators. The only exception so far is Compound A with IC_{50},=0.032 μM (see Fig.9 right) identified by Amgen team using the newly developed assay (Fig.9), however, the core motif will not pass the filters recently described by Baell and Holloway, 2010.

One of disadvantages of enzymatic assay is that despite the apparent specificity, the hits identified in HTS may potentially target other enzymes of the same class. In particular, human genome has more than 70 genes of putative non-heme iron dioxygenases, and there is no principal difference in organization of the active sites of these enzymes. As a rule, the major difference is in the access to the active sites. There are three different forms of HIF (1-3) and three PHD isoforms, and all data reported so far on enzyme specificty using HIF peptides and recombinant enzymes give no clue on the preference for a particular substrate for a PHD isoform. On the other hand, the study of HIF-PHD interaction in yeast two hybrid system indicated principal differences existing among PHD isoforms with respect to recognition of HIF isoforms (Landazuri et al 2006). The latter observations are in agreement with our results obtained with HIF2 ODD-luc and HIF3 ODD-luc reporters showing that HIF3 is not recognized by PHD1 and PHD2. Therefore, running enzymatic assays with PHD2 and HIF peptides does not give a true picture of enzyme specificity and cannot be used for development of isozyme-specific inhibitors.

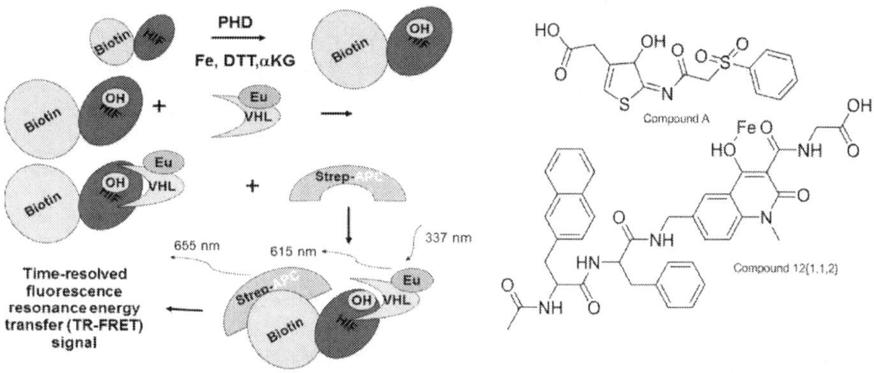

Fig. 9. Schematic presentation of TR-FRET assay (left) developed by Amgen team to monitor the activity of HIF prolyl hydroxylase. The assay employes biotin-labeled HIF, Eu-labeled VHL protein, as well al APC-labeled streptavidin, in addition to the recombinant PHD2 used as a catalyst of the first enzymatic step. The assay was successfully used for HTS purposes: an inhibitor (E)-2-(4-hydroxy-5-(2-(phenylsulfonyl)acetylimino)-4,5-dihydrothiophen-3-yl)acetic acid specific for αKG binding site has been developed (right, Compound A), and later dipeptidyl-quinolones (see compound 12{1,1,2}) specific to PHD1 and 3, and 10-fold less specific to PHD2 (Murray et al 2010).

2.2.2 HIF1 ODD-luciferase reporter construction (Safran et al 2006, Smirnova et al 2010)

Two primary modes of screening for HIF activators have been well described: a recombinant enzyme-based screen for PHD2 inhibitors (used by Fibrogen (Ivan *et al.* 2002), Amgen (Tegley *et al.* 2008, Allen et al 2008)), Procter and Gamble Pharmaceuticals Inc. (Warshakoon *et al.* 2006a, Warshakoon *et al.* 2006b, Warshakoon *et al.* 2006c, Warshakoon et al. 2006d), and other teams (Nangaku *et al.* 2007)); and a cell-based screen using HRE-luciferase reporter construct used by a number of labs including our own.

The cell-based assay with HRE-luc reporter system, a promoter-reporter construct that contained 68 bp of a known hypoxia and HIF-1 regulated gene, enolase, containing a wild type HRE (5'-RCTGT-3'), is a widely used approach for screening of HIF activators with diverse mechanisms of action (Semenza *et al.* 1996). A reporter system is based on transfected immortalized hippocampal neuroblast cell line (HT22) and allows screening for a broad spectrum of compounds that include: activators of HIF transcription; activators of HIF binding to HRE; and effectors of HIF protein stability (PHD inhibitors, pVHL &

proteasome inhibitors). The manual screen of Spectrum library performed in this laboratory using HRE-luc/HT22 line took half a year and resulted in 43 hits. However, in our hands, the cell line's response to positive controls decreases after 7 passages, making the system not suitable for a robotic HTS on 384-well plates.

Taking into account the low specific activity of recombinant enzymes, and the inadequacy of interpretation of the inhibition constant generated using different types of enzyme *in vitro* assays, we developed a cell-based reporter system for HTS of ODD-luc stability, a variant of the cell-based "capture" assay, and accomplished a screen of 85,000 structurally diverse compounds (Smirnova et al 2010). Cell-based assay for HIF1 activators working via inhibition of HIF PHDs employs the same strategy as the one used for screening of Nrf2 activators. The HIF1 ODD-luc reporter system is equivalent to *in vivo* capture assay monitored by consumption of a labeled substrate (ODD-luciferase) (see Fig. 10 left). The reporter system II (Fig. 10 right) consists of the HIF-1α gene fragment encoding the oxygen degradable domain (ODD) containing the key proline residue followed by luciferase gene (*luc*) (Safran et al 2006). The regulation of luciferase protein stability in this reporter system is the same as the physiological activation of HIF: hydroxylation of oxygen-degradable domain (ODD, which contains 530-653 a.a. of HIF1α) results in recognition of the ODD-luc fusion protein by VHL followed by its ubiqutinylation and proteasomal degradation (Fig.10), and as we present below, the approach proved to be productive for HTS purposes.

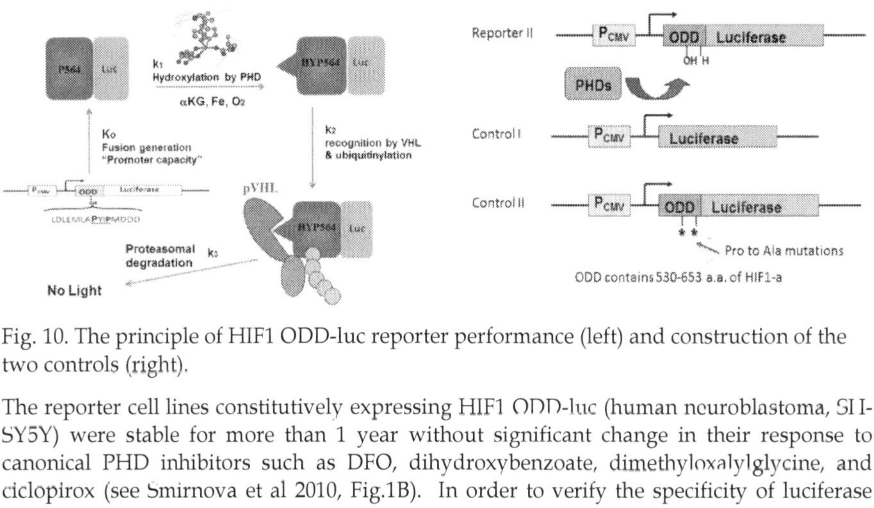

Fig. 10. The principle of HIF1 ODD-luc reporter performance (left) and construction of the two controls (right).

The reporter cell lines constitutively expressing HIF1 ODD-luc (human neuroblastoma, SH-SY5Y) were stable for more than 1 year without significant change in their response to canonical PHD inhibitors such as DFO, dihydroxybenzoate, dimethyloxalylglycine, and ciclopirox (see Smirnova et al 2010, Fig.1B). In order to verify the specificity of luciferase changes as an assay for PHD activity, several control lines were developed: the control line I expressing wild-type luciferase under the control of P_{CMV}-promoter, and the control line II expressing ODD-luc with proline 564 and 567 Mutated to Ala, which generates luciferase fusion that cannot be degraded. Both controls experimentally identify a threshold level of ODD-luc protein attainable in these cells. The background signal for the wild-type HIF ODD-luc line (PYIP) corresponds to approximately 5-6% of the ODD-luc levels in the control lines with wild-type luciferase and AYIA line (double mutant P564A/P567A line) (Fig.10 right). Treatment with 10 μM ciclopirox results in a 10-fold increase of a background signal for the ODD-luc reporter (PYIP line), i.e. reaches almost 50% of the threshold value (see

Smirnova et al 2010, Fig.2). These particular conditions are ideal for HTS as they promote the selection of both weaker and more potent inhibitors than ciclopirox.

2.2.3 Determination of inhibition constants from kinetics of HIF1 ODD-luciferase reporter activation

In accord with validation studies, the HIF ODD-luciferase reporter system is controlled by the rate of PHD-catalyzed reaction: the response of the ODD-luc reporter to canonical HIF PHD inhibitors, and the increased stability of single-point mutant reporters in accord with the predictions (see Smirnova et al 2010), provided confidence that this system could be utilized for screening for novel small molecule HIF PHD inhibitors. From an enzyme kinetics point of view, the HIF ODD-luciferase reporter system is a "capture assay" monitored by the consumption of a substrate, the heterologously expressed HIF ODD-luciferase fusion protein. As we show below, the reporter activation kinetics can be used to determine an apparent inhibition constant for a particular compound. In the kinetic regime, i.e. monitoring the time-course of luminescence changes (Fig.11), the ODD-luc reporter system permits quantitative characterization of promoter capacity (K_o, rate of fusion protein generation), enzyme activity, and inhibition constant determination. The rate of fusion accumulation equals to the rate of its production (K_o) minus the rate of rate-limiting step, controlled by HIF PHDs, which obeys Michaelis-Menten kinetics, as follows:

$$v = d[ODDluc]/dt = K_0 - k_1[PHD][ODDluc]/\{K_m(1+[I]/K_i)+[ODDluc]\} \quad (1)$$

where K_m is the inhibition constant for a competitive inhibitor, k_1 is rate coefficient, [PHD] and [ODD-luc] are the concentrations of the enzyme and substrate, respectively.
The background luminescence signal calibrated with recombinant luciferase allows us to estimate the steady-state concentration of the ODD-luc fusion protein. Under the conditions used the steady-state value of 60 rlu (relative light units) corresponds to 1 pg luciferase protein; dividing this number by the total cell volume taken as a single cell volume (233 μ^3) multiplied by 30,000 cells/well density (numer of cells in a 96 well dish), we get the ODD-luc fusion protein steady-state concentration equal to 2.3 nM, which is way below all reported K_m values for HIF1 (Ivan et al 2002, Tuckerman et al 2004, Koivunen et al 2006). Therefore, we work under non-saturating conditions with respect to HIF substrate, i.e. optimal conditions for selecting inhibitors competitive against HIF substrate. Moreover, as compared to the *in vitro* assay, which uses a 19 amino acid peptide fragment surrounding the oxygen dependent domain (ODD), our ODD-luciferase construct contains 123 amino acid acids, and thus more closely emulates the behavior of native HIF. We can consider the initial concentration of fusion much lower than K_m and ignore it in the rate equation:

$$v = d[ODDluc]/dt = K_0 - k_1[PHD][ODDluc]/K_m(1+[I]/K_i) \quad (2)$$

The capacity of promoter, K_0 can be determined under the conditions of total inhibition of PHD activity by means of complete iron deprivation achieved in the presence of high concentrations of ciclopirox, i.e. when the increase in the ciclopirox concentrations give no further increase in the rate of luciferase signal growth (Fig.11). The intracellular enzyme activity (k_1[PHD]/K_m) can be also determined by dividing the rate of fusion protein accumulation by the steady-state concentration of the fusion protein determined directly from one and the same experiment in luciferase units, without recalculation for the cellular volume, and corresponds to 0.05 min^{-1}. The linear plot of $1/(K_0 - v)$ versus the inhibitor concentration gives the value of the apparent inhibition constant as the intercept on X-axis (Fig.12):

$$1/(K_0 - v) = K_m(1 + [I]/K_i)/k_1[PHD][ODDluc]_0 \qquad \text{(Eq.3)}$$

The apparent inhibition constants determined as an intercept on X-axis for compound 7 and DMOG are 0.0012 mM and 1.3 mM, respectively (see Fig.12), which is in agreement with previous observations on DMOG biological effects exerted in the millimolar range and IC_{50} reported for PHD2 in vitro assay.
The developed approach is good only if the activation effect is significant, at least 3-fold and higher over the background luminescence, otherwise the experimental error of kinetic measurements is too high to perform the above described calculations.

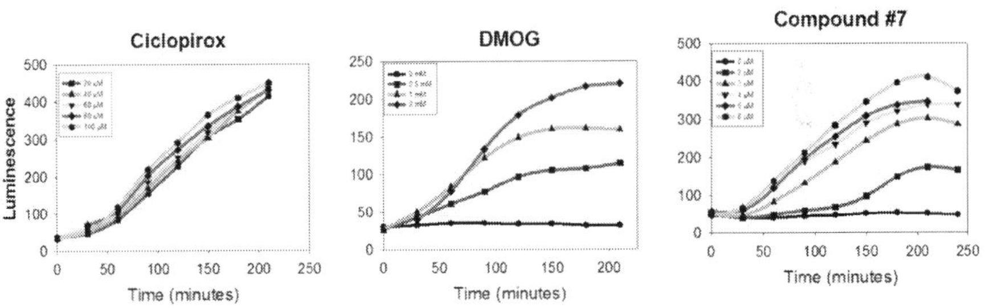

Fig. 11. Experimental kinetics of reporter activation for ciclopirox (complete iron deprivation, which permits determination of the promoter capacity, K_0), dimethyloxalylglycine (DMOG), ketoglutarate analog competing with the latter for the binding in the active center of PHD, and one of the best hits in HTS (Smirnova et al, 2010), compound 7 (formula in Fig.12).

2.2.4 Rationale for discriminating between specific and non-specific PHD inhibition

Since the enzyme controlling the rate-limiting step of reporter activation is iron dependent, any iron chelator will come up as a hit in HTS. To discriminate between the non-specific iron chelation in solution and iron coordination by a chelator in the active site of PHD2 we had to develop a rationale. One of the possibilities to evaluate specificity of the reporter response could be the comparison of concentration titration curves in the presence and absence of extra iron. Only specific PHD inhibitors will act at concentrations lower than that of the added iron. Although this approach may potentially yield specific PHD inhibitors right away, it creates a serious experimental problem: cell lines are extremely sensitive to the presence of more than 2 μM extra iron in the medium, which possibly catalyzes Fenton reaction resulting in cell death within hours of incubation. Another approach is to compare reporter activation parameters with the iron chelation ability in solution for a set of compounds of similar structure. If the iron chelation ability of the inhibitors is linearly proportional to HIF activation parameters, it can be safely concluded that the inhibitors simply inactivate PHDs through their ability to chelate iron non-specifically. If on the other hand activation of HIF and iron chelation ability are not proportional then the inhibitors act on PHD through a more specific mechanism.

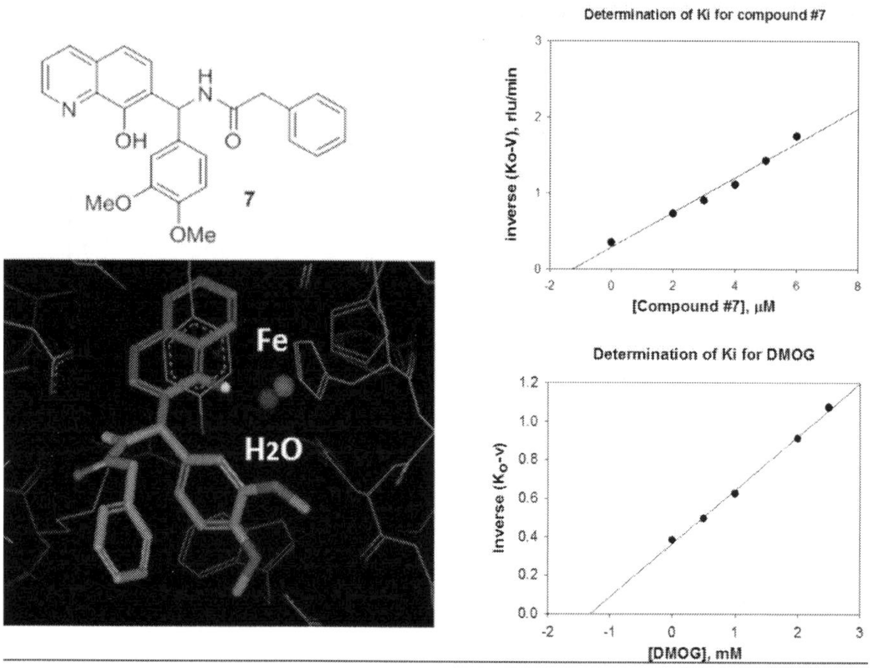

Fig. 12. Calculation of apparent inhibition constants for compound 7 and DMOG using a modified Dixon plot.

To account for iron chelation in solution one should determine the iron binding constant in a model system, for example by displacement of calcein from its complex with iron upon addition of a particular compound monitored by fluorescence (excitation 490 nm, emission 523 nm, cut-off 515 nm) on a Spectramax M5^{e} platereader (Molecular Devices). To linearize the fitting equation we introduce parameter Y as the ratio of calcein-iron complex to free calcein, which can be determined directly from our experiments: Y = *[Fe-Calcein]/[Calcein]*. The apparent binding constant for calcein (ca.50 nM) was determined from Fe titration curve for 1 μM calcein in 5 mM Tris-HCl buffer, pH 7.5 (Fig.13 left). The ratio between the iron binding constant for calcein and a particular compound K_Q/K_{Ca} can be estimated by fitting the titration curve into the dependence of $[Fe]_o$ vs. Y, where $Y=[Ca\text{-}Fe]/[Ca]$ is a ratio of calcein-bound Fe to free (fluorescent) calcein:

$$[Fe]o = K_{Ca}Y + [Ca]oY / (Y+1) + [Q]oY / (Y + K_Q / K_{Ca}) \quad (4)$$

The protocol included addition of 50 µL of Iron in various concentrations 0.5 µM - 2.0 µM to the buffer solution, then the addition of 50 µL calcein so that final concentration of calcein is 1 µM; the addition of 50 µL compound of interest in various concentrations, and then taking end point readings at 20 min incubation. Range of compound concentration was determined through how well the compound liberated calcein from its complex with iron (Fig.13 right). Besides the equilibrium constant, the association rate constant (kinetic coefficient) can be determined as the second order rate constant for calcein displacement kinetics from its

complex with iron (1 μM:1 μM) upon addition of an oxyquinoline (5-20 μM), i.e. calculated from the slope of a linear plot of the initial rate of calcein release *vs.* the concentration of oxyquinoline added. This parameter can be used as a kinetic characteristic of iron binding.
Once the iron binding constants are determined, one can plot the reporter activation parameters versus inverse inhibition constant, or iron association constant. In both cases, IC50 determined from the concentration titration curve is the correct parameter to plot (Fig. 14). The activation magnitude is not a perfect parameter for structure-activity relationship (SAR) studies, because as we wrote earlier, there is a threshold for reporter activation, and if incubation is not short, the reporter hits the plateau, which is one and the same for all hits.

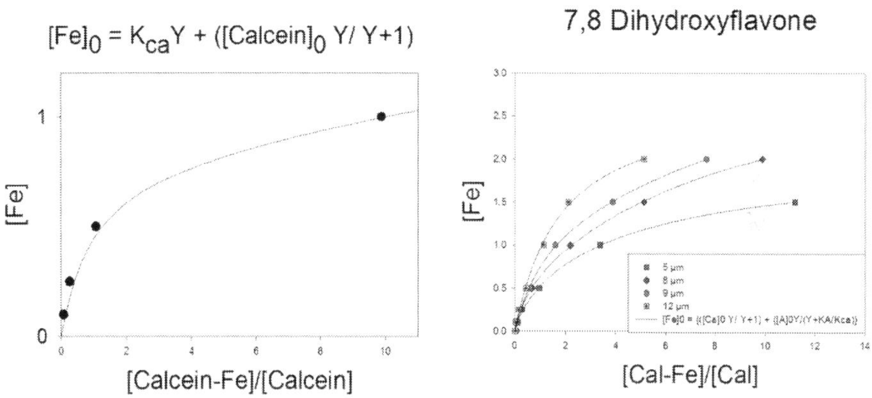

Fig. 13. Determination of iron binding constant for calcein (left) and 7,8 dihydroflavone (right) as an example of iron-binding compound.

As seen in Fig. 14, there is a parallel in iron chelation properties and IC50 for majority of branched oxyquinolines studied, except for 4 compounds which deviate from the linear dependence (##1,4,7,8). All these have a specific branch similar to that shown in Fig. 12 for compounf 7. Compounds 7 and 8 were taken for biological analysis along with compound 10, which was used as a negative control, because despite its iron binding capacity and cell permeability is as good as for compounds 7 and 8, this compound is not a specific PHD inhibitor.
A similar approach can be used to rule out the effect of reducing or oxidative properties (say flavonoids). For this purpose, the rate constant for oxidation/reduction of ferro/ferricyanide, can be measured (not shown). The rate of reduction of dithionitrobenzoic acid can be used to account for disulfide reduction capacity of compounds uder study.

2.2.5 Substrates and substrate specificity of HIF prolyl hydroxylases

The data from the literature and that obtained in this laboratory unequivocally demonstrate that PHDs are important targets for medical intervention. This justifies the necessity of the development of HTS for PHD inhibitors, activators, specific and alternative substrates. The challenge is to develop inhibitors specific for each isoform, since very recently it became clear that the PHD isozymes have their specific substrates.
HIF1 and HIF2 are established substrates for PHD2. PHD1 apparently is specific for Rpb1, the large subunit of RNA polymerase II, which carries the fundamental enzymatic activity

of the complex synthesizing all cellular mRNAs. Rpb1 is ubiquitylated and degraded in response to DNA lesions induced by UV light and high millimolar H_2O_2. Phosphorylation of Ser5 in Rpb1 is a prerequisite for Rpb1 ubiquitylation. It has been discovered that Pro1465 hydroxylation catalyzed by PHD1 is necessary for subsequent Ser5 phosphorylation of Rpb1 in response to oxidative stress. PHD2, in contrast, has an inhibitory effect on this modification (Mikhailova et al 2008). Recently, the Kaelin's group (Zhang et al 2009) demonstrated a link between PHD1 and cyclin D1: PHD1 is estrogen-inducible in breast carcinoma cells and PHD1 inactivation decreases Cyclin D1 levels and suppresses mammary gland proliferation *in vivo*. Regulation of Cyclin D1 is a specific attribute of PHD1 among the PHD proteins and is HIF-independent. Loss of PHD1 (but not PHD2) catalytic activity inhibits estrogen-dependent breast cancer tumorigenesis and can be rescued by exogenous Cyclin D1. PHD1 depletion also impairs the fitness of lung, brain, and hematopoietic cancer lines. These findings support the exploration of PHD1 inhibitors as therapeutics for estrogen-dependent breast cancer and other malignancies. PHD1 appears to be an attractive drug target because PHD1 is not essential in mammals.

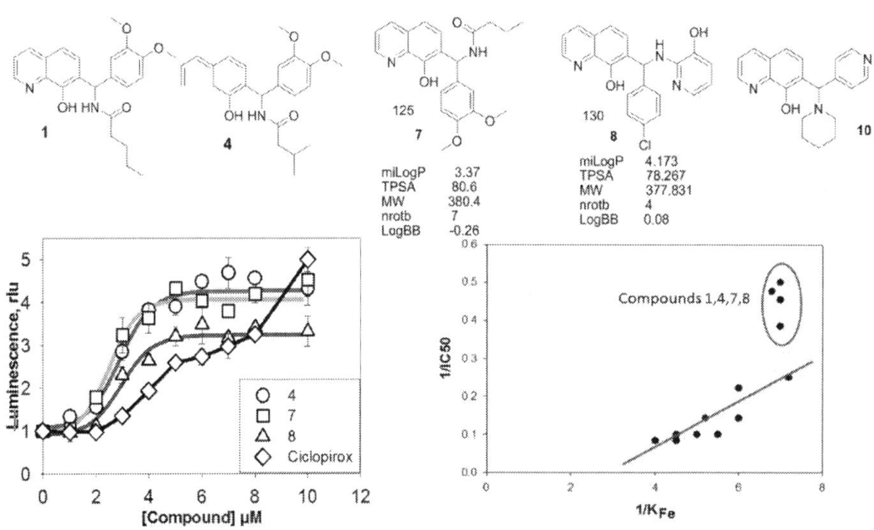

Fig. 14. Evaluation of iron chelation effect on inhibition parameters determined for branched oxyquinolines. Among all compounds of this group tested, only four (compounds 1,4,7,8) showed significant deviation from a linear dependence, and thus are considered as specific PHD inhibitors.

PHD3 hydroxylates β2-adrenergic receptor (β2AR) (Xie et al 2009), the prototypic GPCR that play an important role in the regulation of cardiovascular and pulmonary function, and sustained βAR down-regulation (and dysfunction) is associated with diseases such as heart failure and asthma. β2AR, in particular, enhances bronchodilation and alveolar fluid clearance (which increase O_2 uptake), enhances cardiac output and peripheral vasodilation (which increase O_2 delivery), and enhances cardioprotection and angiogenesis under ischemic conditions, thereby effectively recapitulating the integrated physiological response to hypoxia. Up-regulation of the β2AR in response to hypoxia puts the function of the receptor in new light. The ability of the PHD3-pVHL hydroxylation and ubiquitylation pathway to regulate the β2AR and the implications of that regulation for the response to ischemia and hypoxia suggest previously unidentified targets in the treatment of cardiovascular and respiratory diseases. PHD3 is most abundant in cardiac and smooth muscle, where the β2AR is highly abundant in vivo. PHD3 expression is increased with aging.

On one hand, the disadvantage of the cell-based assay is that there are 3 different isoforms of the enzyme, and reporter activation shows an integral inhibition of all three or the two most abundant (PHD1 and PHD2). On the other hand, the enzymatic assay is sensitive to the isoform-specificity only when the full-size protein substrate (HIF1) is used. The combination of cell-based HIF1 ODD-luc reporter assay with siRNA technique can give an answer on isoform specificity with respect to HIF1 and can be used to clarify the specificity of a particular drug candidate with respect to PHD isoform.

Cell-based HTS is close to the actual reaction conditions in the cell, where concentration of HIF is at below nanomolar level and thus, permits selection of mild inhibitors. Computerized analysis of hits in the case of PHD inhibitors groups hits in accord with their core structure, which obviously is just a mimic of αKG. The average number of hits from 10,000 compound library is on the order of 30-40 compounds, and this low number (in comparison with Neh2-luc screen) permits manual classification. The comparison of the structures of various hit groups from HTS screen of 85,000 compounds demonstrated (1) the presence of a branched motif immediately attached to the iron chelation/coordination core, and (2) the effect of the linker length. As shown in Fig.15, long or rigid branch, immediately attached to the iron-coordinating core, has a profound effect on HIF1 ODD-luc reporter activation. In the case of branched oxyquinolines, we were able to study structure-activity relationship in detail (Smirnova et al 2010), and to demonstrate the specific character of PHD inhibition by branched oxyquinolines (see compound 7 in Fig.12 & compounds 1,4,7,8 in Fig. 14).

Structural analysis of the hits comprised of branched quinolines revealed that the general scaffold consists of three regions: the iron binding motif, linker, and the terminal groups that may serve for surface recognition among the various PHD isozymes (Figure 16). Chemical modification on each of these regions will create a substantial molecular space for exploring the pharmacophoric requirements for PHD inhibitory activity and isoform selectivity with the aim to identify the advanced analogues with requisite physiochemical properties.

Our current research is focused on optimization of the branched portion of 8-hydroxyquinolines to develop isoform-specific PHD inhibitors, as shown in Fig.16. Iron-binding groups can be represented by various iron-coordinating cores, and oxyquinolines are just an example chosen based on the ease of synthetic manipulations. As the iron-binding groups can also contribute to the isozyme selectivity, one may investigate structural alterations in the portion that bears an Fe(II)-binding group by analogy with the known structures of PHD inhibitors mimicking ketoglutarate binding (see Fig.17D). It is known that less flexible structures can mimic bound conformation at the target binding site; moreover, structural rigidification reduces CYP450 interactions and hERG blocking activity, therefore allowing for improvement of ADMET characteristics of the proposed inhibitors. As could be envisioned, the core structure of 8-hydroxyquinoline might be constrained by incorporating

3. Conclusion

The novel approach to HTS of transcription factor activators is extremely promising for the development of specific stabilizers of the corresponding transcription factor, because it is sensitive to the initial step in transcription factor stabilization. The magnitude and sensitivity of reporter assay permits selection of mild activators which provide "fine tuning". The key characteristic of new reporter systems is the possibility to monitor reporter activation in real-time to support structure-activity relationship studies (see Figs. 4 & 11). No other reporter provides such a possibility, and no other reporter provides such sensitivity. For both reporters discussed, this new feature opens a way towards design of specific stabilizers of the corresponding transciption factor.

We were first to predict the possibility of development of isoform-specific PHD inhibitors employing variations in the motif adjacent to the iron binding core based on the results of HTS (Smirnova et al 2010). This prediction was supported by the identified branched oxyquinolines, which were characterized as PHD specific inhibitors and were confirmed to exert the predicted biological effects. Our conclusion on the role of branched portion in recognition of different PHD isoforms has been experimentally confirmed in the recent publication from Amgen group: the branching peptide-like portions attached to the quinolone core (see Compound 12{1,1,2} in Fig.9) resulted in up to 10-fold difference in magnitude of inhibition of PHD2 and PHD1/PHD3 (Murray et al 2010). Hence, isoform-specific PHD inhibitors can be constructed by optimizing the branching portion immediately adjacent to the iron-chelation core. Ongoing work includes synthesis of branched derivatives (Fig. 17) to explore the possibility of developing isoform-specific inhibitors.

We were first to demonstrate the direct effect of gedunins on Nrf2 activation as well as their perfect docking into Keap1 in place of Neh2 peptide. The latter discovery is promising in terms of future identification of non-electrophilic activators working by displacing of Nrf2 from its complex with Keap1, without non-specific oxidation or covalent modification of Keap thiols among other cellular proteins.

The collection of reporters available in the laboratory (HIF1 ODD-luc and its mutants, HIF2 ODD-luc, HIF3 ODD-luc, Neh2-luc) permits their parallel use for HTS purposes, where each reporter plays the role of a control for each other. The new reporter assays combined with secondary biochemical analysis permit selection of drugs working at the first, selective step of transcription factor stabilization.

4. Acknowledgement

The work was funded by the Winifred Masterson Burke Relief Foundation, the Adelson Foundation for Neurorehabilitation and Repair, NYS DOH Center of Research Excellence # CO19772, and Thomas Hartman Foundation for Parkinson's Research.

5. References

Allen, J. R.; Tegley, C. M.; Biswas, K.; Burli, R.; Muller, K. M.; Frohn, M. J.; Golden, J. E.; Mercede, S. J.; Neira, S. C.; Peterkin, T. A. N.; Hungate, R. W.; Kurzeja, R.; Yu, V.; Dao, J. Quinolone based compounds exhibiting prolyl hydroxylase inhibitory activity, and compositions, and uses thereof. WO Patent 2007070359, Apr 3, 2008.

Baell, J.B., and Holloway, G.A. (2010). New substructure filters for removal of pan assay interference compounds (PAINS) from screening libraries and for their exclusion in bioassays. *J Med Chem 53*, 2719-2740.

Balani SK, Miwa GT, Gan LS, Wu JT, Lee FW. (2005).Strategy of utilizing in vitro and in vivo ADME tools for lead optimization and drug candidate selection. *Curr. Topics Med. Chem.* 5, 1033-1038

Bruick, R.K., and McKnight, S.L. (2001). A conserved family of prolyl-4-hydroxylases that modify HIF. *Science* 294, 1337–1340.

Cho, H., Park, H., and Yang, E.G. (2005). A fluorescence polarization-based interaction assay for hypoxia-inducible factor prolyl hydroxylases. *Biochem. Biophys. Res. Commun.* 337, 275–280.

Chowdhury, R., McDonough, M.A., Mecinovic, J., Loenarz, C., Flashman, E., Hewitson, K.S., Domene, C., and Schofield, C.J. (2009). Structural basis for binding of hypoxia-inducible factor to the oxygen-sensing prolyl hydroxylases. *Structure* 17, 981–989.

Cullinan, S.B., Gordan, J.D., Jin, J., Harper, J.W., and Diehl, J.A. (2004). The Keap1-BTB protein is an adaptor that bridges Nrf2 to a Cul3-based E3 ligase: oxidative stress sensing by a Cul3-Keap1 ligase. *Mol. Cell. Biol.* 24, 8477–8486.

Dao, J.H., Kurzeja, R.J., Morachis, J.M., Veith, H., Lewis, J., Yu, V., Tegley, C.M., and Tagari, P. (2009). Kinetic characterization and identification of a novel inhibitor of hypoxia-inducible factor prolyl hydroxylase 2 using a time-resolved fluorescence resonance energy transfer-based assay technology. *Anal. Biochem.* 384, 213–223.

Hewitson, K.S., Schofield, C.J., and Ratcliffe, P.J. (2007). Hypoxia-inducible factor prolyl-hydroxylase: purification and assays of PHD2. *Methods Enzymol.* 435, 25–42.

Hirotsu, Y., Katsuoka, F., Itoh, K., and Yamamoto, M. (2011). Nrf2 degron-fused reporter system: a new tool for specific evaluation of Nrf2 inducers. *Genes Cells 16*, 406-415.

Ivan, M., Haberberger, T., Gervasi, D.C., et al. (2002). Biochemical purification and pharmacological inhibition of a mammalian prolyl hydroxylase acting on hypoxia-inducible factor. *Proc. Natl. Acad. Sci. USA* 99, 13459–13464.

Itoh, K., Wakabayashi, N., Katoh, Y., Ishii, T., Igarashi, K., Engel, J.D., and Yamamoto, M. (1999). Keap1 represses nuclear activation of antioxidant responsive elements by Nrf2 through binding to the amino-terminal Neh2 domain. *Genes Dev.* 13, 76–86.

Kaelin, W.G., Jr. (2005). The von Hippel-Lindau protein, HIF hydroxylation, and oxygen sensing. *Biochem. Biophys. Res. Commun.* 338, 627–638.

Kaspar, J.W., Niture, S.K., and Jaiswal, A.K. (2009). Nrf2:INrf2 (Keap1) signaling in oxidative stress. *Free Radic. Biol. Med.* 47, 1304–1309.

Kobayashi, A., Kang, M.I., Okawa, H., Ohtsuji, M., Zenke, Y., Chiba, T., Igarashi, K., and Yamamoto, M. (2004). Oxidative stress sensor Keap1 functions as an adaptor for Cul3-based E3 ligase to regulate proteasomal degradation of Nrf2. *Mol. Cell. Biol.* 24, 7130–7139.

Koivunen, P., Hirsila, M., Kivirikko, K.I., and Myllyharju, J. (2006). The length of peptide substrates has a marked effect on hydroxylation by the hypoxiainducible factor prolyl 4-hydroxylases. *J. Biol. Chem.* 281, 28712–28720.

Kola I, Landis J. (2004). Can the pharmaceutical industry reduce attrition rates? *Nat. Rev. Drug Discov.* 3, 711-715

Komatsu, M., Kurokawa, H., Waguri, S., Taguchi, K., Kobayashi, A., Ichimura, Y., Sou, Y.S., Ueno, I., Sakamoto, A., Tong, K.I., et al. (2010). The selective autophagy substrate p62 activates the stress responsive transcription factor Nrf2 through inactivation of Keap1. *Nat. Cell Biol.* 12, 213–223.

Landazuri, M.O., Vara-Vega, A., Viton, M., Cuevas, Y., and del Peso, L. (2006). Analysis of HIF-prolyl hydroxylases binding to substrates. *Biochem. Biophys. Res. Commun.* 351, 313–320.

Mikhaylova, O., Ignacak, M.L., Barankiewicz, T.J., Harbaugh, S.V., Yi, Y., Maxwell, P.H., Schneider, M., Van Geyte, K., Carmeliet, P., Revelo, M.P., et al. (2008). The von Hippel-Lindau tumor suppressor protein and Egl-9-Type proline hydroxylases regulate the large subunit of RNA polymerase II in response to oxidative stress. *Mol. Cell. Biol.* 28, 2701–2717.

Moi, P., Chan, K., Asunis, I., Cao, A., and Kan, Y.W. (1994). Isolation of NF-E2- related factor 2 (Nrf2), a NF-E2-like basic leucine zipper transcriptional activator that binds to the tandem NF-E2/AP1 repeat of the beta-globin locus control region. *Proc. Natl. Acad. Sci.* USA 91, 9926–9930.

Moehlenkamp, J.D., and Johnson, J.A. (1999). Activation of antioxidant/electrophile-responsive elements in IMR-32 human neuroblastoma cells. Arch.Biochem. Biophys. 363, 98–106.

Motohashi, H., and Yamamoto, M. (2004). Nrf2-Keap1 defines a physiologically important stress response mechanism. *Trends Mol. Med.* 10, 549–557.

Murray, J.K., Balan, C., Allgeier, A.M., Kasparian, A., Viswanadhan, V., Wilde, C., Allen, J.R., Yoder, S.C., Biddlecome, G., Hungate, R.W., Miranda, L.P. (2010) Dipeptidyl-quinolone derivatives inhibit hypoxia inducible factor-1α prolyl hydroxylases-1, -2, and -3 with altered selectivity. *J Comb Chem.* 12(5), 676-686.

Nangaku, M., Izuhara, Y., Takizawa, S., Yamashita, T., Fujii-Kuriyama, Y., Ohneda, O., Yamamoto, M., van Ypersele de Strihou, C., Hirayama, N., and Miyata, T. (2007). A novel class of prolyl hydroxylase inhibitors induces angiogenesis and exerts organ protection against ischemia. *Arterioscler. Thromb. Vasc. Biol.* 27, 2548–2554.

Price, J.C., Barr, E.W., Hoffart, L.M., Krebs, C., and Bollinger, J.M., Jr. (2005). Kinetic dissection of the catalytic mechanism of taurine:alpha-ketoglutarate dioxygenase (TauD) from Escherichia coli. *Biochemistry* 44, 8138–8147.

Safran, M., Kim, W.Y., O'Connell, F., Flippin, L., Gunzler, V., Horner, J.W., Depinho, R.A., and Kaelin, W.G., Jr. (2006). Mouse model for noninvasive imaging of HIF prolyl hydroxylase activity: assessment of an oral agent that stimulates erythropoietin production. *Proc. Natl. Acad. Sci. USA* 103, 105–110.

Semenza, G.L., Jiang, B.H., Leung, S.W., Passantino, R., Concordet, J.P., Maire, P., and Giallongo, A. (1996). Hypoxia response elements in the aldolase A, enolase 1, and lactate dehydrogenase A gene promoters contain essential binding sites for hypoxia-inducible factor 1. *J. Biol. Chem.* 271, 32529–32537.

Shaw, P., Mead, R., Higginbottom, A., and Barber, S. (2010) Therapeutics for neurological disorders. UK Patent Application #0918626.3 Priority Date 24.10.2008. Publ Date 05.05.2010.

Smirnova, N.A., Rakhman, I., Moroz, N., Basso, M., Payappilly, J., Kazakov, S., Hernandez-Guzman, F., Gaisina, I.N., Kozikowski, A.P., Ratan, R.R., et al. (2010). Utilization of an in vivo reporter for high throughput identification of branched small molecule regulators of hypoxic adaptation. *Chem. Biol.* 17, 380–391.

Smirnova, N.A., Haskew-Layton, R.E., Basso, M., Hushpulian, D.M., Payappilly, J.B., Speer, R.E., Ahn, Y.H., Rakhman, I., Cole, P.A., Pinto, J.T., Ratan, R.R., and Gazaryan, I.G. (2011). Development of neh2-luciferase reporter and its application for high throughput screening and real-time monitoring of nrf2 activators. *Chem Biol 18*, 752-765.

Solomon, E.I., Brunold, T.C., Davis, M.I., Kemsley, J.N., Lee, S.K., Lehnert, N., Neese, F., Skulan, A.J., Yang, Y.S., and Zhou, J. (2000). Geometric and electronic electronic structure/function correlations in non-heme iron enzymes. *Chem. Rev.* 100, 235-350.

Tegley, C.M., Viswanadhan, V.N., Biswas, K., Frohn, M.J., Peterkin, T.A., Chang, C., Bu¨ rli, R.W., Dao, J.H., Veith, H., Rogers, N., et al. (2008). Discovery of novel hydroxy-thiazoles as HIF-alpha prolyl hydroxylase inhibitors: SAR, synthesis, and modeling evaluation. *Bioorg. Med. Chem. Lett.* 18, 3925-3928.

Thompson TN. (2000). Early ADME in support of drug discovery: the role of metabolic stability studies. *Curr. Drug Metab.* 1, 215-241.

Tong, K.I., Katoh, Y., Kusunoki, H., Itoh, K., Tanaka, T., and Yamamoto, M. (2006a). Keap1 recruits Neh2 through binding to ETGE and DLG motifs: characterization of the two-site molecular recognition model. *Mol. Cell. Biol.* 26, 2887-2900.

Tong, K.I., Kobayashi, A., Katsuoka, F., and Yamamoto, M. (2006b). Two-site substrate recognition model for the Keap1-Nrf2 system: a hinge and latch mechanism. *Biol. Chem.* 387, 1311-1320.

Tuckerman, J.R., Zhao, Y., Hewitson, K.S., Tian, Y.M., Pugh, C.W., Ratcliffe, P.J., and Mole, D.R. (2004). Determination and comparison of specific activity of the HIF-prolyl hydroxylases. *FEBS Lett.* 576, 145-150.

Wang, G.L., Jiang, B.H., Rue, E.A., and Semenza, G.L. (1995). Hypoxia-inducible factor 1 is a basic-helix-loop-helix-PAS heterodimer regulated by cellular O2 tension. *Proc. Natl. Acad. Sci. USA* 92, 5510-5514.

Warshakoon, N.C., Wu, S., Boyer, A., Kawamoto, R., Renock, S., Xu, K., Pokross, M., Evdokimov, A.G., Zhou, S., et al. (2006a). Design and synthesis of a series of novel pyrazolopyridines as HIF-1alpha prolyl hydroxylase inhibitors. *Bioorg. Med. Chem. Lett.* 16, 5687-5690.

Warshakoon, N.C., Wu, S., Boyer, A., Kawamoto, R., Sheville, J., Bhatt, R.T., Renock, S., Xu, K., Pokross, M., Zhou, S., et al. (2006b). Design and synthesis of substituted pyridine derivatives as HIF-1alpha prolyl hydroxylase inhibitors. *Bioorg. Med. Chem. Lett.* 16, 5616 5620.

Warshakoon, N.C., Wu, S., Boyer, A., Kawamoto, R., Sheville, J., Renock, S., Xu, K., Pokross, M., Evdokimov, A.G., Walter, R., and Mekel, M. (2006c). A novel series of imidazo[1,2-a]pyridine derivatives as HIF-1alpha prolyl hydroxylase inhibitors. *Bioorg. Med. Chem. Lett.* 16, 5598-5601.

Warshakoon, N.C., Wu, S., Boyer, A., Kawamoto, R., Sheville, J., Renock, S., Xu, K., Pokross, M., Zhou, S., Winter, C., et al. (2006d). Structure-based design, synthesis, and SAR evaluation of a new series of 8-hydroxyquinolines as HIF-1alpha prolyl hydroxylase inhibitors. *Bioorg. Med. Chem. Lett.* 16, 5517-5522.

Wu, J.H., Miao, W., Hu, L.G., and Batist, G. (2010) Identification and characterization of novel Nrf2 inducers designed to target the intervening region of Keap1. *Chem. Biol. Drug Des.* 75, 475-480.

Xie, L., Xiao, K., Whalen, E.J., Forrester, M.T., Freeman, R.S., Fong, G., Gygi, S.P., Lefkowitz, R.J., and Stamler, J.S. (2009). Oxygen-regulated 2-adrenergic receptor hydroxylation by EGLN3 and ubiquitylation by pVHL. *Sci. Signal* 2, 1–10.

Zhang, D.D. (2006). Mechanistic studies of the Nrf2-Keap1 signaling pathway. *Drug Metab. Rev.* 38, 769–789.

Zhang, D.D., Lo, S.C., Cross, J.V., Templeton, D.J., and Hannink, M. (2004). Keap1 is a redox-regulated substrate adaptor protein for a Cul3-dependent ubiquitin ligase complex. *Mol. Cell. Biol.* 24, 10941–10953.

Zhang, Q., Gu, J., Li, L., Liu, J., Luo, B., Cheung, H.W., Boehm, J.S., Ni, M., Geisen, C., Root, D.E., Polyak, K., Brown, M., Richardson, A.L., Hahn, W.C., Kaelin, W.G. Jr, Bommi-Reddy, A. (2009) Control of cyclin D1 and breast tumorigenesis by the EglN2 prolyl hydroxylase. *Cancer Cell* 16(5), 413-24.

Assessment of Cell Cycle Inhibitors by Flow Cytometry

Paolo Cappella and Jürgen Moll
Nerviano Medical Sciences Srl, Nerviano (MI)
Italy

1. Introduction

The main approach used by large pharmaceutical companies for the design of a new drug is based on identifying an initial specific biological target that has been adequately validated. Typically biochemical or cellular assays are used by applying high-throughput screening methods (HTS) to identify hits (HitID) from large chemical libraries in the case of new chemical entities (NCEs) in order to identifying viable parent compounds with pharmacological characteristics.

These compounds are starting points for chemical expansions which result in structure activities relationships (SARs). In the next phase (H2L) identification of a lead compound is the endpoint. Leads are already more drug-like and are expected to have certain activities in a number of biological assays, including cellular assay and hints of in vivo efficacy linked to pharmadynamic biomarker modulation. The optimization of a lead compound (LO phase) are typically properties such as potency and selectivity or activity in animal models, pharmacokinetics (e.g. oral bioavailability). In this phase an initial assessment of toxicological findings and a more systematic investigation in different animal models (e.g. xenograft or transgenic animal models) for demonstrating the therapeutic efficacy performed and ideally result in the selection of the final candidate for potential clinical development (Bleicher et al., 2003).

In the complex process of drug discovery, particularly for inhibitors of the cell cycle, there are two phases in which flow cytometry (FCM) gives major contributions. Firstly, in target validation, in order to demonstrate that inhibition of a specific target determines alteration of the cell cycle, secondly in the usage of cell-based assays in order to characterize compounds to demonstrate that the modulations observed are in line with the expected mechanism of action.

FCM is a major readout the key analysis for studying mechanism of action of drugs that affect proliferation since it is rapid, precise, can be automated with adherent or non-adherent cells.

In this review we want to point out technical and strategic aspects in the cytometric field important for new targeted therapies. In the case where the modulation of a target or treatment with a compound produced, a disturbance in the cell cycle is needed, mono-parametric DNA analysis is recommended, focusing on speed and throughput of samples by automation. Where, instead, the mechanism of action of a drug is the focus of the study, two-parametric analysis such as 5-bromo-deoxyuridine (BrdU) or 5-ethyl-deoxyuridine

(EdU) incorporation is applied (detected by "click chemistry") during the synthesis of DNA can be used.

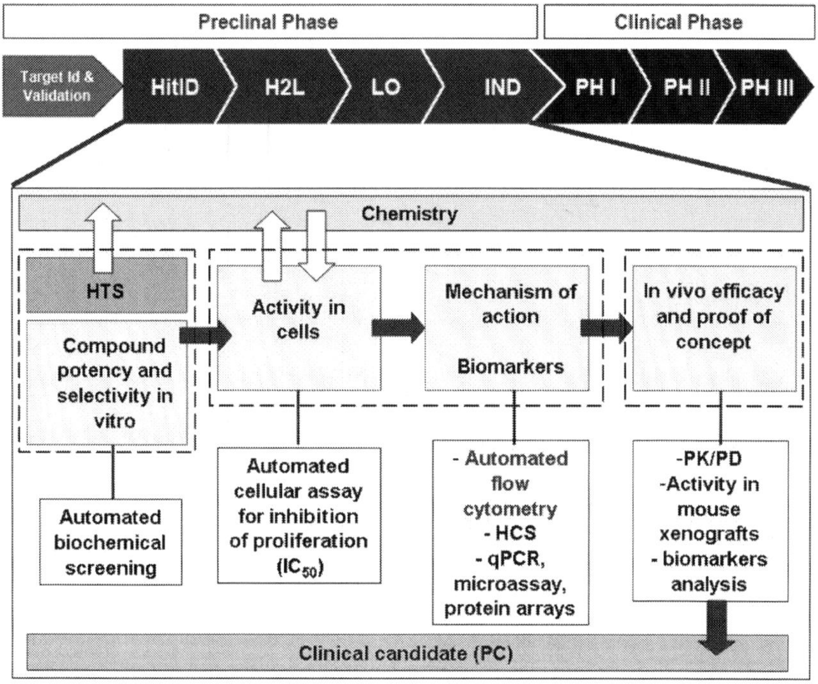

Fig. 1. A typical screening approach used for the identification of small molecule cell cycle inhibitor.

2. Flow cytometry applications for cell cycle analysis

2.1 Mono-parametric analysis of DNA content

Through the use of fluorescent dyes that bind stoichiometrically to DNA such as propidium iodide (PI) the content of cellular DNA can be quantified and the distribution of the cell cycle in a population of asynchronous cells can be determined. After treatment with drugs or SiRNA changes in specific cell cycle stages can be followed.

The profile of DNA content (x-axis, fluorescence of the dye bound to DNA, which is representative of the DNA content and the y-axis, which represents the number of cells) is analyzed using a mathematical model (e.g. Modfit) that determines the percentage of cells in the different phases of the cell cycle. Proliferating cells cycle through three major compartments name by as G1, S-phase and G2/M. The G2 and M phase includes mitosis which contains twice the DNA content before dividing to newborn G1 cells. Fraction of cells with a DNA content below G1 phase, often called "Sub G1" fraction consist of debris and fragmented cells. The degree of polyploidy of cells meaning cells with DNA content higher than G2/M, usually as a result of failure in mitosis.

A typical example is shown in Fig. 2. Human ovarian cancer A2780 cells in exponential growth were analyzed accordingly for their DNA content. Different mechanism of action upon compound treatment can be followed. For example treating A2780 cells in exponential growth with different drugs affecting the cells cycle such as kinase inhibitors show different cell cycle profiles associated with a block before (e.g. CDKs) or after (eg. PLK or Aurora) DNA synthesis (table 1 and Fig. 3).

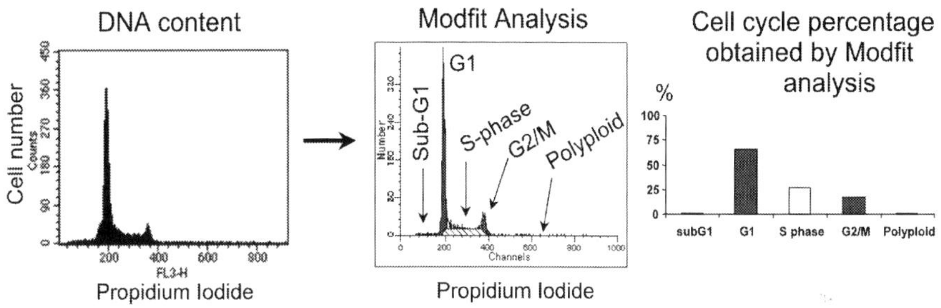

Fig. 2. A2780 cells in exponential growth were analyzed for their DNA content and the percentage of cells in specific stages of the cell cycle percentage was analyzed (X-axis, fluorescence of the dye bound to DNA, representative of the DNA content and y-axis, number of cells to DNA content).

Cell cycle	Small molecule	Major cell cycle phenotype	Reference
G1 and S	CDC-7 kinase inhibitor (PHA-767491), anthracyclins Nemorubicin	Massive cells death detected by sub-G1 due to inhibition of DNA synthesis process	(Albanese et al., 2006; Montagnoli et al., 2008)
	CDKs inhibitor (PHA-848125)	Clear G1 arrest due to CDK inhibition in G1/S transition	(Albanese et al., 2010)
	Camptothecin (irinotecan™, SN-38)	S-phase arrest and cell death	(Cappella et al., 2004)
G2 and M	MPS-1 kinase inhibitor (NMS-P715)	Broad DNA content due to asymmetrical mitosis, cell death by mitotic catastrophe	(Colombo et al., 2010)
	PLK-1 kinase inhibitor (NMS-P937), Eg-5 kinesin spindle protein, Paclitaxel	G2/M arrest due to PLK1 inhibition in mitosis followed by cell death	(Beria et al., 2010; Purcell et al., 2010; Sena et al., 1999)
	Aurora kinase inhibitor (Danusertib™)	Mitotic slippage after G2/M arrest and polyploidy	(Carpinelli et al., 2007; Fancelli et al., 2006)

Table 1. Different cellular phenotypes observed after treatment listed as exemplified for small molecule kinase inhibitors targeting cell cycle kinase or cytotoxic agents.

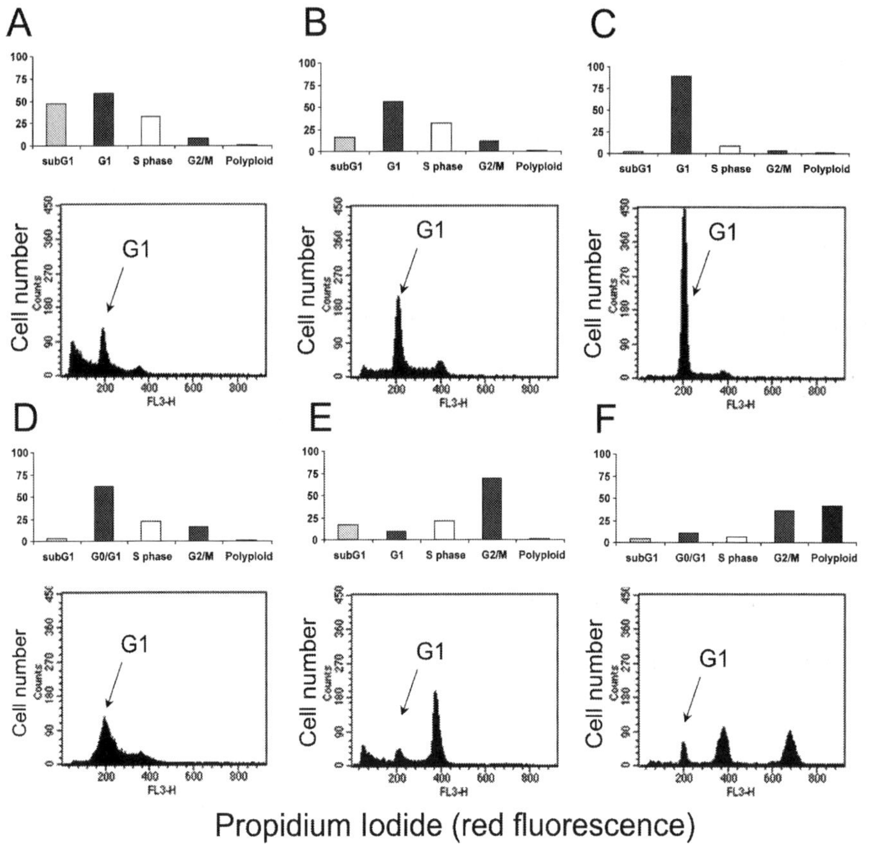

Fig. 3. DNA content and Modfit analysis of A2780 human ovarian cancer cells treated with cell cycle inhibitors at 1μM. A) CDC7 inhibitor NMS-354; B) Nemorubicin; C) CDKs inhibitor PHA-848125; D) MPS1 inhibitor NMS-P715; E) PLK1 inhibitor NMS-P937 and F) Aurora inhibitor Danusertib . DNA content of untreated cells is shown in Fig.2.

For example, Aurora kinase inhibitors such as Danusertib™ results in a specific cell cycle profile due to mitotic slippage that leads to polyploidy. This characteristic cell cycle profile could be used to analyze compound potency and mechanism of action in cells as shown in Fig. 4. Since Aurora kinase inhibitor Danusertib™ was specific on selected kinases panel and not affected G1/S checkpoint (Carpinelli et al., 2007), phenotype changes was related to Aurora A and B inhibition at observed concentrations. In this case, polyploidization process was predominant and the amount of G2/M plus polyploidy cells increased by increasing drug concentration allowing evaluation of ED_{50} by sigmoid model.

Combining ED_{50} by FCM to other mechanism of action bioassay such as antiproliferative and Aurora A and B biochemical assay, these data get compound potency during lead optimization of a putative compound as indicated below.

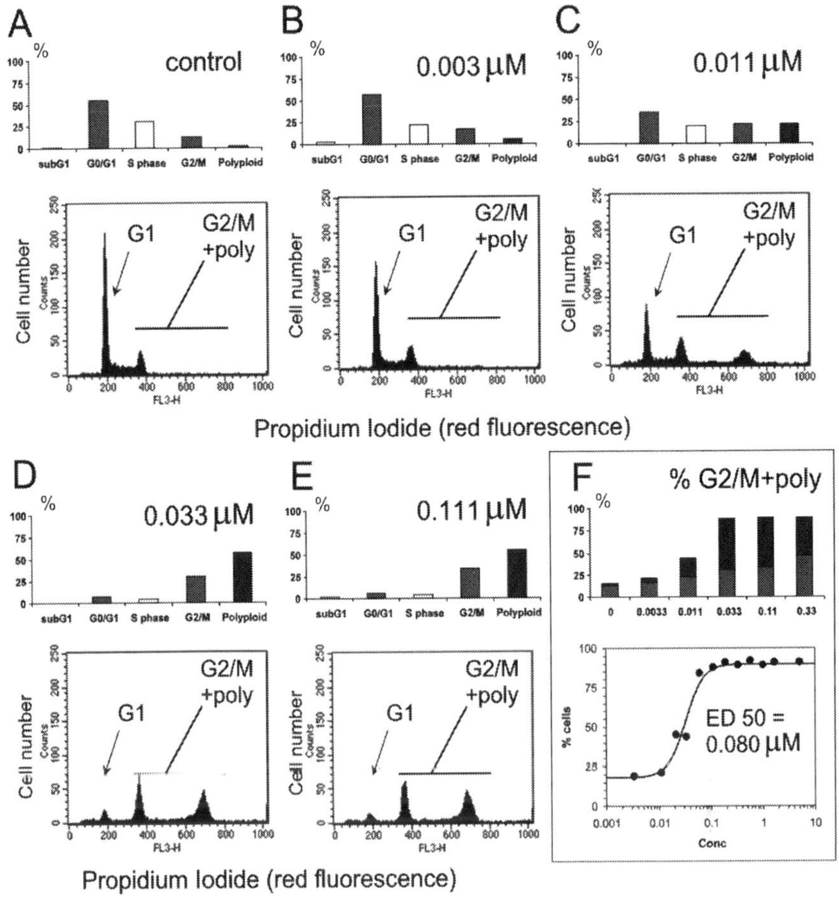

Fig. 4. Human colon cancer HCT-116 cells treated with increasing doses of an Aurora kinase inhibitor. Measurement of cellular potency by counting the number of cells in G2/M or in polyploidy measured by Modfit analysis are shown.

In Fig. 5 we have shown the prototype of classical SAR for cell cycle inhibitor as Aurora inhibitors, pyrrolopyrazole class. Based on this results, compounds endowed with high potency in biochemical and cellular assays as well as acceptable aqueous solubility as showed by compound 5 were selected. Beyond drug discovery, DNA content analysis could be used during target validation process before hit identification.

One of the techniques used for target validation and well established in mammalian cells is to turn off the genes is RNA interference using small interfering RNA (SiRNA) which consist typically of double stranded (21-25mer) oligonucleotides (Colombo & Moll, 2008).

In the outlined experiment, cells were transfected with siRNA and analyzed for up to 72 hours with respect to cell number, colony forming capabilities, DNA content analysis and changes in signal transduction pathways or gene expression pathways.

Cmpd	R′	R″	Aur-A IC_{50}[a]	HCT-116 IC_{50}[b]	HCT-116 FACS ED_{50}[c]
1	H	H	0.13	0.22	0.50
2	F	H	0.009	0.050	0.110
3	OH	H	0.006	0.097	>0.2
4	Me	H	0.024	0.021	0.100
5	**OMe**	**H**	**0.013**	**0.031**	**0.080**

Fig. 5. Structure and Aurora-A Inhibition of substituted-phenylacetyl pyrrolopyrazole.a, Enzyme inhibition IC_{50} μM. b, Antiproliferation IC50 μM. c, FACS ED_{50} evaluated on amount of cells in G2/M and polyploidy. Adapted from (Fancelli et al., 2006) .

In Fig. 6A an example is shown for Eg5 (Purcell et al., 2010) using Eg5 and the corresponding controls to exclude off-target effects.

Since cell lines in culture exhibit different genetic backgrounds, this is reflected in the DNA cell cycle profile after Eg5 siRNA treatment (Fig. 6B). A549 cells are prone to go directly to cell death, while U2-OS cells were blocked in G2/M and H1299 cells became polyploidy.

One dimensional DNA content analysis by FCM is a powerful tool to study the cell cycle as shown for mitotic checkpoints. However it also has its limitations, with respect to resolution and separation of cell cycle stages, in particular for S-phase, if there is a block in DNA synthesis. For this purpose, a second dimension is needed by using BrdU incorporation as readout.

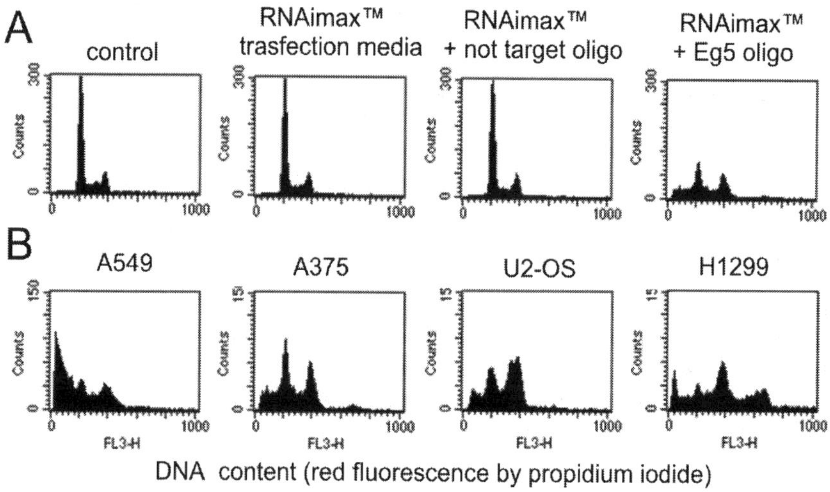

Fig. 6. A. Small RNA interference experiment in A549 cells treated for 72 hrs with 20nM Eg5 oligo, in comparison to not transfected or transfected with a non target oligo. B. Cellular phenotypes observed after RNAi experiments in different cell type;

2.2 DNA CONTENT and Bromo-deoxyuridine (BrdU)

The visualization and quantification of cells actively synthesizing DNA is important for studying the cellular response to drug treatments.

Historically for cell proliferation, incorporation of [$_3$H]-thymidine analogue was used to follow the DNA synthesis (labelling index). The use of radioisotopes ($_3$H β-emitter with a half-life of 12 years) and β-counters is a drawback of this method and technically difficult to analyze.

In 1982, an antibody against 5-bromo-deoxyuridine, BrdU was introduced, capable of binding the labelled DNA as a result of partial denaturation and use of [$_3$H]- labelled thymidine was gradually abandoned in the late 80's after the introduction of BrdU in FCM.

Several methods have been applied to measure the incorporation of BrdU with a need to denature DNA, since only upon denaturising of the double helix, or at least the introduction of specific DNA breaks, where BrdU had been introduced during the synthesis, made recognition by monoclonal anti-BrdU possible (Leif et al., 2004).

This step is the most critical and is achieved by different methods:

1. Heat treatment from 90-100 ° C for 10 min in low ionic strength solutions after partial extraction of histones. This method is less used nowadays because it needs optimization in different cell lines and is particularly destructive to the morphology and cellular constituents. However since DNA denaturation can be performed in 96 wells plate by programmable heater such as PCR apparatus, this method is particular used for HTS applications (Cappella et al., 2010) .
2. Acid or alkali treatments, followed by a neutralization step (Leif et al., 2004). The denaturation of DNA can be varied with time, only partially allowing the use of DNA probes staining such as propidium iodide (PI) , 7-aminoactynomycin D, TOPRO-3, which interacts DNA requiring double helix conformation. The use of acid denaturation may not be the most appropriate method if it is necessary to maintain cellular (scatters) morphology, surface antigenicity or cell constituents such as cyclins (Faretta et al., 1998) or phosphorylation of signaling proteins (Gasparri et al., 2006) during multiparameter analysis.
3. Enzymatic treatment with DNase I / exonuclease III against A-T hypersensitive enzyme sites by digestion at 37 ° C of generate single stranded DNA to exposure incorporated BrdU to monoclonal antibody. This method has proved to be of particular interest for its ability to maintain antigenicity and morphology, allowing to follow additional cellular parameter such as cell signalling events (Gasparri et al., 2006).

Additional methods were reported in the literature using treatment with high-energy radiation for the generation of DNA breaks by photolysis followed by anti-BrdU antibody (Leif et al., 2006).

Regardless of the denaturation method, BrdU incorporation and DNA staining is an accurate method to determinate the cell cycle phase as showed in Fig. 6. Cell cycle analysis by mathematic modelling (Jourdan et al., 2002) by fitting software (e.g,. Modfit™) usually underestimates percentage of cells in S-phase, since G1 and G2/M peaks are fitted by a gaussian model and early and late S-phase are included inside fitted peaks.

An example demonstrating this difference is shown in Fig.7 using the different methods with HCT-116 colon cancer cells, which show 30% vs. 43% of cells in S-phase, depended from the method used.

As explained for Fig. 8A and B, BrdU analysis allows to distinguish and quantify if there is an arrest in DNA synthesis, in which part of S phase and it is possible to separate early S-phase from G1 or late S-phase from G2/M (Cappella et al., 2001).

This advantage is demonstrated in Fig.8A, where HCT116 cells were treated with SN-38, a topoisomerase inhibitor which affects DNA replication. Only by analyzing BrdU incorporation was it possible to detect delays in early (gate E) or late (gate L) S-phase upon SN-38 treatment at 7h (Fig.8B).

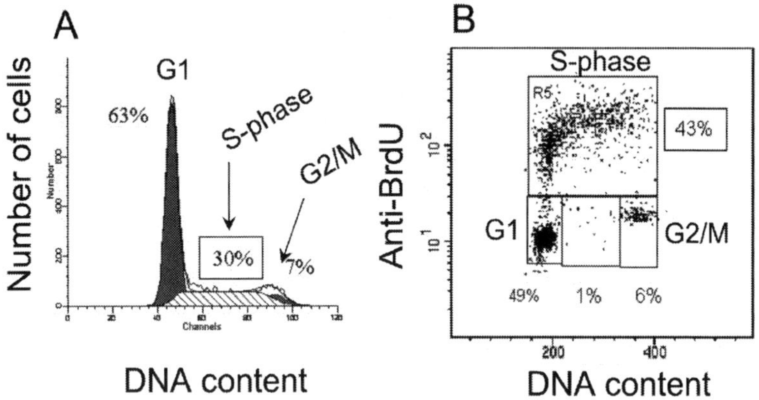

Fig. 7. Profile of DNA content and BrdU incorporation in the same sample. A, DNA content was analyzed by Modfit analysis or B, DNA content by PI (x-axis) and BrdU incorporation (y-axis)

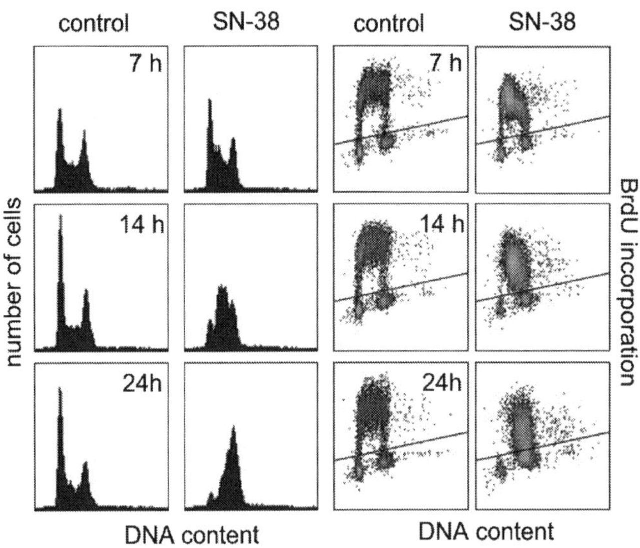

Fig. 8A. Profile of DNA content and BrdU incorporation of HCT-116 cells treated with SN-38 at 10nM for 7, 16 and 24hrs. DNA content by PI (x-axis) and BrdU incorporation (y-axis) are shown. Cells above the line define BrdU positive cells.

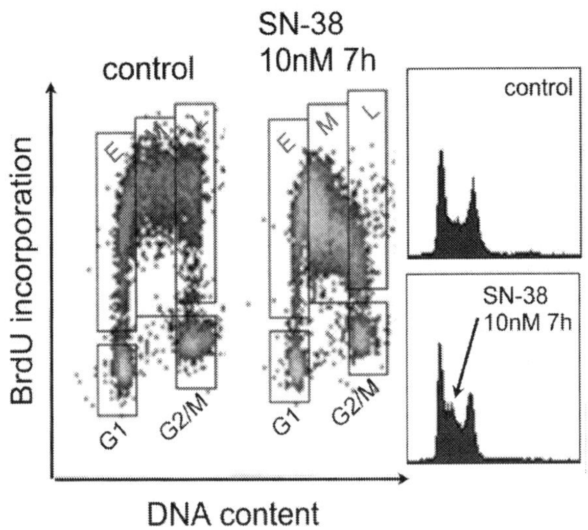

Fig. 8B. BrdU incorporation of HCT-116 cells treated with SN-38 at 10nM for 7h. Gates were set at E, early S-phase; M, middle S-phase; and L, late S-phase. The corresponding DNA content profiles are shown. Arrow indicated impossibility to detect early effects on DNA synthesis. DNA content is quantified by PI (x-axis) and BrdU incorporation (y-axis) by BrdU antibodies staining.

Another advantage is that BrdU incorporation can be performed either *in vitro* or *in vivo*. In Fig. 9 we show an *ex-vivo* analysis of mice bearing HCT-116 xenograft tumors which received intravenous injections of a single dose of irinotecan (60 mg/kg) (Ciomei et al., 2007). After drug administration, BrdU was injected intraperitoneally 2 hours before, and mice were sacrificed. Tumors were removed and disaggregated by pepsin (Terry & White, 2001). By this approach, it was possible to detect cell cycle perturbations of the drug.

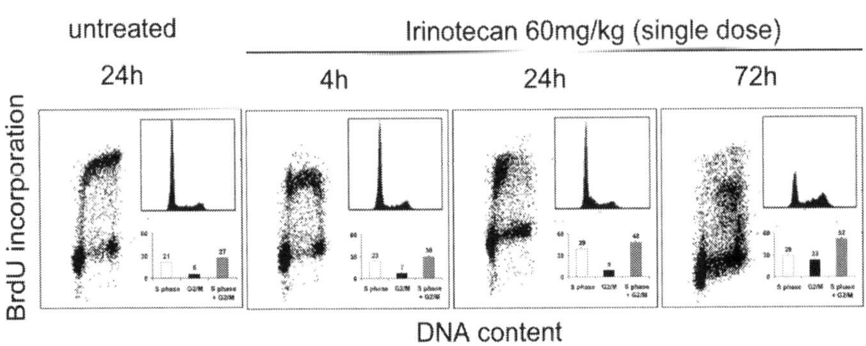

Fig. 9. BrdU incorporation (dot plots) in enzymatically disaggregated HCT-116 tumor cells treated with irinotecan. Cell-cycle profiles (DNA histograms) and percentages of cells in S-phase and/or G2/M are shown as inlets.

Since this drug acted on early DNA replication, initially a delay of G1/S phase (till 24h) was observed whereas at later time points an arrest in S phase and G2/M was more evident. Moreover since DNA synthesis is blocked and cells started to die, BrdU incorporation was abrogated (Cappella et al., 2004).
More recently BrdU incorporation was used for cell sorting of mammalian cells during DNA replication for CGH microarray analysis and for genome-scale analysis of replication timing (Ryba et al., 2011).

2.3 DNA CONTENT and BrdU by click chemistry

Although there is a plethora of methods for the analysis of BrdU incorporation, the major drawbacks are the difficulties related to their full use in the analysis of multi-color FCM and traditional imaging. Thermal denaturation destroys almost all of the antigens and denaturation with "chemicals" such as acids or bases makes the analysis of several antigens impossible (Frank et al., 1995) and therefore alternative methods are needed. In 2001, the term "click chemistry" was coined by Nobel Prize Sharpless to describe reactions with defined criteria and of the most popular reaction that fully meets these criteria is the 1,3-dipolar cycloaddition, also known as the Cu-Catalyzed Azide Alkyne Cycloaddition (CuAAC) between an azide and a terminal alkyne forming a triazole by copper (I) as catalyst (Fig.10) . These systems are very rare in nature and are inert in biological systems and thus particularly important in the "bio-orthogonal" approach where a substrate containing a chemical reporter is introduced in a target (i.e. proteins, sugars, DNA) *in vivo* and then identified by a covalent reaction with a fluorescent probe (Prescher & Bertozzi, 2005).

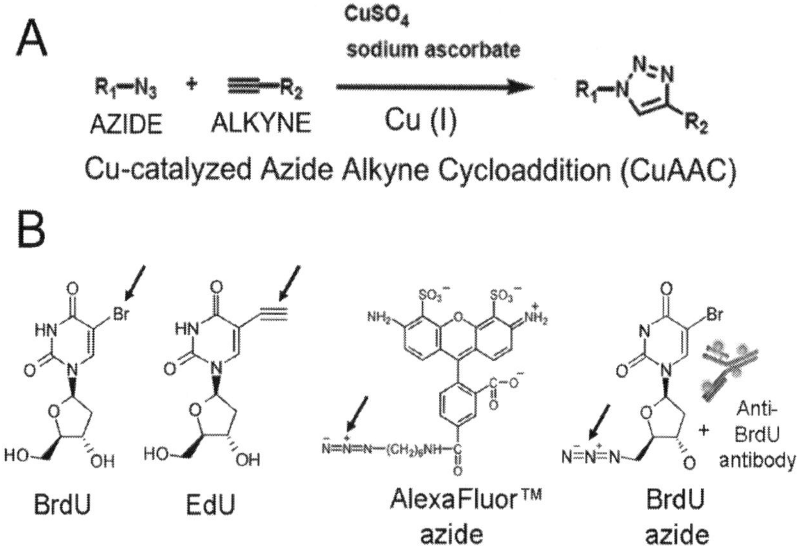

Fig. 10. A) Generic schema for Cu-Catalyzed Azide Alkyne Cycloaddition (CuAAC) between an azide and a terminal alkyne forming a triazole by copper (I), B) Players of bio-orthogonal approach for cell cycle analysis.

It is the case of EdU (5-ethynyl-2′-deoxyuridine) used instead of BrdU for DNA synthesis analysis in FCM. EdU is incorporated into the replication forks of new DNA during S-phase; exposed alkynyl residues can be identified with "click chemistry" reaction using fluorescent azides (AlexaFluor™ 488 Click-IT assay supply by Invitrogen Corp) in presence of copper (I) and cells could be visualized (Darzynkiewicz et al., 2011). One modification of this assay is by replacing dye azide, with a BrdU azide and to detect by BrdU antibody (Fig. 11). As with BrdU, EdU incorporation can also be used *in vivo*. Application and use of this approach is particularly useful in screening compounds that alter the cell cycle when multiparametric readout are needed such as HCS. In this case mild condition for cell treatment is a must in order to conserve antigenic properties and cellular integrity (Cappella et al., 2008).

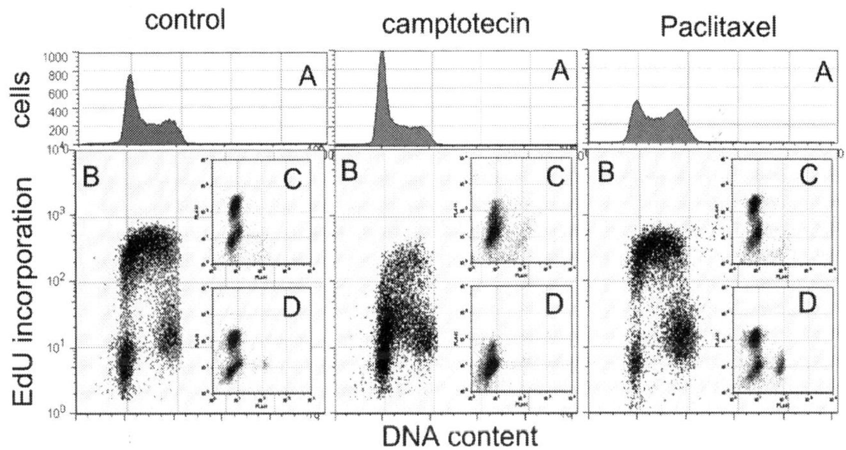

Fig. 11. EdU incorporation as example of multi parametric analysis. Cells were treated with camptotecin or paclitaxel and stained with PI or with corresponding antibodies. A, cell-cycle profiles; B, EdU incorporation and DNA content; C, EdU and cleaved caspase 3; D, EdU and phospho-histone H3 (Cappella et al., 2008).

2.4 DNA CONTENT and sample throughput

Cell cycle analysis by FCM and BrdU incorporation is one of the most powerful techniques to quantitatively distinguish cell cycle phase after treatments, however, high throughput is limited, since most mammalian cells in tissue culture require cell detachment from culture disks. Traditionally, FCM is limited to small-scale laboratory and clinical studies and high throughput methods have recently been developed for drug discovery. Hand-free automations and the introduction of 96 well plate autosamplers have increased throughput capabilities in mammalian or plant cell (Cappella et al., 2010) (Cousin et al., 2009).

Advancements in high throughput FCM have been implemented following the introduction of BD "Multiwell Autosampler" MAS™ and HTS™ , or efficient micro fluidic devices such as "plug-FCM" systems HyperCyt™ have been introduced and whereas traditional autosamplers load samples as single entities, automated sampling systems for FCM allowed individual samples to be assayed sequentially (Black et al., 2010).

Percentages of cells are usually analyzed using appropriate gates. When large numbers of data are generated, in order to visualize the results for an easy readout (Lugli et al., 2010), data can be displayed with cluster software (e.g.Spotfire™) generating heat maps. An example is the profiling of compounds in BrdU experiments regarding percentage of BrdU positive cells, percentage of S-Phase cells and G2/M cells (Fig.12) as derived by Modfit™ analysis from DNA content analysis after drug exposures (Cappella et al., 2010).
Moreover, very recently additional analyses are borrowed from the proteomics and bioinformatics approach. These involve subject classification by principal component analysis (PCA) (Lugli et al., 2007), hierarchical clustering for discovering novel building blocks for imaging probes (Shedden & Rosania, 2010) or scalable analysis (Klinke & Brundage, 2009) using appropriate bioinformatics tools.

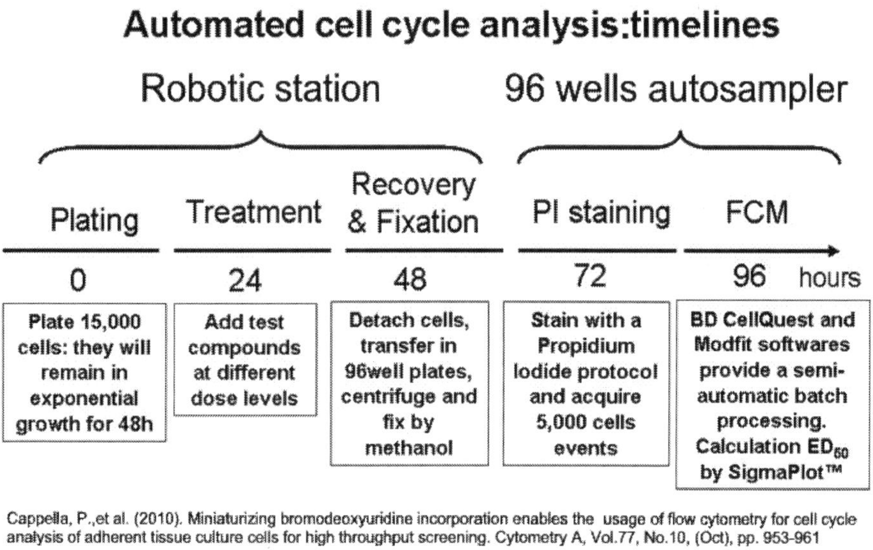

Fig. 12. Example of cell cycle analysis timelines using lab automation.

3. Conclusion

Numerous drugs in oncology affect the cell cycle and therefore cell cycle analysis by FCM is the primary method of choice for measuring compound potency, selectivity or mechanism of action. Most anticancer drugs directly affect cellular proliferation, and their inhibitory effects usually depend on dose and treatment time. Research activities in drugs affecting mitosis, gave characteristic cellular phenotype, and FCM allowed to monitor apoptosis, mitotic arrest, polyploidization or aneuploidy , generating "compound activity fingerprints" useful for mechanism of action studies. The introduction of halogenated nucleotides such as BrdU, or "click chemistry" by EdU has revolutionized the study of cell proliferation.

Moving from tube-based to plate based readout and the recent development of semi automated techniques for staining and analyzing FCM samples has created new challenges. Finally advanced data visualization and analysis such as heat maps has boosted analytical capabilities, necessary for high throughput FCM which can generate very complex datasets.
In this paper we reviewed state-of-the-art DNA analysis for cell cycle studies *in vitro* as *in vivo* and new technologies are emerging ("new-flow methods") which will further facilitate and optimize future analysis.

4. Acknowledgment

Clara Albanese as a part of FCM Unit contributed for critical reading and for *in vivo* experiments. We thank Laura Giorgini and Riccardo Colombo for their practical and theoretical contributions and critical input. The authors as member of target validation team for SiRNA experiments. Authors thank Maurizio Pulici as a part of chemistry department for Aurora project.

5. References

Albanese, C., Alzani, R., Amboldi, N., Avanzi, N., et al. (2010). Dual targeting of CDK and tropomyosin receptor kinase families by the oral inhibitor PHA-848125, an agent with broad-spectrum antitumor efficacy. *Mol Cancer Ther*, Vol.9, No.8, (Aug), pp. 2243-2254, 1538-8514 (Electronic)1535-7163 (Linking)

Albanese, C., Geroni, C., & Ciomei, M. (2006). Nemorubicin and its bioactivation product, PNU-159682, block cell cycle and induce massive apoptosis differently from doxorubicin. *Proceedings of the American Association for Cancer Research*, Vol.2006, No.1, pp. 1096,

Beria, I., Ballinari, D., Bertrand, J.A., Borghi, D., et al. (2010). Identification of 4,5-dihydro-1H-pyrazolo[4,3-h]quinazoline derivatives as a new class of orally and selective Polo-like kinase 1 inhibitors. *J Med Chem*, Vol.53, No.9, (May 13), pp. 3532-3551, 1520-4804 (Electronic)0022-2623 (Linking)

Black, C.B., Duensing, T.D., Trinkle, L.S., & Dunlay, R.T. (2010). Cell-based screening using high-throughput flow cytometry. *Assay Drug Dev Technol*, Vol.9, No.1, (Feb), pp. 13-20, 1557-8127 (Electronic)1540-658X (Linking)

Bleicher, K.H., Bohm, H.J., Muller, K., & Alanine, A.I. (2003). Hit and lead generation: beyond high-throughput screening. *Nat Rev Drug Discov*, Vol.2, No.5, (May), pp. 369-378, 1474-1776 (Print)1474-1776 (Linking)

Cappella, P., Albanese, C., Patton, V.A., Alzani, R., et al. (2004). Effect of edotecarin on cell cycle progression and apoptosis induction in HCT-116 human colon carcinoma model. *Proceedings of the American Association for Cancer Research*, Vol.2004, No.1, pp. 882,

Cappella, P., Gasparri, F., Pulici, M., & Moll, J. (2008). Cell proliferation method: click chemistry based on BrdU coupling for multiplex antibody staining. *Curr Protoc Cytom*, Vol.Chapter 7, (Jul), pp. Unit7 34, 1934-9300 (Electronic) 1934-9297 (Linking)

Cappella, P., Giorgini, M.L., Ernestina Re, C., Ubezio, P., et al. (2010). Miniaturizing bromodeoxyuridine incorporation enables the usage of flow cytometry for cell cycle analysis of adherent tissue culture cells for high throughput screening. *Cytometry A*, Vol.77, No.10, (Oct), pp. 953-961, 1552-4930 (Electronic) 1552-4922 (Linking)

Cappella, P., Tomasoni, D., Faretta, M., Lupi, M., et al. (2001). Cell cycle effects of gemcitabine. *Int J Cancer*, Vol.93, No.3, (Aug 1), pp. 401-408, 0020-7136 (Print) 0020-7136 (Linking)

Carpinelli, P., Ceruti, R., Giorgini, M.L., Cappella, P., et al. (2007). PHA-739358, a potent inhibitor of Aurora kinases with a selective target inhibition profile relevant to cancer. *Mol Cancer Ther*, Vol.6, No.12 Pt 1, (Dec), pp. 3158-3168, 1535-7163 (Print) 1535-7163 (Linking)

Ciomei, M., Croci, V., Stellari, F., Amboldi, N., et al. (2007). Antitumor activity of edotecarin in breast carcinoma models. *Cancer Chemother Pharmacol*, Vol.60, No.2, (Jul), pp. 229-235, 0344-5704 (Print) 0344-5704 (Linking)

Colombo, R., Caldarelli, M., Mennecozzi, M., Giorgini, M.L., et al. (2010). Targeting the mitotic checkpoint for cancer therapy with NMS-P715, an inhibitor of MPS1 kinase. *Cancer Res*, Vol.70, No.24, (Dec 15), pp. 10255-10264, 1538-7445 (Electronic) 0008-5472 (Linking)

Colombo, R., & Moll, J. (2008). Target validation to biomarker development: focus on RNA interference. *Mol Diagn Ther*, Vol.12, No.2, pp. 63-70, 1177-1062 (Print) 1177-1062 (Linking)

Cousin, A., Heel, K., Cowling, W.A., & Nelson, M.N. (2009). An efficient high-throughput flow cytometric method for estimating DNA ploidy level in plants. *Cytometry A*, Vol.75, No.12, (Dec), pp. 1015-1019, 1552-4930 (Electronic) 1552-4922 (Linking)

Darzynkiewicz, Z., Traganos, F., Zhao, H., Halicka, H.D., et al. (2011). Cytometry of DNA replication and RNA synthesis: Historical perspective and recent advances based on "click chemistry". *Cytometry A*, Vol.79, No.5, (May), pp. 328-337, 1552-4930 (Electronic) 1552-4922 (Linking)

Fancelli, D., Moll, J., Varasi, M., Bravo, R., et al. (2006). 1,4,5,6-tetrahydropyrrolo[3,4-c]pyrazoles: identification of a potent Aurora kinase inhibitor with a favorable antitumor kinase inhibition profile. *J Med Chem*, Vol.49, No.24, (Nov 30), pp. 7247-7251, 0022-2623 (Print) 0022-2623 (Linking)

Faretta, M., Bergamaschi, D., Taverna, S., Ronzoni, S., et al. (1998). Characterization of cyclin B1 expression in human cancer cell lines by a new three-parameter BrdUrd/cyclin B1/DNA analysis. *Cytometry*, Vol.31, No.1, (Jan 1), pp. 53-59, 0196-4763 (Print) 0196-4763 (Linking)

Frank, J.D., Manfre, P.D., & Cartwright, M.E. (1995). Effects of Denaturation Agents on Antigenic Expression and Levels of Nonspecific Background Staining for 5-Bromo-2-Deoxyuridine Immunohistochemistry. *Journal of Histotechnology*, Vol.18, No.4, pp. 301-306, 0147-8885

Gasparri, F., Cappella, P., & Galvani, A. (2006). Multiparametric cell cycle analysis by automated microscopy. *J Biomol Screen*, Vol.11, No.6, (Sep), pp. 586-598, 1087-0571 (Print) 1087-0571 (Linking)

Jourdan, M.L., Ferrero-Pous, M., Spyratos, F., Romain, S., et al. (2002). Flow cytometric S-phase fraction measurement in breast carcinoma: Influence of software and histogram resolution. *Cytometry*, Vol.48, No.2, (Jun 1), pp. 66-70, 0196-4763 (Print) 0196-4763 (Linking)

Klinke, D.J., 2nd, & Brundage, K.M. (2009). Scalable analysis of flow cytometry data using R/Bioconductor. *Cytometry A*, Vol.75, No.8, (Aug), pp. 699-706, 1552-4930 (Electronic)1552-4922 (Linking)

Leif, R.C., Stein, J.H., & Zucker, R.M. (2004). A short history of the initial application of anti-5-BrdU to the detection and measurement of S phase. *Cytometry A*, Vol.58, No.1, (Mar), pp. 45-52, 1552-4922 (Print) 1552-4922 (Linking)

Leif, R.C., Vallarino, L.M., Becker, M.C., & Yang, S. (2006). Increasing the luminescence of lanthanide complexes. *Cytometry Part A*, Vol.69, No.8, pp. 767-778, 1552-4930

Lugli, E., Pinti, M., Nasi, M., Troiano, L., et al. (2007). Subject classification obtained by cluster analysis and principal component analysis applied to flow cytometric data. *Cytometry A*, Vol.71, No.5, (May), pp. 334-344, 1552-4922 (Print) 1552-4922 (Linking)

Lugli, E., Roederer, M., & Cossarizza, A. (2010). Data analysis in flow cytometry: the future just started. *Cytometry A*, Vol.77, No.7, (Jul), pp. 705-713, 1552-4930 (Electronic) 1552-4922 (Linking)

Montagnoli, A., Valsasina, B., Croci, V., Menichincheri, M., et al. (2008). A Cdc7 kinase inhibitor restricts initiation of DNA replication and has antitumor activity. *Nat Chem Biol*, Vol.4, No.6, (Jun), pp. 357-365, 1552-4469 (Electronic) 1552-4450 (Linking)

Prescher, J.A., & Bertozzi, C.R. (2005). Chemistry in living systems. *Nat Chem Biol*, Vol.1, No.1, (Jun), pp. 13-21, 1552-4450 (Print) 1552-4450 (Linking)

Purcell, J.W., Davis, J., Reddy, M., Martin, S., et al. (2010). Activity of the kinesin spindle protein inhibitor ispinesib (SB-715992) in models of breast cancer. *Clin Cancer Res*, Vol.16, No.2, (Jan 15), pp. 566-576, 1078-0432 (Print) 1078-0432 (Linking)

Ryba, T., Battaglia, D., Pope, B.D., Hiratani, I., et al. (2011). Genome-scale analysis of replication timing: from bench to bioinformatics. *Nat Protoc*, Vol.6, No.6, (Jun), pp. 870-895, 1750-2799 (Electronic) 1750-2799 (Linking)

Sena, G., Onado, C., Cappella, P., Montalenti, F., et al. (1999). Measuring the complexity of cell cycle arrest and killing of drugs: kinetics of phase-specific effects induced by taxol. *Cytometry*, Vol.37, No.2, (Oct 1), pp. 113-124, 0196-4763 (Print) 0196-4763 (Linking)

Shedden, K., & Rosania, G.R. (2010). Chemical address tags of fluorescent bioimaging probes. *Cytometry A*, Vol.77, No.5, (May), pp. 429-438, 1552-4930 (Electronic)1552-4922 (Linking)

Terry, N.H., & White, R.A. (2001). Cell cycle kinetics estimated by analysis of bromodeoxyuridine incorporation. *Methods Cell Biol*, Vol.63, pp. 355-374, 0091-679X (Print) 0091-679X (Linking)

14

Image-Based High-Content Screening in Drug Discovery

Marjo Götte and Daniela Gabriel
Novartis Institutes for BioMedical Research, Basle, Switzerland

1. Introduction

Immunofluorescence microscopy is a powerful tool for the detection of multiple changes in single cells at sub-cellular level. During the last 10-15 years, confocal and wide-field microscopy have evolved from tedious small scale experiments to medium- or even high-throughput technologies, under the name of high-content screening (HCS). Sample preparation and image acquisition have been automated and several software applications are available for image analysis to obtain quantitative information from the cells. In academia HCS is mainly used in siRNA and cDNA screens to identify genes and proteins involved in specific pathways and processes (Blackmore et al., 2010; Neumann et al., 2010; Pelkmans et al., 2005 as examples). siRNA screens are performed also in pharmaceutical companies for target identification. In addition, in pharmaceutical industry HCS has been adopted as an enabling technology for compound profiling, compound development, secondary screening and even full-deck primary screening (Guzi et al., 2011; Ibig-Rehm et al., 2011; Li et al., 2003; Nadanaciva et al., 2011; Simonen & Gabriel, 2008). The field is still rapidly evolving and new automated cell imagers are coming to the market as well as novel software for image analysis. HCS provides vast amounts of data from each sample and even from each individual cell. During the last years various programs to analyze this data in a multiparametric way have been developed (Gorenstein et al., 2010; Kümmel et al., 2011, Neumann et al., 2010).
Below, the benefits of HCS technology for primary hit finding and secondary screening experiments are discussed. In addition, the technical requirements for high- and medium throughput, the challenges in plate preparation and imaging, image and data analysis and data management are outlined. Examples are provided how to use HCS in primary hit finding campaigns, as well as its use in sophisticated lower-throughput assays using primary cells to generate added value.

2. What are the benefits of high-content screening

Biochemical screens for drug candidates utilize purified proteins in very reductionist assays with the benefit that the compounds can act directly on the target. However, some proteins may not be purified being in their native conformation, sometimes only the catalytic domain of the protein is used in the assay due to problems of producing the full-length protein, and the substrates are often artificial. When a protein functions in a multiprotein complex it might be difficult or impossible to produce all the subunits and to assemble them in an active complex. Sometimes all the components contributing to a cellular reaction are not even known. Typically biochemical screens are performed to identify inhibitors of kinases, proteases, enzymes and protein-protein interactions.

In cellular assays exploiting genetically non-manipulated cells all the components needed for a reaction are usually present, properly assembled and in physiologically correct stoichiometric relations. However, in cellular screens marker or reporter constructs are often used in cells over-expressing the target. In reporter gene assays (RGAs) the readout is usually indirect and can be far downstream of the actual target. Often reporter genes are not in their natural environment in the genome, and they may contain incomplete regulatory regions. Therefore, RGAs are prone to pick up unspecific compounds. Other cellular screening formats for G protein-coupled receptors (GPCRs) like Ca^{2+} flux assays, homogeneous ELISA assays, bioluminescence resonance energy transfer (BRET) and the numerous luminescence-based assays for cell viability and toxicity are robust, easy and fast to perform. Nevertheless, they provide information about a single parameter only, whereas sub-cellular imaging is able to deliver more content. Multiple parameters like cytoplasm shape, size, area, as well as information about nuclear intensity, size, and shape in addition to the target-specific fluorescence readouts can deliver various insights of the compound's mode of action and unspecific effects early on.

In addition to increased content, another benefit of HCS is to enable screening with assays that were earlier impossible in high throughput, such as trafficking of proteins within cells or morphological changes. Sophisticated image analysis in HCS provides more information from the hits than the traditional screens, cytotoxicity being only one additional feature obtained in HCS assays. HCS enables screening for pathways and phenomena without having a specific target in mind, thereby allowing identification of novel targets. Typical examples of phenotypic screens are stimulation of neurite outgrowth, neuronal survival, autophagy or muscle growth. As in standard cellular screens, also in HCS often genetically manipulated cells are used, but HCS assays can be performed with non-manipulated or primary cells by analyzing changes in endogenously expressed cellular components, which makes the assays physiologically more relevant. Compared to traditional biochemical and cellular screening assays HCS is still slower and usually non-homogeneous. Washing steps are generally required in the staining process and image acquisition takes longer than reading fluorescence or luminescence with plate readers, making HCS more time-consuming and expensive.

We have compared variability and sensitivity of HCS and RGA for the screening of inhibitors for PI3K - Akt - Foxo3A pathway. Both assays were equally reproducible, but the HCS assay had a better statistical quality. The HCS assay was more sensitive than the RGA although it was not able to identify additional chemical scaffolds as hits (Unterreiner et al., 2009). However, this study represents only one HCS assay and one RGA, and the picture might change when comparing more assays.

Since 2005 we have used HCS in primary and secondary screening in numerous projects with varying biology and assay set up. Being convinced about the power of HCS we have recently started to perform also full-deck (>1 million compounds) primary screening with the HCS technology.

3. Technical aspects of HCS

3.1 Cells

Not all cells are equally suited for HCS due to the requirements of microscopic images and image analysis. Large cells, not clumping or growing on top of each other are best suited for automated image analysis. The U-2 OS osteosarcoma cells are an example of a cell line well suited for automated image analysis: The nuclei are well separated from each other allowing determination of the accurate cell number, and the cytoplasm of U-2 OS cells is large enabling sub-cellular image analysis (Fig. 1). HEK293 cells, derived from human embryonic kidney cells, are commonly used in cell biology and in cellular screening, but due to their small size they are less suited for sub-cellular analysis. In small-scale experiments high-resolution objectives might be used, therefore the size of the cells does not limit the experiments as much as in higher throughput assays.

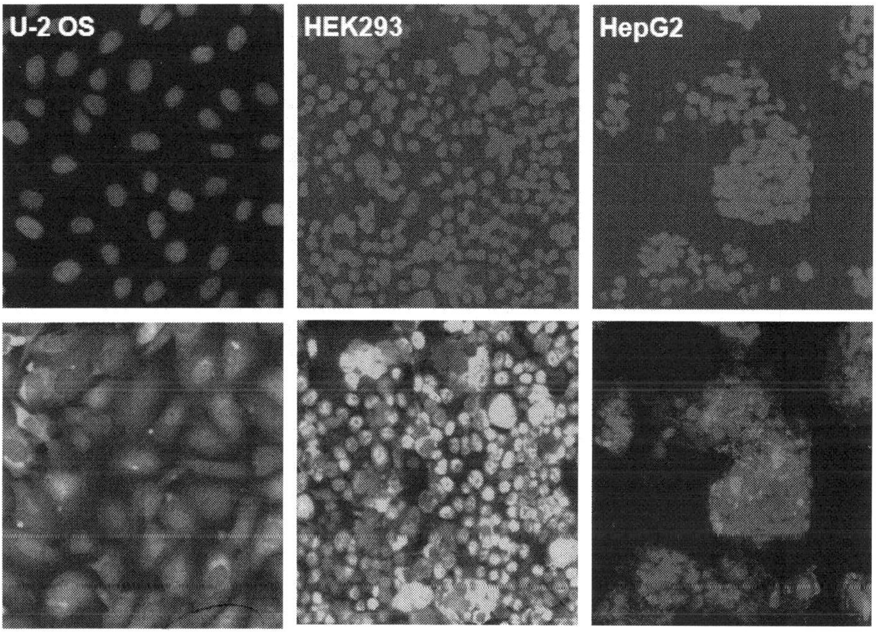

Fig. 1. Examples of some commonly used cell lines with different suitability for HCS. All images are in the same scale and were acquired with IN Cell Analyzer 3000 using the 40x objective. The upper panel images show nuclei stained with different dyes: U-2 OS, red: DRAQ5; HEK293 and HepG2, blue: Hoechst 33342. In the lower panel overlay images are shown using the respective nuclear stain and U-2 OS, green: GFP fusion to a cytoplasmic protein; HEK293, green: cytoplasmic/nuclear protein stained with an antibody; and HepG2, pink: surface receptor stained with an antibody.

For automated image analysis, the cells need to be well separated in order to normalize the signal to cell number to account for changes in cell density by batch to batch variation. Some cells, such as the commonly used hepatocellular carcinoma HepG2 cells, are clumping and it is difficult to determine the cell number based on the nuclear stain. In addition, the HepG2 cells are small in size (Fig. 1). Suspension cells are also not well suited for HCS due to the potential loss of cells by the washing steps of staining processes. In addition, suspension cells are small allowing measurement of changes in fluorescence intensity but analysis of any sub-cellular compartment is hardly feasible. However, depending on the biology, we have used sometimes also small, clumping and even suspension cells in HCS. In these cases the available readouts in image analysis were limited, but by evaluating different methods to stain the cells and to analyze the images acceptable and satisfactory results could be achieved.

Not only established or recombinant cell lines, but also primary cells, as well as embryonic and induced pluripotent stem cells can be used in HCS assays. The benefit of using genetically non-manipulated cells is that the relevant components of the pathway studied are expressed endogenously at proper expression levels and regulated in an authentic way. Fusion of the target to a fluorescent protein, however, is very convenient in HCS assays, since antibody staining can be omitted. Very often transiently or stably transfected cells are used, whereby the expression and regulation of the fusion protein is at least partly under the control of non-natural elements. Creating knock-in cells, where the fusion protein or the marker is in the natural position in the genome most closely mirrors the endogenous expression and regulation. Generation of cells with disease-relevant mutations with this technique provides excellent cell models for screening (Nilles & London, 2007). Until now most of the cells generated with this approach are either cancer cell lines or of mouse origin. However, the technology for induced pluripotent cells is advancing rapidly, making differentiated human cells with natural disease-relevant mutations available (Park et al., 2008).

3.1.1 Live cell analysis versus fixed cells

For kinetic studies living cells are obviously needed. Several large time-lapse high-content screens have been performed in academia. Such screens provide an advantage when processes like apoptosis, where the cells are responding non-synchronously, are studied (Antczak et al., 2009). Also mitosis, which is a rare event at any given time in a cell population, benefits from a time-lapse analysis (Neumann et al., 2010; Schmitz et al., 2010). To follow live cells over time, either fluorescent proteins are used as markers or the cells are stained with dyes that are tolerated by the cells. In order to analyze all samples with the same time intervals good logistics in sample preparation and imaging is required. The different steps in the whole screening process (cell culture and plating, transfection or compound addition, cell incubation and image acquisition) need to function seamlessly which results in reduced batch sizes in live cell screens.

Cell fixation after compound or siRNA treatment enables decoupling sample preparation and image acquisition. Thereby these two processes do not need to function synchronously, and the fixed plates can be stored at 4°C relatively long times (3-5 days generally, depending on the assay also >5 days) without loss of fluorescence signal. Using assays with fixed cells allows higher throughput at a defined end point. However, such assays provide information on the effect of the analyzed compounds only at a single time point that needs to be carefully evaluated for the screen. We have chosen to fix the cells in our screening campaigns, since this allows us more flexibility in the use of the imagers and the plate preparation platforms and an increase of batch size. Also, in case of a technical problems, samples are not lost, and can be imaged after solving the technical issues.

3.2 Sample preparation - automation

HCS assays using fixed cells are non-homogeneous with the need of several washing steps, with the number of washing steps depending on the use of fluorescent fusion proteins or antibody labelling. In our screening unit, the vast majority of projects use antibody staining to visualize the target proteins rather than fluorescent fusion proteins. Therefore, we have built automated platforms for fixation, staining and washing steps required by immunostaining protocols. The first platform (Fig. 2A) serves for compound addition to cell plates followed by an incubation step at 37°C for a defined compound incubation time. Thereafter the cells are fixed by e.g. addition of paraformaldehyde using a dispenser, followed by a washing step with a 1536-well plate washer. On the second platform (Fig. 2B) the plates are further processed by dispense of primary and secondary antibodies, followed by incubation and washing steps. In order to gain flexibility compound addition and fixation steps are decoupled from the antibody staining process on separate platforms.

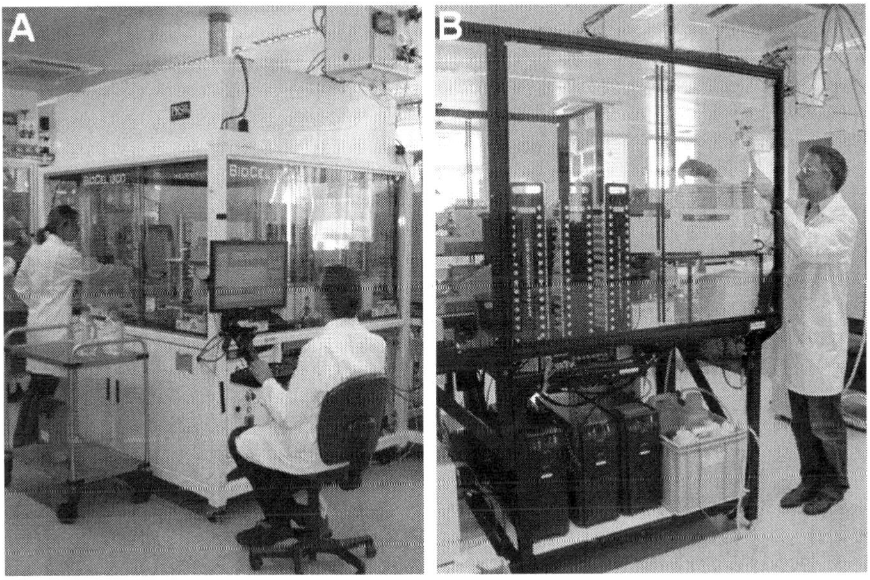

Fig. 2. Plate preparation platforms for automated HCS assays in 384 and 1536-well formats. A) Platform is used for compound addition, incubation and fixation. B) Platform is equipped with robot, dispensers, washers and incubators for automated antibody staining.

When setting up a 1536-well plate high-content assay with an automated plate preparation platform it is critical to test the accuracy (correctness of the transferred volume) and precision (reproducibility) of the plate washers and dispensers, since they have a very high impact on the quality of the HCS assay. Especially for 1536-well dispensers and washers the maintenance and washing procedures are critical to avoid clogging of the pins. The time needed for plate preparation of an immunostaining assay is much longer than in homogenous assays and the higher number of steps can introduce more errors. Therefore, due to the increase of protocol complexity unattended runs are more challenging.

3.3 Cell imagers

In brief, cell imagers for high-content screening are automated microscopes with automated image analysis. The first automated cell imager came to the market 1997 (Giuliano et al., 1997). Since then, numerous confocal and wide-field imagers have become commercially available. Many of them are, or can be optionally equipped with environmental control for live-cell assays. The instruments are usually equipped with autofocus and an image analysis software is included in the package.

For small and medium-scale experiments the throughput of the instrument is not as crucial; however, for high-throughput screening the following features are important: a) the imager should accept 1536-well plates, b) the speed of image acquisition should be high (20-90 min per 1536 well plate), and c) the hard disk of the instrument should be able to store terabytes of data, or alternatively setup for automated data transfer to a dedicated server.

Imaging speed can be enhanced by acquiring two or even three images on different channels simultaneously. This is possible by using imagers equipped with several cameras. However, due to overlapping emission spectra it is rarely possible to acquire more than two images simultaneously. To achieve reasonable statistics, a certain amount of cells need to be analyzed per treatment or well. This can be achieved by acquiring several images per well which, however, will prolong the imaging process. An improvement is the use of cameras with large field of view to capture a decent number of cells in each single image.

Depending on the assay and throughput, different imagers are optimal for high-content screening. In our unit we have used four different HCS instruments. We started HCS using IN Cell Analyzer 3000 (GE) which is a high-resolution confocal imager equipped with 3 laser lines, 3 CCD cameras with a large field of view and on-the-fly image analysis (simultaneous with image acquisition). It is a fast instrument with user-friendly image analysis software, although unable to read 1536-well plates. In order to perform full-deck HCS campaigns in 1536-well format we setup the Opera QEHS (PerkinElmer) which is a confocal imager equipped with 4 lasers and 4 CCD cameras allowing on-the-fly image analysis with sub-cellular resolution. Thus, Opera is the imager of choice for higher throughput screening campaigns with the need of high resolution. For HCS with medium throughput we use IN Cell Analyzer 2000 (GE) which is wide-field imager equipped with a large-chip CCD camera. It can handle 96-1536 well plates; however, image analysis needs to be done after image acquisition. For high-throughput screening campaigns requiring for example fluorescence intensity measurements without sub-cellular resolution, we utilize the Acumen® eX3 (TTP LabTech), a plate scanning device equipped with three lasers. Also Acumen allows analysis of the distribution of fluorescence intensity on-the-fly (in parallel to scanning). In chapter 4 we give examples of different screening campaigns and devices chosen for different assays.

3.4 Image analysis

To efficiently use the wealth of information within the acquired images the automated microscopes are delivered with image analysis software. In addition, several commercially and freely available third party software packages are available to analyze microscope images (Carpenter et al., 2006; Gilbert et al., 2009, Rämö et al, 2009; Wang et al., 2010). The image analysis programs vary from simple, easy-to-use ready-made modules to writing the image analysis scripts by the user (Niederlein et al., 2009; Pepperkok et al., 2006, Swedlow et al., 2003). The former ones make the start of HCS easier for beginners, but the latter offer more flexibility in terms of excluding unwanted structures or defining specific cellular compartments.

For automated image analysis good quality images are required. By size exclusion, dust or larger particles can be filtered out as well as fluorescent particles by fluorescence intensity filter. Sub-cellular analysis is often shown in literature for a single cell as example. When transferred to all cells from a whole well or even to all wells of a 1536-well plate, the algorithm needs to be stable to account for cell populations where size or orientation of the cells may vary. In addition the analysis scripts need to be robust since the intensity of the staining of the cells can vary from well to well due to pipetting procedures.

From a technical point of view, the simplest solution is to use the image analysis software of the imager since no transfer of the images or image conversion step is required. The fastest solution is to analyze images in parallel with image acquisition (on-the-fly image analysis). On-the-fly analysis offers the additional advantage by monitoring the assay quality in a timely fashion that in case of a decreased assay quality, the screener can interact accordingly. Being able to perform image analysis with a computer cluster instead of individual computer(s) would be of great benefit for high-throughput screens to improve analysis speed. Another way to accelerate image analysis is to use multicore computers that can analyze several wells in parallel. However, not all image analysis software packages support multicore analysis.

Not only the provided software coming with the instrument, but also third party software can be used for image analysis. However, each imager creates usually a specific image format with link to metadata (like objective lens used, pixel resolution etc.) which can complicate the use of third party analysis software. Conversion of the images to another format is often required which slows down the whole screening process and usually increases the space needed for image storage. We routinely use the image analysis software provided with the imager, especially for high-throughput campaigns. In few exceptional cases requiring specific algorithms, a third party software with specific features is used for small or medium scale screens.

3.5 Data analysis

To analyse single readouts from HCS campaigns any high-throughput data analysis tool can be used which is able to display heatmaps for plate pattern analysis and to perform dose response curve fitting. The unique requirement for image-based HTS is the generation of a link to the images to rapidly verify whether a hit is a true active or a false positive (Fig. 3). Preferentially the visualization is established in a software package where treatment or compound information is linked.

HCS is able to provide information-rich data sets containing readouts on multiple cellular parameters. In addition to the fluorescence intensity parameters and number of cells, their morphology and the intracellular distribution of cellular proteins can be analysed quantitatively (Loo et al., 2007; Young et al., 2008). To explore the high content of images through multi-parametric data analysis more sophisticated tools are needed. The combination of several parameters can improve the assay quality, however, the statistical parameter, Z′ value, which is commonly used for single readouts needs to be adapted for the analysis of multiple features (Kümmel et al., 2010).

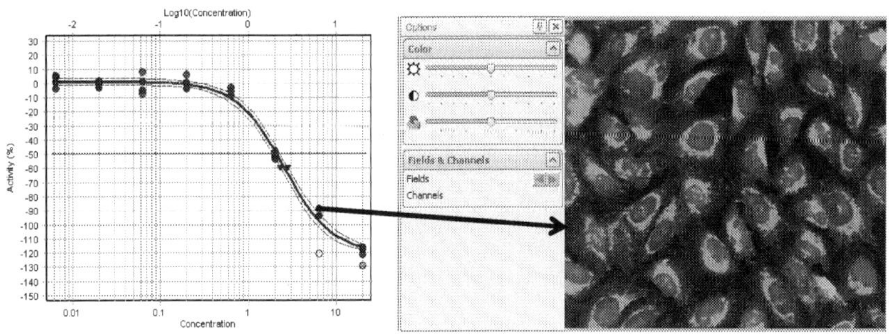

Fig. 3. Example of a concentration response curve fitted in the program to analyze screening data. By clicking an analysis point in a concentration response curve or a well in a heatmap, the respective image is displayed.

In order to enable the analysis of dozens of features in parallel we have generated an in-house software package (Kümmel et al, 2011). Multiple readouts can be either combined to classify samples into hits or inactives or to cluster sample responses into groups similar to control compounds or samples with similar phenotypes (Fig. 4). Such clustering analysis can be used in primary screening for hit identification as well as to cluster hits based on their potency, toxicity or off-target effects.

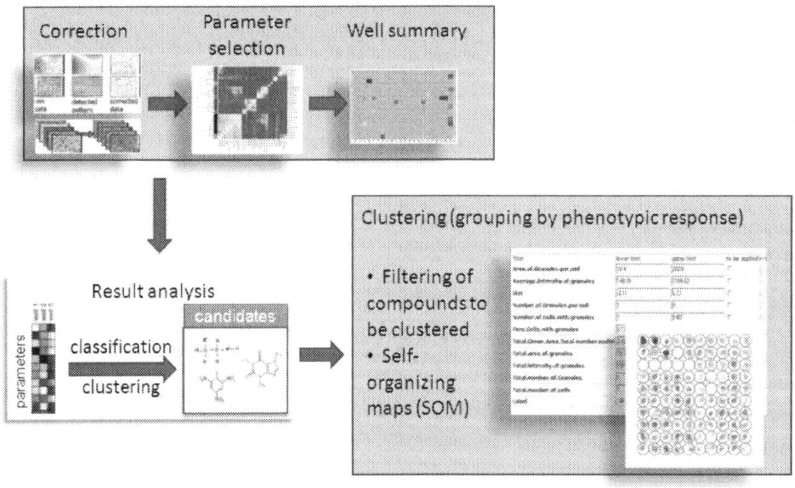

Fig. 4. Analysis of multiparametric HCS data. Data preprocessing consists of correction for plate pattern and plate effects, parameter selection by dimension reduction and well summary. The parameters are being further analyzed by either classification or clustering. Visualization of clustering results in self-organizing maps helps to identify similar phenotypes.

3.6 Data management

Every imager generates its own sometimes proprietary image format, and the format of the data files from each image analysis differs depending on the analysis software used. Therefore, data management and data mining can be problematic when using different imagers or image analysis software packages. With certain image analysis software the data output format might even vary depending on the analysis algorithm applied. To enable the link from image and metadata to the result file can be a challenge due to the variety of formats. In addition, creating software tools enabling the search of plates, compounds, or treatments combined with image and data visualization for comparison of images and data generated by different imagers is still a major challenge.

The high-throughput screening with sub-cellular resolution is focused to specific sites in our company with the consequence of interacting with project teams located in different countries. To allow all team members to view the images irrespective whether they have the specific analysis software or not, we have created a web-based tool to display the images (Fig. 5).

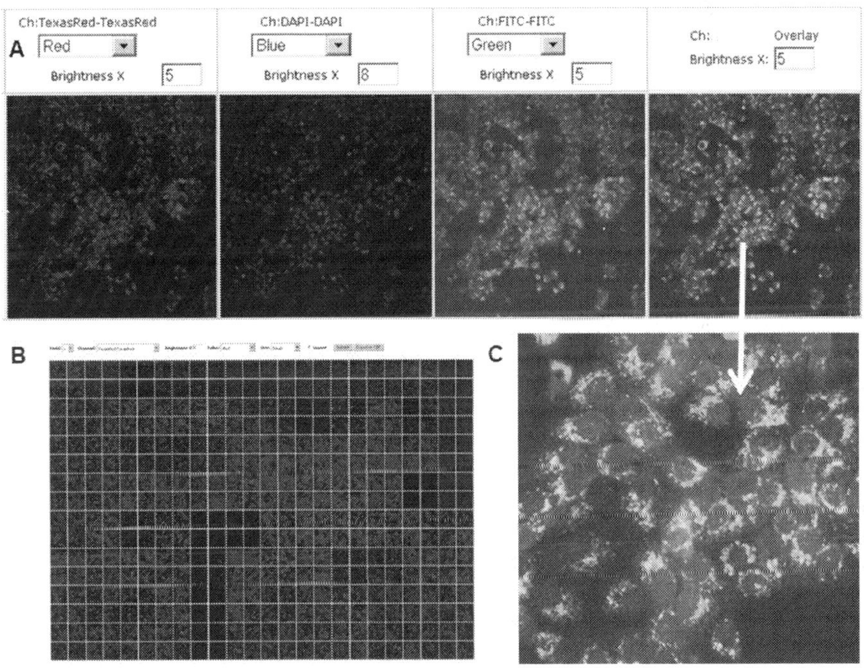

Fig. 5. Visualization of cell images with a web-based tool. Individual wells inspection (A) and whole plate views (B) are possible. In addition images from the respective well or plate view can be explored with higher magnification to visualize details (C).

With this tool individual images as well as an overview of all images on the plate can be visualized, however no analyzed data is being displayed. Currently we are implementing a database where all images and result files are being stored. The visualization in form of heatmaps will be available for different readouts enabling the comparison of the quality of the respective readouts. A direct link from the heatmap will open the image to check the integrity of the well for a quick verification of the results.

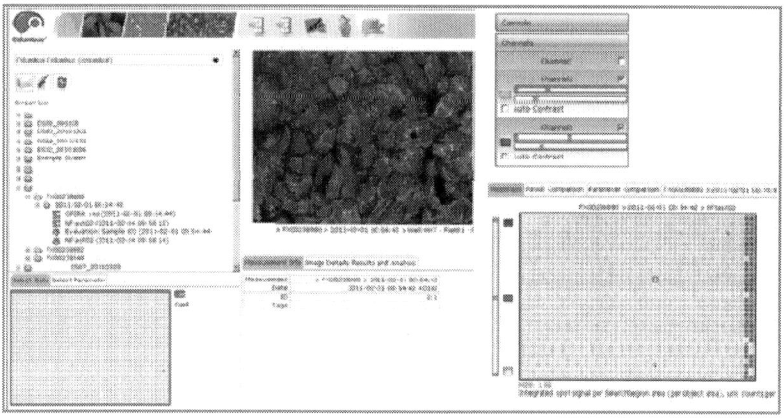

Fig. 6. Visualization of the respective readouts with a link to the images.

4. HCS in primary high-throughput screening

The technologies that have enabled high-content screening in high throughput include plate washers and dispensers for 1536-well plates as well as robot-friendly 1536-well plates suitable for imaging using 10x objectives. Decoupling the plate preparation and imaging processes allows us to exploit all HTS platforms optimally and thereby increase the throughput.

Since we have different instruments in our HCS platform we usually compare image and assay quality and throughput for each project on different readers, and choose the instrument based on the highest quality and throughput. Example projects are described covering high-throughput and medium-throughput campaigns as well as projects with different requirements for resolution.

4.1 HTS for inducers of protein aggregation

As an example, a high-content screening campaign in high throughput to identify compounds inducing protein aggregation within the cytoplasm is described. The sub-cellular analysis of individual cells provided reliable results that could not be reached with any other assay format than high-content imaging. A stable HEK293 cell line was generated overexpressing the protein of interest fused to the HA tag. The detection was based on immunostaining with anti HA antibody followed by a secondary antibody requiring several washing steps. Since HEK293 cells are sensitive to repeated washing steps it was necessary to use poly-D-lysine coated imaging plates which are commercially available.

In this example high-resolution images were needed for the sophisticated image analysis algorithm based on spot detection. Variable spot size with variable intensity was analyzed in the cytoplasmic area which was identified by GFP fluorescence in the cytoplasm. Therefore three colours were imaged with the Opera QEHS, and in order to reach sufficient quality required for HTS two images were acquired per well using a 20x objective. Imaging and simultaneous image analysis summed up to an imaging time of 90 min per plate. According to the setup of the automated plate preparation system, we were able to process >120 x 1536 well plates per week, however, due to the long imaging time, the throughput was limited to 90 plates per weeks.

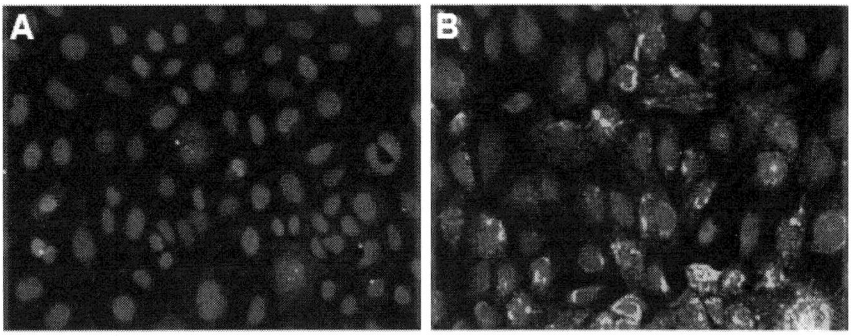

Fig. 7. Protein aggregation in HEK293 cells overexpressing protein of interest tagged with HA-tag (green), nuclear stain Hoechst 33342 (red). A) untreated, B) cells treated with control compound. For better visualization the channel for GFP is not shown and the colours have been changed.

4.2 Medium-throughput screen for granularity

The possibility to quantitatively analyse sub-cellular compartments within the cell is one of the advantages of HCS which makes it for certain projects the unique technique for hit identification. In this example project, the detection of both red and green granules in the cytoplasm of human bladder epithelial cells was aimed for (Fig. 8). For good resolution a 20x objective was required and therefore the use of the laser scanning instrument Acumen was not considered for this project. Long incubation times of the cells made the 1536-well format not suitable and reduced the amount of compounds to be screened to medium throughput.

384-well plates were measured both on the confocal imager Opera QEHS and on the lamp-based imager IN Cell Analyzer 2000 in order to compare image quality and imaging time. Using the 20x objective the image size of Opera images is 430 x 345 µm, whereas the IN Cell Analyzer 2000 has a large field of view camera which results in 760 x 760 µm images. Thus, for imaging the same number of cells two images per well and almost double the imaging time was required with Opera compared to IN Cell Analyzer 2000. Lowering the number of cells imaged had a negative impact on assay quality. Therefore, in this particular assay the imaging time with Opera was 40 min longer per plate already taking into account the ability to acquire images on two channels simultaneously (Table 1).

4.3 Measurement of fluorescence intensity

In most projects high-resolution images are needed for sub-cellular analysis, but in some projects low-resolution images provide adequate results and assay quality. This is especially true for assays where fluorescence intensity is the main readout. In a high-throughput screening campaign we were looking for compounds inhibiting post-translational modification of a protein localized in the nucleus of a prostate cancer cell line. We monitored two different post-translational modifications simultaneously using antibody staining and measuring the fluorescence intensity in the nuclear region. The images taken with Opera QEHS are shown in Fig. 9. The resolution requirements of fluorescence intensity measurement are in general not very high, therefore imaging with the Acumen was considered for this project.

Opera and Acumen provided qualitatively comparable results in 1536-well format in terms of signal to baseline ratio and Z′ values, with the Acumen being much faster with 30 min versus 90 min imaging time with Opera (Table 2). In this specific project the cells needed to be plated at low density, therefore the lower resolution of the Acumen was counterbalanced by the improved statistical quality due to the ability to read the whole well by Acumen (Fig 10).

Primary hit finding was performed using the Acumen whereas the follow-up in concentration-response-curves was done with Opera QEHS to allow the possibility of checking the images for specific compound effects. The reduced imaging time as well as the reduced amount of data storage of the Acumen is an advantage for high-throughput screening in cases where lower resolution is acceptable.

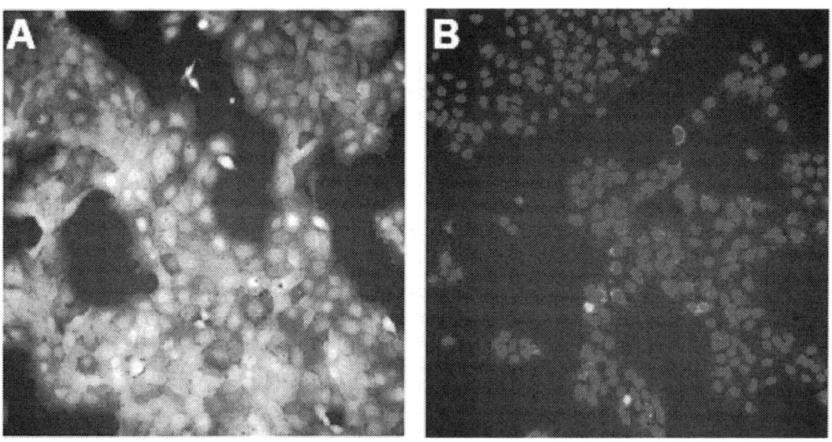

Fig. 8. Granule detection in RT112 cells (human bladder epithelial cells) stably expressing GFP (green) and mCherry fusion proteins (red). Nuclei are stained with Hoechst 33342 (blue). A) untreated, B) cells treated with control compound.

384-well plates, 20x objective, 3 colours	Opera	IN Cell 2000
	2 images / well	1 image / well
Measurement time / plate	100 min	60 min

Table 1. Overview of imaging time of Opera and IN Cell 2000 for granularity measurement

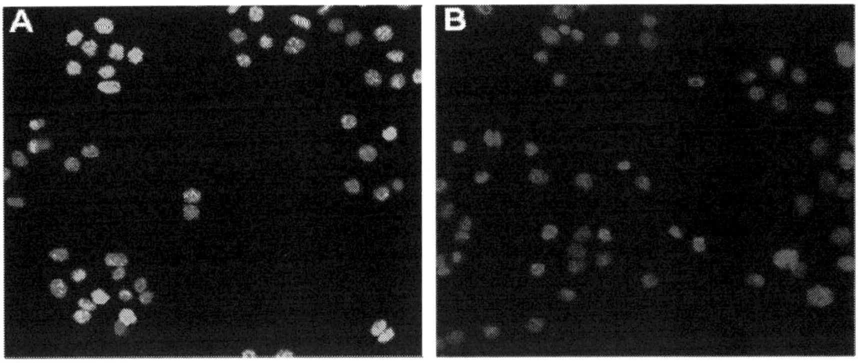

Fig. 9. Images for fluorescence intensity measurement acquired with Opera. DU145 cells (human prostate cancer cells) stained with Antibody B (green), nuclear stain (blue). For better visualization only two colours are shown in the overlay images. A) untreated, B) cells treated with control compound.

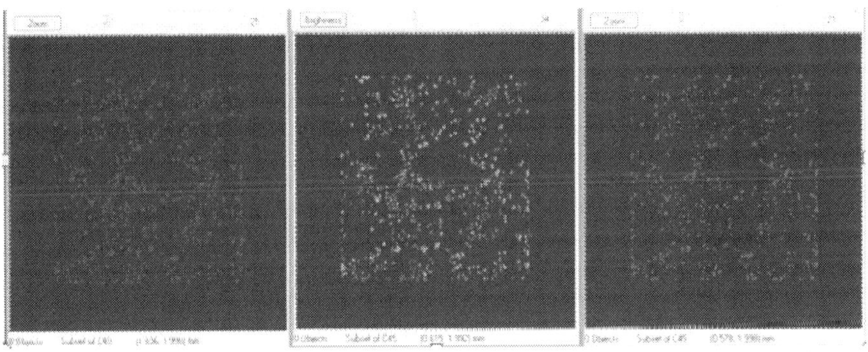

Fig. 10. Fluorescence intensity measurement with Acumen. DU145 cells (human prostate cancer cells) stained with nuclear stain (blue), antibody A (green), antibody B (red).

1536-well plates, 3 colours	Opera	Acumen
	20x objective, 2 images / well	whole well
Measurement time / plate	90 min	30 min

Table 2. Overview of imaging time of Opera and Acumen for fluorescence intensity measurement.

4.4 Analysis of nuclear translocation

Nuclear translocation assays can deliver functional readouts without the side effect of generating many false positives as other conventional assay formats might comprise. Having the advantage of observing the compounds effect on the cells, we decided to screen for small molecules inhibiting the translocation of a protein to the nucleus in U-2 OS cells overexpressing a GFP fusion protein. Since both Opera and Acumen are able to measure nuclear translocation, both were compared for quality and throughput. The assay was quite robust and did not require a very high resolution for the image analysis. Both instruments were able to provide good assay quality in 1536-well format. The plate measurement time was 25 min both with Acumen and with Opera. A 10x objective was used on the Opera and the images were acquired on two channels simultaneously. The applied image analysis on Opera needed longer than the effective imaging time and would have reduced the throughput. However, after streamlining the algorithm, the time of physical imaging and image analysis matched.
Since the confocal images by Opera provide more information on the samples than a plate scanner, the Opera was chosen as the screening instrument for that particular project.

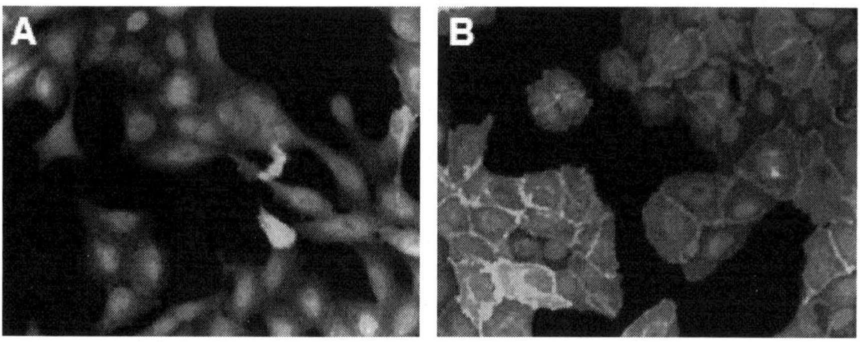

Fig. 11. Translocation of GFP-fusion protein from nuclear region upon small molecule addition. Image analysis is based on the fluorescence intensity in the nuclear area compared to cytoplasm. U-2 OS cells overexpressing GFP fusion protein (green), nuclear stain DRAQ5 (red). A) untreated, B) cells treated with control compound.

4.5 Overview of selected imaging projects

Four different examples are described above with varying requirements for resolution and therefore different choices of imagers for screening. Every assay is optimized for lowest imaging time and highest throughput without loss of quality. Imaging time can vary strongly between 25 to 90 min per 1536 well plate as shown in Table 3.
However, optimizing the imaging time alone is often not sufficient to run a HCS in high throughput; also the immunostaining procedure can be a bottleneck. Antibody staining is much more time consuming than working with GFP fusion proteins since several washing steps are required. To speed up and simplify the staining process the fixative can be added directly to the cell medium, blocking buffer and permeabilization reagent can be combined in one step as well as the nuclear stain added together with the secondary antibody.

Project	Imager	Plate format	Cells	No of compounds screened	Colours	Images/well	Objective	Imaging time/plate (min)
Protein aggregation	Opera	1536	Hek293	>1 mio	3	2	20 x	**100**
Fluorescence intensity	Opera	1536	HEK293	550k	2	2	20 x	**55**
Nuclear translocation	Opera	1536	U-2 OS	>1 mio	2	1	10 x	**25**
Fluorescence intensity	Acumen	1536	DU145	>1 mio	3	whole well	Ca 10x	**30**
Granule detection	IN Cell 2000	384	RT112	20k	3	1	20 x	**60***
Protein aggregation	Opera	384	U-2 OS	25k	2	4	20 x	**30***

Table 3. List of high-throughput assays with different requirements and the effect on the imaging time. * The imaging time needs to be multiplied with 4 in order to compare with imaging of 1536-well plates.

4.6 Technical issues in high-throughput HCS

The time consuming plate preparation process in addition to imaging time (up to several days) can result in delayed quality control measures to detect errors in cell plating or compound distribution. This can be a major issue if undetected failures of batch preparation can only be reported back after a week.

Since the imaging can be of long duration (90 min or more per plate) the 1536-well plates need to be stored in an incubator at 4 °C to prevent evaporation. Nevertheless, before imaging an intermediate step should be calculated to accommodate the plates to room temperature to avoid condensation, therefore we have introduced a 30 min incubation time at room temperature before imaging. Storing fixed and stained plates at 4 °C will allow a later use of the plates for imaging. This decoupled process is beneficial in case of a failure of the plate preparation systems. We observed that although antibacterial agents were added, contaminations can occur with plate storage for longer than two weeks.

Due to small volumes of reagents and the use of common, frequently opened incubators we experienced strong edge effects on 1536-well plates. We were able to compensate that partially with higher volumes of medium or buffer during the incubation steps and using dedicated incubators that are less frequently opened. With a specifically designed 1536-well plate comprising a tightly closing lid (labyrinth lid) evaporation can be mitigated (Pfeifer and Scheel, 2009). In addition, the performance of the plate washers and dispensers needs to be monitored continuously since the washing and dispensing steps are essential for a good performance. The 1536-well dispensing or washing devices have tiny pins which are prone to clogging. Therefore a regular cleaning procedure with detergent, water and ethanol after every use is necessary which leads to a limit in unattended use of the automation systems. Furthermore, working with 1536-well plates often requires shaking to distribute the added reagents evenly. We have added a high-speed shaking step after each reagent addition to our protocol.

5. HCS in small-scale analysis

In contrast to high-throughput assays, where automation-friendly assays and high speed of imaging and image analysis are of utmost importance, in small-scale analysis more complex assay formats are possible. Assay protocols requiring manual or semi-manual steps can be used and precious primary cells, such as neurons, even co-cultures can be used (Anderl et al., 2009). The ability to use primary cells and analyze endogenous proteins can be of great benefit which is enabled by antibody labelling and the sensitivity of confocal imaging. Also several components can be stained in parallel, and to improve the statistical quality of the assay, several images on different channels can be acquired when speed is not the most critical factor. A thorough image and data analysis for also non-expected features can be performed to obtain all possible information from the cells after different treatments.

We have used low and medium-throughput high-content assays to analyze cellular neurotoxicity, neurite outgrowth and neuronal survival. Using primary rat cerebellar granule neurons (CGNs) we developed an imaging assay that has been used in medium throughput to study neurotoxicity (Götte et al., 2010) and neurite outgrowth-promoting activity of low-molecular weight compounds (see below) or proteins (Yan et al,. 2009). The rat cerebellar granule cells can be prepared from a litter of 7-8 pups in 3 h, and the amount of cells obtained allows analysis of 2500 samples in 96-well format and 12.500 samples in 384-well format. The cells can be frozen without loss of viability or ability to grow neurites. Thereby assays with even higher throughput are possible. The intactness of the neuritic network in a high-content assay proved out to be a sensitive measure for cellular neurotoxicity, revealing compound toxicity that was not detected in non-HCS assays or in neuroblastoma cells (Götte et al., 2010). The HCS assay was used to analyze cellular neurotoxicity of compounds whose targets were expressed in the brain.

We have also used the CGNs to study neurite outgrowth in small-scale assays. The neurite outgrowth assay was first developed and validated using the brain-derived neurotrophic factor (BDNF) whose receptor, TrkB, is expressed in the developing CGNs (Segal et al., 1995). Images were acquired with IN Cell Analyzer 3000 and image analysis revealed that BDNF enhanced neurite outgrowth dose-dependently. Additional analysis of the images with a third party software, Neurite Analysis module of HCA-Vision, that is specifically designed to analyze neuronal cultures, revealed that the enhanced neurite outgrowth was rather due to increased branching and increased number of neurites per neuron than increased length of the neurites (Wang et al., 2010). Such detailed information of neuronal morphology can be obtained only from an imaging assay.

We tested the ability of other neurotrophins to promote neurite outgrowth or neuronal survival. Therefore, the CGNs were incubated for 3 days with the neurotrophins, then fixed and stained with the nuclear marker Hoechst 33342 and anti β-tubulin III antibody to specifically label neurons (Lewis and Cowan, 1988). Images were acquired with IN Cell Analyzer 3000 and analyzed with IN Cell 3000 Neurite Outgrowth module for various readouts in respect to neurite area and length (Fig 12). BDNF (10 ng/ml) served as a positive control.

Image analysis revealed that the TrkB ligands, BDNF and NT-4, increased the total number of cells in the culture significantly, suggesting that they have a cell survival-promoting effect (Fig. 12). NT-4 and BDNF enhanced also neurite outgrowth significantly, as seen by the increase of neurite length and neurite area per cell. NT-4 was the most potent neurotrophin enhancing neurite number and branching as analyzed additionally with the HCA-Vision software. NT-3 enhanced neurite outgrowth modestly and only at high concentrations. The preferred receptor for NT-3 is TrkC which is expressed in the CGNs at a lower level than TrkB (Segal et al., 1995), and accordingly, NT-3 had a slight positive effect on cell survival and neurite outgrowth. NT-3 also enhanced the number of neurites at high concentration (Fig. 12) whereas NGF had no effect on either cell survival or neurite outgrowth. This is in accordance with other published data (Courtney et al., 1997; Nonomura et al., 1996), and our own quantitative RT-PCR results indicating very low expression of the NGF receptor, TrkA in the CGNs (not shown). Thus, the high-content assay was able to reveal expected effects of known neurotrophins validating the assay setup.

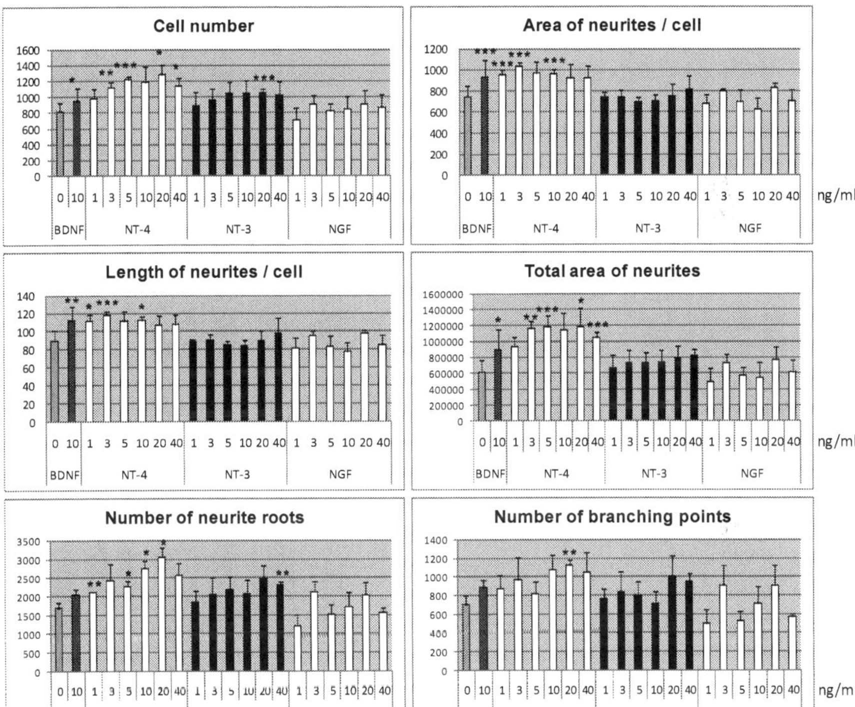

Fig. 12. Effect of neurotrophins NT-4, NT-3 and NGF on cell survival and neurite outgrowth. CGNs from 7 day old rats were incubated with the neurotrophins for 3 days before fixation and staining. Average and standard deviation of triplicate samples are shown. Area and length of neurites are in pixels; pixel size is 0.6 μm. Statistical significance in comparison to DMSO control; ***, p <0.001; ** p<0.01; * p<0.05 in Student' two-tailed paired *t*-test.

The goal was to identify low-molecular weight compounds mimicking the effect of neurotrophins. Several antidepressants have been reported to activate the TrkB pathway *in vivo* (Rantamäki et al., 2007). Therefore, we were interested to test the effect of selected antidepressants on neurite outgrowth of the CGNs expressing TrkB. Three of the nine tested antidepressants enhanced neuronal survival and/or neurite outgrowth significantly. In addition, image analysis was able to reveal differences in the effects among the three active drugs.

Citalopram induced the most pronounced, concentration-dependent neurite outgrowth by enhancing significantly cell survival and the percentage of neuronal cells in the culture (Fig. 13). Neurite outgrowth and percentage of neurons were increased by imipramine up to 1 μM (Fig. 13.), however, at higher concentration neurite outgrowth was reduced, which could indicate cytotoxicity. Fluoxetine did not enhance cell survival but it enhanced neurite outgrowth at low concentrations. At high concentration (10 μM) fluoxetine was toxic reducing total cell number and percentage of neuronal cells and inhibiting neurite outgrowth almost completely.

The advantage of HCS over assays that analyze total amounts of markers, such as β-tubulin III or neurofilament, is that the effect on cell survival and neurite outgrowth can be distinguished. The enhancing effect of fluoxetine on neurite outgrowth, for example, would probably remain undetected in an assay analyzing merely the total amount of β-tubulin due to the fact that fluoxetine slightly reduced the cell number as compared to the DMSO control.

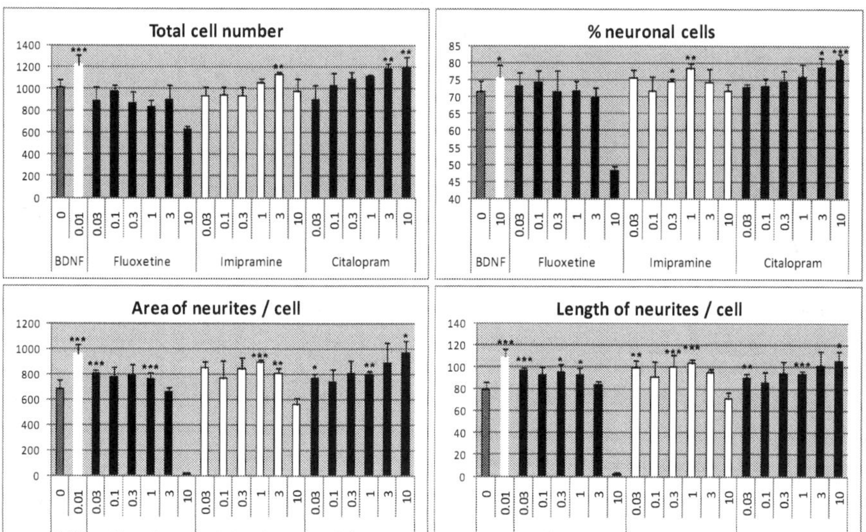

Fig. 13. Effect of fluoxetine, imipramine and citalopram on cell survival and neurite outgrowth. Average and standard deviation of triplicate samples are shown. The concentration of BDNF was 10 ng/ml. The concentrations of the antidepressants are in μM. Area and length of neurites are in pixels; pixel size is 0.6 μm. Statistical significance in comparison to DMSO control; ***, $p < 0.001$; ** $p < 0.01$; * $p < 0.05$ in Student' two-tailed paired *t*-test.

In small-scale experiments, such as the study of the effect of neurotrophic factors and the antidepressants on neurite outgrowth, an extra colour can be afforded to reveal additional effects of the drugs. In our example, the CGN samples were stained additionally with an antibody against TrkB which uncovered an interesting, unexpected phenomenon. TrkB was found to localize to the cell bodies and neurites. TrkB was also found in the tips of the growing neurites but only when the cells were cultivated in the absence of a TrkB ligand. The presence of the TrkB ligands BDNF or NT-4, caused disappearance of the TrkB receptor from the tips (Fig. 14).

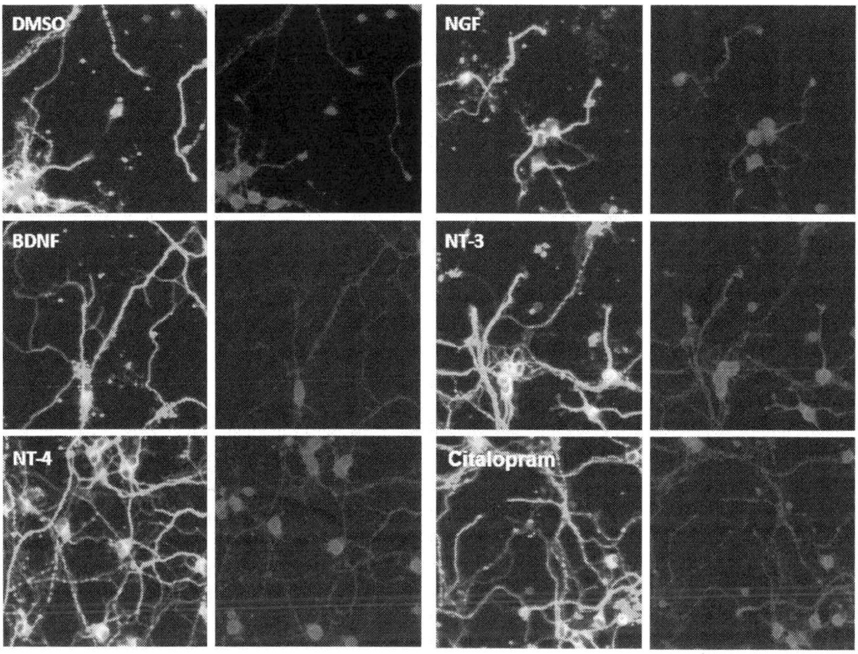

Fig. 14. TrkB ligands and citalopram reduce localization of TrkB to the tips of the neurites. Rat CGNs from 7-8 day old pups were incubated for 3 days with the neurotrophins, DMSO or citalopram, then fixed, stained and images were acquired with IN Cell Analyzer 3000. Red, anti TrkB; green, anti β-tubulin III; blue, nuclei.

In order to quantify TrkB specifically in the tips of the neurites, the neurites were first traced semi-manually with the help of the β-tubulin III staining and using the Imaris® software (Bitplane AG, Zurich, Switzerland). Then the tips were marked as regions of interest (Fig. 15), and the area and intensity of TrkB staining in the marked tips were calculated with a customized MATLAB code. The quantification of TrkB in the tips of the neurites confirmed the visual observation that indeed the TrkB ligands BDNF and NT-4 reduced TrkB in the tips, whereas NGF did not. Surprisingly, also one of the antidepressants, citalopram, caused disappearance of TrkB from tips of the neurites. Whether this is a direct effect of citalopram or whether it stimulates secretion of BDNF which then causes the internalization of TrkB, remains to be studied. Anyhow, this is an example that an additional staining and careful image analysis can reveal unexpected effects of the compounds, and in this special case can help to reveal the mode of action of the active compounds.

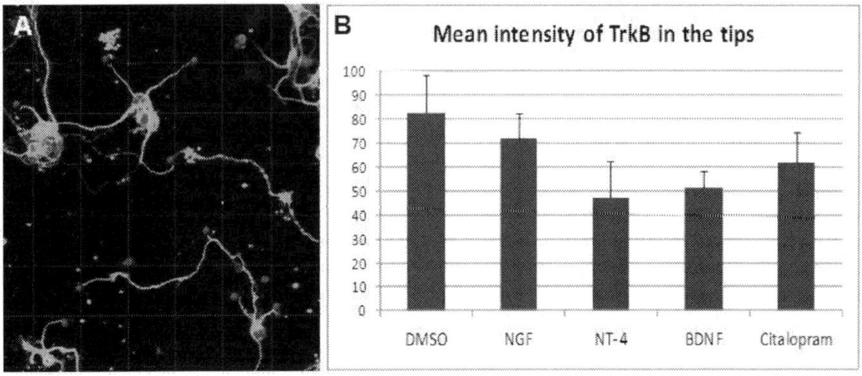

Fig. 15. Quantification of TrkB in the tips of the neurites. A, Image with regions of interest (red) where intensity and area of TrkB staining was measured. Green, β-tubulin staining; blue, nuclei stained with Hoechst 33342. B, intensity of TrkB staining in the tips as analyzed with a MATLAB code. For each condition 29-62 neurites were analyzed.

6. Outlook

The HCS field is developing in two directions. On one hand more sophisticated assays are being developed and more complex biological systems are being exploited, such as stem cells (embryonic, adult, IPS), primary cells, co-cultures, and even tissues and worms like *C. elegans* are quantitatively analyzed. This development is being enabled by improved image analysis software packages for co-cultures or label-free samples.

On the other hand HCS is rendered possible for real high-throughput screening in primary hit finding campaigns through instruments with 1536-well capabilities combining high imaging speed and resolution. Robust assays required for primary hit finding are being developed and sophisticated image analysis packages allow fast, on-the-fly image analysis for real time quality control.

Novel imagers with adjustable confocality and large field of view, which have recently become available, will increase the flexibility and throughput of high-content assays. Hard- and software for sub-cellular imaging are developing for more modular use of the equipment to allow increased diversity of applications, including live-cell imaging with environmental control and even fast kinetics with reagent additions. The analysis of the generated multiparametric data is further emerging and different ways to analyze the vast HCS data are being exploited, with an increasing number of available tools for data visualization.

7. Summary

HCS is an established but still evolving technology in drug discovery. HCS enables in primary screening and compound profiling novel assay formats which were earlier impossible in higher throughput. In addition, sub-cellular imaging is able to deliver more content through multi-parametric data analysis of shape, size, and area in addition to the target-specific fluorescence readouts. There are biological requirements for successful HCS campaigns including well separated cells as well as dedicated algorithms for the respective image analysis. HCS in high throughput requires automated platforms for sample preparation, high-speed imagers and data analysis software with a dedicated IT infrastructure to manage and mine the wealth of data produced. Primary hit finding can be performed in medium to high throughput with a variety of biological readouts based on sub-cellular imaging, including protein aggregation, granularity detection or translocation events. In lower throughput follow-up assays, sub-cellular imaging can be applied to thoroughly analyze compound effects on primary cells and to reveal additional, unexpected effects. At this point it is too early to evaluate the impact of HCS in novel drugs, whether they are improved in having less undesired side-effects, or developed faster, or whether the attrition rate at late phases would be decreased.

8. Acknowledgement

Gabriele Hofmann, Yvonne Ibig-Rehm, Martin Pfeifer, Daniela Siebert and Vincent Unterreiner (Novartis Institutes for BioMedical Research) are acknowledged for performing the HCS assays, Aaron Ponti (FMI) and Patrick Schwarb (FMI) for help in the analysis of TrkB in the tips of the neurites, and Rita Grossenbacher (Novartis Institutes for BioMedical Research) for RT-PCR. Vincent Unterreiner & Stefan Capretta are thanked for automation support, Peter Fürst for managerial support, Anne Kümmel and Paul Selzer for multiparametric data analysis tool, and John Lin for image visualization.

9. References

Anderl, J.L., Redpath, S. & Ball, A.J. (2009) A neuronal and astrocyte co-culture assay for high content analysis of neurotoxicity. *J. Vis. Exp.* Vol. 5, No. 27, p. 1173.

Antczak, C., Takagi, T., Ramirez, C.N., Radu, C. & Djaballah, H. (2009) Live-cell imaging of caspase activation for high-content screening. *J. Biomol. Screen.*, Vol. 14, No. 8, pp. 956-969.

Blackmore, M.G., Moore, D.L., Smith, R.P., Goldberg, J.L., Bixby, J.L. & Lemmon, V.P. (2010) High content screening of cortical neurons identifies novel regulators of axon growth. *Mol. Cell. Neurosci.*, Vol. 44, No. 1, pp. 43-54.

Carpenter, A.E., Jones, T.R., Lamprecht, M.R., Clarke, C., Kang, I.H., Friman, O., Guertin, D.A., Chang, J.H., Lindquist, R.A., Moffat, J., Golland, P. & Sabatini, D.M. (2006) CellProfiler: image analysis software for identifying and quantifying cell phenotypes. *Genome Biol.*, Vol. 7, No. 10, pp. R100-R100.11.

Courtney, M.J., Åkerman, K.E.O. & Coffey, E.T. (1997) Neurotrophins protect cultured cerebellar granule neurons against the early phase of cell death by a two-component mechanism. *J. Neurosci.*, Vol. 17, No. 11, pp. 4201-4211.

Gilbert, D.F., Meinhof, T., Pepperkok, R., & Runz, H. DetecTiff©: A novel image analysis routine for high-content screening microscopy. (2009) *J. Biomol. Screen.*, Vol. 14, No. 8, pp. 944-955.

Giuliano, K., DeBiasio, R., Dunlay, T., Gough, A., Voloska, J., Zock, J., Pavlakis, G.N. & Taylor, D.L. (1997) High-content screening: a new approach to easing key bottlenecks in the drug discovery process. *J. Biomol. Screen.* Vol. 2, No. 4, pp. 249-259.

Gorenstein, J., Zack, B., Marszalek, J.R., Bagchi, A., Subramaniam, S., Carroll, P. & Elbi, C. (2010) Reducing the multidimensionality of high-content screening into versatile powerful descriptors. *Biotechniques*, Vol. 49, No. 3, pp. 663-665.

Götte, M., Hofmann, G., Michou-Gallani, A-I., Glickman, J.F., Wishart, W. & Gabriel, D. (2010) An imaging assay to analyze primary neurons for cellular neurotoxicity. *J. Neurosci. Methods*, Vol. 192, No. 1, pp. 7-16.

Guzi, T.J., Paruch, K., Dwyer, M.P., Labroli, M., Shanahan, F., Davis, N., Taricani, L., Wiswell, D., Seghezzi, W., Penaflor, E., Bhagwat, B., Wang, W., Gu, D., Hsieh, Y., Lee, S., Liu, M. & Parry, D. (2011) Targeting the Replication Checkpoint Using SCH 900776, a Potent and Functionally Selective CHK1 Inhibitor Identified via High Content Screening. *Mol. Cancer Ther.*, Vol. 10, No. 4, pp. 591-602.

Ibig-Rehm, Y., Götte, M., Gabriel, D., Woodhall, D., Shea, A., Brown, N.E., Compton, T. & Feire, A.L. (2011) High-content screening to distinguish between attachment and post-attachment steps of human cytomegalovirus entry into fibroblasts and epithelial cells. *Antiviral Res.*, Vol. 89, No. 3, pp.246-256.

Kümmel, A., Gubler, H., Gehin, P., Beibel, M., Gabriel, D. & Parker, C.N. (2010) Integration of Multiple Readouts

into the Z' Factor for Assay Quality Assessment. *J. Biomol. Screen.*, Vol. 15, No. 1, pp. 95-101.

Kümmel, A., Selzer, P., Beibel, M., Gubler, H., Parker, C.N. & Gabriel, D. (2011) Comparison of multivariate data analysis strategies for high-content screening. *J. Biomol. Screen.*, Vol. 16, No. 3, pp. 338-347.

Lewis, S.A., Cowan, N.J. (1988) Complex regulation and functional versatility of mammalian alpha- and beta-tubulin isotypes during differentiation of testis and muscle cells. *J. Cell. Biol.*, Vol. 106, No. 6, pp. 2023-2033.

Li, Z., Yan, Y., Powers, E.A., Ying, X., Janjua, K., Garyantes, T. & Baron, B. (2003) Identification of gap junction blockers using automated fluorescence microscopy imaging. *J. Biomol. Screen.*, Vol. 8, No. 5, pp. 489-499.

Loo, L. H., Wu, L. F. & Altschuler, S. J. (2007) Image-based multivariate profiling of drug responses from single cells. *Nat. Methods.*, Vol. 4, No. 5, pp. 445–453.

Nadanaciva, S., Lu, S., Gebhard, D.F., Jessen, B.A., Pennie, W.D. & Will, Y. (2011) A high content screening assay for identifying lysosomotropic compounds. *Toxicol. In Vitro*, Vol. 25, No. 3, pp. 715-723.

Neumann, B., Walter, T., Hériché, J.K., Bulkescher, J., Erfle, H., Conrad, C., Rogers, P., Poser, I., Held, M., Liebel, U., Cetin, C., Sieckmann, F., Pau, G., Kabbe, R., Wünsche, A., Satagopam, V., Schmitz, M.H., Chapuis, C., Gerlich, D.W., Schneider, R., Eils, R., Huber, W., Peters, J.M., Hyman, A.A., Durbin, R., Pepperkok, R. & Ellenberg, J. (2010) Phenotypic profiling of the human genome by time-lapse microscopy reveals cell division genes. *Nature*, Vol. 464, No. 7289, pp. 721-727.

Niederlein, A., Meyenhofer, F., White, D. & Bickle, M. (2009) Image analysis in high-content screening. *Comb. Chem. High Throughput Screen*. Vol. 12, No. 9, pp. 899-907.

Nilles, K.M. & London, B. (2007) Knockin animal models of inherited arrythmogenic diseases: what have we learned from them ? *J. Cardiovasc. Electrophysiol.*, Vol. 18, No. 10, pp. 1117-1125.

Nonomura, T., Kubo, T., Oka, T., Shimoke, K., Yamada, M., Enokido, Y. & Hatanaka, H. (1996) Signaling pathways and survival effects of BDNF and NT-3 on cultured cerebellar granule cells. *Dev. Brain Res.*, Vol. 97, No. 1, 42-50.

Park, I.H., Arora, N., Huo, H., Maherali, N, Ahfeldt, T., Shimamura, A., Lensch, M.W., Cowan, C., Hochedlinger, K. & Daley, G.Q. (2008) Disease-Specific Induced Pluripotent Stem Cells. *Cell*, Vol. 134, No. 5, pp. 877-886.

Pelkmans, L., Fava, E., Grabner, H., Hannus, M., Habermann, B., Krausz, E. & Zerial M. (2005) Genome-wide analysis of human kinases in clathrin- and caveolae/raft-mediated endocytosis. *Nature*, Vol. 436, No. 7047, pp. 78-86.

Pepperkok, R., & Ellenberg, J. (2006) High-throughput fluorescence microscopy for systems biology. *Nature Rev Mol Cell Biol*, Vol. 7, No. 9, pp.690-696.

Pfeifer, M.J. & Scheel, G. (2009) Long-term storage of compound solutions for high-throughput screening by using a novel 1536-well microplate. *J. Biomol. Screen.*, Vol. 14, No. 5, pp. 492-498.

Rämö, P., Sacher, R., Snijder, B., Begemann, B., Pelkmans, L. (2009) CellClassifier: supervised learning of cellular phenotypes. Bioinformatics, Vol. 25, No. 22, pp. 3028–3030.

Rantamäki, T., Hendolin, P., Kankaanpää, A., Mijatovic, J., Piepponen, P., Domenici, E., Chao, M.V., Männistö, P.T. & Castrén, E. (2007) Pharmacologically diverse antidepressants rapidly activate brain-derived neurotrophic factor receptor TrkB and induce phospholipase-Cγ signalling pathways in mouse brain. *Neuropsychopharmacol.*, Vol. 32, No. 10, pp.2152-2162.

Schmitz, M.H., Held, M., Janssens, V., Hutchins, J.R., Hudecz, O., Ivanova, E., Goris, J., Trinkle-Mulcahy, L., Lamond, A.I., Poser, I., Hyman, A.A., Mechtler, K., Peters, J.M. & Gerlich, D.W. (2010) Live-cell imaging RNAi screen identifies PP2A-B55alpha and importin-beta1 as key mitotic exit regulators in human cells. *Nat. Cell Biol.*, Vol. 12, No. 9, pp. 886-893.

Segal, R.A., Pomeroy, S.L. & Stiles, C.D. (1995) Axonal growth and fasciculation linked to differential expression of BDNF and NT3 receptors in developing cerebellar granule cells. *J. Neurosci.*, Vol. 15, No. 7, pp. 4970-4981.

Simonen, M. & Gabriel, D. (2008) High-content screening as improved lead finding strategy. *Eur. Pharm. Rev.*, Vol. 13, No. 2, pp. 46-53.

Swedlow J.R., Goldberg, I., Brauer, E., & Sorger, P.K. (2003) Informatics and quantiative analysis in biological imaging. *Science*, Vol. 300, No. 5616, pp.100-102.

Unterreiner, V., Ibig-Rehm, Y., Simonen, M., Gubler, H. & Gabriel, D. (2009) Comparison of variability and sensitivity between nuclear translocation and luciferase reporter gene assays. *J. Biomol. Screen.*, Vol.14, No. 1, pp. 59-65.

Wang, D., Lagerstrom, R., Sun, C., Bishof, L., Vallotton, P. & Götte, M. (2010) HCA-Vision: Automated neurite outgrowth analysis. *J. Biomol. Screen.*, Vol.15, No. 9, pp. 1165-1170.

Yan, W.K., Goette, M. Hofmann, G., Zaror & I. Sim, J. (2009) High-level soluble expression, purification and characterization of active human midkine from Escherichia coli. *Protein Expr. Purif.*, Vol. 70, No. 2, pp. 270-276.

Young, D. W., Bender. A., Hoyt, J., McWhinnie, E., Chirn, G. W., Y; et al. (2008) Integrating high-content screening and ligand-target prediction identify mechanism of action. *Nat. Chem. Biol.*, Vol. 4, No. 1, pp. 59-68.

15

Recent Advances in Biotherapeutics Drug Discovery and Development

Xiaotian Zhong[1], Peter Neumann[2], Michael Corbo[3] and Evan Loh[3]
[1]*Pfizer Global Biotherapeutics Technologies, Cambridge, MA*
[2]*Institute for Clinical Research and Health Policy Studies, Tufts Medical Center, Boston, MA*
[3]*Pfizer Biotherapeutics Development and Strategic Operation, Collegeville, PA USA*

1. Introduction

Biotherapeutics drugs, such as antibodies, Fc-like fusion proteins, and therapeutic replacement enzymes, constitute the most rapidly growing drug class, and have become a major clinical success of human therapeutics over the past decade. These therapeutics of large-molecule have revolutionized the treatment of a variety of diseases in areas such as oncology, inflammatory and autoimmune diseases, hemophilia, cardiovascular disease, infectious diseases, and rare genetic diseases. In comparison with small-molecule therapeutics, biotherapeutics have a higher approval success rate and a similar development phase length. Physician and patients have accepted biotherapeutics drugs even though most of these products are administrated via injection. Many new biotherapeutics candidates are filling the pre-clinical and clinical pipelines of major Biopharmaceutical companies. The aim of this chapter is to provide a review on recent advances in Biotherapeutics drug discovery and development. Action mechanisms, tools for biotherapeutics generation, design processes, issues like safety and side effects, will be described. In addition, pharmacoeconomics and strategies to provide affordable biotherapeutics drugs will be discussed.

2. An overview of biotherapeutics drug discovery and development

Since the first recombinant-DNA-derived drug human insulin was approved for Eli Lilly by the UK and the US regulators in 1982, more than 170 biotherapeutics products have been launched to benefit quality of life of millions of patients worldwide. These biotherapeutics drugs compose of various types of biological molecular entities, and have revolutionized the treatment of a variety of human diseases ranging from cancer and autoimmune diseases to rare genetic disorders over the past three decades.

Biotherapeutics drugs can be generally classified into three big groups (Table I), based on their physiological properties and mode of actions. The first group is peptides and small protein therapeutics which include growth factors, hormones, and cytokines. This category has been traditionally a major engine for the growth of biotherapeutics drugs, exemplified by insulins, epoetin alpha (Epogen, Aranesp), and granulocyte colony-stimulating factor (Neupogen, Neulasta).

Drug Classes	Examples
1) Peptides and small therapeutic proteins	
A. Growth factors	erythropietins, granulocyte colony-stimulating factors
B. Hormones	insulin, human growth hormone, glucagon-like peptide analogs
C. Cytokines	Interferon-α, β,γ, Interleukins (Neumega, anakinra)
2) Non-immune proteins	
A. Therapeutic replacement enzymes	Naglazyme, Myozyme, Elaprase
B. Blood factors	Factor VIII; factor VIIa, factor IX
C. Anticoagulants	Tissue plasminogen activator, recombinant hirudin, activated protein C
3) Therapeutic antibodies and Fc-like fusion proteins	
A. Therapeutic antibodies	rituximab, adalimumab, cetuximab, trastuzumab
B. Fc-Fusion proteins	etanercept, CD2-Fc, abatacept, Nplate

Table 1. Drug classes of Biotherapeutics drugs

The second group is non-immune therapeutic proteins which include therapeutic replacement enzymes, blood factors, and anticoagulants. This category typically includes recombinant proteins used for treatment of rare genetic disorders, i.e. Naglazyme for Maroteaux-Lamy syndrome, Myozyme for Prompe disease, and Elaprase for Hunter syndrome. Though relatively small, this is a rapidly growing sector of Biotherapeutics drugs.

The third group is therapeutic antibodies and Fc-like fusion proteins. This category ranks the most rapidly growing group of biotherapeutics drugs, propelled by the success of the "big 6": Enbrel, Remicade, and Humira for autoimmune diseases; Rituxan, Herceptin, and Avastin for treatment of several types of cancers. By 2010, at least 11 products from this group have reached global sales of exceeding 1 billion US dollars.

Over the past 10 years, biotherapeutics drugs have become the fastest growing class of therapeutic agents. The total sales of biotherapeutic drug in the US alone reached close to $50 billion in 2010 (Aggarwal 2010). Novel biotherapeutics molecules, i.e. monoclonal antibodies and fusion proteins especially, have been entering clinical study at a rate of over 40 per year since 2007 (Reichert 2011). Hundreds of antibodies and fusion proteins are undergoing clinical evaluation. By the end of 2010, over 30 of this kind of drug candidates were in Phase2/3 or Phase 3 clinical studies, representing a substantial proportion of the late stage therapeutics pipeline. In addition, biotherapeutics drugs have a significantly higher likelihood of being a first-in-class therapy compared with small molecule drugs, considering their novelty and quality. The pharmaceutical and biotechnology industry has therefore been investing increasingly substantial resources in the discovery and development of biotherapeutics products.

Clearly, the process of the discovery and development of a biotherapeutics drug poses challenges that are different from those set by a traditional small molecule drug. In general, biotherapeutics drugs are designer drugs whose mode of action in an underlying disease pathophysiology is usually better understood than those targeted by small-molecule drugs. The data derived from relevant models can support a more rational clinical development program, facilitating better predictions of dosing, efficacy and safety profiles in comparison with small molecule therapeutics. Biotherapeutics drugs therefore have a higher approval success rate, though a similar development phase length, compared with those of small molecule drugs (Reichert 2010). However, as proteins or peptides produced from living cells, biotherapeutics agents require more complicated manufacturing and characterization process to minimize product variation among bath-to-batch. They must be well characterized with regards to potency, identity, quality, purity, and stability.

Advancements in biotherapeutics engineering technologies, and a deeper understanding of mechanism for biotherapeutics action, their safety and side effects in human, have been in action in producing a new generation of biotherapeutics drugs. Experience gained through current biotherapeutics has helped guide future development process via strength building, limitation overcoming, and opportunity seizing. Details of these scientific and technologic knowledges are reviewed in the following sections. By examining the cost issue associated with biotherapeutics drugs, insights into the strategies for affordable biotherapeutics drugs are also discussed.

3. Mechanisms for biotherapeutics action

Diverse mechanisms have been employed by biotherapeutics drugs to achieve therapeutic efficacy and disease modulation. These include direct enzyme replacement, stimulation of biological signal responses, enzymes inhibition, effector functions, Toxin conjugation, cytokine and growth factor blockade.

A. Direct enzyme replacement

Insulin for diabetes control is considered to be the oldest example for enzyme replacement therapy since its breakthrough discovery more than 80 years ago (Hirsch 2005). The development of recombinant insulin in early 1980 eliminates side effects posted by bovine and porcine extracted products. Since then, new generations of insulin analogues such as rapidly-acting analogues and long-acting analogues have been produced. A more recent example for enzyme replacement drugs is the treatment of rare disease disorders such as Lysosomal storage disorders. Gaucher disease and Prompe disease are caused by the lack or dysfunction of an enzyme in the lysosome. Imiglucerase (Genzyme), a recombinant version of glucocerebrosidase, can rescue the deficiency of the disease when this replacement drug is injected regularly throughout patients' lives. After the medical and commercial success in Gaucher disease, a number of enzyme replacement therapies have been approved for several different diseases. Agalsidase β (Genzyme) and agalsidase α (Shire) are for Farbry disease; Laronidase (BioMarin/Genzyme) for Hurler-Schcic syndrome; Idursulphase (Shire) for Hunters Syndrome; Alglucosidase α (Genzyme) for Pompe disease; galsuphase (BioMarin) for Maroteaux-Lamy syndrome. All these products are in orphan diseases group. Recombinant Factor VIII, VIIa, and IX play an important role in blood clotting and are used for people who are genetically deficient (Hemophilia A & B) or have undergone blood loss during a surgery or trauma.

B. Effector functions

The Fc portion of an antibody, composed of the hinge and constant domains, can communicates with the immune system once the antibody binds its target. The communication is through effector functions which include antibody-dependent cellular cytotoxicity (ADCC), antibody-dependent cellular phagocytosis (ADCP), and complement-dependent cytotoxicity (CDC). ADCC and ADCP are through the interaction between Fc and FcγR receptors expressed on a variety of immune cells such as natural killer cells, monocytes, neutrophils and macrophages. CDC is mediated via the interaction of Fc with complement proteins such as C1q. Several antibody therapeutics, including rituximab, adalimumab, cetuximab, trastuzumab and alemtuzumab support ADCC and CDC in vitro, which might also contribute to the therapeutic efficacy in clinical setting such as the destruction of tumor cells or viral infected cells.

C. Cytokine and growth factor blockage.

Tumor necrosis factor (TNF) antagonists, such as therapeutic antibody infliximab, adalimumab, golimumab, certolizumab, and Fc fusion protein etanercept, are presently the most successful class of biotherapeutics drugs for inflammatory diseases. One major mode of action for these antagonists are blocking either soluble TNF or membrane associated factor. Other biotherapeutics drugs with a similar mechanism include canakinumab (Anti-IL-1β antibody) for the treatment of cryopyrin-associated periodic syndrome and ustekinumab (anti-IL-12/IL-23 antibody) for the treatment of psoriasis.

D. Receptor blockage and modulation

Therapeutics antibody can target receptors to block ligand-receptor interaction, which also down-regulate surface expression of the targeted receptor. These antibodies include tocillizumab (targeting IL-6 receptor), efalizumab (targeting αL integrin [CD11a/LFA1]), and natalizumab (targeting α4 subunit of α4β1 & α4β7 integrin). However, targeting surface receptors can potentially result in antigen-induced clearance of therapeutic antibody and decrease its serum half-life. This mechanism can also theoretically have a greater risk for triggering immunogenic response, as antigen-dependent internalization can increase MHC class II antigen processing.

E. Toxin conjugation

To enhance monoclonal antibody utility in the clinical treatment of cancer, cytotoxic drugs such as doxorubicin, calicheamicin, auristatins, and maytansinoids, have been conjugated with monoclonal antibodies (Senter 2009). Targeted site-specific and intracellular delivery of toxins into tumor cells elicits potent antitumor activity in both preclinical and clinical studies. Currently there are one approved antibody conjugated molecule (Gemtuzumab ozogamicin, Mylotarg) and several in late-stage clinical trials (Trastuzumab-DM1, Inotuzumab Ozogamicin).

F. Stimulation of biological signal responses

Romiplotim, a peptide -Fc fusion protein of thrombopoietin analogue, activates Tie2 receptor for the platelet regeneration to treat chronic idiopathic thrombocytopenic purpura. Exenatide mimics a natural peptide (Glucagon-like peptide 1) but is resistant to degradation by protease DPP4 for diabetes control. Erythropietins trigger red blood cell regeneration for anemia. Granulocyte colony-stimulating factors set off white blood cells regeneration for neutropenia; Neumega (recombinant IL-11 receptor agonist) stimulates biological signaling response for chemotherapy-induced thrombocytopenia.

G. Enzymes inhibition

Ecallantide (Dyax), a Kunitz domain-based scaffold, targets human plasma kallikrein for the treatment of attacks of hereditary angioedema. Recombinant hirudin is an inhibitor of thrombin, and activated protein C also has anti-thrombic activity.

4. Tools for biotherapeutics generation

The success of biotherapeutics drugs is attributed to the great technology and tool development for biotherapeutics generation over the past three decades. Various selection technologies, multiple protein engineering platforms, a profusion of biotherapeutics formats and scaffolds, new production systems, and new methods for increasing stability and aggregation resistance, have blossomed into a next wave of therapeutic candidates. The following is a summary of early tools and recent developments.

A. Hybridomas

Mouse hybridomas generated from the stable fusion of immortalized myeloma cells with B cell from immunized mice is the first developed and most widely used technology for the generation of monoclonal antibodies (Kohler and Milstein 1975). This technology has a ubiquitous use and a broad success in drug discovery research. However due to mouse antibodies' high immunogenicity in humans, the weak interaction with human complement and FcγRs, and short half-life with no binding to human salvage receptor FcRn, they have a very low clinical success rate. These limitations have been largely overcome by chimerization and humanization in the current era of antibody therapeutics.

B. Chimerization and humanization

Chimerization of an antibody is joining the variable domains of a mouse monoclonal antibody to the constant domains of a human antibody (Boulianne et al. 1984; Morrison et al. 1984). This tool utilizes a detailed understanding of the structure and function of immunoglobulin domains as well as the determinants of antigen binding. The humanization strategies involve transferring the complementary-determining regions (CDRs, the antigen-binding loops) from a mouse antibody to a human IgGs, and additional mutagenesis of one or more framework-region residues back to the parent mouse antibody.

C. Human antibodies from transgenic mice

A growing number of antibodies entering clinical trials and the market are completely human. Some of them are derived from transgenic mice that express human immunoglobulin genes (Lonberg 2005). Mice that are transgenic for human immunoglobulin genes and have disrupted mouse immunoglobulin heavy-chain and Igκ light-chain can be immunized with target-antigens to produce human antibodies. B cells that express specific human antibodies can be cloned for hybridomas, similar to the generation of mouse monoclonal antibodies. The binding affinity of these transgenic-mouse-generated antibodies is often high, likely due to the in vivo affinity maturation process and therefore obviating the in vitro affinity optimization steps. Human IgG1 output from transgenic mice and the direct use of hybridomas cell lines for human antibody production can allow early screening for biological function and for pre-clinical development. One challenge to use transgenic mice is to derive antibodies that are crossreactive with mouse antigens. It is often desirable to evaluate biological function of the species-crossreactive antibodies in animal models of disease. In transgenic mice, self-reactive antibody-producing cells are selected against by the processes of immune tolerance induction.

D. Human antibodies from phage-display libraries

Phages encoding a single-chain V-domain antibody fragment(scFv) on their surface and selective recovery of phage on the basis of antigen binding were first reported by McCafferty et al (McCafferty et al. 1990). Diverse human immunoglobulin-heavy-chain V (VH) gene segments and light-chain V (VL) gene segments were prepared from peripheral-blood lymphocytes of non-immunized donors by PCR, and scFvs genes were made by randomly combining VH and VL gene segments using PCR. The combinatorial library (up to ~10^{11} genes) can be cloned for display on the surface of phage and used to identify scFvs that bind target antigens. Further progress in phage-display technology has included display of Fabs and high-throughput screening methods adapted from small-molecule drug discovery. A particular strength of phage-display libraries, in contrast to hybridomas technology, is the direct selection for specific binding properties, such as species crossreactivities. In addition, phage-display technology has a capability to provide very large collections of antibodies, which allows the identification of high potency antibodies or with rare combinations of properties.

E. Glycoengineering

Glycoengineering is changing protein-associated carbohydrate to alter pharmacokinetic property or biological function of therapeutic proteins, because of the ability to manipulate DNA sequences. Glycoengineering can increase molecular stability, solubility, serum half-life, in vivo biological activity, and reduce immunogenicity. One well known example of this technology is the discovery of darbepoetin alfa, a hyperglycosylated analogue of erythropoietin that contains two additional N-linked carbohydrates (Elliott et al. 2003). The introduction of new N-linked glycosylation consensus sequences into desirable position in the peptide backbone can increase sialic acid containing carbohydrate, thereby increasing serum half-life. Another aspect of glycoengineering is generating various glycoforms of a glycoprotein. An engineered CHO cells with overexpressing galactosyltransferase and sialyltransferase can maximize sialic acid content of recombinant glycoproteins produced (Weikert et al. 1999). A fucosyl-transferase knock-out cell line produce antibody protein with fucose-free glycan attached at Asn 297 in the IgG-Fc region, which possess a significantly increased ADCC activity (Niwa et al. 2004; Shields et al. 2002). Another glycoengineering approach involves in vitro treatment of a purified glycoprotein with glycosidases or glycotransferases. Cerezyme, the recombinant glucocerebrosidase, has been treated with neuraminidase, β-galactosidase and β-hexosaminidase, to trim outer oligosaccharide to expose core mannose residues underneath for macrophage targeting (Brady and Barton 1994; Hoppe 2000).

F. Multispecific antibodies

Bispecific antibodies that are capable of strong and specific binding with two different antigens have been on the scene for decades. They can target two or more disease mechanisms as a single agent and provide a unique alternative to combination therapies. More importantly, bispecific antibodies can achieve some therapeutic strategies that are not feasible with conventional monospecific monoclonal antibody combination. For instance, by targeting both immune effector cells surface molecules and tumor cell surface markers, bispecific antibodies could preferentially recruit activating effector cells to kill tumor cells (Chames and Baty 2009). Bispecific antibodies have been used for the site-specific targeting insulin and transferring receptors on the blood-brain barrier (BBB) as transporter and anti-amyloid-β targeting binding across BBB is significantly increased (Boado et al. 2010). Bispecific antibodies can be generated via several approaches, including cell fusion-based quadromas and triomas(Nisonoff and Rivers 1961), chemical cross-linking-based approach (Graziano and Guptill 2004), and recombinant technology-based approaches, such as using Ig hetero-oligomerization domain(Muller et al. 1998; Ridgway et al. 1996), non-Ig hetero-oligomerization domains, scFv-based bispecific, and single variable domain-based bispecific (Holt et al. 2003), dual-variable domain immunoglobulin(Wu et al. 2007).

G. Intrabodies

Intrabodies are antibodies that are designed to be expressed intracellularly against different target antigens present in cytosol, nucleus, endoplasmic reticulum, mitochondria, peroxisomes, and plasma membrane (Lo 2008; Williams and Zhu 2006). Though Introbodies have the potential of interfering with intracellular biosynthetic pathways, the major obstacle of Intrabodies is the absence of efficient in vivo delivery method to live target cells(Stocks 2006). Current attempts are using recombinant adenovirus and vaccinia virus vetors or immunoliposomes (Williams and Zhu 2006).

H. Protein engineering,

Molecular biology techniques such as site-directed mutagenesis and error-prone PCR have been routinely used for biotherapeutics generation. Computational modeling and structure-based drug design with three-dimentional structural information are widely applied to protein engineering. Screening technologies such Peptide Phage-display Libraries, "Peptides on Plasmids" libraries, Ribosome display, mRNA display, CIS display, and DNA display, have also been utilized for biotherapeutics lead generation (McGregor 2008).

5. Design processes for biotherapeutics

Biotherapeutics-based drug development is driven by unmet medical needs. Designing a successful biotherapeutics requires understanding of several critical areas.

First is the understanding of disease biology. Human diseases are complex and heterogeneous that multiple redundant and distinct mechanisms determine the final disease outcome and contribute to multifaceted, distinct disease symptoms (acute versus chronicle) and pathologies. It is important to evaluate if there are good preclinical models and understand the limitation of the predictive power of these animal models. Translational medicine helps define good biomarkers for disease progress and designing clinical trials with appropriate end points that reflect the role of the specific targeted mechanism in a complex disease.

Second is the understanding of target biology. It is critical to determine which target should be chosen in a defined mechanism. Targeting either soluble ligands or surface receptors, serving as agonist or antagonist, need to be determined. An overall target biology within the context of the disease (specific aspects of the disease that are driven by the target) need to be understood. Typically drug targets can be classified into three groups. The first group is so-called "clinically validated targets" because of their proof-of-activity shown in humans. This validated approach has a high probability of success, but the competition is crowded and freedom to operation is decreased. The second group is experimentally- validated targets, whose importance for disease mechanisms have been demonstrated by a vast literature. Most cytokines and associated receptors for immunological disorders and tyrosine kinases receptors in oncology fall into this category, as the mechanisms driving these disorders are reasonably well known. The third group of targets is those new or less well studied target proteins that might be involved in pathogenic disorders. More extensive and careful validation is required. They are with a greater potential for new therapeutic breakthroughs, but carrying out a greater risk of development failures.

Lastly is the advancement of biotherapeutic technologies. We need to understand affinity and potency, specificity and cross-reactivity, physicochemical properties, immunogenicity, expression and purification, solubility and stability, pharmacokinetics and pharmacodynamics, and formulability and manufacturability. In short, we need to know what features a good biotherapeutic protein must possess by incorporation of lessons learned over the years, as well as identify key issues critical for technology advancement.

6. Safety and side effects of biotherapeutics

Administration of biotherapeutics carries the risk of immune response and numerous adverse effects that are related to their specific targets and organ-specific adverse events (Giezen et al. 2008; Hansel et al. 2010). The following discuss a range of adverse effects encountered with biotherapeutics, some of which have been fatal, and strategies to minimize these events. These events include those documented for licensed biotherapeutics as well as examples of side effects found during exploratory clinical studies. Some of the severe adverse effects are not anticipated from currently available preclinical screening tools and animal models. These lessons can provide new strategies and guidelines needed for the development of safer and more efficacious biotherapeutics.

A. Acute Immune reactions

Biotherapeutics can induce acute infusion reactions either due to their mechanism of action and/or their foreign nature of the molecule and/or co-purified impurities that result in acute reactions either via innate immunity or due to the reaction with pre-existing, or induced IgE antibodies. Clinical magnification can range from local skin reactions at the injection site through acute anaphylaxis and systemic inflammatory response syndrome. For rituximab (Coiffier et al, 2002), first dose infusion reactions combine serum sickness, tumor lysis syndrome and cytokine release syndrome, primarily as a result of its mechanism of action. These initial reactions can be minimized by appropriate hydration and

premedication, and cautious incremental increases in the rate of infusion. Acute anaphylactic and anaphylactoid reactions are commonly described for cetuximab which has been attributed to pre-existing IgE antibodies against galactose-α1,3-galactose which is expressed on the cetuximab molecule (Chung et al. 2008).

B. Immunogenicity

The development of immunogenicity, or anti-drug antibodies, has important clinical ramifications. The development of immunogenicity could lead to a number of important clinical implications, including alternation in PK and loss of efficacy through neutralization, an increase in adverse events associated with drug-antibody interactions, and, dependent upon the nature of the biotherapeutic, the potential for cross reactivity of antibodies with endogenous ligands. As such, the assessment of immunogenicity and the assessment of ADA's clinical implications is a crucial part of biotherapeutics development. The development and appropriate validation of anti-drug antibody assays is a fundamental necessity in understanding ADA. Interference by a parent drug and existing antibodies must be evaluated. In addition, a comprehensive assessment of the clinical implications of the ADA must be assessed in the clinical setting to evaluate both safety and efficacy, as well as any reasonable cross-reactive effect.

C. Infections

A well documented side effect of biotherapeutics is infection, which is generally due to removal of the therapeutic targets that have a protective function in the normal immune system. An increased risk of tuberculosis infection has been associated with TNFα-specific biotherapeutics (Schneeweiss et al. 2007). Progressive multifocal leukoencephalopathy (PML) is a rapidly progressive demyelinating disease that is due to reactivation of the infection in the central nervous system with the polyoma virus John Cunningham virus (JCV), though most healthy people are seropositive for JCV. The risk of PML is about 1 in 1,000 multiple sclerosis patients treated with natalizamab (Yousry et al. 2006). A number of PML cases are found for rituximab (Carson et al. 2009) and efaliziumab (Molloy and Calabrese 2009).

D. Autoimmune diseases

Biotherapeutics such as monoclonal antibodies have the capacity through their immunomodulatory actions to cause various autoimmune conditions (Mongey and Hess 2008), such as Lupus-like syndromes and drug-related lupus, Thyroid disease, and autoimmune colitis. For instance, the treatment of TNFα specific monoclonal antibodies has been found associated with the development of anti-nuclear antibodies and anti-bodies to double-stranded DNA as well as with lupus-like syndromes (Mongey and Hess 2008). When used in multiple sclerosis, anti-CD52 immunosuppressive monoclonal antibody alemtuzumab was found to cause antibody-mediated thyroid autoimmunity in almost 25% of study patients (Coles et al. 1999).

Other agents have observed autoimmune events as a result of their direct mechanism of action. Anti-Cytotoxic T-lymphocyte-antigen 4 (CTLA4) specific monoclonal antibodies such as ipilimumab and tremelimumab increase T-cell stimulation and has been shown antitumor activity (Maker et al. 2005), but also cause an autoimmune enterocolitis and other immune-related adverse events such as rash and hepatitis (Peggs et al. 2006).

E. Cancer

Some antibody therapeutics such as infliximab and ustekinumab (Rennard et al. 2007; Weiss et al. 2007) have even been found inducing tumorigenicity in auto-immune patients.

F. Platelet and thrombotic disorders

Drug-induced immune thrombocytopaenia is a decrease in the number of circulatory platelets in the blood caused by medications such as biotherapeutics (Aster and Bougie 2007). An acute severe, self-limiting thrombocytopaenia has been found with the treatment of infliximab (TNFα-specific), efalizumab [CD11a-specific; (Tamhane and Gurm 2008)] and rituximab (CD20-specific), but the mechanisms of action remain unknown.

G. Dermatitis

The EGFR-specific antibodies such cetuximab and panitumumab can commonly cause a skin rash on the face and upper torso (Perez-Soler and Saltz 2005). The dermatitis is thought to be part of the pharmacodynamic action of these agents, because EGFR is widely expressed on epithelial cells (Bianchini et al. 2008).

H. Cardiotoxicity

Trastuzumab, a humanized monoclonal antibody targeting HER2, has been used to treat HER2-positive metastatic breast cancer (Hudis 2007). However in the trials, cardiotoxicity as an unexpected adverse event was discovered (Force and Kerkela 2008). This cardiac dysfunction caused by trastuzumab is target-related, because blocking HER2 signaling causes mitochondrial outer membrane permeabilization and eventually apoptosis of cardiac muscle cells with impaired contractility and ventricular function (Kuramochi et al. 2006).

I. Cytokine storm

Cytokine storm is an uncontrolled hypercytokinaemia that causes multiple organ damage. It is a prominent side effect with CD3 specific [muromonab; (Plevy et al. 2007)], CD52 specific [alemtuzumab; (Wing et al. 1996; Wing et al. 1995)] and CD20 specific [rituximab; (Winkler et al. 1999)]. A fully humanized monoclonal antibody TGN1412 triggered an immediate and severe cytokine storm when given to six healthy male volunteers (Suntharalingam et al. 2006).

7. Pharmacoeconomics and strategies to provide affordable biotherapeutics drugs

Biotherapeutics are distinctive from traditional small molecule pharmaceuticals in terms of administration mode, relatively high prices, and significant disease modification. The high development cost and high financial risk are associated with the complex process of biotherapeutics drug discovery and development as seen in the previous sections. However the new and effective biotherapeutics drugs present society a fundamental question about how to make these promising drugs more affordable. One example is Orphan drugs whose prices are often substantially higher than those of other drugs, and might occur at the expense of common diseases if more orphan drugs are approved (Tambuyzer 2010). In UK, due to the high treatment cost relative to patient benefit, National Institute of Clinical Excellence did not approve reimbursement for several cancer drugs including monoclonal antibody Avastin (Raftery 2009). In US, some health plans require more than 30% co-insurance and some biotherapeutics can cost as high as $100,000, the financial burden on patients is significant. A concern has been raised for society how to pay for these innovative drugs (Zhong 2010).

Pharmacoeconomic evaluation and value-based analysis, which serve to guide optimal healthcare resource allocation, have been used for new drug reimbursement and coverage (Cohen and Wilson 2009; Neumann 2009). But the direct application of these evaluation in health policy recommendation and formulation remains highly debated (Neumann and Weinstein 2010). It has been argued that weeding out inefficiencies may be more effective in controlling cost than denying reimbursement. From research and development standpoints, decreasing costs and increasing success rate for the drug approval is a critical part of achieving this mission.

Clinical testing in human for new biotherapeutics drugs entails a large sum of financial investment. Though biotherapeutics have higher probabilities of clinical success, they have a higher attrition rate in phase III trials than small-molecule drugs (Grabowski 2008), indicating that the failure results are known only after high development cost have been incurred. Improving trial designs with biomarker identification and proper patient selection is the key to decreasing trial attrition rate. One good example is the EGFR-targeted therapy of colorectal cancer. Even though EGFR is widely overexpressed in tumor cells from most of patients, only those with a wild type KRAS phenotype will benefit from EGFR-specific cetuximab or panitumumab treatment (Walther et al. 2009).

Besides increasing productivity, lowering production and processing cost is another important factor to provide affordable biotherapeutics treatments. Recent breakthroughs in production yields of mammalian cells, shortening production time, and improving purification and formulation for antibody production, are critical features for cost reduction. In addition, non-mammalian production systems such as engineered yeast and plant cells are being used for biotherapeutics production, which could be a substantial saving for the removal of costly viral inactivation validations step.

Increasing expenditures and the high prices of biotherapeutics have highlighted the need of lower-cost generic substitutes for off-patent biotherapeutics drugs, usually called biosimilars (Ledford 2010).

Biosimilars terminology stems from the inherent variability in the production of complex proteins in a living organism. As such, the innovator, or reference product has a range of critical quality attributes that affect the overall properties of the molecule. These attributes range from the fundamental amino acid sequence, through complex glycosylation. Given the complexity of these molecules, the determination of biosimilarity is a broad assessment of similarity, encompassing advanced analytical techniques, and nonclinical and clinical assessments. It is the confluence of these data that allow for the assessment of biosmilarity. Typically, the biosimilar process begins with the reverse engineering of the reference innovator product. While the amino acid sequence may be published, variability must be confirmed. Additionally, post-translational modification, such as glycosylation profile must be determined analytically as these are dependent upon the cell line, fermentation conditions and purification process. The glycoforms on the protein often contribute not only to their pharmacokinetics, but their inherent activity. Once the critical quality attributes are determined, cell line development is used to determine an appropriate cell line and subclone to produce a molecule within the desired attribute framework. While molecule dependent, it is likely that some nonclinical and clinical work will be necessary to demonstrate biosimilarity. Clinical experience may be required to ensure the safety and efficacy of the biosimilar. The level of clinical experience may range from human bioequivalence up through and including non-inferiority/equivalence studies based upon efficacy. Additionally, the post market surveillance of biosimilars will be important in understanding their long term safety profile relative to the innovator molecule.

The regulatory requirements for biosimilar approval should be sufficiently high to ensure that patient safety and efficacy are assured so that these important treatments can be used with confidence.

At this point in time, at least 12 biosimilar products, encompassing human growth hormone, erythropoietin, and granulocyte colony-stimulating factors, have been authorized for marketing. Some complex biotherapeutics such as antibody of rituximab are approved locally in India, China, and South Korea. The US Food and Drug Administration has been developing guidelines that will expand the development of biosimilars since it received the authority to approve biosimilars as part of President Barack Obama's health-care reforms. The introduction of biosimilars will make a number of biotherapeutics drugs significantly affordable when their patents expire. The EMEA has published biosimilar guidelines, as have other countries. Additionally, the World Health Organization (WHO) has developed a position paper on the development of biosimilars.

8. Conclusions and perspectives

Tremendous progress has been made in the research and development of biotherapeutics drugs. Much has been learnt from the scientific and clinical experiences of these biological molecules. New technologies and new discoveries are always emerging, yet many challenges remain. Identifying and validating new targets, addressing oral delivery of biotherapeutics drugs, and improving phase III success rate, are a few to be named. The advent of age of biosimilars will surely make biotherapeutics drugs more accessible and economical. The key is striking a balance between the incentives for cost saving and rewarding innovation.

9. Acknowledgement

This book chapter is dedicated to the centenary of the late Prof. Haoran Jian (1911-2011) (by X.Z.).

10. References

Aggarwal S. 2010. What's fueling the biotech engine-2009-2010. Nat Biotechnol 28(11):1165-71.

Aster RH, Bougie DW. 2007. Drug-induced immune thrombocytopenia. N Engl J Med 357(6):580-7.

Bianchini D, Jayanth A, Chua YJ, Cunningham D. 2008. Epidermal growth factor receptor inhibitor-related skin toxicity: mechanisms, treatment, and its potential role as a predictive marker. Clin Colorectal Cancer 7(1):33-43.

Boado RJ, Lu JZ, Hui EK, Pardridge WM. 2010. IgG-single chain Fv fusion protein therapeutic for Alzheimer's disease: Expression in CHO cells and pharmacokinetics and brain delivery in the rhesus monkey. Biotechnol Bioeng 105(3):627-35.

Boulianne GL, Hozumi N, Shulman MJ. 1984. Production of functional chimaeric mouse/human antibody. Nature 312(5995):643-6.

Brady RO, Barton NW. 1994. Enzyme replacement therapy for Gaucher disease: critical investigations beyond demonstration of clinical efficacy. Biochem Med Metab Biol 52(1):1-9.

Carson KR, Evens AM, Richey EA, Habermann TM, Focosi D, Seymour JF, Laubach J, Bawn SD, Gordon LI, Winter JN and others. 2009. Progressive multifocal leukoencephalopathy after rituximab therapy in HIV-negative patients: a report of 57 cases from the Research on Adverse Drug Events and Reports project. Blood 113(20):4834-40.

Chames P, Baty D. 2009. Bispecific antibodies for cancer therapy: the light at the end of the tunnel? MAbs 1(6):539-47.

Chung CH, Mirakhur B, Chan E, Le QT, Berlin J, Morse M, Murphy BA, Satinover SM, Hosen J, Mauro D and others. 2008. Cetuximab-induced anaphylaxis and IgE specific for galactose-alpha-1,3-galactose. N Engl J Med 358(11):1109-17.

Cohen J, Wilson A. 2009. New challenges to medicare beneficiary access to mAbs. MAbs 1(1):56-66.

Coiffier B, Lepage E, Briere J, Herbrecht R, Tilly H, Bouabdallah R, Morel P, Van Den Neste E, Salles G, Gaulard P and others. 2002. CHOP chemotherapy plus rituximab compared with CHOP alone in elderly patients with diffuse large-B-cell lymphoma. N Engl J Med 346(4):235-42.

Coles AJ, Wing M, Smith S, Coraddu F, Greer S, Taylor C, Weetman A, Hale G, Chatterjee VK, Waldmann H and others. 1999. Pulsed monoclonal antibody treatment and autoimmune thyroid disease in multiple sclerosis. Lancet 354(9191):1691-5.

Elliott S, Lorenzini T, Asher S, Aoki K, Brankow D, Buck L, Busse L, Chang D, Fuller J, Grant J and others. 2003. Enhancement of therapeutic protein in vivo activities through glycoengineering. Nat Biotechnol 21(4):414-21.

Force T, Kerkela R. 2008. Cardiotoxicity of the new cancer therapeutics--mechanisms of, and approaches to, the problem. Drug Discov Today 13(17-18):778-84.

Giezen TJ, Mantel-Teeuwisse AK, Straus SM, Schellekens H, Leufkens HG, Egberts AC. 2008. Safety-related regulatory actions for biologicals approved in the United States and the European Union. JAMA 300(16):1887-96.

Grabowski H. 2008. Follow-on biologics: data exclusivity and the balance between innovation and competition. Nat Rev Drug Discov 7(6):479-88.

Graziano RF, Guptill P. 2004. Chemical production of bispecific antibodies. Methods Mol Biol 283:71-85.

Hansel TT, Kropshofer H, Singer T, Mitchell JA, George AJ. 2010. The safety and side effects of monoclonal antibodies. Nat Rev Drug Discov 9(4):325-38.

Hirsch IB. 2005. Insulin analogues. N Engl J Med 352(2):174-83.

Holt LJ, Herring C, Jespers LS, Woolven BP, Tomlinson IM. 2003. Domain antibodies: proteins for therapy. Trends Biotechnol 21(11):484-90.

Hoppe H. 2000. Cerezyme--recombinant protein treatment for Gaucher's disease. J Biotechnol 76(2-3):259-61.

Hudis CA. 2007. Trastuzumab--mechanism of action and use in clinical practice. N Engl J Med 357(1):39-51.

Kohler G, Milstein C. 1975. Continuous cultures of fused cells secreting antibody of predefined specificity. Nature 256(5517):495-7.

Kuramochi Y, Guo X, Sawyer DB. 2006. Neuregulin activates erbB2-dependent src/FAK signaling and cytoskeletal remodeling in isolated adult rat cardiac myocytes. J Mol Cell Cardiol 41(2):228-35.

Ledford H. 2010. 'Biosimilar' drugs poised to penetrate market. Nature 468(7320):18-9.

Lo A, Zhu, Q. Marasco, WA, editor. 2008. Intracellular antibodies (intrabodies) and their therapeutic potential. Berlin, Heidelberg: Springer-Verlag. pp.343-373 p.

Lonberg N. 2005. Human antibodies from transgenic animals. Nat Biotechnol 23(9):1117-25.

Maker AV, Attia P, Rosenberg SA. 2005. Analysis of the cellular mechanism of antitumor responses and autoimmunity in patients treated with CTLA-4 blockade. J Immunol 175(11):7746-54.

McCafferty J, Griffiths AD, Winter G, Chiswell DJ. 1990. Phage antibodies: filamentous phage displaying antibody variable domains. Nature 348(6301):552-4.

McGregor DP. 2008. Discovering and improving novel peptide therapeutics. Curr Opin Pharmacol 8(5):616-9.

Molloy ES, Calabrese LH. 2009. Therapy: Targeted but not trouble-free: efalizumab and PML. Nat Rev Rheumatol 5(8):418-9.

Mongey AB, Hess EV. 2008. Drug insight: autoimmune effects of medications-what's new? Nat Clin Pract Rheumatol 4(3):136-44.

Morrison SL, Johnson MJ, Herzenberg LA, Oi VT. 1984. Chimeric human antibody molecules: mouse antigen-binding domains with human constant region domains. Proc Natl Acad Sci U S A 81(21):6851-5.

Muller KM, Arndt KM, Pluckthun A. 1998. A dimeric bispecific miniantibody combines two specificities with avidity. FEBS Lett 432(1-2):45-9.

Neumann PJ. 2009. Are mAbs different?: a comment on Cohen and Wilson. MAbs 1(1):29-30.

Neumann PJ, Weinstein MC. 2010. Legislating against use of cost-effectiveness information. N Engl J Med 363(16):1495-7.

Nisonoff A, Rivers MM. 1961. Recombination of a mixture of univalent antibody fragments of different specificity. Arch Biochem Biophys 93:460-2.

Niwa R, Shoji-Hosaka E, Sakurada M, Shinkawa T, Uchida K, Nakamura K, Matsushima K, Ueda R, Hanai N, Shitara K. 2004. Defucosylated chimeric anti-CC chemokine receptor 4 IgG1 with enhanced antibody-dependent cellular cytotoxicity shows potent therapeutic activity to T-cell leukemia and lymphoma. Cancer Res 64(6):2127-33.

Peggs KS, Quezada SA, Korman AJ, Allison JP. 2006. Principles and use of anti-CTLA4 antibody in human cancer immunotherapy. Curr Opin Immunol 18(2):206-13.

Perez-Soler R, Saltz L. 2005. Cutaneous adverse effects with HER1/EGFR-targeted agents: is there a silver lining? J Clin Oncol 23(22):5235-46.

Plevy S, Salzberg B, Van Assche G, Regueiro M, Hommes D, Sandborn W, Hanauer S, Targan S, Mayer L, Mahadevan U and others. 2007. A phase I study of visilizumab, a humanized anti-CD3 monoclonal antibody, in severe steroid-refractory ulcerative colitis. Gastroenterology 133(5):1414-22.

Raftery J. 2009. NICE and the challenge of cancer drugs. Bmj 338:b67.

Reichert JM. 2010. Metrics for antibody therapeutics development. MAbs 2(6):695-700.

Reichert JM. 2011. Antibody-based therapeutics to watch in 2011. MAbs 3(1):76-99.

Rennard SI, Fogarty C, Kelsen S, Long W, Ramsdell J, Allison J, Mahler D, Saadeh C, Siler T, Snell P and others. 2007. The safety and efficacy of infliximab in moderate to severe chronic obstructive pulmonary disease. Am J Respir Crit Care Med 175(9):926-34.

Ridgway JB, Presta LG, Carter P. 1996. 'Knobs-into-holes' engineering of antibody CH3 domains for heavy chain heterodimerization. Protein Eng 9(7):617-21.

Schneeweiss S, Setoguchi S, Weinblatt ME, Katz JN, Avorn J, Sax PE, Levin R, Solomon DH. 2007. Anti-tumor necrosis factor alpha therapy and the risk of serious bacterial infections in elderly patients with rheumatoid arthritis. Arthritis Rheum 56(6):1754-64.

Senter PD. 2009. Potent antibody drug conjugates for cancer therapy. Curr Opin Chem Biol 13(3):235-44.

Shields RL, Lai J, Keck R, O'Connell LY, Hong K, Meng YG, Weikert SH, Presta LG. 2002. Lack of fucose on human IgG1 N-linked oligosaccharide improves binding to human Fcgamma RIII and antibody-dependent cellular toxicity. J Biol Chem 277(30):26733-40.

Stocks M. 2006. Intracellular antibodies: a revolution waiting to happen? Curr Opin Mol Ther 8(1):17-23.

Suntharalingam G, Perry MR, Ward S, Brett SJ, Castello-Cortes A, Brunner MD, Panoskaltsis N. 2006. Cytokine storm in a phase 1 trial of the anti-CD28 monoclonal antibody TGN1412. N Engl J Med 355(10):1018-28.

Tambuyzer E. 2010. Rare diseases, orphan drugs and their regulation: questions and misconceptions. Nat Rev Drug Discov 9(12):921-9.

Tamhane UU, Gurm HS. 2008. The chimeric monoclonal antibody abciximab: a systematic review of its safety in contemporary practice. Expert Opin Drug Saf 7(6):809-19.

Walther A, Johnstone E, Swanton C, Midgley R, Tomlinson I, Kerr D. 2009. Genetic prognostic and predictive markers in colorectal cancer. Nat Rev Cancer 9(7):489-99.

Weikert S, Papac D, Briggs J, Cowfer D, Tom S, Gawlitzek M, Lofgren J, Mehta S, Chisholm V, Modi N and others. 1999. Engineering Chinese hamster ovary cells to maximize sialic acid content of recombinant glycoproteins. Nat Biotechnol 17(11):1116-21.

Weiss JM, Subleski JJ, Wigginton JM, Wiltrout RH. 2007. Immunotherapy of cancer by IL-12-based cytokine combinations. Expert Opin Biol Ther 7(11):1705-21.

Williams BR, Zhu Z. 2006. Intrabody-based approaches to cancer therapy: status and prospects. Curr Med Chem 13(12):1473-80.

Wing MG, Moreau T, Greenwood J, Smith RM, Hale G, Isaacs J, Waldmann H, Lachmann PJ, Compston A. 1996. Mechanism of first-dose cytokine-release syndrome by CAMPATH 1-H: involvement of CD16 (FcgammaRIII) and CD11a/CD18 (LFA-1) on NK cells. J Clin Invest 98(12):2819-26.

Wing MG, Waldmann H, Isaacs J, Compston DA, Hale G. 1995. Ex-vivo whole blood cultures for predicting cytokine-release syndrome: dependence on target antigen and antibody isotype. Ther Immunol 2(4):183-90.

Winkler U, Jensen M, Manzke O, Schulz H, Diehl V, Engert A. 1999. Cytokine-release syndrome in patients with B-cell chronic lymphocytic leukemia and high lymphocyte counts after treatment with an anti-CD20 monoclonal antibody (rituximab, IDEC-C2B8). Blood 94(7):2217-24.

Wu C, Ying H, Grinnell C, Bryant S, Miller R, Clabbers A, Bose S, McCarthy D, Zhu RR, Santora L and others. 2007. Simultaneous targeting of multiple disease mediators by a dual-variable-domain immunoglobulin. Nat Biotechnol 25(11):1290-7.

Yousry TA, Major EO, Ryschkewitsch C, Fahle G, Fischer S, Hou J, Curfman B, Miszkiel K, Mueller-Lenke N, Sanchez E and others. 2006. Evaluation of patients treated with natalizumab for progressive multifocal leukoencephalopathy. N Engl J Med 354(9):924-33.

Zhong X. 2010. Paying for a long-fighting war: The healthcare dilemma of cancer medicines. Pharmaceutical Medicine 24(2):83-88.

16

Drug Discovery by Aptamers in Protozoan Infectious Diseases

Carsten Wrenger[1] and Henning Ulrich[2]
[1]*Department of Parasitology, Institute of Biomedical Science, University of Sao Paulo, Sao Paulo*
[2]*Department of Biochemistry, Institute of Chemistry, University of Sao Paulo, Sao Paulo*
Brazil

1. Introduction

In the last decades the need for novel diagnostic and chemotherapeutic tools became apparent. The increasing population and upcoming diverse disease patterns are leading to a synergistic effect, which emphasises the required demand for new types of pharmacological agents. Additionally, newly gained knowledge such as completing the human genome and on-going transcriptome and proteome projects identified novel targets for therapeutic intervention. However the upcoming number of diseases as well as their variety force medical science to accelerate the process of drug discovery by employing sophisticated methodologies for chemical synthesis of biological active compounds and time- and cost-sparing screening assays to develop novel drugs. These diseases are not only related to cancer or insights from the human genome project but become more prominent by time, since they are derived from human external sources such as infectious agents causing serious disease of mankind. For instance, approximately a quarter of the entire population is living in malaria endemic areas and is thereby daily exposed to lethal pathogens such as *Plasmodium falciparum* (WHO).
Due to novel chemical synthesis procedures, approaches using combinatorial libraries followed by high-throughput screenings for biological activity are the current method of choice to increase the procession time and decrease application costs in the search for possible drug candidates. Subsequently possible drug targets are identified by *in vitro* assays, which test their biological relevance, and validated in animal models. Rational drug design, natural product or combinatorial library approaches have been employed to identify possible lead compounds for drug development. In order to compensate for the high demand of new drugs novel high-throughput strategies for screening high numbers of compounds were developed, which also decreased the production time (Fernandes, 1998). Most promising drug candidates are often subject to chemical modifications to improve their synthesis parameters as well as their toxicity profile and stability under physiological conditions. This procedure has been employed for several generations of drug development which were afterwards verified in animal models before clinical studies were applied (Faria and Ulrich, 2002, Majumder et al. 2009). The design of specific inhibitors against proteins involved in disease mediation is one of the primary objectives in pharmacological research.

The identification level of possible drug candidates for therapeutic applications has been increased by using a variety of screening strategies for active compounds in combinatorial libraries. In general, the suitability of combinatorial library approaches for drug design is based on the probability that a member of a high quantity population consisting of different molecules and structures, like peptides, carbohydrates and/or oligonucleotides, binds to the respective target of choice. For the discovery of specific ligands with binding capabilities to a desired target peptide- and oligonucleotide-based libraries were of particular interest since the library and thereby identified binders can be replicated by enzymatic catalysis. The SELEX technique (systematic evolution of ligands by exponential enrichment), was developed in parallel by Tuerk and Gold (1990) and Ellington and Szostak (1990) and is based on an oligonucleotide combinatorial library containing a vast number (around 10^{13}) of different sequences and structural motifs for the *in vitro* selection of DNA or RNA molecules with binding specificity to their respective targets. The selected high affinity binders are called aptamers (from *aptus* (Latin) = to fit). Functional DNA or RNA molecules were identified as specific binders to a number of different targets including nucleotides (Sassanfar and Szostak, 1993, Meli et al., 2002), biologically active peptides and soluble proteins (Jellinek et al., 1993, Ruckman et al., 1998, Williams et al., 1996, Proske et al., 2002) and complex targets such as membrane-bound receptors (Ulrich et al. 1998) and blood vessels (Blank et al. 2001). However, due to degradation processes of nucleic acids in biological systems, aptamers were not ideal drug candidates. This limitation was overcome by chemical improvements in oligonucleotide synthesis which prolonged the stability of the molecules in biological tissues as well as their pharmacokinetics (Trujillo et al., 2007, Ni et al., 2011). New skills in oligonucleotide modification and lower synthesis costs extended the investigation of protein interactions from *in vitro* to *in vivo* applications and also the design of new compounds for pharmaceutical applications. The deriving aptamer properties are evoked by their respective tertiary structure providing unique features for these oligonucleotides to bind with nanomolar or even picomolar dissociation constants to their target proteins being higher than most of the natural occurring ligands or inhibitors. Moreover, aptamers possess numerous advantages over antibodies in many applications due to their non-peptide character and flexibility to interact with even to hidden targets with characteristics of small molecule binding. Further advantages of aptamers include the simplicity of synthesis and the ability of chemical modification of the nucleotides or backbones, their stability against thermal denaturation and nuclease degradation, the lack of immunogenicity and rapid penetration of tissues. Moreover, aptamers posses the ability to interact with functional protein domains such as ligand-binding domains mainly due to molecule-size advantages compared to antibodies or natural ligands (Ulrich et al., 2006).

As already outline above aptamers can be subject to a variety of changes to enhance their stability especially for *in vivo* applications. These modifications can be introduced by using T7 RNA polymerase which accepts, for instance nucleotides like 2'-F-pyrimidines as substrates (Pestourie et al., 2005; Ulrich et al., 2006). By adding phosphorothioate based nucleotides to DNA- or 2'-F or 2'-amino-substitution of 2'OH groups of riboses to RNA-libraries a nuclease resistant oligonucleotide library will be produced.

In contrast to 2'-amino-pyrimidine substitution – 2'-fluoro-pyrimidine modifications lead to higher thermal stability (Aurup et al., 1994; Cummins et al., 1995) resulting in a theoretically increased affinity of aptamers to their targets (Eaton et al., 1995). In order to improve pharmacokinetics and the bioavailability, high molecular weight or/and lipophilic moieties like polyethylene glycol are fused to the respective ends of the aptamers increasing aptamers' half-life in plasma up to nine hours in contrast to a few minutes observed with unmodified aptamers (Willis et al., 1998). However, on the back site, aptamer applications face some diagnostic and/or pharmaceutical limitations in terms of their incapacity to pass biological membranes hindering intracellular aptamer applications (reviewed in Rimmele 2003).

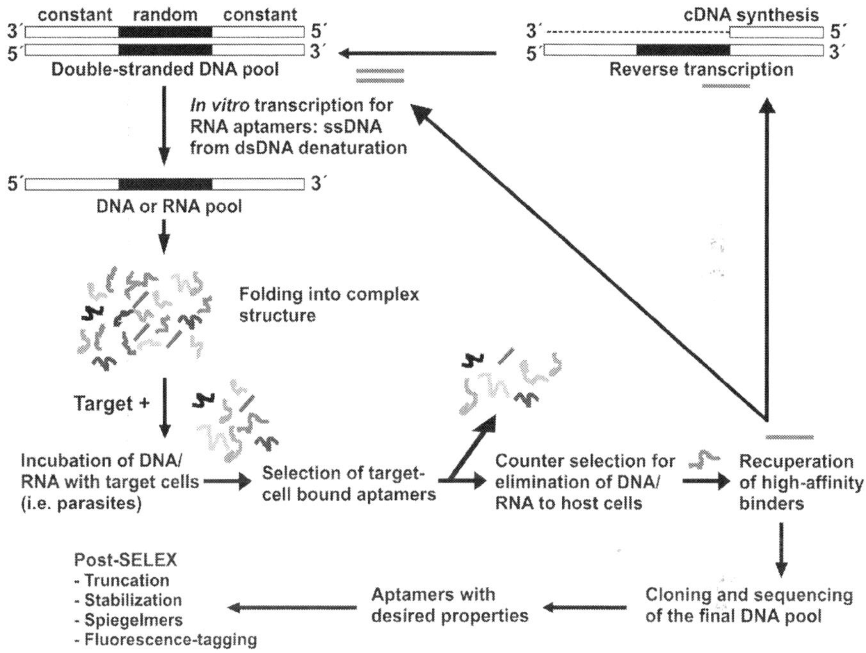

Fig. 1. *In vitro* selection of aptamers as high-specificity binders to target cell epitopes.

RNA or single-stranded (ss)-DNA-libraries for *in vitro* selection are obtained from a double-stranded DNA template containing a random region flanked by two constant sequences for PCR amplification (and *in vitro* transcription in case of RNA aptamers). Libraries are stabilized against nuclease activity by chemical modifications of the nucleotides. DNA or RNA libraries are generated by *in vitro* transcription or thermal denaturation followed by single-strand purification. The random oligonucleotide pool is exposed to its target cell (i.e. an erythrocyte expressing *P. falciparum* derived proteins on its cell surface), followed by elution of bound RNA/DNA molecules. Subsequently, these oligonucleotides are incubated with uninfected erythrocytes. All DNA/RNA molecules bound to these healthy cells are discarded, while unbound oligonucleotides are used for PCR amplification and generation of the DNA pool for the next selection cycle. The Cell SELEX process continues until the combinatorial oligonucleotide pool is purified to a homogeneous population binding with high affinity and specificity to their respective targets. Aptamers are identified by DNA sequencing and characterized for their binding affinities. Post-SELEX modifications are performed for optimization of aptamers for diagnostic and *in vivo* applications.

The modality of Cell SELEX, where aptamers are selected on the basis of binding to specific cell surface epitopes of disease cells, i.e. cancer cells or cells infected by pathogens (a positive selection step), followed by exposure of the library to a healthy somatic cell type, where all DNA/RNA molecules binding to common cell surface epitopes are discarded (negative selection step) has further broaden possible applications of the SELEX technique (see Figure 1 for details). The final library following various cycles of positive and negative selection ideally contains one or more aptamers binding to differentially expressed cell surface markers. In many cases, these aptamers were able to detect a differential expression pattern on the cell surface, also named a molecular signature of the cells, not expressed by other cells. These features have made aptamers potent tools for targeting cancer cells and therapeutic agents for delivering a toxic load or an RNAi construct interfering with cancer cell replication or metabolism. The combination of improved synthesis protocols towards industrial scale and novel chemical modifications techniques was beneficial for the development of aptamer-based tools for diagnosis and therapy. We foresee that aptamers as nucleic acid based drugs will soon become of major pharmacological relevance in both, diagnostics and therapeutics.

2. Applying the SELEX technique on protozoan parasites

Parasite-caused diseases affect millions of people in the entire world. Parasitic infections are not only restricted to humans, they also play a major role in animal health. Just a few years ago infectious diseases were classified as an issue of the past. However, due to the increasing level of drug resistance of pathogens the need for new treatments or even more important vaccines has become apparent. Unfortunately, these infectious diseases which are responsible for a level of mortality and morbidity are particular endemic in developing countries (Renslo and McKerrow, 2006). A variety of these parasitic diseases, including the so called neglected Chagas disease, leishmaniasis, sleeping sickness, schistosomiasis, elephantiasis, or onchocerciasis and of course malaria, are transmitted by vectors and, therefore, attempts to combat transmission vectors became prominent. Due to the continuously increasing human population and rising resistances of human pathogenic agents towards current treatment, there is an urgent need for novel diagnostic and therapeutic tools to tackle the foreseeable problems of the next generation. High attention is not only drawn to the development of new tools and their fast application but also to the commercial value in terms of their maintaining and application costs. In this chapter we summarize the current status of SELEX applications in human infectious diseases caused by protozoan pathogens.

3. SELEX applications in *Leishmaniasis*

The sandflies of the *Phlebotomus* genus are responsible for the transmission of the protozoan flagellate *Leishmania*. Infection with this parasite causes leishmaniasis, which can cause death in the absence of treatment. Specially, visceral leishmaniasis (kala azar), caused by *L. donovani/infantum* infection, is responsible for a high level of mortality if untreated. Muco-cutaneous leishmaniasis (*L. braziliensis* infection) or cutaneous leishmaniasis (*L. major/mexicana* infection) are not considered to be lethal, however the latter can result in unaesthetic stigmata (Herwaldt, 1999). The major intention of the treatment is prevention from death after infection by *L. donovani*. Due to this high potency the antimonials Pentostam® and Glucantime® were the therapeutics of choice for antileishmanial therapy since decades. However, these drugs revealed a number of disadvantages in terms of their mode of administration, the long duration of treatment, the high cost and the serious side effects. Therefore, the traditional drugs Amphotericin B and pentamidine were resurrected although they are known for causing irreversible toxic effects. However, new formulations and adapted dosages made these drugs applicable (Berman, 1997, Berman, 1999). The first oral drug, miltefosine was introduced by the Indian government for treatment of visceral leishmaniasis in 2002. Despite cure rates of up to 98% (Roberts, 2005, Berman, 2008), the drug also evokes serious side effects such as vomiting, diarrhea and can cause abnormalities. In order to discover novel therapeutics to tackle leishmaniasis without such serious side effects, the SELEX technology has been applied on the parasite *L. infantum* which is responsible for the most severe visceral leishmaniasis. Gonzales and co-workers were focussing on peculiarities such as gene expression and organisation in *Leishmania* (Ramos et al., 2007 and 2010). *Leishmania* does not condense its chromatin during mitosis which might be caused by the respective histones. Although histones are extremely conserved proteins in all livestock, high sequence divergences have been identified in the N- and C-terminal protein regions as targets for diagnostic and/or therapeutic intervention. Ramos et al. developed aptamers against the recombinantly expressed histone antigens H2A and H3 and even, despite of the sequence homology of histone proteins, the generated aptamers were highly selective for the parasite proteins. Aptamers were also directed against the *L. infantum* kinetoplastid membrane protein-11 (KMP-11) which is a major component of the cell membrane of kinetoplastid parasites (Moreno et al., 2003). Since KMP-11 is a cytoskeleton-associated protein it is believed that its function lies in mobility or is related to the flagellar structure. The SELEX technique has also been employed in gaining cellular knowledge on how the tRNA import into the mitochondrion of *L. tropica* is achieved (Bhattacharyya et al., 2002). However, approaches towards the development of therapeutic have yet to be carried out due to missing biological activity of the selected aptamers or difficulties in accessing target proteins. Therefore, current applications of aptamers to *Leishmania* are mainly restricted investigative or diagnostic tools.

4. SELEX applications towards treatment of *Trypanosoma* infections

In the last century infectious diseases caused by the tropical protozoan parasites *Trypanosoma* became more prominent due to their medical importance. Infections are caused by the pathogens *Trypanosoma cruzi*, the causative agent of Chagas' disease occurring in Latin America, and *T. brucei ssp.*, the African trypanosomes, which are responsible for sleeping sickness and Nagana in cattle. These infectious diseases are accountable for relevant health and socioeconomic problems in endemic countries such as Latin America, sub-Saharan Africa, and tropical and other subtropical areas in Africa and America. The current medication is known for its toxicity, poor activity in immune-suppressed patients and long term treatment combined with high costs. Moreover, vaccines are not foreseeable in the near future. Therefore, the current treatment is just relying on chemotherapeutics. The treatment of Chagas' disease is based on two nitroheterocyclic drugs, nifurtimox and benznidazole, which are administered as pro-drugs and become intracellularly activated. However, both drugs occasionally reveal serious side effects, but no other compound is near preclinical or clinical development for the treatment of Chagas´ disease. The human African trypanosomiasis (also called sleeping sickness) is caused by *T. brucei*, which is transmitted to humans by infected Tsetse flies. Human sleeping sickness is triggered by two sub-species *T. b. rhodesiense* is responsible for acute infections and *T. b. gambiense* leading to more chronic infections. The parasites proliferate in the lymph, blood as well as in peripheral organs and invade the central nervous system, instigating serious neurological disorders (Barrett et al., 2003).

Without treatment the disease is lethal. In the human host, African trypanosomes sustain extracellularly and face the exposure to the human immune system. The parasites circumvent the human immune response mainly by antigenic variation of their variant surface glycoprotein coat (VSG) (Vickerman, 1978). However, the parasite also displays invariant surface proteins, but they are inaccessible to the host's immune response.

Prior to infesting the central nervous system by the parasites, medication is carried out with suramin and pentamidine against the *rhodesiense* and *gambiense* forms of the disease, respectively. Afterwards first-line treatment is mediated by melarsoprol, although the drug often induces serious, sometimes fatal side effects. Originally developed for cancer chemotherapy, eflornithine was also effective against the *gambiense* form. Eflornithine is an inhibitor of the ornithine descarboxylase (ODC) leading to a depletion of the parasites' polyamine levels (Docampo and Moreno, 2003). Interestingly, the drug shows similar affinity to both the mammalian and parasite's enzymes; however the trypanosomal ODC has a shorter half-life than its mammalian counterpart which makes the parasite's metabolism more susceptible resulting in growth arrested. The parasite does not differentiate into the non-dividing stumpy forms and become sensitive to host immune system, since these forms are not able to undergo antigenic variation of their VSG (Wang, 1995). Surface proteins, such as the VSG coat of the African trypanosomes, were also targeted by aptamers. Three aptamer families were isolated with binding affinities in the nanomolar and subnanomolar range (Lorger et al., 2003). Since RNA aptamers are subject to rapid degradation in serum they need to be modified in order to prolong their half-life from a few seconds to several hours (Ulrich et al. 2004). Chemical modification of the anti-*T. brucei* aptamer led to nuclease resistance (Lorger et al., 2003). However, as per definition the VSG coat is variable and thereby modified by the parasite in time to escape the immune response of the human host, attention was drawn to other surface proteins of *T. brucei*. In particular, invariant surface glycoproteins (ISGs), which comprise receptor complexes and transporters (Overath et al., 1994), were targeted by RNA aptamers using a combinatorial selection process on live trypanosomes. The selected RNA aptamers bound to a single 42 kDa protein located within the flagellar pocket of the parasite which might be ESAG 7, a transferrin receptor subunit (Homann and Goringer, 1999). These results were very promising since the aptamer bound to an invariant trypanosomal surface protein enabling the selective targeting of the non VSG coat. Even further, Homann and Goringer could demonstrate that at increased temperature, the terminal ends of the aptamer were degraded and became rapidly engulfed into the parasite and incorporated into the lysosome by vesicular transportation. Proof-of principle experiments were carried out with biotin labelled aptamers which were visualized by immune fluorescence microscopy using anti-biotin antibodies (Goringer et al., 2003). The obtained results demonstrate that the specific RNAs could be exploited as so called 'piggy backs' molecules to traffic aptamer-coupled drugs into the lysosomal compartment of the parasite. Such aptamers might have the potential to act as novel drugs against African trypanosomiasis. SELEX applications were not only restricted to T. brucei; this technology was also applied on American trypanosomiasis caused by T. cruzi. As already outlined the causing agent of Chagas' disease depends on invasion of host cells to complete its life cycle. Thereby the parasite needs to build up parasite-host cell adhesion for initiation of the invasion process (Alves and Colli, 2008). Macromolecules on host cell surfaces such as laminin, thrombospondin, heparan sulfate, and fibronectin are believed to be involved in parasite-host cell contact (Ulrich et al., 2002, Simmons et al., 2006). Approaches have been undertaken to selectively interfere with parasite host cell receptors in order to inhibit the cellular invasion process of *T. cruzi*. The SELEX technology was employed to evolve nuclease-resistant RNA aptamers which block *in vitro* receptor-ligand interactions between *T. cruzi* trypomastigotes and epithelial monkey kidney LLC-MK(2) cells and thereby partially inhibit cell invasion by the parasite (Ulrich et al., 2002). Aptamers were identified with binding affinities in the nanomolar range to parasite receptors expressed by infective trypomastigote and not by insect epimastigote forms for the host cell matrix molecules fibronectin, heparan sulphate, laminin and thrombospondin (Ulrich et al., 2002; Alves and Colli, 2008). Reduction in the infection rate *in vitro* of up to 70 percent was observed at a low micromolar aptamer concentration.

5. SELEX approaches have also been undertaken to other protozoan parasites such as the malaria pathogens

The parasitic disease malaria represents one of the most serious threats to human health worldwide with an enormous impact on the mortality and morbidity, especially in sub-Saharan Africa. More than 2000 million people are exposed to the infection with malaria leading to estimated 500 million clinical cases and more than one million deaths per annum; mostly young children in Africa. A vaccine is not available and the control of the disease depends solely on the administration of a small number of drugs. Malaria is presently undergoing resurgence and the fight against *Plasmodium falciparum* -the most virulent species accounting for over 90% of deaths- has become a significant problem (Greenwood et al., 2008). Due to the high mutational rate of the parasite and its resulting rapid adaptation to environmental changes, its drug resistance and geographic distribution are increasing. Further aspects such as socio-economic factors, increasing migration patterns, failing health care systems and the rapid development and dispersal of the respective insecticide resistant forms of the mosquito vector are contributing to the problem. Currently, only one drug, Artemesinin, is still effective against the malaria parasite. However, the first evidence of drug resistance against Artemisinin and combinations has been reported at the Cambodian/Thailand border from where resistance against the most cost-effective drug, chloroquine, has also spread to the rest of the world (Wangroongsarb et al., 2011). Therefore continuous discovery and development of new drugs are urgently needed. In the past the discovery of novel antimalarials was mainly directed towards chemotherapeutic interventions and vaccines (Alonso et al., 2011). As far as drugs are concerned, major focus was drawn on the peculiarities occurring in the malaria parasite such as the folate metabolism, haemoglobin degradation and subsequently the polymerisation of heme into the chemically inert "malaria" pigment, hemozoin. Chloroquine is believed to interfere with the heme detoxifying biochemical pathway which leads to parasites' death. In a recent report aptamers were used to prevent hemozoin formation in a proof-of-concept study to demonstrate that oligonucleotide-based drugs are exploitable to modulate essential biochemical pathways in *P. falciparum* (Niles et al., 2009). Indeed hemozoin formation was significantly inhibited by heme-binding aptamers in parasite extract. Even further, a growth inhibitory effect could be shown in aptamer preloaded human erythrocytes (Niles et al., 2009). However, *in vivo* assays have yet not been performed in order to evaluate whether these aptamers are also applicable as drugs. In another approach RNA aptamers were generated binding to the major parasite derived surface protein embedded in the erythrocytic membrane - the *var*-gene encoded *P. falciparum* erythrocyte membrane protein 1 (*Pf*EMP1) (Barfod et al., 2009). *Pf*EMP1 is involved in cytoadherance to human cells, such as endothelial cells of blood vessels or in spontaneous binding of uninfected erythrocytes to *P. falciparum*-infected red blood cells (rosetting). The secretion of this protein is proposed to accentuate the symptoms of malaria by preventing the clearance of infected erythrocytes in the spleen (Buffet et al., 2011). While doing so the parasite would become susceptible to the human immune system. However the genome of the parasite encodes about 60 var-genes and the parasite is able to switch expression to another gene of this family, leading to a different *Pf*EMP1 protein. Due to antigenic variation the parasite can avoid interference with the host immune response (Flick and Chen, 2004). Recently, Barfod and co-workers selected aptamers against the recombinantly expressed N-terminal DUFFY-binding like domain (DBL1a) of the *Pf*EMP1 protein. Subsequently, the isolated aptamers were tested on cellular level by screening against populations of infected and non-infected erythrocytes (Barfod et al., 2009). The set of biological active aptamers inhibited the rosetting progress which is indicative for the functionality of the RNA ligands and promising for further evaluation of their activity *in vivo*.

6. Conclusion

Aptamers are able to identify individual epitopes within a complex mixture of potential targets and can also be used for ligand-mediated target purification (Nery et al., 2009, Ulrich and Wrenger, 2009). It has been demonstrated that aptamers evolved against human membrane proteins bind specifically to previously unidentified target proteins (Morris et al., 1998). The same methodology (deconvolution SELEX) was used to stain rat brain tumor vessels and identify the endothelial regulatory protein pigpen as aptamer-target protein (Blank et al., 2001). These works resulted in the conclusion that each cell type differs from others by its molecular signature exposed on the cell surface. The fact that aptamers can distinguish between small differences in the molecular signature of cell-surface antigens emphasizes the feasibility of the chosen technology. Even further highly specific aptamers distinguishing between host cell proteins are capable to selectively bind and thereby interfere with parasite-derived proteins in order to stop proliferation of these deadly human parasites.

7. References

Alonso PL, Brown G, Arevalo-Herrera M, Binka F, Chitnis C, Collins F, Doumbo OK, Greenwood B, Hall BF, Levine MM, Mendis K, Newman RD, Plowe CV, Rodríguez

MH, Sinden R, Slutsker L, Tanner M (2011). A research agenda to underpin malaria eradication. PLoS Med. 8:e1000406.

Alves MJ, Colli W (2008). Role of the gp85/trans-sialidase superfamily of glycoproteins in the interaction of Trypanosoma cruzi with host structures. Subcell. Biochem. 47:58-69.

Aurup H, Tuschl T, Benseler F, Ludwig J, Eckstein F (1994) Oligonucleotide duplexes containing 2'-amino-2'-deoxycytidines: thermal stability and chemical reactivity. Nucleic Acids Res. 22:20-24.

Barfod A, Persson T, Lindh J (2009) In vitro selection of RNA aptamers against a conserved region of the Plasmodium falciparum erythrocyte membrane protein 1. Parasitol. Res. 105:1557-1566.

Bhattacharyya SN, Chatterjee S, Adhya S (2002). Mitochondrial RNA import in Leishmania tropica: aptamers homologous to multiple tRNA domains that interact cooperatively or antagonistically at the inner membrane. Mol. Cell. Biol. 22:4372-4382.

Berman JD (1997) Human leishmaniasis: clinical, diagnostic, and chemotherapeutic developments in the last 10 years. Clin. Infect. Dis. 24:684-703.

Berman JD (1999) U.S Food and Drug Administration approval of AmBisome (liposomal amphotericin B) for treatment of visceral leishmaniasis. Clin. Infect. Dis. 28:49-51.

Berman JJ (2008). Treatment of leishmaniasis with miltefosine: 2008 status. Expert Opin. Drug Metab. Toxicol. 4:1209-1216.

Blank M, Weinschenk T, Priemer M, Schluesener H. (2001) Systematic evolution of a DNA aptamer binding to rat brain tumor microvessels. selective targeting of endothelial regulatory protein pigpen J. Biol. Chem. 276:16464-16468.

Buffet PA, Safeukui I, Deplaine G, Brousse V, Prendki V, Thellier M, Turner GD, Mercereau-Puijalon O (2011). The pathogenesis of Plasmodium falciparum malaria in humans: insights from splenic physiology. Blood 117:381-392.

Cummins LL, Owens SR, Risen LM, et al. 1995. Characterization of fully 2'-modified oligoribonucleotide hetero- and homoduplex hybridization and nuclease sensitivity. Nucleic Acids Res. 23:2019–2024.

Docampo R, Moreno SN (2003). Current chemotherapy of human African trypanosomiasis. Parasitol. Res. 90 Supp 1:S10-13.

Eaton BE, Gold L, Zichi DA. (1995). Let's get specific: the relationship between specificity and affinity. Chem. Biol. 346:818–822.

Ellington AD, Szostak JW. (1990). In vitro selection of RNA molecules that bind specific ligands. Nature 346:818-822.

Faria, M.; Ulrich, H. (2002) The use of synthetic oligonucleotides as protein inhibitors and anticode drugs in cancer therapy: accomplishments and limitations. Curr. Cancer Drug Targets 2:355-368.

Fernandes PB. (1998) Technological advances in high-throughput screening. Curr Opin Chem Biol. 2:597-603.

Flick K, Chen Q (2004) Var genes, PfEMP1 and the human host. Mol. Biochem. Parasitol. 134:3-9

Göringer HU, Homann M, Lorger M (2003). In vitro selection of high-affinity nucleic acid ligands to parasite target molecules. Int. J. Parasitol. 33:1309-1317.

Greenwood BM, Fidock DA, Kyle DE, Kappe SH, Alonso PL, Collins FH, Duffy PE (2008) Malaria: progress, perils, and prospects for eradication. J. Clin. Invest. 118:1266-1276.

Herwaldt BL (1999). Leishmaniasis. Lancet. 354:1191-1199.

Homann M, Göringer HU (1999) Combinatorial selection of high affinity RNA ligands to live African trypanosomes. Nucleic Acids Res. 27:2006-2014.

Jellinek D, Lynott, CK, Rifkin DB, Janjic, N. (1993) High-affinity RNA ligands to basic fibroblast growth factor inhibit receptor binding. Proc. Natl. Acad. Sci. USA, 1993, 90, 11227-11231.

Lorger M, Engstler M, Homann M, Göringer HU (2003). Targeting the variable surface of African trypanosomes with variant surface glycoprotein-specific, serum-stable RNA aptamers. Eukaryot. Cell. 2:84-94.

Majumder P, Gomes KN, Ulrich H. (2009) Aptamers: from bench side research towards patented molecules with therapeutic applications. Expert Opin. Ther. Pat. 19:1603-1613.

Meli M, Vergne J, Decout JL, Maurel MC. (2002). Adenine-aptamer complexes: a bipartite RNA site that binds the adenine nucleic base. J. Biol. Chem. 277, 2104-2111.

Moreno M, Rincón E, Piñeiro D, Fernández G, Domingo A, Jiménez-Ruíz A, Salinas M, González VM. (2003). Selection of aptamers against KMP-11 using colloidal gold during the SELEX process. Biochem. Biophys. Res. Commun. 308:214-218.

Morris KN, Jensen KB, Julin CM, Weil M, Gold L (1998). High affinity ligands from in vitro selection: complex targets. Proc. Natl. Acad. Sci. USA 95:2902-2907.

Nery AA, Wrenger C, Ulrich H. (2009). Recognition of biomarkers and cell-specific molecular signatures: aptamers as capture agents. J. Sep. Sci. 32:1523-1530.

Ni X, Castanares M, Mukherjee A, Lupold SE (2011). Nucleic Acid Aptamers: Clinical Applications and Promising New Horizons. Curr. Med. Chem. (in press).

Niles JC, Derisi JL, Marletta MA (2009). Inhibiting Plasmodium falciparum growth and heme detoxification pathway using heme-binding DNA aptamers. Proc. Natl. Acad. Sci. USA 10:13266-13271.

Overath P, Steverding D, Chaudhri M, Stierhof YD, Ziegelbauer K (1994) .Structure and function of GPI-anchored surface proteins of Trypanosoma brucei. Braz. J. Med. Biol. Res. 27:343-347.

Pestourie C, Tavitian B, Duconge F (2005). Aptamers against extracellular targets for in vivo applications. Biochimie. 87:921-930.

Proske D, Gilch S, Wopfner F, Schatzl HM, Winnacker EL, Famulok, M (2002). Prion-protein-specific aptamer reduces PrPSc formation. Chembiochem. 3, 717-725.

Renslo AR, McKerrow JH (2006). Drug discovery and development for neglected parasitic diseases. Nat. Chem. Biol. 2:701-710.

Ramos E, Piñeiro D, Soto M, Abanades DR, Martín ME, Salinas M, González VM. (2007). A DNA aptamer population specifically detects Leishmania infantum H2A antigen. Lab. Invest. 87:409-416.

Ramos E, Moreno M, Martín ME, Soto M, Gonzalez VM. (2010). In vitro selection of Leishmania infantum H3-binding ssDNA aptamers. Oligonucleotides 20:207-213.

Rimmele M. 2003. Nucleic acid aptamers as tools and drugs: recent developments. Chembiochem. 4:963–971.

Roberts MT. (2005). Current understandings on the immunology of leishmaniasis and recent developments in prevention and treatment. Br. Med. Bull. 75-76: 115-130.

Ruckman J, Green LS, Beeson J, Waugh S, Gillette WL, Henninger DD, Claesson-Welsh L, Janjic N (1998). 2'-Fluoropyrimidine RNA-based aptamers to the 165-amino acid form of vascular endothelial growth factor (VEGF165). Inhibition of receptor binding and VEGF-induced vascular permeability through interactions requiring the exon 7-encoded domain. J. Biol. Chem. 273, 20556-20567.

Sassanfar M. Szostak JW (1993). An RNA motif that binds ATP. Nature 364, 550-553.

Simmons KJ, Nde PN, Kleshchenko YY, Lima MF, Villalta F (2006). Stable RNA interference of host thrombospondin-1 blocks Trypanosoma cruzi infection. FEBS Lett. 580:2365-2370.

Trujillo CA, Nery AA, Alves JM, Martins AH, Ulrich H (2007). Development of the anti-VEGF aptamer to a therapeutic agent for clinical ophthalmology. Clin. Ophthalmol. 1:393-402.

Tuerk C, Gold L. (1990). Systematic evolution of ligands by exponential enrichment: RNA ligands to bacteriophage T4 DNA polymerase. Science 249:505-510.

Ulrich H, Magdesian MH, Alves MJ, Colli W. (2002). In vitro selection of RNA aptamers that bind to cell adhesion receptors of Trypanosoma cruzi and inhibit cell invasion. J. Biol. Chem 277:20756–20762.

Ulrich H, Martins AH, Pesquero JB (2004). RNA and DNA aptamers in cytomics analysis. Cytometry A. 59:220-231.

Ulrich H, Trujillo CA, Nery AA, Alves JM, Majumder P, Resende RR, Martins AH (2006). DNA and RNA aptamers: from tools for basic research towards therapeutic applications. Comb. Chem. High Throughput Screen 9:619-632.

Ulrich H, Wrenger C (2009) Disease-specific biomarker discovery by aptamers. Cytometry A. 75:727-733.

Vickerman K (1978). Antigenic variation in trypanosomes. Nature 273:613-617.

Wangroongsarb P, Satimai W, Khamsiriwatchara A, Thwing J, Eliades JM, Kaewkungwal J, Delacollette C (2011). Respondent-driven sampling on the Thailand-Cambodia border. II. Knowledge, perception, practice and treatment-seeking behaviour of migrants in malaria endemic zones. Malar J. 10:117.

Williams DL Jr, Murphy KL, Nolan NA, O'Brien JA, Lis EV Jr, Pettibone DJ, Clineschmidt BV, Krause SM, Veber DF, Naylor EM, Chakravarty PK, Walsh TF, Dhanoa DM, Chen A, Bagley, SW Fitch KJ, Greenlee WJ. (1996) Pharmacology of L-744,453, a novel nonpeptidyl endothelin antagonist. Life Sci. 58, 1149-1157.

Willis MC, Collins BD, Zhang T, Green LS, Sebesta DP, Bell C, Kellogg E, Gill SC, Magallanez A, Knauer S, Bendele RA, Gill PS, Janjić N. (1998). Liposome-anchored vascular endothelial growth factor aptamers. Bioconjug. Chem. 9:573-582.

17

Streamlining ICH Q6B Analytical Testing of Biotherapeutics

Elizabeth Higgins, Elisabeth Kast and Amy Lachapelle
GlycoSolutions Corporation, USA

1. Introduction

ICH Q6B is a useful guide for determining appropriate analytical testing of a biotherapeutic. This document describes an approach to streamlining this testing by selecting a short list of the most powerful analytical methods early in development and the use of universal methods. Universal methods are designed to provide useful data for the majority of protein therapeutics. Some of these universal methods include size exclusion chromatography for the determination of aggregation and degradation products, ion exchange HPLC for the determination of charge variants and oligosaccharide profiling for glycosylated therapeutics. This allows for more testing earlier without spending time and money optimizing methods for a particular drug.

The authors discuss how to determine what testing is required in early development, how to know when more testing is required and when more optimization of the universal methods is warranted. Data will be shown to demonstrate how the same assay can be used from initial lot-to-lot comparisons through assay validation and a full characterization of the therapeutic. For example, N-linked oligosaccharide profiling by HPLC is a relatively quick and simple means of evaluating the glycosylation of a biotherapeutic using chromatographic peak areas. Understanding the heterogeneity of the glycosylation early in product development from lot -to- lot comparisons, along with bioassay, in vivo and pre-clinical testing, is an effective way of defining the window for the product's critical quality attributes. Further along in development, the N-linked profiling assay can be used to quantitate the heterogeneity of the glycosylation and the oligosaccharide peaks can then be collected and identified by mass spectrometry, glycosidase sequencing and other methods.

2. Guiding principles for characterization throughout drug development

The methods will change, assays may be added, and some assays eliminated during product development. However, as a drug moves from Pre-Clinical to Clinical to Marketing Approval there are certain points to keep in mind starting with the earliest lot to ensure a solid characterization package for your drug.

Scientific Literature: For many drugs there is very little information on how the structure of the molecule impacts the function of the molecule. However, when there is information on the molecule or similar molecules, this information can be used to select the quality attributes of your molecule most likely to affect the efficacy or safety of your drug. These attributes are worth monitoring over the course of development so that they can be used to define the design space for your drug—variation that is acceptable because it has been demonstrated to have no affect on the safety and efficacy of the drug.

Retains: Assays evolve and new ones may be developed throughout the characterization process. It is important to be able to retrospectively analyze your drug. This is especially true for any clinical or key pre-clinical lots. The more lots you have to test, the easier it is to confidently set assay specifications.

Reference Material: Beyond retains, it is important to establish Reference Materials. These are drug lots that are set aside to demonstrate that future lots are comparable to previous material and that the drug is not changing. These can also ensure that an assay is delivering consistent results over time.

Stability: Drug lots that are not comparable to historical lots, whether these changes are coincident with decreased biological activity or not, are extremely valuable for understanding the relationship between activity and drug heterogeneity—what heterogeneity is acceptable and what heterogeneity negatively impacts the safety and/or efficacy of the drug product. It is important to identify assays that detect these critical quality attributes and the early in development. When changes in the product do not occur naturally, it is possible to force these changes using accelerated stability/degradation studies where the drug is stressed and forced to degrade.

Release Tests/Assay Validation:

It is always important to keep in mind that some assays will become Release Tests and will need to be validated. It is wise to remember this when choosing and designing assays to avoid trouble in the future when they need to be validated and transferred to a QC laboratory.

3. Pre-clinical evaluation of sample heterogeneity

Numerous lots of drug are prepared throughout development of a therapeutic. These are first used in animal studies, followed by preclinical studies and finally clinical studies. Throughout the course of these studies, valuable information regarding the heterogeneity of the drug can be determined early on using some basic analytical assays. These studies can help to define a window of acceptable product variation. "If a consistent pattern of product heterogeneity is demonstrated, an evaluation of the activity, efficacy, and safety (including immunogenicity) of individual forms may not be necessary" (ICHQ6B). For example, oligosaccharide profiling, IEX-HPLC and SEC-HPLC are universal assays usually requiring little methods development and are relatively quick and easy to perform. These assays are also easily transferred to a QC environment, can be validated and used as lot release assays. Performing these assays early in the development process helps to identify the extent of heterogeneity routinely seen in a sample. Performed routinely, these assays can identify stability issues (oxidation/deamidation or aggregation/degradation during storage) or critical process parameters (glycosylation changes with process change). Understanding the product variants at an early stage aids in optimizing the types of assays required for the determination of product identity later on in development. For example, if charge variants are present in a sample, the IEX-HPLC assay may need to be further optimized for resolution of these variants. Further, these variants can be isolated and subjected to peptide mapping techniques so that the site of oxidation can be determined and the peptide map optimized to resolve the variant peptides. It is often possible to force degradation of the drug using accelerated stability or degradation pathway studies where the drug is stressed by changing parameters such as the pH of the formulation and storage temperature. This helps to identify critical quality attributes of the drug and determine whether the assays are able to detect these critical changes. It also allows for determining which changes in the drug impact the biological activity.

During early stage development, there should be an adequate focus placed on determining the appropriate analytical tests for the identity, purity and concentration or activity of the drug.

4. Phase I: Determination of physicochemical properties

Determination of the physicochemical properties of the drug substance is a critical step in the development of suitable identity tests. These properties include the purity, concentration and/or activity, molecular weight and size of the sample as well as charge, hydrophobicity and post-translational modifications (PTMs).

4.1 Purity and molecular weight determination

Purity and molecular weight analyses are most easily evaluated by SDS-PAGE/CE-SDS (native and denaturing) along with Western blot analysis. SDS-PAGE/CE-SDS allows for the visualization of the protein species in a sample and can be quantitative depending on the detection method. Comparison of native versus denatured sample by gel electrophoresis or CE analysis can also confirm the presence of 3-dimensional structure such as disulfide bonding and oligomerization. Further analysis of the gel by Western blotting with various antibodies identifies the presence of drug substance degradation products along with process specific contaminants. If molecular weight variants such as aggregates or degradation products occur in a product, size exclusion chromatography can be a valuable tool for the routine detection and quantitation of these variants. SEC-HPLC is a universal method and can be run with minimal development work. SEC columns can separate over a wide range of molecular weights, and optimization of the column conditions need not take place until later in the product development stage if the method is not separating molecular weight variants identified in the product through orthogonal methods. SEC-HPLC can be preparative and used as an initial step for a two-dimensional analysis of size variants. The variant peaks can be isolated for characterization by MALDI-TOF MS to confirm the size or analyzed by peptide mapping for identity, etc. Once the purity of the sample is ascertained by these methods, the molecular weight of the drug substance should be confirmed by MALDI-TOF analysis. This type of multidimensional analysis is illustrated in work by Kotia et al. (Kotia, 2010). In this work, truncated fragments of a monoclonal antibody heavy and light chain are detected by CE-SDS. These truncated fragments were correlated to heavy and light chain peptide maps and sequence identity was confirmation by N-terminal sequencing. Multidimensional analysis of product degradation utilizing both SEC-HPLC and CEX-HPLC followed peptide mapping with MS-ESI detection is shown in work by Lau et al. and Kim et al. (Lau H., 2010) (Kim, 2010)

4.2 Protein content and extinction coefficient determination

Protein content needs to be determined early in development since many other assays are dependent upon it. It is important to use an assay that is precise, i.e. gives reproducible

results. For instance, the results of potency and bioassays are reported based on protein concentration. Reporting these results based on inconsistent protein determinations yields inconsistent results that may not accurately reflect the activity of the drug. Determination of protein content is not as straightforward as it would seem. Colorimetric assays such as the Bradford assay or bicinchoninic acid assay rely on the use of an external reference standard for protein determination. However, different proteins will have different molar ratios of reactive sites and the same amount of one protein can give a different absorbance than the same amount of the reference standard used. Amino acid analysis can also be used for quantitative analysis of protein content, but this assay also has its difficulties. Different proteins can hydrolyze differently under the same conditions and many amino acids are not stable to acid hydrolysis. Numerous studies have been conducted by the ABRF to determine the precision and accuracy of colorimetric protein assays and quantitative amino acid analysis. These studies report high variability between test sites and variability in the accuracy of measuring different proteins as well. Summarizing the results from the AARG2003 study (Alterman *et al.*), 28 laboratories were given five protein samples at a concentration of 2.5 mg/mL. Excluding the results from the fetuin sample (average determined concentration = 1.18 mg/mL) the average yield of all four proteins was 1.69 ± 0.24 mg/mL. This indicates a substantial bias (32%) in the determination of protein content, although some of this bias could be due to initial sample handling and salt content. In our hands, we see an assay bias of 13% for our BSA standard (N= 94) with an average yield of 1.75 ± 0.47 mg/mL from a 2.01 mg/mL standard solution.
Theoretical extinction coefficients can be easily determined from the amino acid sequence (e.g. using the ProtParam tool at www.ExPaSy.org). However, the extinction coefficient needs to be confirmed experimentally using a suitably determined protein concentration as protein conformation can have an effect on the measured absorbance.

4.3 Charge and hydrophobicity variants

Charge and hydrophobicity variants are most easily analyzed by ion-exchange and reversed-phase HPLC. These assays are highly sensitive and selective, both being able to detect changes at a single site in the protein sequence. Both assays are an excellent starting point for multi-dimensional analysis as the methods are quantitative and scalable. Variant peaks can be isolated for characterization by mass spectrometry methods or peptide mapping. Hydrophobicity variants can consist of single point amino acid substitutions. Charge variants can include oxidized, deamidated, phosphorylated, and sulfated species as well as variation in the extent of sialylation. More than likely these variants will need to be characterized using in-depth identity tests.
Ion exchange chromatography can easily pick up low levels of charge variants. The assay is very quick and in general, requires only a small amount of purified protein. Running this analysis early on allows for the early identification of charge variants. Early identification of the extent, or percent modification, can be used to set product specifications. These assays can also be used throughout process development to determine which process changes affect product variation. Ion exchange HPLC is an excellent starting point for further investigation into the identification of the variants. Vlasek et al. describe the use of cation exchange chromatography for characterization of a monoclonal antibody in which two lysine variants were separated using CEX-HPLC as well as two acidic variants. (Vlasak, 2009). The initial use of ion-exchange HPLC allowed for isolation and extensive characterization of the variant

peaks, such as preparation of Fab fragments from the variants as well as preparation of heavy and light chains, followed by mass spectrometry analysis, Edman degradation, DSC to evaluate stability and CD spectroscopy for higher order structure analysis.

4.4 Glycosylation

Glycosylation of biotherapeutics is now routinely analyzed early in development and typically drug lots are assayed as they are manufactured for lot-to-lot consistency in their glycosylation. We have already covered this topic in detail in a review article (Higgins, 2010). Although monosaccharide composition analysis was historically used to monitor glycosylation (releasing monosaccharides from oligosaccharides using acid and then quantifying each monosaccharide) this method has now been mostly replaced by oligosaccharide profiling. Oligosaccharide profiling involves releasing intact N- and/or O-linked oligosaccharides from the protein and then analyzing them by HPLC or mass spectrometry. Oligosaccharide profiling can be used to monitor the population of oligosaccharides present on the glycoprotein and most importantly determine whether the heterogeneity is the same from lot-to-lot. Mass spectrometry of the released pool of oligosaccharides can be used to characterize the types of oligosaccharides present (oligomannose, complex, and antennarity). Both HPLC and MS can be used to quantify the relative ratio of different oligosaccharides, however, MS often requires the use of radioactive labels. The ratio is valuable when these methods are used for lot release.

Monosaccharide composition analysis is now mostly utilized in situations where additional testing is warranted: process qualification lots, lots for reference material or comparability testing. It is also used when a particular monosaccharide is critical to a drug (e.g. the amount of fucose) or could impact safety (a monosaccharide not commonly found on human proteins but found in the expression system used to produce the drug). Sialic acid analysis can also be a useful assay since the level of sialylation is often a critical quality attribute as it affects the plasma clearance of many glycoproteins.

5. Phase II/III: Development and characterization of identity tests

5.1 Determination of primary amino acid sequence and peptide mapping

The primary amino acid sequence of a protein is determined using a combination of analytical techniques. Complete sequence information is often difficult to obtain. The N and C terminal amino acids need to be confirmed. N-terminal sequencing can be performed by Edman degradation or MALDI-PSD analysis. MALDI-PSD analysis has the advantage in that it can also be used to identify the C-terminal amino acids in a protein or a peptide. Otherwise, C-terminal sequencing involves the use of a specific C-terminal protease followed by separation and identification of the released amino acids by HPLC. Full sequence determination is generally performed using a combination of peptide mapping following peak identification by Edman degradation or MS/MS.

Development of a good peptide map is critical for the development of appropriate identity tests. Once the purity of the product has been established the identity of the protein should be determined by peptide mapping. Peptide mapping involves cleaving a protein into smaller peptides, generally using enzymes that cleave the protein at specific amino acids to generate peptides that can be predicted from the peptide sequence. These peptides are then separated by reversed-phase HPLC followed by detection using UV and/or MS. At the start, if the protein is known to contain N-linked oligosaccharides or disulfide bonds, comparative peptide maps of deglycosylated and non-reduced protein should be generated to evaluate the extent of variability in these regions and to begin identifying the disulfide linked peptides and the glycopeptides. A good peptide map will resolve most of the peptides in the mixture to baseline. Well resolved peaks can then be identified by N-terminal sequencing using Edman degradation or LC-MS. Both methods are commonly used.

5.2 Disulfide and glycopeptide mapping

If a protein contains disulfide bonds, it is necessary to cleave the disulfide bond with a suitable reducing agent such as dithiothreitol followed by blockage of the free cysteine with an agent such as iodoacetamide or iodoacetic acid to prevent the random reformation of the bonds. Reduction of the disulfide bonds is necessary to confirm the amino acid sequence of the peptide, as mixed peptides will not correlate to the known amino acid sequence. Peptides involved in disulfide linkages can be identified by comparison of the reduced and alkylated peptide map with a peptide map generated from the non-reduced protein (see Figure 1). Additional identification of the peptides involved in the disulfide bridging can be confirmed by MALDI-TOF analysis using a reducing matrix. These matrices will break the disulfide bonds on target, generating masses of the disulfide linked peptide along with the masses of each of the released peptides. Examples of the peptide mapping for the determination of disulfide bonding in antibodies can be found in Bloom (1997) and Wypych (2008)(Bloom, 1997).

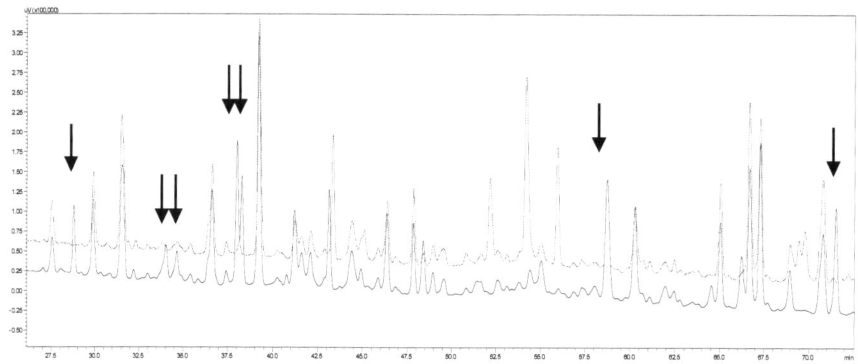

Fig. 1. Disulfide Peptide Map of Fetuin. The tryptic peptide map is enlarged to show the region of the map containing the most changes. Arrows indicate the generation of new peaks in the peptide map when fetuin is reduced and alkylated prior to trypsin digest. The top (red) chromatogram represents fetuin tryptic peptides generated from non-reduced fetuin. The bottom (black) chromatogram represents fetuin tryptic peptides generated from reduced and alkylated fetuin.

Comparison of peptide maps generated from glycosylated and deglycosylated drug substance can be used to identify glycosylated peptides (see Figure 2). Identification of these peptides can be performed by LC-MS, LC-MALDI or N-terminal sequencing. Further, glycosylated peaks can be isolated and for the purpose of attempting to determine the type of glycosylation on the peptide. Examples of approaches to the identification of glycopeptides by glycopeptide mapping can be found in (Rohrer, 1993) (Ohta, 2002)Ohta (2002) and Rohrer (1993).

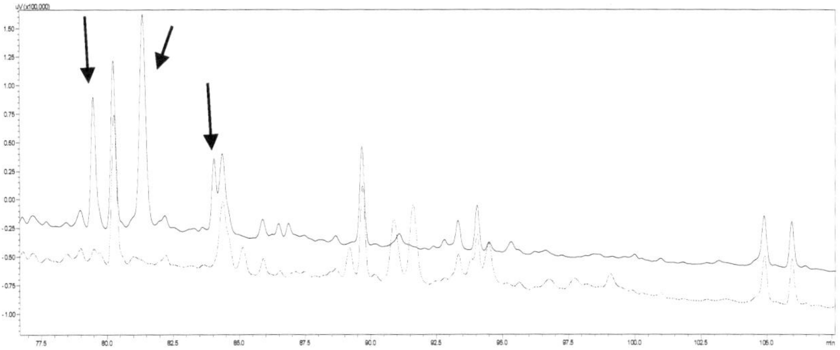

Fig. 2. Glycopeptide Map of Fetuin. The tryptic peptide map is enlarged to show the region of the map containing the most changes. The top (black) chromatogram represents fetuin peptides deglycosylated using PNGase F prior to reversed-phase chromatography. The bottom (red) chromatogram represents the same, untreated tryptic peptides. Arrows indicate the deglycosylated glycopeptides.

5.3 Site-specific glycosylation

Site-specific glycosylation analysis gives detailed data on the relationship between peptide and glycosylation heterogeneity. A review by An et al (2009) describes current methods used. The most challenging part of site-specific analysis is the enrichment of glycopeptides, a necessary step due to the relative low abundance of glycopeptides in comparison to non-glycosylated peptides. Such methods as lectin affinity columns, HILIC (Hydrophilic Interaction Chromatography) or ERLIC (Electrostatic Repulsion-Hydrophilic Interaction Chromatography) columns are employed, to varying degrees of success.

Lectins will bind oligosaccharides and different lectins show a preference for different types of oligosaccharides. Lectin affinity columns can therefore be used to bind glycopeptides and/or separate glycopeptides into groups with differences in their oligosaccharides. HILIC enrichment is based upon the proposed increase in hydrophilicity of glycopeptides versus non-glycosylated peptides due to the polysaccharide moiety. ERLIC operates in a similar fashion as HILIC, with the addition of electrostatic interactions to the binding mechanism. Both HILIC and ERLIC utilize gradients of high organic solvent to low organic solvent, where HILIC is generally performed using a polar chromatographic matrix and ERLIC utilizing an ion exchange matrix. Glycopeptides will bind more strongly than most non-glycosylated peptides, allowing for the removal of non-glycosylated peptides from a mixture. While these methods can enrich the glycopeptide content of a peptide mixture, the separation of the two has not been optimized. Some glycopeptides will be found in the early eluting fractions, and complex mixtures of glycopeptides can be seen to elute over a wide concentration of decreasing organic solvent along with some non-glycosylated peptides. Due to the heterogeneous nature of glycosylation, one peptide might contain many different glycoforms, leading to challenges in separation and identification.

5.4 Characterization of the oligosaccharide profile

Characterization of the oligosaccharide profile is critical for understanding the heterogeneity of glycosylation. By having a well-characterized oligosaccharide profile, changes in glycosylation are easier to track. A summary of characterization options is shown in Figure

3. Oligosaccharide profiling is commonly done by HPLC coupled with fluorescent detection (after oligosaccharide derivatization with a fluorescent label such as 2-aminobenzoic acid or 2-aminobenzamide), in-line LC-MS (typically using electrospray ionization (ESI) as the MS ion source) or standalone MS (either permethylated, derivatized, or native glycans using either MALDI or ESI).

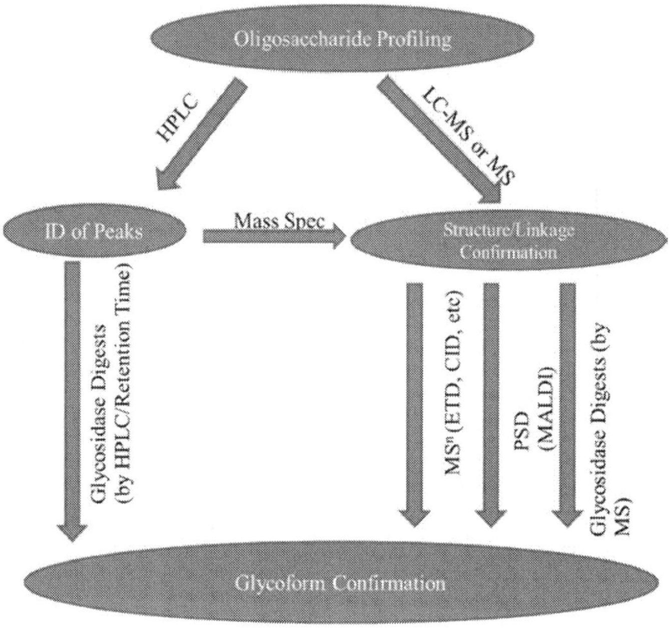

Fig. 3. A flowchart of possible approaches for characterization of the oligosaccharide profile.

When working from an HPLC fluorescent profiling method, fractions must be collected for further characterization. After fractions are collected, glycoforms can be identified either through glycosidase sequencing, which relies on highly specific enzymes and shifts in retention times to confirm linkage and composition, or through further mass spectrometric analysis. An example of HPLC profile characterization of the N- and O-linked oligosaccharides of fetuin using fraction collection followed by MALDI-TOF-MS identification is shown in Figure 4. Additional mass spectrometric analysis may include post source decay using MALDI-TOF-MS, MSn using such fragmentation techniques as electron transfer dissociation (ETD) or collision induced dissociation (CID), or glycosidase sequencing using shifts in mass to identify losses from the parent mass. A review by Geyer and Geyer (2006) contains further information. Often, multiple approaches are needed to fully characterize an oligosaccharide profile, as seen in Qian et al (2006).

While MS-MS and MSn are powerful tools, analysis of mass spectrometric data can be complicated and time-consuming, requiring database searches and knowledge of glycobiology to successfully narrow down potential structures. While several groups have sought to automate the process, in the authors' experience the results often contain inaccurate structures, not likely to be found in nature, which makes data analysis more complex.

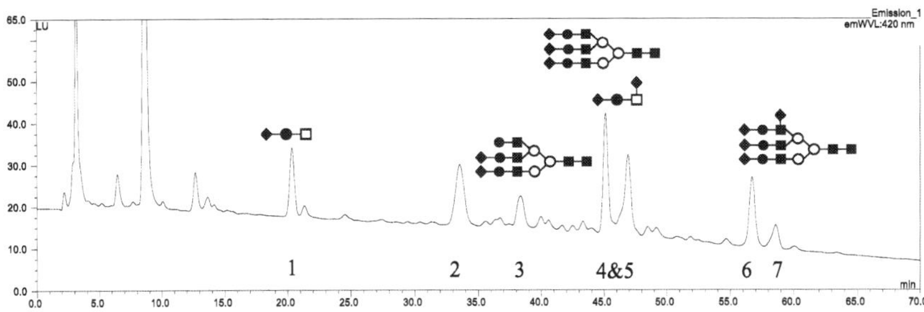

Fig. 4. N- and O-linked Oligosaccharide Profile of Fetuin. The selected fractions were collected and analyzed by negative ion mode MALDI-TOF-MS to determine peak identity. Linkages were not confirmed; however, the results are strongly correlated to the literature on fetuin. Symbols: ■ N-acetylglucosamine (GlcNAc); □ N-acetylgalactosamine (GalNAc); ● galactose; O mannose, △ fucose and ♦ sialic acid.

6. Marketing approval: Lot release assays

Many assays can be used to characterize a drug during development. Some will continue to be used to trouble shoot production problems and demonstrate comparability through process changes and a subset of these assays will become release assays. The list will include release assays common to most, if not all, biotherapeutics such as concentration, purity, peptide mapping and oligosaccharide profiling. Additionally, any assays determined during process development which monitor critical quality attributes specific to the drug will become a release assay. These assays could include quantification of sialic acid, assays used to evaluate the truncation of the amino acid sequence and assays which identify post-translational medications such as phosphorylation or gamma carboxylation.

Unlike assays used for characterization, the release assays will need to be validated and transferred to QC laboratories. Some of these assays such as concentration or activity are so important for moving the product into the clinic that they will need to be validated early and used for lot release on earlier lots. Other assays, like peptide mapping and oligosaccharide profiling might not be validated until later (but before marketing approval). This allows more time for the extensive work often required to identify the peptides/oligosaccharides in the peaks and collect data on any variation seen in these separations from many drug lots before setting specifications.

7. Conclusions

An approach to characterization of a therapeutic has been presented in which analytical testing is simplified by initially focusing on the assays required early in development for all therapeutics (purity, molecular weight, activity and/or concentration). Next, the drug is evaluated using assays that are routinely used for release testing such as peptide mapping and oligosaccharide profiling. Incorporating these assays earlier in development allows for better tracking of lot-to-lot variation in the product and collection of more data before setting assay specifications. Finally, assays will need to be added or existing assays modified, to track variation in the drug that is detected during development (changes such as truncation of the protein or post-translational modifications). Tracking any heterogeneity in the drug is most critical if it is likely to affect the safety or efficacy of the drug.

The authors believe that it is important to use universal methods. Universal methods do not require extensive assay development work and are sensitive to certain physicochemical properties of the drug such as molecular weight or charge. It is better to obtain more data earlier in development using these universal methods than to spend time early in drug development optimizing assays specific for your protein before understanding the heterogeneity naturally present in your drug and how it is likely to degrade.

8. References

International Conference on Harmonisation; Guidance on Specificatons: Test Procedures and Acceptance Criteria for Biotechnological/Biological Products. (1999). Federal Register, 64.

Alterman, M. C. (n.d.). AARG2003 Study: Quantitation of proteins by Amino Acid Analysis and Colorimetric Assays.

An, J. A.; Froehlich, J.W.; Lebrilla, C. B. (2009). Determination of Glycosylation Sites and Site-specific Heterogeneity in Glycoproteins. Current Opinions in Chemical Biology 13, 421-426.

Bloom, J. M. (1997). Intrachain disulfide bond in the core hinge region of human IgG4. Protein Science, 6, 407-415.

Geyer, H; Geyer, R. (2006). Strategies for analysis of glycoprotein glycosylation. Biochemica et Biophysica Acta, 1764, 1853-1869.

Higgins, E. (2010) Carbohydrate Analysis Throughout the Development of a Protein Therapeutic. Glycoconjugate Journal, 27, 211-225.

Kim, J. J. (2010). Characterization of a unique IgG1 mAb CEX profile by limited Lys-C porteolysis/CEX separation coupled with mass spectrometry and structuratl analysis. Journal of Chromatography B, 878, 1973-1981.

Kotia, R. R. (2010). Analysis of monoclonal antibody product heterogeneity resulting from alternate cleavage sites of signal peptide. Analytical Biochemistry, 399, 190-195.

Lau H., P. D. (2010). Investigation of degradation processes in IgG1 monoclonal antibodies by limited proteolysis coupled with weak cation-exchange HPLC. Journal of Chromatography B, 878, 868-876.

Ohta, M. K. (2002). Usefulness of Glycopeptide Mapping by Liquid Chromatography/Mass Spectrometry in Comparability Assessment of Glycoprotein Products. Biologicals, 30, 235-244.

Qian, J.; Liu, T.; Yang, L.; Daus, A.; Crowley, R.; Zhou, Q. (2007). Structural characterization of N-linked oligosaccharides on monoclonalantibody cetuximab by the combination of orthogonal matrix-assisted-laser desorption/ionization hybrid quadrupole–quadrupole time-of-Xight tandem mass spectrometry and sequential enzymatic digestion. Analytical Biochemistry, 364, 8-18.

Rohrer, J. C. (1993). Identification, Quantitation and Cahracterization of Glycopeptides in Reversed-Phase HPLC Separations of Glycoprotein Proteolytic Digests. Analytical Biochemistry, 212, 7-16.

Vlasak, J. B.-R.-H. (2009). Identification and Characterization of asparagine deamidation in the light chain CDR1 or a humanized IgG1 antibody. Analytical Biochemistry, 392, 145-154.

Wypych, J. L. (2008). Human IgG2 Antibodies Display Disulfide-mediated Structural Isoforms. The Journal of Biological Chemistry, 283(23), 16194-16205.

18

Biomarkers in Drug Development: A Useful Tool but Discrepant Results May Have a Major Impact

Abdel-Baset Halim
Daiichi-Sankyo Pharma Development
USA

1. Introduction

The high costs incurred when drugs fail during clinical trials has prompted interest in biomarkers as biological indicators for progress of disease, effect of therapeutic interventions, and/or drug-induced toxicity. One of the goals is to reduce attrition of drugs during the clinical, and probably preclinical, phases of drug development, and hence, the overall cost of drug development.

The role of biomarkers has been exponentially increasing in guiding decisions in every phase of drug development, from drug discovery and preclinical evaluations through each phase of clinical trials and into post-marketing studies. In early phases of drug development, biomarkers are used to evaluate activity in animal models, prove mechanism of action and concept of an investigational entity, bridge pre-clinical and clinical pharmacology, and evaluate safety in animal models and humans. In late stages of drug development, biomarkers can be used to make decisions in the evaluation of dose-response and optimal regimen for desired pharmacologic effect and safety, and some biomarkers can be used as a surrogate endpoint for efficacy and/or toxicity. Also, biomarkers can predict patients' response to compound-enabling patient enrichment strategies by identifying certain patient populations that are more likely to respond to the drug therapy or to avoid specific adverse events. This shift toward "personalized medicine," in which the patient receives a treatment based on his/her genetic makeup as well as medical profile, is helping the drug industry achieve the goal of quick and cost-effective research, especially in poorly served areas such as neurodegenerative disorders and cancer.

Biomarker assays range from exploratory type of assays performed on a fit-for-purpose basis to rigorously validated assays when a biomarker is used as a surrogate end point, for patient selection, or for randomization into different arms. Validation of biomarker assays should be considered a continuous and evolving process. It is imperative that biomarker development be accelerated along with therapeutics. Assay validation is essential, but of equal or even greater importance is the monitoring of assay performance and level of quality during production.

Despite all of the potential benefits of using biomarkers to advance pharmaceutical research and development, discrepant results can pose a threat to development programs by triggering false decisions.

This chapter will address the following topics;

1. Biomarker classes and their potential utility in drug development.
2. Pre-analytical, analytical, or post-analytical laboratory sources of errors.
3. Biomarkers in personalized medicine, and ideal path for drug and companion diagnostic co-development.
4. The major reasons behind discrepant results from biomarkers laboratories with real-life examples, their impact on the pharmaceutical industry, and how to mitigate them.

2. Biomarker definition

A biomarker is a characteristic that is objectively measured and evaluated as an indicator of normal biologic processes, pathogenic processes, or a pharmacologic response to a therapeutic intervention (Atkinson, 2001). According to the FDA's definition, a biomarker is a measurable endpoint that can be used as an indicator of a particular disease or some other physiological state of an organism (FDA, 2011a). With these definitions, biomarkers include imaging (CT, MRI, PET, x-ray) or clinical laboratory testing which can span a whole range of laboratory testing including simple serum chemistries (e.g. blood glucose), immunochemistry, cell surface protein expression, drug metabolizing isoenzyme phenotype, blood pressure, psychometric testing, pain scales, microbial culture, pulmonary function tests, electrocardiogram, bone density, single gene mutations or global mutation scanning, gene amplification, targeted and global gene-expression, or protein and phosphoprotein signatures.

3. Some historical background

Medical practice in ancient times was performed mainly by physical examination and observation of the patient. However, testing of biological fluids for diagnostic and predictive purposes started around 6000 years ago with the analysis of human urine (Armstrong 2007). Prior to Hippocrates (460 - 370 BC), Babylonian, Egyptian and Far Eastern cultures were familiar with the diagnostic utility of urine. Urine assessments by Sumerian and Babylonian physicians were documented in as far back as 4000 BC, when they first discovered that something other than physical evidence of disease could be utilized to make a clinical decision. In those days, whenever a patient was diagnosed with a serious disease, they would ask him/her to breathe into a sheep's nose. The animal would then be slaughtered and the liver removed and carefully inspected for evidence of disease. The resulting observation was to be used to predict the outcome of the patient's case and its treatment. The Babylonians based this diagnostic art on their theory that the liver was the center of the human body's organs and that the whole of human physiology occurred there, which aligns with our modern perception of the metabolic importance of hepatic cells.

One of the earliest recorded diagnostic tests for hormones in body fluids was documented in the time of Ikhnaton and Cleopatra, when Egyptian pharaohs tested for pregnancy by adding a patient's urine to a bag containing wheat and barley seeds. If the seeds germinated the woman was pregnant. If the barley seeds germinated first, it was an indication that the unborn infant was male, but if the wheat seeds germinated first then it indicated that the woman was carrying a female fetus. Testing of this pregnancy theory in 1963 showed 70% predictive value. Over the centuries, pregnancy testing became more sophisticated. In the early twentieth century scientists in several laboratories across Europe independently described the presence of a substance that promotes ovary development and growth in rabbits and mice, and they recognized that the substance was a specific hormone, now known as human chorionic gonadotropin (hCG). In 1928 German scientists Aschheim and Zondek developed the first bioassay for hCG in urine by injecting a woman's urine into an immature rat and looking for an estrous reaction; hyperemia of the ovaries and growth of the follicles.

Another ancient diagnostic test was documented in Hindu cultures, utilizing the sweetness of urine and its ability to attract black ants to diagnose diabetes mellitus. (Winsten, 1969; Haber, 1988; Leavitt, 2006; Armstrong, 2007; Eknoyan, 2007; and NIH, 2011). Urine was once, and still is to a degree, regarded as a powerful fluid in many cultures. Towards the end of the 18th century, doctors with an interest in chemistry turned their attention to the scientific basis of urine analysis and to its use in practical medicine. To serve this interest, Boehringer Manheim launched the first urine dipstick in the mid-20th century.

Over the last four decades, the importance of biomarkers in clinical trials and patient management has increased exponentially. The following graph (Figure 1) shows the number of publications listed on PubMed over the past 40 years for the keywords *biomarker, clinical trial,* and *biomarkers & clinical trials*. The number of hits increased 251-fold (from 325 to 81545) for *biomarker* and 3045-fold (2 to 6089) for *biomarker & clinical trial,* versus 21-fold (4932 to 105533) for *clinical trial* from 1971/1972 to 2009/2010. These data indicate the significant growth in interest in biomarkers and their association with clinical trials over time.

4. Brief biomarker laboratory regulatory aspects

CLIA (Clinical Laboratory Improvement Act) certification and CAP (College of American Pathologists) accreditation have become a customary element of laboratory capability presentations. As a consequence of media coverage and public concern regarding false-negative Pap smears in detecting cervical cancer, congressional hearings were held in 1976 and again in 1988 on medical laboratory practices. Congress passed the Clinical Laboratory Improvement Amendments of 1988 (CLIA 1988) to ensure accuracy and reliability of laboratory testing. This legislation, for the first time, extended federal regulation to all laboratories (hospital, independent, and physician office laboratories, etc.) that perform microbiological, serological, chemical, hematological, immunohematological, immunological, toxicological, cytogenetical, exfoliative cytological, histological, pathological or other examinations performed on materials derived from the human body, for the purpose of diagnosis, prevention of disease, and treatment of patients. The Centers for Medicare & Medicaid Services (CMS) have primary responsibility under CLIA for regulating approximately 195,000 labs that are certified under CLIA. Since 1988, the CMS, along with the Food and Drug Administration (FDA) and the Centers for Disease Control and Prevention (CDC), has been working to improve the quality of laboratory testing through a variety of research, educational and enforcement activities. Of these quality enhancement measures, certified labs performing moderate and high complexity tests have been required, since 1994, to participate successfully in approved proficiency testing (PT) programs, which provide an external evaluation of the accuracy of each laboratory's test results. These surveys may be conducted by the CLIA program, a State survey agency under contract with CMS, or private CMS-approved agencies such as Commission on Office Laboratory Accreditation (COLA), the Joint Commission on Accreditation of Healthcare Organizations (JCAHO), or CAP.

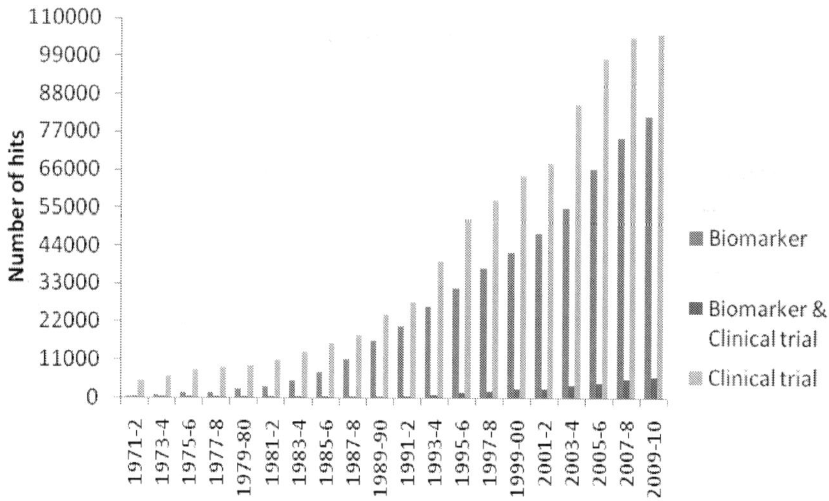

Fig. 1. Number of hits for "biomarker", "clinical trial", and "biomarker + clinical trial" in PubMed.

CAP is the largest PT provider in the world, and is also the largest laboratory-accrediting agency in the United States. Through the PT program, the CAP provides individual laboratories with multiple specimens, usually three to five, for testing on three different occasions per year. The participants analyze the specimens and return results to the CAP for evaluation. Consequently, each participating laboratory receives a report of their performance along with a report summarizing the results of all participating laboratories in a peer group format. The CAP believes that by comparison to the most relevant instrument/reagent combinations, a laboratory's performance is accurately assessed (www.CAP.org). The CAP automatically forwards results for analytes regulated for proficiency testing to the CMS for laboratories that are accredited by the US government under the CLIA.

Of the tens of thousands of biomarker assays applied for different purposes in clinical trials, only 88 analytes (biomarkers) are regulated by CLIA-- 9 hematology, 17 general immunology, 1 diagnostic immunology, 5 immunohematology, 25 routine clinical chemistry, 7 endocrinology, 15 toxicology and therapeutic drug monitoring, and 9 microbiology. For all other 'non-regulated' analytes, CLIA dictates that the laboratory must have a quality assurance plan that establishes the accuracy and reliability of the testing at least twice per year. Proficiency testing programs offer a wide array of products to conveniently assist laboratories in fulfilling this requirement (www.CAP.org). The CAP offers proficiency testing for more than 1,000 analytes. (CLIA, 1988; CMS, 2006; Paxton, 2007; Howerton et al, 2010; Benneyan, 2011; and CAP, 2011).

5. Utility of biomarkers in clinical trials

High attrition rates are a critical issue in drug development, especially within oncology (Walker and Newell, 2009). The overall attrition rate for developing a drug was calculated to be 10,000:1. From an average of 10,000 new chemical entities presented to pharmacology and safety testing, only about 10% (1000) would pass the criteria of activity and lack of toxic side effects. Of the 1,000 entities approved for clinical study, only 1% would show the combined safety and efficacy required by the clinic. Last but not least, out of the 10 NDA submissions to the FDA, only 10% of these (1 drug), on average, passes the review process (Network Science, 2011). This high attrition rate adds to the expensive and lengthy process of developing new medication, resulting in stagnation in the development of new compounds (Bowalekar, 2011).

One of the options for the pharmaceutical industry to improve the high attrition rate during drug development is to move away from treat-and-see testing of new drugs in patients and focus on generating translational biomarkers early in the research process to enable more predictive evaluation of drug action in clinical trials (Gool et al, 2010). As a form of encouraging guidance, the FDA released a critical path initiative document in 2004, emphasizing the need for developing innovative trial designs. One of the innovations suggested was to use biomarkers to evaluate safety and effectiveness, predict effectiveness, provide informative links between mechanism of action and clinical effectiveness, connect animal and human studies, and serve as surrogate endpoints. New imaging technologies and emerging techniques of pharmacogenomics and proteomics show great promise in this respect, but much developmental work and standardization of the biological, statistical, and bioinformatics methods must occur before these techniques can be easily and widely applied (FDA, 2004).

6. Classes of biomarkers in clinical trials

Clinical laboratory measurements are an essential component of most drug studies to demonstrate safety and efficacy.

6.1 Safety biomarkers

Application of the most sensitive procedures to identify toxicity as early as possible in clinical development before engagement into expensive phase III trials is essential. Thus, at phases 1 and 2, careful selection of the correct tests should be mandatory, and the selection of those tests should be based on the compound profile and pre-clinical toxicology data (Craig, 2004). In addition to physical examination, vital signs, and electrocardiogram (ECG), constantly monitored safety lab biomarkers can act as common vital organ function tests applied across different therapeutic areas or as specialized testing applied to detect unique toxicities. Safety testing can be classified as follows:

6.1.1 Liver safety tests

The liver's unique position between the gastrointestinal tract and the rest of the body, in addition to its vast capability to perform diverse functions essential for life, dictate its enormous role in maintaining metabolic homoeostasis of the body and turn it into the first resort for drugs and other toxicants. The most common tests applied in clinical trials are serum aspartate transaminase (AST), alanine transaminase (ALT), alkaline phosphatase (ALP), gamma-glutamyl transferase (GGT), and bilirubin. Changes observed in different liver tests depend on the significance of the liver's involvement. ALT is located mainly in the cell cytosol but AST is located mainly in the mitochondria, which makes ALT quicker in release after acute hepatocellular injury. Also, ALT elevation lasts longer than AST's, and it is a more liver-specific enzyme for which serum elevation is rarely observed in conditions other than parenchymal liver damage. ALP and GGT are membrane-bound enzymes. ALP significantly increases in conditions that cause biliary obstruction but only moderately elevates in parenchymal cell damage. Although renal tissue has the highest content of GGT, the primary source of serum GGT is believed to be of hepatobilairy origin. Release of GGT into serum is caused by the toxic effect of alcohol or some drugs on the microsomal structures of hepatic cells. Bilirubin is a marker of the excretory liver functions, and both conjugated and unconjugated bilirubin increase in obstructive liver damage (Craig, 2004 and Balistreri and Rej, 1994). Albumin and prothrombin time can be used to assess changes in the synthetic functions of the liver but significant changes may only happen with chronic hepatocellular damage.

According to the FDA's guide, drug-induced liver injury (DILI) is predominantly hepatocellular damage that can be revealed by the rise in serum ALT or AST. The ability to cause some hepatocellular injury, however, is not a reliable predictor of a drug's potential for severe DILI. Many drugs that cause transient rises in serum amino transaminases (AT) activity do not cause progressive or severe DILI, even if drug administration is continued. Severe DILI are induced by those drugs that can cause hepatocellular injury extensive enough to reduce the liver's ability to clear bilirubin from the plasma or to synthesize prothrombin and other coagulation factors (FDA, 2009).

6.1.2 Renal dafety tests

In addition to its homeostatic and endocrine functions, the kidneys' excretory function is essential for life, ridding the body of most of the present undesirable end products and toxicants. Blood urea nitrogen (BUN), serum creatinine, glomerular filtration rate (GFR), creatinine clearance, serum electrolytes (sodium, potassium, chloride, and bicarbonate), and complete urine analysis (color, pH, specific gravity, glucose, proteins, ketone bodies, and microscopic exam for blood, leukocytes, casts) are the traditional renal toxicity tests in clinical trials. Cystatin-c, β_2-microglobulin, uric acid, clusterin, N-acetyl-beta-d-glucosaminidase, neutrophil gelatinase-associated lipocalin (NGAL), N-acetyl-β-d-glucosaminidase (NAG), and kidney injury molecule-1 (KIM-1) have been used as nephrotoxic biomarkers and some of them were found to be superior to BUN and creatinine in detecting glomerular and tubular injury (Craig, 2004, Balistreri et, 1994, Tonomura et al, 2010, Prozialeck et al, 2009, Guha et al, 2011, Alkhalaf et al, 2010, Vaidya et al, 2009, Dharnidharka et al, 2002, Dieterle et al, 2010, van Timmeren et al, 2007).

6.1.3 Hematology safety biomarkers

Bone marrow is a primary target for toxicity caused by many classes of drugs including cytotoxic compounds, and the effect can be reflected by changes in peripheral blood components. Complete blood count, one of the fundamental safety indices in drug development, includes total hemoglobin, hematocrit, red cell count, mean red cell volume, mean cell hemoglobin, red cell distribution width%, mean cell hemoglobin concentration, total white cell count, differential white cell count (Neutrophils, lymphocytes, basophils, esinophils, and monocytes), and platelets (Craig, 2004).

6.1.4 Bone safety biomarkers

Bone is a living connective tissue constantly undergoing a process of remodeling, which includes a degradation stage of bone resorption by the action of osteoclasts and a building stage of formation mediated by the action of osteoblasts. Serum calcium and inorganic phosphates have been traditionally used as bone biomarkers in clinical trials.

6.1.5 Basic metabolic dafety biomarkers

Blood glucose, triglycerides (TG), total cholesterol, low density lipoprotein cholesterol (LDL-c), and high density lipoprotein cholesterol (HDL-c).are commonly used within the safety biomarker panel but can be used as efficacy biomarkers too.

6.1.6 Other specific safety biomarkers

Other target organ or compound mechanism of action-driven biomarkers may include serum immunoglobulin levels, C-reactive protein (CRP), fibrinogen, thyroid stimulating hormone (TSH), thyroxine, testosterone, insulin, lactate dehydrogenase (LDH), creatine kinase (CK) and its isoenzymes, cardiac troponin (cTn), and methemoglobin can be used as markers for specific toxicities (Craig, 2004; Reagan, 2010 and Subramaniam et al, 2010).

6.2 Efficacy biomarkers

The purpose of efficacy testing differs fundamentally from safety monitoring in that biomarkers are being used to demonstrate a change in all, or at least a good proportion of treated subjects; in other words, the more positive the biomarker, the higher the efficacy of a drug. Efficacy biomarkers can be classified into the following groups: surrogate, predictive, pharmacodynamic (PD), and prognostic biomarkers.

Figure (2) illustrates different classes of biomarkers; drug metabolizing enzyme, drug receptor, and intermediary pathway substrate polymorphisms as predictive of a drug response, an intermediary signal produced from the interaction of a drug with its receptor as a PD biomarker, and a surrogate biomarker to demonstrate the final drug action. The diagram shows that panels 1 and 4 have similar pharmacological pathway components, in terms of quality and quantity, but the magnitude of the endpoints' action can be significantly affected by the rate of converting the inactive drug to an active one). Panels 2 and 3, compared to Panel 1, show that two subjects may have the same efficiency of drug metabolizing enzymes but, due to mutations in the drug receptor or downstream intermediary protein substrate, the drug does not perform its intended final action.

6.2.1 Surrogate biomarkers

A surrogate endpoint is a laboratory or physical measurement used in clinical trials to indicate a drug's response and can be used in place of a clinical endpoint (Lonn, 2001). A clinical endpoint is a characteristic or variable that reflects a patient's health status, usually related to efficacy, and is usually acceptable as evidence of efficacy for regulatory purposes. A surrogate biomarker can be used to assess the benefit of or harm from a therapeutic agent, based on epidemiologic,

Table (1) summarizes the basic biomaker safety panel recommended for each trial, which looks very similar to the basic standard-of-care lab profile:therapeutic, pathophysiologic, or other scientific evidence that links the biomarker to the clinical outcome (Woodcock, 2011). Surrogate biomarkers are hugely beneficial when substituted for clinically significant endpoints, also known as patient-oriented outcomes, which can be very time consuming and expensive to prove, for example, blood pressure (BP) for stroke or myocardial infarction. Other examples of surrogate biomarkers are cholesterol, LDL-c, triglycerides, blood glucose, glycosylated hemoglobin (HbA1c), arterial plaque thickness, CD4 count or viral load for HIV response, HCV RNA viral load for HCV response, bacterial count, tumor size, and bone mineral density (Temple, 2009, Woodcock, 2011). Even if evidence for surrogacy is not enough, such types of biomarkers are useful in proving the concept for which a candidate drug is to be used, such as the inhibition of platelet aggregation by an antithrombotic agent (Temple, 2009).

AST
ALT
ALP
Bilirubin
GGT
Urea
Creatinine
Sodium
Potassium
Uric acid
Glucose
Cholesterol
Total protein
Albumin
Calcium
CRP
Thyroxine
TSH
Complete blood count with platelets
Complete urinalysis

Table 1. Basic safety biomarker panel in clinical trials

6.2.2 Predictive biomarkers

Predictive biomarkers can stratify patient populations into responders and non-responders, predict whether or not a drug will have the intended effect, or forecast the extent to which a drug can be effective and/or toxic in different patient populations. The discovery of Cytochrome P450-2D6 (CYP2D6) polymorphism in 1977 (Mahgoub et al, 1977 and Tucker et al, 1977) opened the door for research on the impact of such metabolizing enzyme's genetic variability on the efficacy and toxicity of drugs. However, 34 years after this discovery, only 76 genetic and genomic biomarkers, mainly CYP2D6 followed by CYP2C19, are on FDA labels of 70 approved drugs, mainly for oncology and psychiatry followed by antiviral and cardiovascular drugs (Figure 3). Drug label information on genomic biomarkers can describe drug exposure and clinical response variability, risk for adverse events, genotype-specific dosing, mechanisms of drug action, polymorphic drug target and disposition genes, and precautions- interactions, contraindications, patient counseling, nutritional management (FDA, 2011b).

6.2.2.1 Predictive biomarkers in personalized medicine

Completion of the human genome project about a decade ago enormously facilitated our understanding of human genetics and the associated biology, and it has become increasingly clear that patients with different genetic makeup manifest diseases differently and respond to medication differently - in terms of both efficacy and safety. Also, there is a rapidly spreading notion that uncertainty about which patients might respond positively or negatively to a particular treatment regimen has significant consequences on patient health and attrition rate in drug discovery, that empirical drug development is unsustainable, and that biomarkers can provide guidance and help with these issues. In this respect, the personalization of medicine, via targeting the right population, offers the potential for mitigating the problem of universalizing therapy into a single, all-encompassing solution. If two populations with genetic and biological makeup similar to Panels 1 and 2 depicted above in Figure (2) use the same drug, Panel 1's population would observe the desired effect while the population in Panel 2 would only be exposed to the side effects of the drug. The population depicted by Panel 4 will need to double the dose used for Panel 1 to get same value. Figure (4) illustrates the concept of predictive biomarkers and personalized medicine. In graph (A), the use of biomarker had no impact, while graph (B)'s biomarker-positive population responded significantly better to a target drug, as measured by survival rate, than the biomarker- negative population when treated with the same drug or the control arm (marker-positive or -negative) receiving the standard therapy.

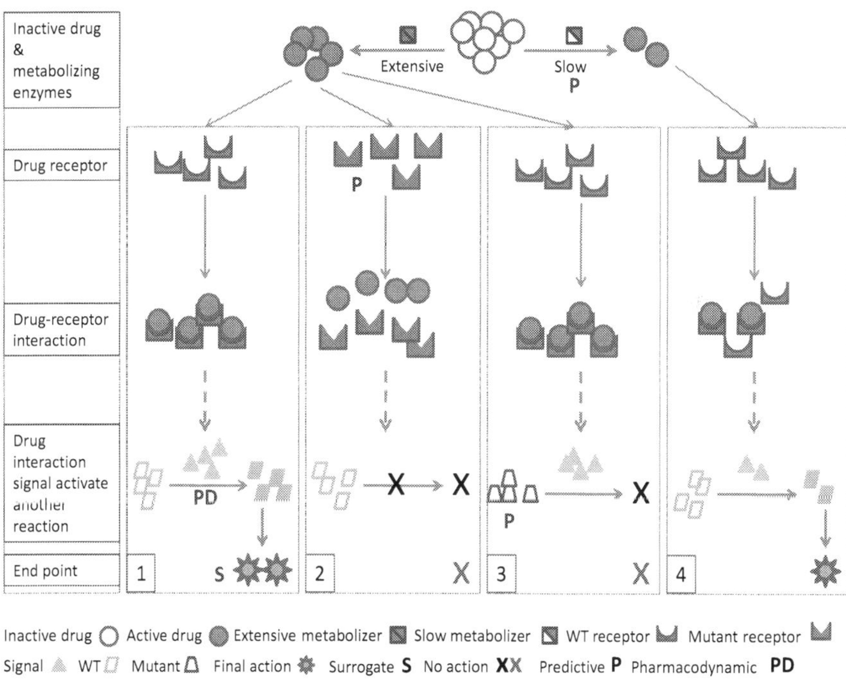

Fig. 2. Illustration of surrogate, predictive, pharmacodynamic (PD) biomarkers.

6.2.2.2 Personalized medicine and companion diagnostics (CDx)

Recent advances in cancer research have focused on drug candidates with specific molecular targets including mutated genes in cancer cells. To achieve the greatest benefit from such types of therapeutic agents, populations that are positive for the target should be identified and exclusively treated, and, in order to do that, an in-vitro diagnostic test (IVD) should be readily available. This IVD can be an existing test for a biomarker that is classified by the FDA as "known valid;" in other words, the biomarker is accepted by the scientific community at-large as a predictor of clinical outcomes, such as LDL-c, HbA1c, and CYP2C19. When a biomarker appears to have predictive value but is not yet replicated or widely accepted, it is classified by the FDA as "probable valid," as in the cases of EGFR and KRAS mutations. These types of biomarkers can be used in targeted therapies to demonstrate the efficacy or toxicity of an agent during a drug's clinical development, and then become "known valid" when treatment is approved (Frueh, 2006). This approach mandates co-development of an IVD with a drug- a companion diagnostic (CDx).

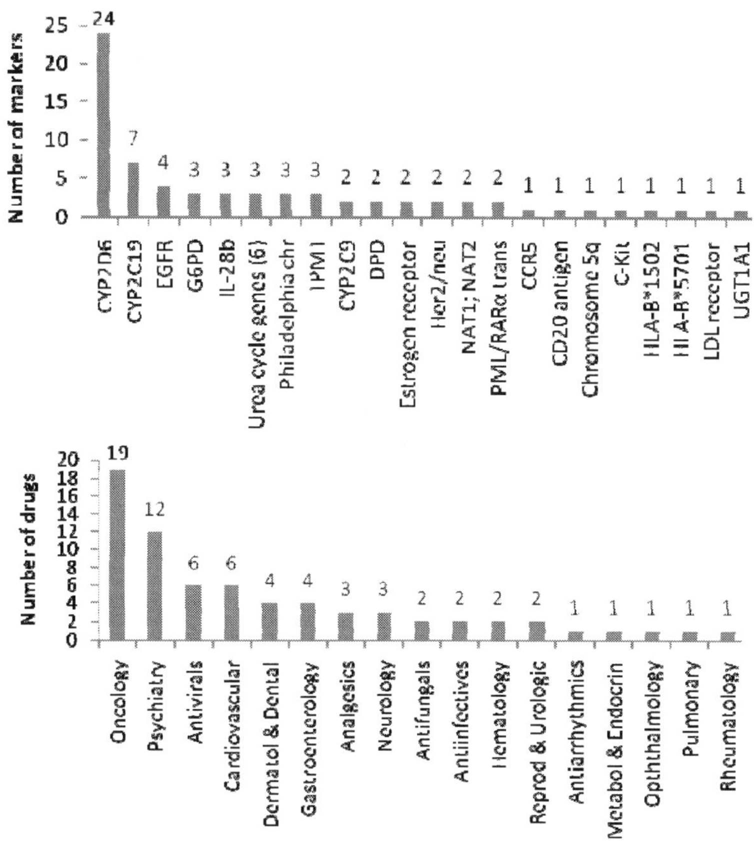

Fig. 3. Biomarkers (A) listed on labels of FDA-approved drugs (B).

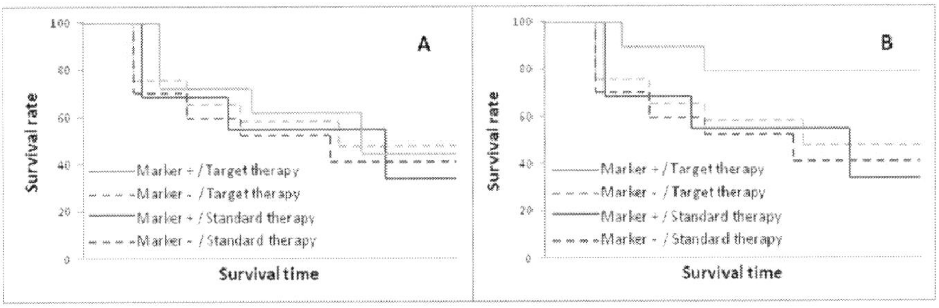

Fig. 4. Depiction of how a biomarker can predict response to a medication: the biomarker is predictive in Panel B but not in Panel A.

Co-development can occur during any stage of drug development but, ideally, a biomarker should be integrated early in the drug's development program so that trial data will support both drug and test approval. Clinical qualification of a biomarker should be prospective, but the retrospective path remains a possibility. Under any circumstances, the biomarker assay should be analytically validated before testing clinical samples. As shown by the following table (Table 2), only a few oncology drugs and IVD have been approved thus far (Datamonitor, 2011). Despite of the biological, analytical, clinical, regulatory, and project management hurdles, co-development of drugs and IVD appears to be the future in facilitating the personalized medicine approach. Figure (5) depicts the ideal path for drug-IVD co-development. After the end of phase II and prior to initiation of pivotal phase III trial, in which the predictive biomarker will be used for patient randomization, both CDER (the Center for Drug Evaluation and Research; the branch of FDA responsible for drug approval) and CDRH (the Center for Devices and Radiological Health; the branch of FDA responsible for approval of medical devices), should approve the approach of co-development. Figure (6) illustrates the process of qualifying a predictive biomarker in pivotal phase III.

Drug	Indication	Biomaker/CDx
Imatinib (Gleevec)	CML	BCR-ABL (PCR), c-KIT IHC
Erlotinib (Tarceva)	NSCLC, pancreatic	EGFR and KRAS mutation
Gefitinib (Iressa)	NSCLC	EGFR and KRAS mutation
Cetuximab (Erbitux)	Colorectal cancer; head and neck cancer	EGFR and KRAS mutation
Panitumumab (Vectibix)	Colorectal	EGFR and KRAS mutation
Trastuzumab (Herceptin)	Breast cancer, gastrointestinal	HER2 ISH, IHC, ELISA

Table 2. Approved oncology drugs with diagnostic tests

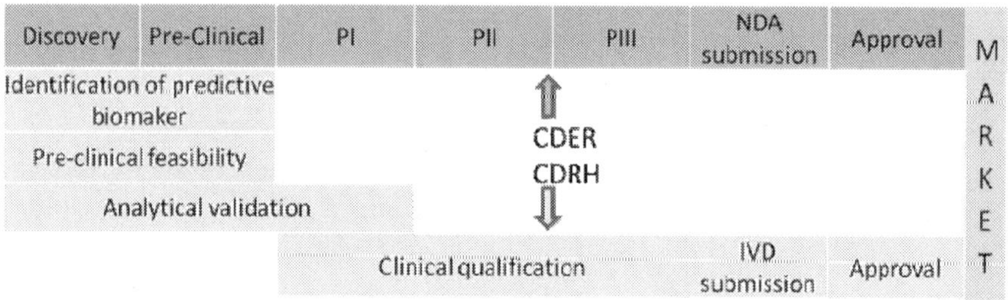

Fig. 5. Ideal path for drug-IVD co-development. Blue; drug development, pink; IVD development. CDER; the Center for Drug Evaluation and Research (the branch of FDA responsible for drug approval), CDRH; the Center for Devices and Radiological Health (the branch of FDA responsible for approval of medical devices).

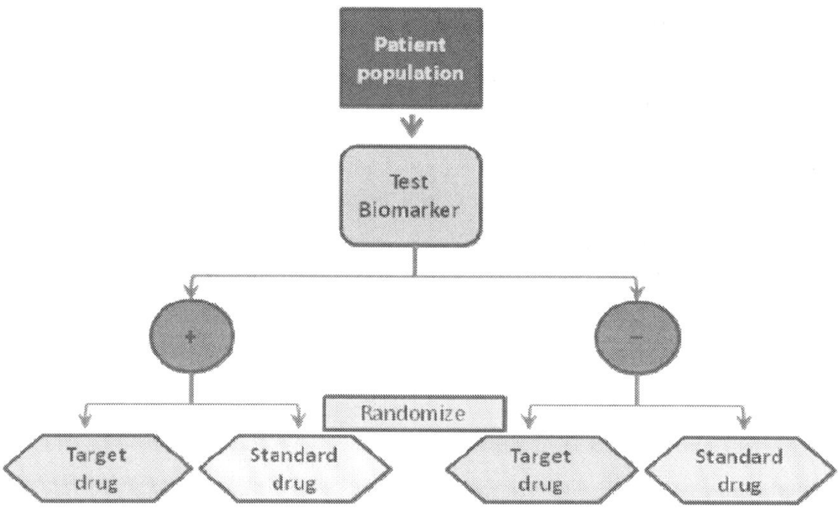

Fig. 6. Qualification of a predictive biomarker in pivotal phase III trial

6.2.3 Pharmacodynamic (PD) biomarkers

These are the biomarkers which demonstrate that a drug hits its target and impacts its biochemical pathway. Such types of biomarkers are necessary to demonstrate proof of the drug's mechanism of action (POM), i.e. markers of pharmacological response. This class constitutes the majority of biomarkers in early phases of drug discovery (preclinical, phase I, and, probably, phase II). In correlation with pahrmacokinetic (PK) measurements, this class of biomarkers can help to determine effective dose and dose schedule. The biomarker illustration in Figure (2) shows that detection of an intermediary signal can indicate that the drug hit its target and the magnitude of the signal can reflect the efficacy of the interaction.

The contribution of biomarkers to the goals of 87 phase I oncology trials was analyzed to reveal that biomarkers supported the proposed mechanism of action in 39% of the trials, contributed to dose selection for subsequent phase II studies in 13%, contributed to the selection of dosing schedule for phase II studies in 8%, and biomarkers were considered by the authors to be potentially useful for selecting a patient population in subsequent studies in 19% of the trials. These biomarkers were determined in serum (36.8% of total), tumor tissue (25.6%), peripheral blood mononuclear cells (22.7%), normal solid tissue (3.7%), and cerebrospinal fluid (0.2%), in addition to 10.9% by special in-vivo imaging. The non-imaging biomarkers included proteins, cytokines, and enzyme activity in serum, CSF, or tissue lysates, proteins by immunohistochemistry (IHC), and DNA and RNA gene expression (Goulart et al, 2007).

6.2.4 Prognostic biomarkers

Prognostic biomarkers can predict the risk or outcome of a disease in patient population without the involvement of therapy. For example, a population that tested positive for a given prognostic biomarker can survive longer or live better than another that tested negative. Figure (7) depicts the concept of a biomarker's ability to predict overall survival in Panel A but not Panel B. In addition to its predictive power, prognostic biomarkers may help enrich a clinical trial by choosing people more likely to respond to treatment. Examples of prognostic biomarkers include prostatic specific antigen to predict survival in prostatic cancer patients (D'Amico et al, 2004 and Kelloff et al, 2004), Preoperative CA125 to predict metastatic disease in patients with uterine carcinoma (Gupta et al, 2011), and CRP as a risk factor in cardiovascular events (Ridker et al, 2008 and Abd et al, 2011), CRP to predict reduced overall and disease-free survival breast cancer (Allin et al, 2011), and serum LDH to predict overall survival in metastatic brain tumors (Eigentler et al, 2011). The number of circulating tumor cells (CTC) was shown to predict overall and progression-free survival in patients with metastatic breast and ovarian cancers (FDA, 2005 and Poveda et al, 2011), and to predict the effect of treatment earlier than imaging (Nakamura et al, 2010). Also, HER2-positive CTC was suggested as a prognostic value in metastatic breast cancer (Hayashi et al, 2011).

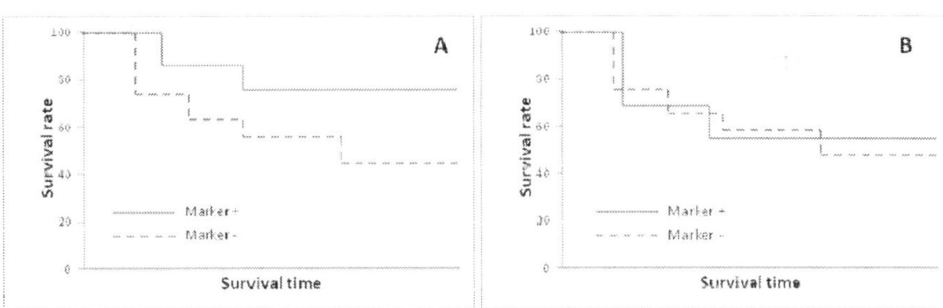

Fig. 7. Illustration of a prognostic biomarker. A biomarker can predict clinical outcome (survival) in Panel A but not in Panel B.

7. Discrepant results and its major impact on clinical trials

7.1 Types of laboratory errors

Despite all of the potential benefits of using biomarkers to advance pharmaceutical research and development and to fully implement the concept of personalized medicine, discrepant results can be a threat to development programs by triggering false decisions. Many tools and strategies have been adopted to enhance laboratory quality, including internal quality control (QC) procedures, external quality assessment programs, certification and accreditation, licensing of lab professionals, continuing education programs, and the regulation of lab services. Despite these quality measures, some imminent sources of error still require urgent intervention.

Most errors affecting laboratory test results occur in the pre-analytical phase, where they account for more than 90% of the errors currently encountered within the entire diagnostic process, and the positive trends towards the reduction of laboratory errors over the past decade (predominantly those in the analytical phase) have hardly affected the pre-analytical phase (Lippi et al, 2006a; Lippi et al, 2006b and Lippi, 2009). Those variables often result in sub-optimal or poor specimen quality with the impact of producing incorrect results. Laboratory errors can be classified as pre-analytical, analytical, or post-analytical.

7.1.1 Pre-analytical

Pre-analytical errors occur between the test order and the analytical phase, and may affect sample integrity and its suitability for analysis.

Patient preparation for the test

- Nutritional status and diet influencing test results.
- Physical activity prior to sampling.
- Emotional distress prior to or during sampling.
- Smoking.
- Alcohol intake.
- Menstruation and pregnancy in females.
- Medications or suppliments that interfere with measured analytes.
- Some clinical procedures and other diagnostic intervention.

Phlebotomy-related

- Wrong test ordered or incorrect timing of sampling.
- Missing or wrong patient ID.
- Posture of the patient during sampling.
- Unsuitable tube or anticoagulant.
- Incorrect source of blood (arterial versus venous).
- Blood supply is not enough to collect adequate sample, e.g. collapsed vein.
- Contamination from skin wipes.
- Dilution of specimen from venous infusion or incorrect ratio of blood to liquid anticoagulant.
- Hemoconcentration due to long application of tourniquet, especially at high pressure.
- Improper mixing of anticoagulant which may produce partial clotting.
- Hemolysis due to usage of small needle, vigorous mixing, or pneumatic tube systems with many curves.
- Air bubbles.
- Nonhomogenous blood sample due to partial clotting during collection from heel or finger sticks.
- Wrong order of blood draw tubes. The recommended order is blood culture bottles, citrate, serum, heparin, EDTA, and then fluoride-containing tubes.

Sample processing, storage, and shipping-related

- Inadequate coagulation time for serum separation.
- Lag time between sampling and analysis.
- Wrong centrifugation temperature, speed, or time.
- Storage temperature or wrong freezer, e.g. automatic freeze-thaw.
- Necrotic tissue/fluid or wrong tissue collected via fine needle biopsy.
- Inappropriate acquisition and handling of fresh frozen tissue for RNA, proteins, or phosphoproteins analyses.
- Inappropriate fixation and embedding of tissue biopsies into paraffin blocks.
- Wrong thickness of tissue sections for histopathology, IHC, FISH, etc.
- Unsuitable shipping conditions.

Table (3) lists the most common pre-analytical variables that may impact biomarker results.

These variables are the result of broad heterogeneity in several pre-analytical processes, mainly due to the lack of reliable guidelines (Lippi et al, 2006a, Lippi et al, 2006b, and Lippi, 2009). Assurance of availability of appropriate lab instruments (mainly centrifuges and freezers) during clinical site qualification, along with clear, concise, illustrative lab manuals, well-trained phlebotomists, good techniques for tissue biopsy, and onsite training are essential tools in mitigating the pre-analytical lab errors.

7.1.2 Post-analytical

Post-analytical errors may occur after a sample has been processed and analyzed by an instrument, as listed in Table (4) below.

- Improper documentation of test results, wrong manual transcription, or questionable interface between analyzing instrument and database.
- Incorrect patient identification information entered at time of test. Patients' results may be mixed with one another.
- Failure to recognize and act on abnormal results, e.g. repetition of samples with unexpected results or panic values.

Table 4. List of most common post-analytical variables

Although uncommon, post-analytical errors can be very serious, especially when producing alarming values without verification, e.g. very low platelet count from a sample which was inappropriately collected or mixed. To mitigate this class of errors, the central lab has to implement an effective process for sample identification and acquisition, proper interface of testing device with the database, and a process for identification and repeat of analysis, and probably recollection, of samples with unexpected abnormal values especially those with panic results. A pharmaceutical company needs to take the proper measures to ensure error-free post-analytical phase and reporting.

7.1.3 Analytical

With momentous efforts from lab professionals and in-vitro diagnostic partners, clinical laboratory errors due to analytical issues have been significantly reduced over time with the evolution of innovative technologies and the implementation of a number of quality control and quality assurance (QC&QA) check points, including internal (electronic) QC, liquid QC, calibration, delta checks, method comparison, and proficiency testing, among other measures. Figure (8) illustrates the two types of analytical errors: random (A) and systematic (B), where random error can affect a sample or a few samples within an analytical run while systematic error affects all samples analyzed after an error has occurred and until it is fixed. Each biomarker assay has a "default" imprecision, oscillation of values from the same sample, when measured multiple times, around the average of observations. Typically, a clinical lab considers an assay to be well-performing if results from a quality control sample are nicely distributed around the average and within "Average ± 2SD" as shown in Figure (8). Results scattered outside the 2SD limits in panel (A) denote random error, while panel (B) shows consistent drift or bias (systematic error). Random error is usually caused by the pipetting of wrong volumes, air bubbles, small clots, or inadequately mixed samples. Systematic error can affect a single analytical run or even just a part of a run, a few runs, or can have a longitudinal impact which may span the entire life of a testing device. Figure (8B) illustrates a short-term systematic error which may occur following inappropriate calibration of a device or an improperly qualified new lot of reagents. Figure (9) demonstrates a real example of the difference between results from splits of 43 samples analyzed for ALP on two different chemistry analyzers in two labs, where 9A shows that the actual values were remarkably higher in Lab B than Lab A, and 9B shows that the percent difference (% bias) of lab B from lab A ranged between 150 and 350% across different levels of ALP.

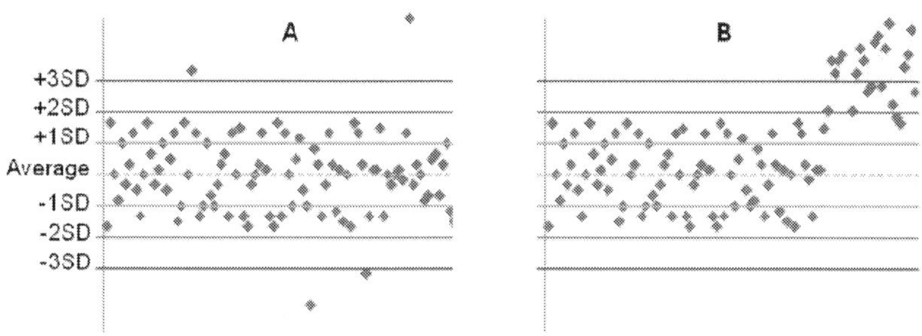

Fig. 8. Illustration of random (A) and systematic error (B).

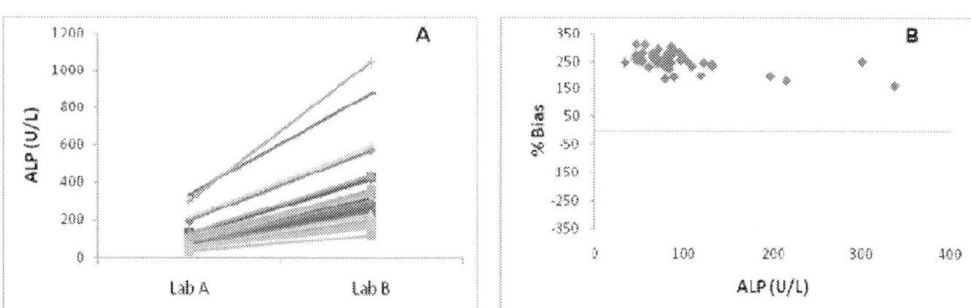

Fig. 9. Systematic error in ALP between two analytical devices used at two different labs; (A) Actual ALP values from 43 split samples, and (B) is Bland-Altman plot for the percent of bias of Lab B from Lab A.

7.2 Lack of traceability as a major source of systematic errors

The overall quality of clinical laboratory results can be compromised by the lack of traceability; absence of true method-to-method or platform-to-platform, or even between different reagent lots for an assay, standardization; or at least harmonization of test results. If assays or technologies are properly validated via proper method-to-method and lab-to-lab comparison, lack of traceability aspects, except reagent lot-to-lot variability, can be easily highlighted. Assay validation is always completed using the same lot or a few lots of reagent at best, which cannot detect low-performing lots afterwards. This is not only the problem of "sophisticated" biomarker assays, e.g. IHC, ISH, genotyping, etc., it also impacts supposedly well-standardized chemistry assays that have been used for decades as standard-of-care.

In past publications (2009, 2011a, and 2011b), I emphasized the gravity of the problem. For one sample analyzed by more than 4,000 laboratories using different types of instruments and thromboplastin reagents, the INR (international normalized ratio of prothrombin time) values ranged between 2.9 and 7.6. When another sample was analyzed for activated partial thromboplastin time (aPTT), thrombin time (TT), and anti-FXa assay (Heparin test) in different labs employing different platforms and methodologies, the ratio of maximum to minimum reported results was up to 4-fold, 40-fold, and 50-fold, respectively. For yet another sample analyzed for ALP and LDH, the ratio was 4-fold. In other instances, percent difference between maximum and minimum HDL-c reported results from a sample analyzed on different platforms was up to 47%; and when another sample (with a target value of 152mg/dl as estimated by a standard procedure) was analyzed on different platforms for LDL-c, the reported results from different labs were between about 120 and 202 mg/dl.

Lack of traceability between different lab platforms or methodologies, even for well-established technologies like chemistry or immunochemistry analyzers employed by central labs, is mainly due to unavailability of primary or secondary standards to calibrate devices or methodologies across different brands. Also, there is no "gold standard" device or methodology to use as a predicate even for well established lab analyzers. While greater automation and innovation has, in general, improved laboratory performance over the last decade, it is also a double-edged sword as, in the absence of a gold standard approach; this seems to contribute significant systematic bias between different devices and reagents. The way the FDA (2011) approves analytical devices or methodologies based on substantial equivalence to legally marketed devices (precedent devices) should be drastically revised.

7.2.1 Impact of lack of traceability on clinical trials

This long term systematic source of error is commonly overlooked and is often aggravated by the disconnect between clinical laboratory services on the one side, and clinicians, and drug developers on the other, and the misinterpretation of test results by following general clinical guidelines per test rather than using a reference range or set cut-off values for medical decisions for specific platforms/reagents. Considering the widely applicable INR therapeutic target range for Warfarin (2.0 to 3.0 units), a result from the sample mentioned above can be within the therapeutic target, indicate slight anticoagulation, or demonstrate dramatic anticoagulation which may need immediate medical intervention. The difference between maximum and minimum results from the anti-FXa example can be more than 23-fold the unfractionated heparin (UFH) therapeutic range (0.35-0.70 U/ml). Following the National Cholesterol Education Program (NCEP) guidelines, a clinician may interpret the results from the LDL-c example as near optimal, borderline high, high, or very high and will treat his/her patient accordingly.

The problem can impact decision making by pharmaceutical developers if they use absolute biomarker values to compare the outcomes of different studies on a drug's efficacy and/or toxicity, or employing biomarkers to bridge between different drug candidates belonging to a particular class of compounds. Also, global clinical trials may be impacted where different specialty or safety biomarker labs are employed. It is not uncommon for different lab locations within a global organization (or even within one lab location) to use different platforms interchangeably to analyze samples from the same trial.

A pharmaceutical development program may take as long as 10 years or more, thus switching biomarker vendors is likely, using multiple platforms or changing platforms by a lab is common, and employing different lots of reagents and calibrators is definite. Without paying close attention to these variables, results from different platforms, even from the same lab, may lead to erroneous go/no-go decisions and make compatibility of results from different studies almost impossible. Also, unless appropriately understood and interpreted, if such lab tests are used as an efficacy or toxicity biomarker, the drug may be inappropriately labeled. The inter-laboratory discrepancies in results could be even higher than those included in my articles, because data were gathered from "well-controlled" laboratories for theoretically standardized tests used to manage patients' health and as surrogate biomarkers in clinical trials. Until global standardization or harmonization approaches are employed, the pharmaceutical industry needs to monitor biomarker data rigorously and understand these challenges for better interpretation of biomarker results.

7.3 Impact of discrepant results on personalized medicine

As explained earlier, companion diagnostics (CDx) are essential in enabling target therapeutic products to achieve their expected safety and efficacy. Therefore, the risk from failure of CDx is equal to the risk of wrongly using therapeutic products. It has been reported that BCR-ABL (leukemia biomarker and approved CDx) gene transcripts have been analyzed at over 150 hospitals and labs and results were non-comparable, where the number of transcripts reported from 6 CLIA-certified, reliable labs (two commercial and 4 cancer institutions) varied by more than 2Logs. The introduction of common primers/reagents/calibrators, which was difficult to achieve, improved comparability (Jessup, 2011).

In addition to the adverse effect of incorrect test results on patient management, the use of loosely validated assays may spoil a trial outcome and impose a wrong go/no-go decision, especially if the rate of target mutation is relatively small as shown by figure (10). For example, suppose the rate of a mutant gene is 20%, and the rate of response to a therapeutic agent is 70% and 10% in patients with mutant and wild type (WT) genes, respectively, such as tyrosine kinase inhibitors in mutant and WT EGFR (Mitsudomi and Yatabe, 2007), if the biomarker assay is 90% sensitive and 90% specific, which can be considered acceptable or good by some professionals, it would have two implications:

1. In the clinical trial, the efficacy signal will be diluted, as instead of the two arms (WT and M) being cleanly separated (100% WT and 100% M in the corresponding arms) and the efficacy in the M arm clearly demonstrated, the signal in the M arm would be diluted by the carryover from the WT falsely identified as M. In this case, the average efficacy signal, or overall survival, will be less than the 100% M if identified by the 100%

specific assay. The signal in the WT arm would erroneously increase due to the carryover from M falsely identified as WT because of the 10% false negative, but as the majority is still WT, the impact is not as substantial as in the M arm. In this example, the average efficacy signal would be 0.52 and 0.12 in the M and WT arms instead of 0.70 and 0.10 had the assay been 90% sensitive and 90% specific versus 100% and 100%. This means that the ratio of efficacy signal (in M arm to WT arm) would be reduced from 7.0 to 4.4. Using the same model, such reduction in efficacy signal due to an assay's low performance would change the efficacy signal in the target population of any given drug, such as Herceptin, where the average overall survival for patients with high levels of HER2 and control arm would change from 16 and 11.8 months (Roche, 2010) to 14.7 and 11.9 months, respectively, decreasing the efficacy signal from 1.4 to 1.2.

2. If the biomarker is used as a CDx to qualify a patient for treatment after drug approval, two out of the 20 M will not be given the drug (10%), and 8 out of 80 subjects with WT (10%) will be wrongly treated with the drug.

8. Conclusion

There is no doubt that biomarkers can play a vital role in drug development as tools to monitor drug toxicity, prove a compound mechanism of action, prove the concept for which a drug will be used, and predict efficacy and toxicity. Biomarker hypothesis-driven drug development and personalized medicine seem to be the future of drug industry. However, despite the enormous enhancement in biomarkers laboratories' level of quality, some sources of errors still pose an imminent risk to drug development. Due to lack of standardization, even for well trusted safety biomarker assays, a major source of error is the discrepant results from different laboratories or even from the same lab employing different platforms or methodologies. This source of error is commonly overlooked and is often aggravated by the disconnect between clinical laboratory services on the one side, and clinical guidelines, clinicians, and drug developers on the other. Results from the same sample can vary substantially, even for trusted standardized tests from "well-controlled" laboratories, with consequent impact on drug developers' decisions and patient management including personalized medicine approach.

It may be expensive for pharmaceutical companies to operate and maintain in-house laboratories if assets are underutilized, due to a global shortage of good laboratory and QA professionals, a resulting difficulty in acquiring and maintaining laboratory certification and licensure, and rapidly evolving technologies. Therefore, outsourcing the lab services can be an attractive option. Using contract research organization or academic institution laboratory services may reduce overhead and operating costs and provide pharmaceutical companies with access to new technologies as needed. While greater automation has, in general, improved laboratory performance over the last decade, it is also a 'double-edged sword'. The increase in automation combined with consolidation of instrument/reagent/calibration manufacturers has resulted in many suppliers oversimplifying technology and electronically locking-out laboratories from using competitors' reagents or independent calibrators so as to increase sales and profits. Thus, laboratories have become deeply dependent on suppliers for their quality and are often forced to change methods, instruments, calibrators and reference ranges at the whim of suppliers. This has been further compounded by many laboratories attempting to cut costs by reducing experienced and educated laboratory professionals (doctoral level and even master's level) who have the knowledge and experience to maintain stable calibration and optimal accuracy and precision. In fact, some labs have gone further by reducing bench level personnel from 4-year degree certified medical technologists to 2-year associate degree laboratory technologists or lower.

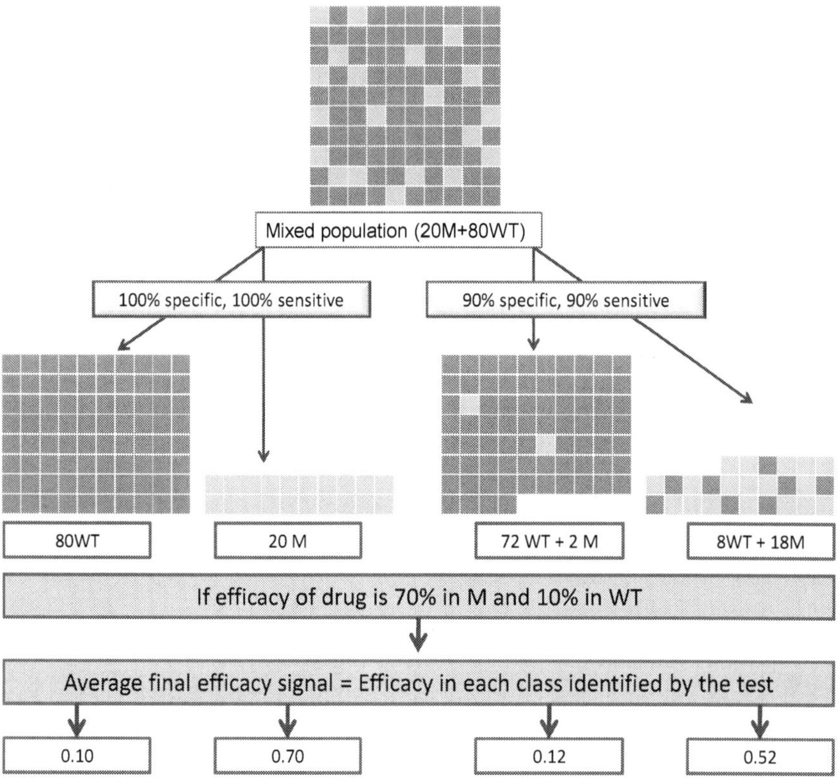

Fig. 10. Impact of low sensitivity and sensitivity of a biomarker assay on the outcome of stratification of patients according to the status of a gene mutation.

$$\text{Average efficacy signal in each arm} = \frac{[\#\text{ of WT x efficacy of the drug in the WT}]+[\#\text{ of M x efficacy of the drug in the M}]}{\text{Total number of subjects in each arm}}$$

Regulatory and laboratory accrediting agencies need to pay more attention, find resources, and implement a road map to fix the major challenge in biomarker laboratory; lack of traceability between different technologies. Meanwhile, it remains the responsibility of drug developers to assure that a biomarkers lab has the right tools and skills to analyze samples from a clinical trial, the assay validation is at the level of the decision to be made, and that biomarker data are properly interpreted.

9. References

Abd, TT, Eapen, DJ, Bajpai, A, Goyal, A, Dollar, A, and Sperling, L. (2011). The role of C-reactive protein as a risk predictor of coronary atherosclerosis: implications from the JUPITER trial. *Curr Atheroscler Rep,* 13(2):154-61.

Alkhalaf, A, Klooster, A, van Oeveren, W, Achenbach, U, Kleefstra, N, Slingerland, RJ, Mijnhout, GS, Bilo, HJ, Gans, RO, Navis, GJ, Bakker, SJ. (2010). A double-blind, randomized, placebo-controlled clinical trial on benfotiamine treatment in patients with diabetic nephropathy. *Diabetes Care,* 33(7):1598-601.

Allin, KH, Nordestgaard, BG, Flyger, H, and Bojesen, SE. (2011). Elevated pre-treatment levels of plasma C-reactive protein are associated with poor prognosis after breast cancer: a cohort study. *Breast Cancer Res,* 13(3):R55.

Armstrong, JA. (2007). Urinalysis in Western culture: A brief history. *Kidney International,* 71:384-387.

Atkinson, AJ, Colburn, WA, DeGruttola, VG, DeMets, DL, Downing, GJ, Hoth, DF, Oates, JA, Peck, CC, Schooley, RT, Spilker, BA, Woodcock, J, and Zeger SL. (2001). Biomarkers and surrogate endpoints: Preferred definitions and conceptual framework- Biomarkers Definitions Working Group. *Clin Pharmacol Ther,* 69:89-95.

Balistreri, WF, and Rej R. (1994). *Tietz Textbook of Clinical Chemistry* (Second Edition), W.B. Saunders, Philadelphia.

Benneyan, JC. (2011). Optimal Policies for Clinical Laboratory Quality Control, AHCPR Grant # R0S HS09329-01, In: *Northeastern University,* accessed June 30, 2011, Available from:
<http://www1.coe.neu.edu/~benneyan/papers/ahcpr_summary.pdf>

Bowalekar, S. (2011). Adaptive designs in clinical trials. *Clin Res Method, 2:23-27.*

CAP. (2011). CLIA-regulated analytes, updated June 4, 2010, In: *CAP,* accessed June 30, 2011, Available from: <http://www.cap.org>

CLIA. (1988). Clinical and environmental laboratories, public health and safety- Clinical Laboratory Improvement Amendments of 1988. Vol 42 C.F.R. 263a; 1988:PL 100-578, In: *CDC,* accessed June 30, 2011, Available from:
<http://wwwn.cdc.gov/clia/docs/fr22mr02n.htm>

CMS. (2006). Initiatives to improve quality of laboratory testing under the CLIA program, July 2006, In: *CMS,* accessed June 30, 2011, Available from: <http://www.cms.gov/CLIA/downloads/060630.Backgrounder.rlEG.pdf>

Craig, A. (2004). *Stephens' Detection of New Adverse Drug Reactions,* Fifth Edition, John Wiley & Sons, Ltd, Retrieved from:
< http://dyahperwitasari.files.wordpress.com/2009/12/booktextstefen05.pdf>

Datamonitor. (2011). Case Study: Personalized Cancer Therapy- The era of biomarker identification and companion diagnostic co-development. Reference Code: HC00048-001. Publication Date: 03/2011, *Datamonitor,* accessed June 30, 2011, Available from:
http://www.datamonitor.com/store/Product/case_study_personalized_cancer_therapy_the_era_of_biomarker_identification_and_companion_diagnostic_co_development_?productid=HC00048-001

D'Amico, AV, Chen MH, Roehl, KA, and Catalona WJ. (2004). Preoperative PSA Velocity and the Risk of Death from Prostate Cancer after Radical Prostatectomy. *N Engl J Med,* 351:125-135.

Dharnidharka, VR, Kwon, C, and Steven, G. (2002). Serum cystatin C is superior to serum creatinine as a marker of kidney function: A meta-analysis. *Am J Kidney Dis*, 40(2): 221-226.

Dieterle, F, Perentes, E, Cordier, A, Roth, DR, Verdes, P, Grenet, O, Pantano, S, Moulin, P, Wahl, D, Mahl, A, End, P, Staedtler, F, Legay, F, Carl, K, Laurie, D, Chibout, SD, Vonderscher, J, and Maurer, G. (2010). Urinary clusterin, cystatin C, beta2-microglobulin and total protein as markers to detect drug-induced kidney injury. *Nat Biotechnol*, 28(5):463-9.

Eigentler, TK, Figl, A, Krex, D, Mohr, P, Mauch, C, Rass, K, Bostroem, A, Heese, O, Koelbl, O, Garbe, C, and Schadendorf, D. (2011). Number of metastases, serum lactate dehydrogenase level, and type of treatment are prognostic factors in patients with brain metastases of malignant melanoma. *Cancer*, 117(8):1697-703.

Eknoyan, G. (2007). Looking at urine: The renaissance of an unbroken tradition. *Am J Kid Dis*, 49:865-872.

FDA. (2004). Innovation or Stagnation: Challenge and Opportunity on the Critical Path to New Medical Products. Challenges and Opportunities Report - March 2004, In: *FDA*, accessed June 30, 2011, Available from: http://www.fda.gov/ScienceResearch/SpecialTopics/CriticalPathInitiative/CriticalPathOpportunitiesReports/ucm077262.htm

FDA. (2005). CellSearch CTC 510k clearance, In: *FDA*, accessed June 30, 2011, Available from: <http://www.accessdata.fda.gov/cdrh_docs/pdf5/K050245.pdf >

FDA. (2009). Guidance for Industry Drug-Induced Liver Injury: Premarketing Clinical Evaluation, In: *FDA*, accessed June 30, 2011, Available from: http://www.fda.gov/downloads/Drugs/GuidanceComplianceRegulatoryInformation/Guidances/UCM174090.pdf

FDA (2011a)-TRACK Research Glossary, In: *FDA*, accessed June 30, 2011, Available from: <http://www.fda.gov/AboutFDA/Transparency/track/ucm252974.htm>

FDA. (2011b). Table of Pharmacogenomic Biomarkers in Drug Labels, In: *FDA*, accessed on June 26, 2011, Available from: <http://www.fda.gov/drugs/scienceresearch/researchareas/pharmacogenetics/ucm083378.htm>

FDA. (2011). Device Approvals and Clearances, In: *FDA*, accessed June 30, 2011, Available from: <http://www.fda.gov/MedicalDevices/DeviceRegulationandGuidance/HowtoMarketYourDevice/PremarketSubmissions/PremarketNotification510k/ucm134571.htm>

Frueh, WF. (2006). Challenges in Biomarker and Drug Challenges in biomarker and drug co-development and regulation: the regulatory view for drugs. AACC Annual Meeting, Chicago, IL -July 24, 2006, In: *FDA*, accessed July 3, 2011, Available from: <http://www.fda.gov/downloads/Drugs/ScienceResearch/ResearchAreas/Pharmacogenetics/ucm085613.pdf>

Goulart, BH, Clark, JW, Pien, HH, Roberts, TG, Finkelstein, S and Chabner, BA. (2007). Trends in the Use and Role of Biomarkers in Phase I Oncology Trials. *Clin Cancer Res*, 13:6719-6726. 2007.

Guha, M, Heier, A, Price, S, Bielenstein, M, Caccese, RG, Heathcote, DI, Simpson, TR, Stong, DB, and Bodes, E. (2011). Assessment of biomarkers of drug-induced kidney injury in cynomolgus monkeys treated with a triple reuptake inhibitor. *Toxicol Sci*, 120(2):269-83.

Gupta, D, Gunter, MJ, Yang, K, Lee, S, Zuckerwise, L, Chen, LM, Goldberg, GL, and Huang, GS. (2011). Performance of serum CA125 as a prognostic biomarker in patients with uterine papillary serous carcinoma. *Int J Gynecol Cancer*, 21(3):529-34.

Haber, MH. (1988). Pisse Prophecy: a brief history of urinalysis. *Clin Lab Med*, 8:415-430.

Halim, AB. (2009). Impact of discrepant results from clinical laboratories on patients and pharmaceutical trials: Evidence from proficiency testing results. *Biomarkers Med, 3(3): 231-8 (2009).*

Halim, AB. (2011). Discrepant results from clinical laboratories are a potential source of risk to patients under therapy with heparin or anti-thrombin agents: Evidence from proficiency testing data. *Biomarkers Med, 5(2): 211-8.*

Halim, AB. (2011). Proficiency testing: A Useful Tool for Monitoring Global Lab Performance and for Identifying Discordances. *Lab Med,* Accepted for publication.

Hayashi, N, Nakamura, S, Tokuda, Y, Shimoda, Y, Yagata, H, Yoshida, A, Ota, H, Hortobagyi, GN, Cristofanilli, M, and Ueno, NT. (2011). Prognostic value of HER2-positive circulating tumor cells in patients with metastatic breast cancer. *Int J Clin Onco,* Online print accessed 2011 Jun 26.

Leavitt, SA. (2006). "A private little revolution": The home pregnancy test in American culture. *Bull Hist Med*, 80:317-345.

Howerton, D, Krolak, JM, Manasterski, A, and Handsfield, JH. (2010). Proficiency testing performance in US laboratories: results reported to the Centers for Medicare & Medicaid Services, 1994 through 2006. *Arch Pathol Lab Med*, 134(5):751-8.

Jessup, JM. (2011). The NCI clinical assay development program (CADP): A resource to support molecular diagnostic development for management of cancer patients. *Biomaker World Congress*, Philadelphia, May 2-4, 2011.

Kelloff, GJ, Bast, RC Jr, Coffey, DS, D'Amico, AV, Kerbel, RS, Park, JW, Ruddon, RW, Rustin, GJ, Schilsky, RL, Sigman, CC, and Woude, GF. (2004). Biomarkers, Surrogate End Points, and the Acceleration of Drug Development for Cancer Prevention and Treatment: An Update Prologue. *Clin Cancer Res*, 10:3881-3884.

Lippi, G, Guidi, GC, Mattiuzzi, C, and Plebani, M. (2006a). Preanalytical variability: the dark side of the moon in laboratory testing. *Clin Chem Lab Med*, 44(4):358-65.

Lippi, G. (2009). Governance of preanalytical variability: travelling the right path to the bright side of the moon? *Clin Chim Acta*, 404(1):32-6.

Lippi, G, Montagnana, M, and Giavarina, D. (2006b). National survey on the pre-analytical variability in a representative cohort of Italian laboratories. *Clin Chem Lab Med*, 44(12):1491-4.

Lonn, E. (2001). The use of surrogate endpoints in clinical trials: focus on clinical trials in cardiovascular diseases. *Pharmacoepidemiol Drug Saf*, 10(6):497-508.

Mahgoub, A, Idle, JR, Dring, DG, Lancaster, R, and Smith, RL. (1977). Polymorphic hydroxylation of debrisoquine in man. *Lancet*, 2:584–586.

Mitsudomi, T and Yatabe, Y. (2007). Mutations of the epidermal growth factor receptor gene and related genes as determinants of epidermal growth factor receptor tyrosine kinase inhibitors sensitivity in lung cancer. *Cancer Sci*, 98: 1817-1824.

Nakamura, S, Yagata, H, Ohno, S, Yamaguchi, H, Iwata, H, Tsunoda, N, Ito, Y, Tokudome, N, Toi, M, Kuroi, K, and Suzuki, E. (2010). Multi-center study evaluating circulating tumor cells as a surrogate for response to treatment and overall survival in metastatic breast cancer. *Breast Cancer*, 17(3):199-204.

National Institute of Health (2011). A timeline of pregnancy testing, In: *NIH*, accessed June 30, 2011, Available from:
<http://history.nih.gov/exhibits/thinblueline/timeline.html>

Network Science. (2011). Drug Development: The Short Story- Attrition Rate, In: *Network Science Corporation*, accessed June 30, 2011, Available from: <http://www.netsci.org/Courseware/Drugs/Intro/slide06.html>

Paxton, A. (2011)PT approach for non-regulated tests sets higher bar, In: *CAP TODAY*, accessed June 30, 2011, Available from: <http://www.cap.org/apps/cap>

Poveda, A, Kaye, SB, McCormack, R, Wang, S, Parekh, T, Ricci, D, Lebedinsky, CA, Tercero, JC, Zintl, P, and Monk, BJ.. (2011). Circulating tumor cells predict progression free survival and overall survival in patients with relapsed/recurrent advanced ovarian cancer. *Gynecol Oncol,* Online print accessed 2011 Jun 26.

Prozialeck, WC, Edwards, JR, Vaidya, VS, and Bonventre ,JV. (2009). Preclinical evaluation of novel urinary biomarkers of cadmium nephrotoxicity. *Toxicol Appl Pharmacol,* 238(3):301-5.

Reagan, WJ. (2010). Troponin as a biomarker of cardiac toxicity: past, present, and future. *Toxicol Pathol,* 38(7):1134-7.

Ridker, PM, Danielson, E, Fonseca, FA, Genest, J, Gotto, AM Jr, Kastelein, JJ, Koenig, W, Libby, P, Lorenzatti, AJ, MacFadyen, JG, Nordestgaard, BG, Shepherd, J, Willerson, JT, and Glynn, RJ. (2008). Rosuvastatin to prevent vascular events in men and women with elevated C-reactive protein. *N Engl J Med,* 359(21):2195-207.

Roche. (2010). Herceptin Media Release, In: *Roche*, accessed Jul 5, 2011, Available from: <http://www.roche.com/med-cor-2010-01-28>

Subramaniam, A, Corallo, C, and Nagappan, R. (2010). Dapsone-associated methaemoglobinaemia in patients with a haematologic malignancy. *Anaesth Intensive Care,* 38(6):1070-6.

Temple, RJ. (2009). FDA Perspective on the Use of Biomarkers. CMOD BM & SE SymposiumOctober 20, 2009, In: *FDA*, accessed 2011 June 26, Available from: <http://www.cmod.org/assets/2009_Secure_Files/Oct_2009/16%20CMOD%20Oct%202009%20Temple.pdf>

Tonomura, Y, Tsuchiya, N, Torii, M, and Uehara, T. (2010). Evaluation of the usefulness of urinary biomarkers for nephrotoxicity in rats. *Toxicology,* 273(1-3):53-9.

Tucker, GT, Silas, JH, Iyun, AO, Lennard, MS, and Smith, AJ. (1977). Polymorphic hydroxylation of debrisoquine in man. *Lance,* 2:718.

Vaidya, VS, Ford, GM, Waikar, SS, Wang, Y, Clement, MB, Ramirez, V, Glaab, WE, Troth, SP, Sistare, FD, Prozialeck, WC, Edwards, JR, Bobadilla, NA, Mefferd, SC, and Bonventre, JV. (2009). A rapid urine test for early detection of kidney injury. *Kidney Int,* 76(1):108-14.

van Gool, AJ, Henry, B, and Sprengers, ED. (2010). From biomarker strategies to biomarker activities and back. *Drug Discov Today,* 15(3-4):121-6.

van Timmerem, MM, van den Heuvel, MC, Bailly, V, Bakker, SJL, van Gor, H, and Stegeman, CA. (2007). Serum cystatin C is superior to serum creatinine as a marker of kidney function: A meta-analysis. *J pathol,* 212(2):209-217.

Walker, I and Newell, H. (2009). Do molecularly targeted agents in oncology have reduced attrition rates? *Nat Rev Drug Discovery,* 8:15-16.

Whelton, A, Watson, AJ, and Rock, RC. (1994). *Tietz Textbook of Clinical Chemistry* (Second Edition), W.B. Saunders, Philadelphia.

Winsten, S. (1969). The skeptical chemist. *Clin Chem,* 15:737-744.

Woodcock, J. (2011). Biomarkers: Physiological & Laboratory Markers of Drug Effect, In: FDA, accessed June 26, 2011, Available from: < http://www.cc.nih.gov/training/training/principles/slides/Biomarkers-2010-2011-3slides.pdf>

Part 4

Drug Delivery

19

Nanotechnology Based Targeted Drug Delivery: Current Status and Future Prospects for Drug Development

Sadhna Sharma and Amandeep Singh
Department of Biochemistry,
Postgraduate Institute of Medical Education and Research, Chandigarh,
India

1. Introduction

Nanotechnology mediated delivery of therapeutic agents is one of the rapidly emerging fields today that has gained significant commercial and academic attention. It is a promising approach to alleviate the drawbacks of conventional therapy and major limitations associated with drug development like poor water solubility, low bioavailability, drug toxicity etc. Nano-scale drug-delivery systems can be devised to tune and regulate release pharmacokinetics, pharmacodynamics, solubility, immunocompatibility, cellular uptake, biodistribution and to minimize toxic side effects, thus enhancing therapeutic index of traditional pharmaceuticals (Emerich & Thanos, 2007). They can be used to deliver both small-molecule drugs and various classes of biomacromolecules such as peptides, proteins, plasmid DNA and synthetic oligodeoxynucleotides. Nanoparticle mediated drug delivery, thus has the potential to contribute significantly in the drug development process which has relied on conventional formulation strategies that are often inadequate. An underlying concept in drug development process is to establish a link between in vitro potency, physicochemical properties and absorption, distribution, metabolism, excretion and toxicity characteristics of a drug candidate which is often cited as a major contributing factor in the failure of drug development. While the nanoparticle mediated sustained release of drugs offers an obvious therapeutic advantage, the targeted delivery of drugs in the body is required to prevent the release of therapeutics at non-specific sites and unwanted side-effects. The conjugation of targeting moieties with drug-loaded nanoparticles can be used for receptor-mediated and targeted delivery. Such targeted nanoparticles have the characteristics of a perfect drug delivery system that tends to maximize the therapeutic activity while minimizing the toxic side effects of drugs.

2. Nanotechnology mediated drug delivery systems

Drug delivery systems are defined as supramolecular assemblies incorporating agents intended to treat a disease. They are intended to overcome the shortcomings of the conventional drugs, such as unfavorable pharmacokinetics, poor solubility, instability, high toxicity, drug resistance and low cellular uptake. Since the discovery of liposomes (Bangham &

Horne, 1964), there has been extensive research towards the development of new drug delivery systems. Liposomes and emulsions dominated the drug delivery field for some period. With the renewed interest in nanotechnology, new nano-sized formulations and nanomaterials have been developed. These new materials include polymeric nanoparticles, solid lipid nanoparticles, liposomes, nanoemulsions, cyclodextrins and dendrimers.

Polymeric nanoparticles: Nanoparticles are solid, colloidal particles consisting of macromolecular substances varying in size from 10 to 1000 nanometers. A drug can be dissolved, entrapped, adsorbed, attached or encapsulated into a nanoparticle. Depending on the method of preparation, nanospheres or nanocapsules can be developed with different properties and different release characteristics for the encapsulated therapeutic agent. For nearly three decades, polymeric nanoparticles have been studied extensively because of their unique and valuable physicochemical and biological properties. Indeed, nanoparticles can protect the drug from degradation (physical stability during storage and in biological fluids), enhance its transport and distribution (possibility of drug targeting by modification of surface charge with inserted ligands, such as antibodies, surfactants, polymers and others) and prolong its release; hence, the plasma half-life of the drug entrapped can be improved (Allemann et al., 1993). As some nanoparticle characteristics such as particle size and surface charge can be modulated by modifying some process parameters, they can be used in various applications involving different routes of administration. Although polymers are the most widely used materials nanoparticles consist of a variety of materials, including polymers, proteins and lipids. The polymers used include natural and synthetic materials and the main characteristics required are biodegradability and biocompatibility. In general, synthetic polymers (polyesters and their copolymers polyacrylates and polycaprolactones) offer greater advantages than natural ones (albumin, gelatin, alginate, collagen and chitosan) because they can be tailored to have a wider range of properties. The advantage of using polymeric nanoparticles as colloidal carriers for advanced drug delivery is mainly their small size, which allows nanoparticles to penetrate even small capillaries and be taken up within cells, allowing efficient drug accumulation at targeted sites in the body. Also, the biodegradable polymers used for their preparation allow for sustained drug release at the targeted site over a period of days or even weeks after administration (Vinogradov et al., 2002). Biodegradable polymer nanoparticles have been extensively investigated as therapeutic carriers (Moghimi et al., 2001). Polymeric nanoparticles have been formulated to encapsulate either hydrophilic or hydrophobic small drug molecules, as well as macromolecules such as proteins and nucleic acids (Perez et al., 2001). The release of encapsulated drugs occurs at a controlled rate in a time or environment dependent manner. More importantly, the rate of drug release can be controlled by modification of the polymer side chain, development of novel polymers or synthesis of copolymers (Wang et al., 2008). In general, these biodegradable polymer systems can provide drug levels at an optimum range over a longer period of time than other drug delivery methods, thus increasing the efficacy of the drug and maximizing patient compliance, while enhancing the ability to use highly toxic, poorly soluble or relatively unstable drugs. Poly(d,l-lactic acid), poly(d,l-glycolic acid), poly(ε-caprolactone) and their copolymers at various molar ratios diblocked or multiblocked with polyethylene glycol (PEG) are the most commonly used biodegradable polymers (Wang et al., 2008). For instance, poly lactide-co-glycolide (PLGA) encapsulated antibiotics have been investigated for the treatment of tuberculosis using murine models (Pandey & Khuller, 2006). Nanoparticles being compact are well suited to traverse cellular membranes to mediate drug or gene delivery. It is also expected that due to small size and high surface/volume ratio, nanoparticles will be less susceptible to reticuloendothelial system clearance and will have better penetration into tissues and cells, when used in vivo (Nimesh et al., 2006). Thus, PLGA has generated tremendous interest due to its excellent biocompatibility, biodegradability, and mechanical strength.

Solid Lipid Nanoparticles: Solid lipid nanoparticles (SLNs) are nanocrystalline structures made of fatty acids that are solid or semisolid at room temperature (Jenning et al., 2002). A wide variety of high melting-point lipids and methods can be used to prepare and stabilize the SLNs (Muller et al., 2000). Besides, their surface characteristics can be altered by coating with hydrophilic molecules which tends to improve plasma stability, biodistribution and subsequent bioavailability of drugs entrapped (Uner & Yener, 2007). Sustained drug release and site specificity for drug delivery can be achieved by altering the properties of SLNs, such as their lipid composition, size, and surface charge. SLNs offer several advantages such as relative ease of production, sterilization, and scale-up, without the use of organic solvents, low-cost excipients, and biocompatibility. As compared to nanoemulsions which are liquid-lipid encapsulations of the drug, SLNs containing the lipid in the solid state impart greater drug stability and better control over drug-release kinetics (Mallipeddi & Rohan, 2010).

Liposomes: Liposomes are lipid vesicles consisting of phospholipid bilayers. They are spherical vesicles that contain a bilayered membrane structure composed of natural or synthetic amphiphilic lipid molecules (Zhang & Granick, 2006; Torchilin, 2005). Their biocompatible and biodegradable composition, as well as their unique ability to encapsulate both hydrophilic and hydrophobic therapeutic agents, makes liposomes excellent therapeutic carriers. They have an aqueous core which can be used to encapsulate hydrophilic drugs while hydrophobic and amphiphilic drugs can be solubilized within the phospholipid bilayers. Liposomes are of three types, i.e. small unilamellar vesicles, large unilamellar vesicles, and multilamellar vesicles. Liposomes in their native form are taken up by the reticuloendothelial system and are quickly cleared from the circulation. This property has been exploited for the macrophage delivery of antiretrovirals. Since liposomes are typically constructed from naturally occurring phospholipids, they tend to pose a lower risk of eliciting unwanted toxic or antigenic reactions when used as drug carriers. Liposomes can also be coated with biocompatible moieties such as PEG to prolong their circulation half-life (Torchilin, 2005). The polymer coating of the liposomes can also be engineered to carry a functional group, which can be used for targeting ligand conjugation. Liposomes have been used widely as pharmaceutical carriers in the past decade, with 11 formulations approved for clinical use and many more in clinical development. Some of the commonly used therapeutics include liposomal amphotericin, liposomal doxorubicin and liposomal daunorubicin (Wang et al., 2008).

Dendrimers: Dendrimers are a versatile class of regularly-branched macromolecules with unique structural and topologic features that are 2.5 - 10 nm in size (Svenson & Tomalia, 2005). They consist of repeatedly branched polymeric macromolecules with numerous arms extending from a center, resulting in a nearly-perfect three-dimensional geometric pattern. Small size, narrow molecular weight distribution, and relative ease of incorporation of targeting ligands make them attractive candidates for drug delivery. Dendrimers have minimal polydispersity and high functionality. Similar to polymers, they are obtained by attaching several monomeric units, but unlike the conventional polymers, they have a highly branched three-dimensional architecture. Dendrimers are characterized by the presence of three different topologic sites, i.e., a polyfunctional core, interior layers, and multivalent surface (du Toit et al., 2010). The polyfunctional core, surrounded by extensive branching has the ability to encapsulate several chemical moieties. The core may be surrounded by several layers of highly branched repeating units such as polyethers, porphyrins, polyamidoamines, polyphenyls, and polyamino acids. The properties of the dendrimers are predominantly based on the multivalent surface, which has several functional groups that interact with the external environment. The precise physicochemical properties of dendrimers can be controlled during synthesis by controlling the core groups, the extent of branching, and the nature and/or number of functional groups on the surface (Svenson & Tomalia, 2005). They are synthesized from either synthetic or natural building blocks such as amino acids, sugars and nucleotides. Their characteristics as carriers of therapeutics include nanoscale spherical architecture, narrow polydispersity, multifunctional surface chemistry and large surface area. Many dendrimer families have been reported (Bosman et al., 1999) and amongst them, polyamidoamine (PAMAM) and poly(propylenemine) (PPI) families have been most widely used for biomedical applications. The specific molecular structure of dendrimers enables them to carry various drugs through their multivalent surfaces by covalent conjugation or electrostatic adsorption. Alternatively, dendrimers can be loaded with drugs, by using the cavities in their cores through hydrophobic interaction, hydrogen bonding or chemical linkage. Their surface can be engineered to provide precise spacing of surface molecules and to conjugate targeting molecules. Other remarkable properties of dendrimers include the availability of terminal surface groups which can be customized for bioconjugation of drugs, signaling groups or targeting moieties. They possess unique surfaces that may be designed with functional groups to augment or resist trans-cellular, epithelial or vascular biopermeability. Their surface groups can be modified to optimize biodistribution receptor mediated targeting, therapy dosage or controlled release of drug from the interior space (Tomalia et al., 2007)

3. Nanotechnology and cancer

3.1 Limitations of the current chemotherapeutic agents

Cancer is one of the leading causes of morbidity and mortality globally (World Health Organization, 2009). The conventional treatments for cancer include the use of chemotherapeutic drugs, radiotherapy and interventional surgery. Breast cancer is the most common type of malignancy diagnosed in women and almost one third of all cancers diagnosed in women are breast cancer (Jemal et al., 2008). The main objectives of the treatment strategies are to prolong the survival and improve the quality of life. Despite availability of few new drugs (Newman & Singletary,2007; Guarneri & Conte, 2004), breast cancer treatment is still unsatisfactory. Amongst active drugs, Taxanes (paclitaxel and docetaxel) (Miele et al., 2009) have proved to be fundamental in the treatment of advanced and early-stage breast cancer. Paclitaxel has demonstrated significant antitumor activity in clinical trials against a broad range of cancers (Singla et al., 2002). These drugs, however, do have a few limitations. The main limitation is their highly hydrophobic nature. Owing to this, lipid-based solvents (mixture of Cremophor and ethanol) or surfactants like polysorbate 80 (Tween® 80) are used as a vehicle for taxanes. Cremophor EL® (CrEL) is a non-ionic surfactant polyoxyethylated castor oil (Rowinsky et al., 1990). Polyoxyethylated castor oil is toxic itself as it can leach plasticizers from standard intravenous tubing releasing di (2-ethylhexyl) phthalate (DEHP). It stimulates the release of histamine with consequent well-described hypersensitivity reactions, including anaphylaxis in patients (Rowinsky & Donehower, 1995). Besides, intravenous administration of the current Cremophor EL-based formulation in a non-aqueous vehicle may lead to some serious side effects in some patients such as hypersensitivity, neurotoxicity, nephrotoxicity & hyperlipidemia (Gelderblom et al., 2001). Polysorbate 80 is also associated with hypersensitivity reactions, although less frequently than CrEL. Polysorbate 80 may cause irreversible sensory and motor neuropathies and may alter the membrane fluidity (Vaishampayan et al., 2001). More importantly, CrEL and polysorbate 80 may limit tumor penetration as polar micelles of CrEL-paclitaxel in the plasma compartment entraps the drug and can lead to non-linear pharmacokinetics due to decreased drug clearance as well as volume of distribution. Most of other current chemotherapeutic agents in the market are low molecular weight agents with high pharmacokinetic volume of distribution both of which may contribute to their cytotoxicity. Because of their low molecular weight, they are readily excreted from the body, hence requiring a higher concentration that may be toxic. The most important fact is that most of these drugs lack specificity and cause significant damage to normal tissues, eventually leading to serious unwanted side effects such as bone marrow suppression, alopecia, and the sloughing of the gut epithelial cells (Lou & Prestwich, 2002). The use of nanocarriers can help alleviate these problems and allow for the preparation of low water soluble cancer medications. The nanoscale dimension of these carriers enables the drug to accumulate in the tumor mass by passively crossing fenestrations in the diseased vasculature and avoiding the perfusion of normal tissues. These nanoparticles have the potential to cross the inter-endothelial junctions and diffuse within the extravascular compartment, addressing all the possible therapies in a more specific manner. In addition, such carriers can be optimized and modified to target the tumor cells particularly. This helps to deliver the drug specifically to neoplastic tissues, sparing the normal ones, thereby reducing systemic toxicity. The modifications include chemical binding of specific moieties or ligands on these nanocarriers. Tumor-specific high affinity ligand like folate (Farokhzad et al., 2006) enhance the interaction of nanoparticles with tumor cells, greatly improving biodistribution and bioavailability of the concerned drug. Perhaps the most important and vast utilization of nanotechnology mediated drug delivery has been in cancer chemotherapy and presently, approximately 150 drugs in development for cancer treatment are based on nanotechnology (Jain, 2010).

3.2 Nanodrug delivery systems for anti-cancer agents

A large number of researchers have used different approaches and techniques for formulating nanoparticles for anti-cancer agents. Some of these studies along with their prominent findings are mentioned here. Paclitaxel has been the focus of many drug delivery approaches to alleviate the side effects of its conventional formulation. Several approaches have been employed till date, and one of the most successful of them is Albumin-bound paclitaxel (ABI-007, Abraxane®; Abraxis BioScience and AstraZeneca). Albumin has a number of biological characteristics that make it an attractive drug vehicle in oncology. It is a natural carrier of endogenous hydrophobic molecules such as vitamins, hormones and other water-insoluble plasma substances (Hawkins et al., 2008). Moreover, albumin seems to help endothelial transcytosis of protein-bound and unbound plasma constituents through binding to a cell-surface (John et al., 2003; Minshall et al., 2003). Besides, osteonectin, also known as secreted protein acid rich in cysteine (SPARC) has been shown to bind albumin because of a sequence homology with gp60. SPARC, as caveolin-1, is often present in some neoplasms (breast, lung, and prostate cancer), leading to the accumulation of albumin in some tumors and thus facilitating intra-tumor accumulation of albumin-bound drugs (Hawkins et al., 2008). Albumin-bound paclitaxel ABI-007 is a nanovector application for breast cancer. It represents one of the strategies developed to overcome the solvent-related problems of paclitaxel and it has been recently approved by the US Food and Drug (FDA) Administration for pre-treated metastatic breast cancer patients. ABI-007 is a novel, albumin-bound, 130-nm particle formulation of paclitaxel, free from any kind of solvent (Miele et al., 2009). It is used as a colloidal suspension derived from the lyophilized formulation of paclitaxel and human serum albumin diluted in saline. Albumin tends to stabilize the drug particle and prevents any risk of capillary obstruction and does not require any specific infusion systems or steroid/antihistamine premedication before the infusion (Desai et al., 2006). Preclinical studies, conducted in athymic mice with human breast cancer demonstrated that ABI-007 has a higher penetration into tumor cells with an increased anti-tumor activity, compared with an equal dose of standard paclitaxel (Desai et al., 2006). A phase I clinical trial on patients with solid tumors and breast cancer showed a maximum tolerated dose of ABI-007 about 70% higher than that of CrEL paclitaxel formulation. ABI-007 was administered intravenously with no premedication, in shorter infusion periods and with a standard infusion device. The toxicities observed were sensory neuropathy, stomatitis, and ocular toxicity. None of the patients experienced hypersensitivity reactions. Moreover, the pharmacokinetic parameters showed a linear trend (Ibrahim et al., 2002). A consequent phase II trial confirmed that ABI-007 has significant antitumor activity in patients with metastatic breast cancer, with a good overall response rate and less side effects (Ibrahim, 2005). A micellar nanoparticle formulation of paclitaxel (NK105) was also developed to reduce its toxicity and increase the antitumor activity of paclitaxel (Hamaguchi et al., 2005). Paclitaxel was incorporated into the inner core of the micelle system by physical entrapment through hydrophobic interactions between the drug and the block copolymers for paclitaxel. When compared to free paclitaxel, NK105 increased plasma AUC by approximately 90-fold together with a 25-fold higher tumor AUC. NK105 showed potent antitumor activity against a human colorectal cancer cell line HT-29 xenograft compared with paclitaxel owing to its enhanced accumulation in the tumor and its sustained release from micellar nanoparticles. Neurotoxicity was significantly decreased with NK105 as evidenced by both histopathological and physiological assessments. Although these current vehicles employed hold promise to replace the Cremophor EL-based vehicle for paclitaxel delivery, their role to overcome multi-drug resitance (MDR) of tumor cells to paclitaxel still remains unsolved. Therefore, another challenge is to develop a new delivery system that consists of aqueous-based vehicles and possesses ability to overcome the MDR of tumor cells for paclitaxel delivery. Poly(ethylene glycol)-block-poly(propylene glycol)-block-poly(ethylene glycol) (PEO-block-PPO-block-PEO) micelles have been commonly used for solubilization of hydrophobic drugs (Kabanov et al., 2002). It is found that Pluronics could interact with MDR cancer cells resulting in drastic sensitization of these tumors with respect to doxorubicin and other anticancer agents (Minko et al., 2005). In addition, inclusion of paclitaxel in liposomal formulations (LEP-ETU) has proved to be a good approach to improve the drug's antitumor efficacy (Zhang et al., 2005). Endostatin, a

20 kDa internal fragment of the carboxy terminus of collagen XVIII, has the potential to inhibit the growth of a variety of human tumors by inhibiting neovascularization (Zhuo et al., 2010). However, most available endostatins are either unstable or expensive, which limits their clinical application. Endostar, a novel recombinant human endostatin, has been expressed and purified in *E.coli*. It has been approved by the Chinese State Food and Drug Administration for the treatment of non-small cell lung cancer in 2005 and has a broad spectrum of activity against solid tumors. Endostar has been shown to inhibit endothelial cell proliferation, migration, and vessel formation (Zhuo et al., 2010). Nanoparticles containing endostar were formulated from modified (PEG-PLGA) and they could maintain adequate concentrations of endostar in plasma and tumor, thereby improving its antitumor effect. Compared with endostar, endostar-loaded PEG-PLGA nanoparticles had a longer elimination half-life and lower peak concentration, caused slower growth of tumor cell xenografts, and prolonged tumor doubling time. The nanoparticles changed the pharmacokinetic characteristics of endostar in mice and rabbits, thereby enhancing anticancer activity. Endostar-loaded PEG-PLGA nanoparticles were observed to have a better anticancer effect than conventional endostar (Sanyuan et al., 2010). CPX-1 is another novel liposome-encapsulated formulation of irinotecan and floxuridine designed to prolong in vitro optimized synergistic molar ratios of both drugs following infusion. Phase I studies in patients with advanced solid tumors showed that CPX-1 was well tolerated, and had significant antitumor activity (Batist et al., 2009). MCC-465 is an immunoliposome-encapsulated doxorubicin which is tagged with polyethylene glycol (PEG) and the F(ab) fragment of human mAb GAH (goat anti-human), which positively reacts to >90% of cancerous stomach tissues but negatively to all normal tissues. In preclinical studies, MCC-465 showed superior cytotoxic activity against several human stomach cancer cells compared with doxorubicin or doxorubicin- incorporated PEG liposomes. A phase I clinical trial showed that MCC-465 was well tolerated (Matsumura et al., 2004). Polymeric micelles can be utilized to increase the accumulation of drugs in tumor tissues utilizing the enhanced permeability and retention (EPR) effect and to incorporate various kinds of drugs into the inner core by chemical conjugation or physical entrapment with relatively high stability. There are several anticancer drug-incorporated micelle carrier systems under clinical evaluation, these include a CDDP (cisplatin)-incorporated micelle, NC-6004, and Paclitaxel incorporated micelle, NK105 for stomach cancer. Phase I studies of polymer doxorubicin (PK1) showed signs of activity coupled with five-fold decreased anthracycline toxicity in chemotherapy-refractory patients. Phase II studies were conducted using a similar material in patients with breast cancer, non-small cell lung cancer and colorectal cancer (Seymour et al., 2009). The results showed an increased efficacy with limited side effects, supporting the concept that polymer-bound drugs can improve anticancer activity. The anti-tumor activity of SP1049C, a novel P-glycoprotein targeting micellar formulation of doxorubicin consisting of doxorubicin and two non-ionic block copolymers, has been evaluated in patients with advanced adenocarcinomas of the esophagus and gastroesophageal junction and showed good tolerability (Valle et al., 2010). These results thus demonstrate superior antitumor activity of SP1049C compared with doxorubicin in a standard formulation. Phase III clinical trials are now in progress (Jain, 2010). In a study, 5-fluorouracil (5-FU) loaded and polyethylene glycol-poly(γ-benzyl-L-glutamate (PEG-PBLG) nanoparticles (5-FU/PEG-PBLG) were formulated. These nanoparticles exhibited favorable pharmacokinetic characteristics, including sustained drug release, prolonged drug half-life, and increased tissue retention. In vivo, 5-FU/PEG-PBLG nanoparticles had good anti-tumor activity against colon cancer xenografts and oral squamous cell carcinoma xenografts. The results

imply that PEG-PBLG nanoparticle delivery system for 5-FU may be able to effectively reduce adverse side effects of 5-FU therapy and improve the therapeutic index of 5-FU (Su et al., 2008).

Dendrimers have been extensively used for delivering anti-cancer drugs. Polyamindoamine (PAMAM) dendrimers have been used to formulate doxorubicin conjugates which led to significantly increased nuclear accumulation of doxorubicin from the PAMAM-hyd-DOX conjugates and thus exhibited higher cytotoxicity to tumor (Kwon, 2003). Polyester-based dendrimer-PEO-doxorubicin conjugate was observed to substantially inhibit the progression of DOX-insensitive C-26 tumor subcutaneously implanted in BALB/c mice. This dendrimer-PEO-doxorubicin conjugate also showed the ability to eliminate the tumors at certain doses and was found to be equally effective to a liposomal formulation of doxorubicin (Martin, 1998). PAMAM dendrimers have also been conjugated to cisplatin to form a fairly water soluble nanoformulation with the ability to release cisplatin slowly in vitro. This formulation showed superior activity over conventional cisplatin when injected intraperitoneally into mice bearing B16F10 tumor cells. Also, when administered intravenously to treat a subcutaneous B16F10 melanoma, the dendrimer-cisplatin displayed additional antitumor activity whereas cisplatin was inactive (Nishiyama & Kataoka, 2006). In another study, dendrimer-based stealth nanoparticles were designed to encapsulate anastrozole, which is a drug used to treat breast cancer after surgery and for metastases in both pre and post-menopausal women. It was demonstrated that stealth nanoparticles composed of a PAMAM dendrimers core and a poly-ethylene glycol (PEG) layer could encapsulate anastrozole, hence causing improved water solubility of anastrozole. A sustained release of anastrozole was achieved, implicating an increased therapeutic index (Sarkar, 2008).

3.3 Tumor-specific targeting with nanocarriers

Tumors have unique features, which make them distinct from normal tissues. These include leaky tumor blood vessels and defective lymphatic drainage, that promote the delivery and retention of particles, a phenomenon recognized as the enhanced permeability and retention (EPR) effect. Nanoformulation can more easily enter and accumulate within tumor cells. This implicates that higher doses of the drug can be delivered, increasing its anticancer effects while decreasing the side effects associated with systematic chemotherapy. However, there are many variable factors, such as clearance of nanoparticles in the circulation by kidneys and uptake by reticuloendothelial cells, that affect the amount of anticancer nanoparticles retained in the tumor. One way to overcome some of these variables is targeted drug delivery. Targeted delivery of therapeutic agents to cancer has important implications for detection, diagnosis and therapy of cancer. Biomarkers that differentiate cancerous tissue from normal tissues can be used as targets for this purpose.

3.4 Ligands employed for tumor-specific targeting

Folate is nonimmunogenic and folate nanoparticles are rapidly internalized by receptor-bearing cancer cells (Sudimack & Lee, 2000) in a manner that bypasses cancer cell multi-drug-efflux pumps (Goren et al.. 2000). The folate receptor is expressed on human ovarian, endometrial, colorectal and lung cancers but is largely absent from normal tissues (Sudimack & Lee 2000). Folate receptor, a cell membrane associated glycosylphosphatidylinositol anchored glycoprotein involved in human growth and development, cell division and DNA synthesis, has been explored to target therapeutics in cancer cells due to its over expression on malignant cancer cells. Binding of folic acid to folate receptor (FR-α and FR-β) initiates receptor-mediated endocytosis and internalization of folic acid. Most human tissues lack the folate receptor, except the placenta, choroids plexus, lungs, and kidneys; however, cellular activation and proliferation leads to over expression of high-affinity folate receptors in many cancers. Thus, folate-mediated targeting has been used to deliver protein toxins, low-molecular weight chemotherapeutic agents, liposomes containing chemotherapeutic drugs and immunotherapeutic agents to cancer cells (Xiang, 2008). Many studies have been carried out to prove the enhancement of anticancer activity via folate mediated targeting. Folate-conjugated nanoparticles have been used on human cervical carcinoma cells and found no cellular uptake of folate-conjugated nanoparticles in A549 cells which lacks folate receptor (Zhang, 2010). It was demonstrated that uptake of folic acid conjugated doxorubicin by HeLa cells showed greater cytotoxicity compared to non-folate-mediated nanoparticles (Zhang, 2010). Another characterized ligand to be exploited for targeting tumor cells is transferrin which plays an essential role in iron homeostasis and cell growth. Inherent characteristic of some cancer cells is over expression of transferrin receptor. However, high expression of transferrin receptor is seen in hypothalamus and medulla oblongata compared to other parts of brain and many in vivo studies showed that transferrin increases brain delivery of nanoparticles (Hänninen et al., 2009). Uptake of transferrin into cells is mediated by transferrin receptors which are cell membrane associated glycoproteins. Binding of transferrin to transferrin receptor initiates receptor mediated endocytosis and internalization of transferrin. Whereas in presence of inhibitors, transferrin mediated nanoparticles interact with the cells in a specific manner and enter the cells via the caveolae pathway (Chang et al., 2009). Many studies have been carried out to prove the enhancement of anticancer activity via transferrin mediated targeting. The anticancer activity of transferrin conjugated solid lipid nanoparticles of curcumin on MCF-7 breast cancer cells has also been studied and results showed that the cell uptake and cytotoxicity increased considerably with transferrin conjugated solid lipid nanoparticles compared to curcumin solution. Transferrin conjugated nanoparticles enhance the antitumor activity via active target mechanism and also contributes to the photo stability and sustain release of drug (Mulik, 2010).

Another attractive molecular target is vasoactive intestinal peptide receptors (VIP-R). In vitro studies using human breast cancer tissues and cells have shown the presence of high densities of VIP receptors, with high affinity and specificity for VIP. It is well known that angiogenesis is vital for tumor growth (Naumov et al., 2006).Studies in breast cancer patients have showed that angiogenesis positively correlates with the degree of metastasis, tumor recurrence and shorter survival rates, thus demonstrating the value of angiogenesis as a prognostic cancer marker (Weidner et al., 1992; Weidner et al., 1992). There is an up regulation of angiogenic cytokines and growth factors, most notably the vascular endothelial cell growth factor (VEGF) and angiopoietin (Ang) families, as well as integrins (Desgrosellier & Cheresh, 2010). It is hence not surprising that these molecules are often targeted in both experimental and clinical cancer settings. Development of anti-angiogenesis therapy is based on either drugs that prevent the formation of new blood vessels supplying to the tumor (e.g. TNP-470, endostatin, angiostatin), or drugs that damage existing blood vessels (e.g. combretastatin) (Folkman, 2003). Specifically targeting tumor vasculature significantly lowers the side effects associated with the drug. It has been shown that polymer-conjugated angiogenesis inhibitor TNP-470 (caplostatin) accumulates selectively in the tumor vessels by the EPR effect and inhibits hyperpermeability of tumor blood vessels (Satchi-Fainero et al., 2005; Satchi-Fainero et al., 2004). Nanoparticle-conjugated chemotherapeutic agents such as doxorubicin (Chaudhuri et al., 2010) and angiogenic small molecule inhibitors (Harfouche et al., 2009) can preferentially home into tumors by the EPR effect, resulting in selective vascular shutdown and inhibition of tumor growth. It should be noted that EPR alone is not always sufficient in targeting the tumor sites and hence is often used in conjunction with active targeting. This combination ensures that nanoparticles are retained in the tumor tissues following their extravasation from leaky vessels. Active targeting of tumor tissues is achieved by chemically arraying ligands on the surface of nanoparticles that can recognize and selectively bind to receptors specifically expressed on tumor cells and vessels. The high surface area to volume ratio of the nanoparticles leads to high local density of ligands for targeting. Nanoparticle mediated active targeting of the tumor vasculature in anti-angiogenic therapy has been achieved by targeting the VEGF receptors (VEGFRs), avb3 integrins, and other angiogenic factors. Integrin avb3 has been the most widely used targeting moiety on nanovectors due to its pleitropic up regulation in a variety of tumors (Anderson et al., 2000; Park et al., 2004), some of which have been successfully translated into several clinical trials (Desgrosellier & Cheresh, 2010). Tumor-homing peptides have been used to target abraxane, a clinically approved paclitaxel-albumin nanoparticle to tumors in mice. The targeting was accomplished with two peptides, CREKA, and LyP-1 (CGQKRTRGC). LyP-1-abraxane produced a statistically highly significant inhibition of tumor growth compared to untargeted abraxane. CREKA (cysteine-arginine-glutamic acid-lysine-alanine) is a pentapeptide that binds to clotted plasma proteins and homes to tumors because interstitial tissue of tumors (Dvorak et al., 1985) and the vessels wall contain clotted plasma proteins, while the vessels in normal tissues do not. LyP-1 is a cyclic 9-amino-acid peptide (Cys-Gly-Gln-Lys-Arg-Thr-Arg-Gly-Cys) that provided the first demonstration that lymphatic vessels in tumors can differ molecularly from normal lymphatics (Laakkonen et al., 2002). A protein known as p32 or gC1qR receptor (Ghebrehiwet et al., 1992) is the target molecule for the LyP-1 peptide and, in addition to overexpression in tumors, it also exhibits aberrant cell surface expression in tumor lymphatics, tumor cells, and, a subset of myeloid cells which contributes to the tumor specificity of LyP-1 homing (Fogal et al., 2008). The results showed that synthetic particles coated with LyP-1 extravasate and spread into tumor tissue.

Various other polymeric nanoparticles have been used for targeted delivery of cancer therapeutics. PLGA copolymers have been extensively used in the field of cancer research, owing to their biodegradability and bio-compatibility, resulting in their FDA approval. In a study targeting the MAPK signaling pathway, the use of PLGA copolymer for chemically conjugating PD98059, a selective MAPK inhibitor has been reported (Basu et al., 2009). The resulting nanoparticles selectively resulted in melanoma regression in a mouse model. In a novel strategy, temporal targeting of tumor cells and the tumor vasculature was achieved using a nanoscale delivery system that comprised of a core PLGA nanoparticle encapsulated within a (PEG)-linked lipid envelop (Sengupta et al., 2005). PEGylation of a molecule renders the latter non-toxic and non-immunogenic, and is an FDA approved method (Veronese & Pasut, 2005). PLGA nanoparticles have also been utilized for delivering natural products like curcumin, thought to have anti-cancer effects. Curcumin-loaded PLGA nanoparticles were reported to successfully suppress tumor necrosis factor (TNF)-regulated expression of VEGF, culminating in reduced tumor metastasis (Anand et al., 2010). In a study, chitosan nanoparticles have shown significant inhibition of tumor growth and induction of tumor necrosis in a mouse hepatocellular carcinoma xenograft model (Xu et al., 2009). The anti-tumor activity of these nanoparticles was found to be related with their anti-angiogenic activity, which was linked to significant reduction in the levels of VEGFR-2 expression and subsequent blockage of VEGF-induced endothelial cell activation. In a study, doxorubicin-loaded solid lipid nanoparticles on MCF-7/ADR cells (doxorubicin-resistant breast cancer cell line) showed that doxorubicin-loaded solid lipid nanoparticles efficiently enhanced apoptotic cell death through the higher accumulation of doxorubicin in MCF-7/ADR cells in comparison with free doxorubicin (Kang et al., 2010). Doxorubicin, when conjugated with polymeric dextrans of various molecular weights, its cytotoxicity was significantly higher than free doxorubicin when studied on human carcinoma KB-3-1 cells and its multidrug-resistant subclone KB-V-1 cells (Lam et al., 2000). Similarly, it has been demonstrated that paclitaxel nanocrystal formulation using D-α-tocopheryl polyethylene glycol 1000 succinate have significant advantages over Taxol in achieving better therapeutic effect in Taxol-resistant cancer cells both in vitro and in vivo (Liu, 2010).

4. Nanodelivery of therapeutics to central nervous system (CNS)

The blood-brain barrier (BBB) is one of the stringent and efficient barriers present in human body. BBB allows only a restricted exchange of compounds between the plasma and CNS, which include hydrophilic molecules, small proteins, and charged molecules. This barrier consists of a layer of endothelial cells connected by tight junctions, which circumferentially surround the entire cell margin at the brain capillaries (Butte et al., 1990). The luminal blood-brain barrier (BBB) is comprised of tight junction bound endothelia that serve to retard brain entry of most high molecular weight and/or hydrophilic therapeutics. Principal mechanisms involved in limited uptake of drugs by BBB include: a) absence of paracellular openings, b) lack of pinocytocis and c) significant protein mediated efflux. The deficiency in pinocytic vesicles and the high metabolic capacity of cerebral endothelial cells (Reese & Karnovsky, 1967) also contribute to limiting the exchange of anticancer agents between the plasma and the CNS. Furthermore, the cerebral endothelium has a high level of ATP-binding cassette (ABC) transporters such as P-glycoprotein involved in drug efflux mechanisms (Golden & Pollack, 2003). Thus the BBB prevents the uptake of all large-molecule and more than98% of pharmaceutical small-molecule drugs (Pardridge, 2001). Only small (<5000Da), lipid-soluble, electrically neutral molecules and weak bases are able to diffuse passively across the BBB (Abraham et al., 1994). Therefore, significant research is dedicated to develop methods and technologies to circumvent the BBB for brain drug delivery (Smith, 2003).Previous technologies for brain delivery of drugs (i.e. BBB circumvention) includes drug or BBB manipulation. Manipulation of the BBB chiefly consists of temporary disruption of tight junctions to allow paracellular movement of the molecule from plasma to brain. This methodology has indeed proven to be efficacious (Kroll et al., 1998; Remsen et al., 2000), yet there are concerns regarding significant toxicity of free CNS drug (Remsen et al., 1995; Fortin et al., 2000). These physiological characteristics of the BBB hence offer a substantial hinderance for delivery of drugs to the CNS. Theoretically, there are two strategies to overcome this: either the barrier integrity can be altered or drug characteristics can be altered. However, interventional methods do have their drawbacks.
Such non-specific opening of the barrier by either mechanism allows the entry of toxins and unwanted molecules, potentially resulting in significant damage (Greig, 1989). The primary

disadvantage is the requirement of extremely invasive neurosurgery, thus limiting their potential. Besides, diffusion of the drug from the injection site may occur. Owing to such risks associated with altering of the BBB physiology, modifying the drugs or their mode of delivery is a much better option. Nanoparticle mediated drug delivery may be superior to both of these techniques, since no manipulation of the barrier or the drug is necessary. Furthermore, native carriers and receptors expressed at the BBB can be used for targeted delivery. Such native carriers as lipoproteins can deliver hydrophilic and large compounds across the barrier. Nanoparticles may cross the BBB either by passive diffusion or receptor-mediated endocytosis. One significant benefit of tumor therapy with nanoparticles as a drug carrier is the prolong of mean residence time in the body. Whereas this benefit may increase the exposure of the tumor to the chemotherapeutic agent, it also prolongs the exposure of the remainder of the body to the drug potentially increasing toxicity. Using high-affinity ligands for these transporters along with nanoparticles can lead to site-directed delivery of drugs. Increased uptake of polysaccharide nanoparticles cross-linked with phosphate (anionic) and quaternary ammonium (cationic) ligands, with a surrounding lipid bilayer has been demonstrated (Fenart et al., 1999). It was observed that lipid bilayer containing dipalmitoyl phosphatidyl choline and cholesterol coating on the charged nanoparticles leads to a 3–4 fold increase in brain uptake. In addition, the nanoparticles remained intact as they crossed the BBB, without altering BBB integrity at the same time. Another drug, amitriptyline, when adsorbed onto polybutylcyano-acrylate nanoparticles, using polysorbate-80 as a surfactant, led to a 10-fold increase in its levels in brain (Schroder et al., 1998). This was attributed to an increased of the plasma concentration of the drug resulting in a larger gradient at the BBB and thus greater concentrations of the drug entering the brain by passive diffusion (Alyautidin et al., 1995). Cellular endocytosis has been suggested to be the transport mechanism of polybutyl-cyanoacrylate nanoparticles coated with polysorbate-80 across the BBB, when the nanoparticles were not coated with surfactants, the particles remained in the blood vessels (Kreuter et al., 1995).It is postulated that apolipoprotein-E (apo-E) adsorbs onto nanoparticles coated with polysorbates thereby causing endocytosis at the BBB (Kreuter, 2001). A number of studies have been done to improve the brain drug distribution of anesthetic agents such as dalagrin, kytorphin, and the neuromuscular blocking agent tubocurarine. These anesthetics show therapeutic effects only when given directly to the brain, as they do not cross the BBB appreciably from the plasma. Tubocurarine (a myoparalytic, quaternary ammonium compound) when adsorbed onto polybutylcyanoacrylate particles coated with polysorbate-80 was efficiently transported at BBB. Otherwise, Tubocurarine, when given intravenously, is a found in negligible concentrations in the cerebrospinal fluid and does not affect spontaneous and evoked bioelectric activity of the brain. On the other hand, with peripherally administered nanoparticles, seizure electroencephalograph patterns were observed (Alyautdin et al., 1998). In addition, most of the chemotherapeutic drugs used for brain tumours are polar molecules and do not readily penetrate the BBB. This is further complicated by the need to maximize time and exposure concentration of the chemotherapeutic agent to the cancer cells. However, when these two factors are maximized to provide therapeutic efficacy, plasma concentrations are high, resulting in significant systemic toxicity. Nanoparticles as chemotherapeutic carriers have been studied as a solution to these issues (Lockman, 2002). In the case of brain tumors, however, the proliferation and invasion of tumoral cells generally cause a local disruption of the BBB (Gururangan & Friedman, 2002). Cancer cells produce various mediators such as arachidonic acid, leukotrienes, prostaglandin E and

thromboxane B2, thus increasing the permeability of the capillary endothelium (Wahl et al., 1993). Moreover, the tumor secretes proangiogenic factors including a basic fibroblast growth factor and a vascular endothelial growth factor inducing the formation of new blood vessels in the tumor (Folkman, 1995). These capillaries, characterized by frequent fenestrations, also improve the permeability of the blood–tumor interface and consequently the penetration of drugs. But the disruption of the BBB does not occur in the healthy tissue surrounding the main tumor and thus the desired anticancer agents cannot reach the adjacent tumors located in the normal tissue. The choroid plexus forms a second barrier separating the blood from the cerebrospinal fluid (CSF) (Wolburg et al., 2001). The blood–CSF barrier is functionally and morphologically different from the BBB. The choroid epithelial cells form tight junctions and are responsible for the barrier function. These cells show a low resistance in comparison with the endothelial cells of the BBB (Saito & Wright, 1983). The capillary endothelium in the choroid plexus is fenestrated, allowing the diffusion of small molecules (Pappas & Tennyson, 1962). Despite its permeability the blood–CSF barrier does not significantly increase the penetration of drugs into the brain, its surface being 1000-fold smaller than the surface area of the BBB (Pardridge, 1997). Active targeting of the BBB represents a promising non-invasive strategy for improving drug delivery to brain tumors. It consists in using the various influx transport systems expressed within the cerebral endothelial, including carrier-mediated transport, receptor-mediated endocytosis and adsorptive-mediated endocytosis. These transport systems are usually overexpressed on tumors. More than 20 transporters have been identified, all highly expressed on the cerebral capillaries of the BBB. Amogst them, GLUT1 transporter is of significant importance. It promotes the transport of D-glucose from the blood to the brain and mediates the passage of substances exhibiting similar structures, including 2-deoxyglucose, galactose, mannose, and glucose analogs through the BBB (Pardridge,1995). Its capacity to transport glucose through the BBB is considerably higher than other nutrient transporters (Tsuji, 2005). Besides, the GLUT1 transporter is differentially regulated in human brain tumors, for example it is overexpressed in cerebral hemangioblastoma but under expressed in glioblastoma multiforme (Tsukamoto et al., 1996). Usually the predominant glucose transporter in high-grade gliomas is the GLUT3 isoform, which is also expressed on neurons in the healthy brain (Boado et al., 1994). Thus, considering their affinity for the GLUT1 transporter, mannose derivatives were incorporated on the surface of liposomes. Mannose-liposomes prepared from p-aminophenyl, a mannoside were able to cross the BBB via the glucose transporter, to finally reach the mouse brain (Umezawa & Eto, 1988). The choline transporter consists of an anionic-binding area which interacts with positively charged quaternary ammonium groups or simple cations (Lockman, 2002). It plays a major role in the brain uptake of choline, acting as a precursor for the neurotransmitter acetylcholine and as an essential component of membrane phospholipids (phosphatidylcholine) (Allen & Smith, 2001). Moreover, the choline transporter also interacts with other quaternary ammoniums such as carnitine (Cornford et al., 1978) and thiamine (Kang et al., 1990). No saturation of this carrier was observed under physiological concentration, allowing the transport of other components without affecting the choline delivery to the brain (Allen & Smith, 2001). Besides, the concentration of choline containing components is increased in brain tumors (Tedeschi et al., 1997), suggesting a high choline transport activity in cerebral cancerous cells. The nanoparticles coated with choline were able to cross an in vitro model of the BBB. Their passage through the endothelial cell monolayer was three or four fold higher than that of uncoated nanoparticles, without any modification of paracellular permeability (Fenart et al., 1999). In another instance, nanoparticles were coated with thiamine. Endogenous serum/blood ligands such as insulin and tranferrin have gained much attention (Pardridge, 2002). Folic acid also represents a promising site-specific ligand for brain targeting. The main advantage of these endogenous ligands is their high affinity for both brain and tumoral cells. Moreover, they are biocompatible and non-immunogenic (Vyas & Sihorkar, 2000). Transferrin is a monomeric glycoprotein that can transport one or two iron atoms (Daniels et al., 2006). Transferrin receptor is overexpressed on the brain capillary endothelium (Jefferies et al., 1984) and at the surface of proliferating cells such as brain tumor cells (Hall, 1991). In contrast, a low level of transferrin receptor is observed on normal tissues. However, transferrin receptor can be saturated under physiologic conditions due to a high endogenous plasma concentration of transferrin. The useful properties of transferrin have been exploited for the delivery of various drugs to the brain. Transferrin has been used as an endogenous cellular transport system for the delivery of diphteria toxin (CRM 107) to malignant brain tumors (Laske et al., 1999). Diphtheria toxin conjugated with transferrin produced tumor responses without any systemic toxicity in patients with cerebral tumors refractory to conventional therapy. In another study, beta-endorphin peptides were successfully delivered to the brain after conjugation with cationized albumin (Pardridge et al., 1990). Ligands such as peptidomimetic monoclonal antibodies (MAbs) have been developed, which can bind to the endothelium (Pardridge, 1999). The MAb known as OX26 recognizes an extracellular domain on the transferrin receptor, distinct from the transferrin binding site and thus does not interfere with endogenous transferrin binding. Other studies have shown targeting of OX26 on the brain capillary endothelial cells and its ability to reach the cerebral parenchyma (Pardridge et al., 1991). This antibody has also been used as a neurodiagnostic agent for the early detection of brain cancers (Kurihara & Pardridge, 1999). Transferrin has been coupled to pegylated liposomes and a significant increase of the brain uptake for transferrin-PEG-liposomes in comparison with PEG-liposomes was observed (Hatakeyama et al., 2004). Doxorubicin, an antineoplastic agent, was encapsulated in liposomes coupled to transferrin (Eavarone et al., 2000). In vitro studies revealed a four-fold increase of pegylated transferrin-liposome uptake by glioma cells in comparison with non-targeted liposomes. Transferrin-liposomes used for the delivery of antimetabolic drug 5-fluorouracil (5-FU) to the brain were also investigated (Soni et al., 2005). In vivo experiments revealed that their accumulation was higher than that of non-modified liposomes. The cytotoxicity against cancer cells of doxorubicin packaged within this targeted micellar system was significantly improved (Lai et al., 2005). Folates such as folic acid and 50-methyltetrahydrofolic acid (MTFA) are also transported across the cell membranes (Zhao et al., 1997). The folate receptor is expressed in a limited number of normal tissues such as the thyroid, kidney, choroid plexus (Ross et al., 1994) and the BBB (Wu et al., 1999) It has been identified as a tumor marker due to its overexpression in a large number of tumors such as ovarian carcinomas and brain tumors (Weitman et al., 1992). In addition, immediately after binding with its ligand, the folate receptor is internalized in an early endosome and after a conformational change at acidic pH, the folate molecule is released (Lee et al., 1996). The folate receptor expressed at the BBB has been postulated to mediate the transport of MTFA and folic acid through the BBB (Wu & Pardridge, 1999). Folate-conjugated nanocarriers have been used to selectively target the cells expressing the folate receptor. Enhanced uptake of doxorubicin-loaded folic acid liposomes into C6 glioma has been demonstrated. The amount of doxorubicin internalized into these tumoral cells was sufficient to limit cell growth (Saul et al., 2003). Furthermore, this preferential binding of folic acid-PEG-liposomes was observed through in vitro and in vivo experiments for cancer cells expressing high levels of FR such as murine lung carcinoma, human epidermal carcinoma and lymphoma (Shmeeda et al., 2006). Folate-coupled copolymeric micelles have been widely used for the tumor-specific drug delivery (Nishiyama & Kataoka, 2006). Doxorubicin-loaded folic acid-PEG-PLGA micelles showed a significant accumulation of drugs in the tumor tissue in mice (Yoo & Park, 2004). Paclitaxel-loaded PCL/MPEG micelles decorated with folic acid exhibited a higher cytotoxic effect on cancer cells such as MCF-7 and HeLa cells (Park et al., 2005). Folate targeting was also developed from PEG poly (cyanoacrylate) nanoparticles (Stella et al., 2003). In addition to BBB functional permeation limiting characteristics, brain microvasculature endothelia also presents an electrostatic barrier at physiologic pH. The negative electrostatic charge is created by surface expression and adhesion of the glycocalyx residues: proteoglycans, sulfated mucopolysaccharides, and sulfated and sialic acid-containing glycoproteins and glycolipids (Poduslo & Curran, 1996). This anionic nature of the edndothelium repels anionic molecules (Vorbrodt et al., 1990) and cationic molecules have been shown to occupy anionic areas at the BBB endothelium (Nagy et al., 1983) and increase BBB permeability via presumed tight junction disruption (Hardebo & Kahrstrom, 1985). Transport of cationized albumins and cationized immunoglobulins to the cerebral parenchyma was hence significantly improved in comparison with native proteins (Pardridge et al., 1990). Similar electrostatic interactions between nanoparticles and BBB endothelia have been demonstrated. Cationized NPs have an increased brain distribution compared to anionic and neutral NPs, owing to this interaction (Fenart et al.., 1999). Such cationic NPs have been shown to have immediate toxic effects at brain microvasculature endothelium (Lockman et al., 2004). Anionic sites are located on the luminal surface of brain capillaries due to the sialic acid residues of glycoproteins (Vorbrodt, 1989). The active targeting of drugs has been used for cationized albumin (Pardridge et al., 1987; Kumagai et al., 1987) and evaluated in isolated brain capillaries and in rat brain. In comparison with native protein, it was noted that there was an enhanced uptake of positively charged albumin by the brain capillaries. In vivo studies in rats on cationized albumin transport through the BBB were also carried out (Triguero et al., 1990). About 15% of the cationized protein detected in the whole brain was located in the post-capillary extracellular space. Cationization was shown to improve the accumulation of the protein in brain tissues (Pardridge et al., 1990). Cationized heterologous proteins have more immunogenic properties than homologous proteins (Muckerheide et al., 1987). In another study, it was demonstrated that the beta-endorphin, a non-transportable chimeric peptide, when covalently coupled to cationized albumin was able to reach the cerebral parenchyma (Pardridge et al., 1990). Cationized bovin serum albumin (CBSA) has been conjugated to pegylated liposomes and these liposomes were specifically taken up when in contact with isolated brain capillary endothelial cells (BCEC) and a monolayer of porcine BCEC (Thole et al., 2002). These results showed the ability of CBSA nanoparticles to pass through the BBB to reach the cerebral parenchyma. The coating of nanoparticles using hydrophilic surfactants has proved promising for the delivery of drugs to the brain. However, their targeted effect depends on the chemical structure, physicochemical and biochemical parameters of the surfactant. Only a few polysorbates have been reported to interact with the brain endothelium (Kreuter et al., 1997). Another approach uses the adsorption of plasma proteins such as apolipoproteins (apo) on the surface of coated nanoparticles after intravenous administration. Because apoE is involved in the transport of low-density lipoprotein to the brain nanocarriers coated with polysorbate mimic LDL after apoE adsorption. This protein is expressed at a high level in brain tumors such as astrocytomas and glioblastomas (Murakami et al., 1988). The effects of nanoparticles made of PBCA coated with polysorbates such as polysorbate 80 have been widely investigated (Kreuter et al., 1995). Polysorbate 80-coated PBCA nanoparticles were taken up into human and bovine endothelial cells rapidly and in an amount 20-fold higher than with conventional nanocarriers (Ramge et al., 2000). The pharmacokinetic behavior of doxorubicin packaged within coated PBCA nanoparticles was significantly enhanced after intravenous injection in healthy rats. This formulation allowed a considerable accumulation of the drug in the brain (Gulyaev et al., 1999). The therapeutic potential of doxorubicin-loaded PBCA nanoparticles coated with polysorbate 80 was evaluated for the treatment of glioblastoma intracranially implanted in rats (Steiniger et al., 2004; Gelperina et al., 2002). Antitumor efficiency, based on the increase of the median survival time as compared to doxorubicin, was improved with coated nanoparticles in comparison with uncoated nanocarriers. Coating in a hydrophilic surfactant have been applied to more biocompatible nanocarriers such as lipid colloidal systems for drug delivery to the brain. The SLN surface was coated in various hydrophilic surfactants (Goppert & Muller, 2005) and polysorbate-coated in SLN showed a specific adsorption of plasma proteins such as apoE. Polysorbate 80-coated atovaquone-loaded SLN were used for the treatment of toxoplasmic encephalitis (Scholer et al., 2001). The role of polysorbate 80 in the brain targeting of PLA nanoparticles was also investigated (Sun et al., 2004). In another study, dipalmitoylated apoE-derived peptides, characterized by a high lipid affinity, were anchored on liposomes (Sauer et al., 2006) and taken up within BCEC. Doxorubicin is a polar molecule that does not normally cross the BBB. When doxorubicin adsorbed on polybutylcyanoacrylate nanoparticles with polysorbate-80 as a surfactant was given intravenously, therapeutic concentrations of doxorubicin could be achieved (Gulyaev et al., 1999). Besides, nanoparticles containing doxorubicin administered intravenously to rats led to a significant cure of glioblastomas. Another lipophilic anticancer drug camphotericin when adsorbed on solid lipid nanoparticles led to an increased bioavailability of the drug in brain (Yang et al., 1999). Nanoparticle mediated brain drug delivery has also been used successfully for dalargin (Kreuter et al., 1995), the hydrophilic antitrypanosomal drug diminazene diaceturate (Olbrich et al., 2004) and paclitaxel (Feng et al., 2004; Koziara et al., 2004).

5. Nanotechnology and pulmonary drug-delivery systems

Pulmonary delivery of chemotherapeutic entities is one of the highly desired aspects of drug delivery and the application of polymeric nanoparticles to the pulmonary routes is widely recognized now. The lungs offer a non-invasive route for the delivery of various dugs as they demonstrate relatively high permeability to hydrophilic macromolecules and express relatively low peptidase/protease activity (Wall, 1995). The lungs are an attractive target for drug delivery as they provide high systemic bioavailability, avoid first-pass metabolism, enhance the onset of therapeutic action and provide huge surface area (Yang et al., 2008, Patton & Byron, 2007). It should be noted that if the lungs are to be considered for the systemic delivery, a high percentage of the dose must be delivered to the lungs and the site of deposition should be as peripheral as possible (Colthorpe et al.., 1992). An approach to improve the pulmonary delivery of drugs would be to produce much smaller drug particles, as they offer high penetration and deposition of the aerosol (Burch et al., 1986). Nanocarrier systems in pulmonary drug delivery have the potential to achieve relatively uniform distribution of drug dose among the alveoli. They can also help to achieve enhanced solubility of the drug than its own aqueous solubility while maintaining the sustained-release of drug which consequently reduces the dosing frequency, with improved patient compliance (Bailey & Berkland, 2009). Due to their biocompatibility, surface modification capability and sustained-release properties, polymeric nanoparticles are intensively studied using various important drugs. The pulmonary drugs include anti-asthmatic drugs (Stark et al., 2007), antituberculosis drugs (Pandey et al., 2003; Zahoor et al., 2005), pulmonary hypertension drugs (Kimura, 2009), and anticancer drugs (Azarmi et al., 2006). However, there are some obstacles to the successful delivery of drugs to the lungs. These include degradation by the proteases in the lung, which tends to reduce their overall bioavailability, the limitations posed by barrier between capillary blood and alveolar air that eventually hinders direct exposure of the drugs to lungs. To overcome these limitations, the design (size, shape, and aerodynamic properties) of the dosage forms (nanocarriers) is a rational option. Nanoparticle dispersions consisting of small particles of 10–400 nm diameter show great promise as carriers in pulmonary drug delivery systems. Drugs can be trapped in the core of a micelle and transported at concentrations even greater than their intrinsic water solubility. In addition, a hydrophilic shell can form around the micelle, effectively protecting the contents and it may prevent recognition by the reticuloendothelial system and prevent early elimination from the bloodstream (Smola et al., 2008). Such polymeric micelles are able to evade the mononuclear phagocytic system due to their bulky hydrophilic outer shell and lead to a sustained release of the drug (Marsh et al., 2003). In this direction, beclomethasone dipropionate loaded polymeric micelles were designed which were directly administrable to the lung in nanoparticle sizes in inhalation dosage form intended to be an effective means of treating asthma and chronic pulmonary obstructive disease. Among the various drug delivery approaches for lungs, liposomes are one of the most extensively investigated systems for controlled delivery of drug to the lung (Zeng et al., 1995). Liposomes seem particularly appropriate for delivery of therapeutic agent to lung, as these vesicles can be prepared from compounds endogenous to the lungs such as the components of lung surfactant and these properties make liposomes attractive candidates as drug delivery vehicles (Justo & Moraes, 2003). The first pharmaceutical liposomal products in market include the synthetic lung surfactant Alveofact® for pulmonary instillation for the treatment of respiratory distress syndrome (Muller et al., 2000). Typically, liposomal formulations have been delivered to the lung in the liquid state, and nebulizers have been used extensively for the aerosol delivery of liposomes in the liquid state (Schreier et al., 1993). Liposomal drug formulations for aerosol delivery have their own potential advantages, including aqueous compatibility, sustained pulmonary release to maintain therapeutic drug levels and facilitated intra-cellular delivery particularly to alveolar macrophages (Schreier et al. 1993). Perhaps more importantly, liposomes may prevent local irritation and reduce toxicity both locally and systematically (Gonzalez-Rothi & Schreier 1995). Increased potency with reduced toxicity is characteristic of many drug-liposomal formulations (Cullis et al. 1989). Liposomal aerosols have proven to be non-toxic in acute human and animal studies (Waldrep et al., 1997). These results suggest that drug-liposome aerosols are more effective for delivery, deposition and retention of water-insoluble, hydrophobic, lipophilic compounds in contrast to water soluble compounds (Taylor & Farr, 1993). In another study, non-phospholipid vesicles loaded with beclomethasone dipropionate were fabricated with non-ionic surfactant, polysorbate 20 (Terzano et al., 2005). Levonorgestrel encapsulated liposomes were instilled intratracheally in rats and were compared with the plain drug suspension. The results clearly demonstrated the superiority of pulmonary drug delivery with regards to maintenance of effective therapeutic concentration of the levonorgestrel in the plasma over a longer period and also to reduce frequency of dosing and systemic side effects associated with oral administration of levonorgestrel (Shahiwala & Misra, 2004). Much interest has also been focused on cationic liposomes for pulmonary delivery which have additional advantages like evasion from complement inactivation after in vivo administration (Densmore, 2006). Moreover, liposomes conjugated with cell-penetrating peptides are recognized as potential nanocarrier systems for intracellular delivery of macromolecules to the lung. Liposomes modified with cell-penetrating peptides, antennapedia, the HIV-1 transcriptional activator, and octaarginine have been reported to enhance the cellular uptake of liposomes to airway cells (Cryan et al., 2006). Liposomes of EYPC-cholesterol (CHOL) incorporating dexamethasone palmitate (DEXP) were studied (Benameur et al., 1995), the DEXP incorporated into the liposomes kept its biological activity. It has been shown that a 30 minutes after the instillation the pulmonary concentration of glucocorticoids was twice higher when the drug is encapsulated into liposomes compared to the solubilized drug (Suntres & Shek, 1998). Particles composed of biocompatible and bio-degradable polymers have also been studied for the targeting of drugs by pulmonary route (Zeng et al. 1995; Li et al., 2001). Synthetic polymers are much more frequently used than natural polymers. Solid lipid nanoparticles (SLN) combine the advantages of the biocompatibility of lipids and the possibility of industrial scale up of nanoparticles. The advantages of drug release from SLNs in the lung are controlled drug release profile, a faster in vivo degradation compared to particles made from PLA or PLGA. In addition, SLNs proved to possess a higher tolerability in the lungs compared to particles made from some polymeric materials (Muller et al., 2000) Besides, toxicological profile of SLNs when using physiological lipids, is expected to be better than that of polymer-based systems, because physiological lipids have little or no cytotoxicicity.(Muller et al., 1997) It is feasible that aqueous suspensions and perhaps dry powder formulations of SLN can be used for pulmonary inhalation aerosol administration of drugs using nebulizers and dry powder inhalers (Muller et al., 2000). Several studies have been published on the pulmonary applications of SLNs as local delivery carriers for small molecules (Pandey & Khuller, 2005) or as systemic delivery carriers for macromolecules (Liu et al., 2008). Drugs like prednisolone, diazepam and camptotecin have been incorporated into SLN for pulmonary applications (Muller et al. 2000). Pandey and Khuller studied the chemotherapeutic potential of SLNs incorporating rifampicin, isoniazid and pyrazinamide against experimental tuberculosis and observed the slow and sustained-release of drugs from the SLNs in vitro and in vivo (Pandey & Khuller, 2005). Novel nebulizer-compatible SLNs containing insulin have been examined for pulmonary delivery (Liu, 2008). In this case, SLNs were successful as a pulmonary carrier system for insulin. Deposition and clearance of SLNs after inhalation of aerosolized insoluble particles showed that after deposition, inhaled material began to translocate to regional lymph nodes (Videira et al., 2006) indicating that inhalation can be an effective route to deliver drug-containing lipid particles to the lymphatic systems and lipid particles can be used as potential drug carriers for lung cancer therapy (Videira, 2006). Dendrimers have also been assessed for pulmonary delivery. In a study, low molecular weight heparin (LMWH)–dendrimer complex was formulated using various PAMAM dendrimers, then evaluated for safety and the efficacy in preventing deep vein thrombosis, concluding that cationic dendrimers can be used as pulmonary delivery carriers for a relatively large molecular weight anionic drug (Bai, 2007).

Later, pegylated dendrimers (mPEG-dendrimer) were formulated to increase the pulmonary absorption and circulation time of the drug, with significant positive results showing increased half-life and absorption of the drug. These results also implicated that LMWH loaded in the mPEG-dendrimer could potentially be used as noninvasive delivery system for the treatment of thromboembolic disorder (Bai, 2009). Nanoparticles based on lecithin have also shown promising deposition profile for hydro-fluoroalkanes (HFAs) (Dickinson et al. 2001). Liposomes functionalized with lecithins have shown to improve their binding to human alveolar cells (Abu-Dahab et al., 2001). Pulmospheres™ have been successfully formulated using phospholipids to be dispersed into HFAs and have been demonstrated to release uniform amounts of drugs when aerosolized (Dellamary et al. 2000). Anticancer drug 9-nitrocamptothecin (9NC) has been encapsulated into DLPC-liposomes, which prevented the loss of drug by albumin and the amount of effective 9NC contained in the liposomes was 10–50 times lower than that used by other routes of administration (Knight et al. 2000). The greater therapeutic effectiveness is a result of rapid absorption in the respiratory tract and more specifically, in the pulmonary tissues and penetration into the organ and tumor sites. One of the highly desired objectives of pulmonary drug delivery is the targeted, specific delivery to the alveolar macrophages. Targeting drugs to alveolar macrophages has the distinct advantage of delivering high concentrations of drug to a cell that plays a central role in the progression of disease (tuberculosis) and in immune responses. Microspheres have been shown to target alveolar macrophages without eliciting a pulmonary inflammatory response in vitro (Ng et al. 1998), and were non-toxic. Lectins are non-immunological glycoproteins that have the capacity to recognize and bind to glycoproteins exposed at the epithelial cell surface. Mucoadhesive nanoparticles, coated with mucoadhesive polymers such as poly(acrylic acid) or chitosan demonstrated a slower elimination rate, indicating that chitosan-nanospheres adhere to the mucus in the trachea and in the lung tissues as a result of the mucoadhesive properties of chitosan (Takeuchi et al., 2001). Perhaps the most important application of drug delivery for pulmonary disease has been the chemotherapeutics of tuberculosis. Tuberculosis treatment is lengthy and often leads to poor patient compliance. Poly-lactide-co-glycolide (PLGA), alginate and solid lipid nanoparticles nanoparticles have been successfully used to achieve a significant sustained release in vivo. Not only were the drugs available in the plasma and tissues of experimental animals for a longer time, less frequent dosing with nanoparticle loaded drugs was equally effective as free drugs. These drug loaded nanoparticles were even effective at much lower concentrations than free drugs and were completely non-toxic (Ahmad & Khuller, 2008; Ahmad et al., 2006; Sharma et al., 2004; Ahmad et al., 2007).

6. Nanoparticle mediated antiretroviral therapy

Acquired immunodeficiency syndrome (AIDS) is one of the biggest global threats today. Despite standard therapy, the disease is still far from being under control. The current clinical therapy, known as 'highly active antiretroviral treatment' (HAART), has made significant contribution towards reducing mortality (Richman et al., 2009). HAART, however, is not as effective, owing to a few drawbacks. First and foremost, these drugs are unable to eliminate human immunodeficiency virus (HIV) from resting CD4+T cells in the blood (Chun et al., 2007). Most of the drugs under HAART have various limitations. Didanosine has poor stability in the gastric environment and low bioavailability owing to hepatic first pass. Zidovudine has a short half-life, variable bioavailability and hematological toxicity. Tenofovir can cause renal toxicity, including acute renal failure, Fanconi syndrome and proteinuria (Cihlar & Ray, 2010). Efavirenz has a very low solubility, low absorption and limited biodistribution. Etravirine also has low solubility (Sosnik et al., 2009). The protease inhibitors (saquinavir, indinavir, ritonavir, lopinavir, nelfinavir, amprenavir, fosamprenavir, atazanavir, tipranavir and darunavir) too have a poor oral bioavailability (Hochman, 2000) and limited penetration into the lymphatic system and CNS (Li & Chan, 1999). In addition, other associated problems such as adverse drug effects, poor drug regimen compliance and drug interactions are associated with antiretroviral therapy (Richman et al., 2009). Nanotechnology based drug delivery has the potential to overcome nearly all of the shortcomings mentioned above. Nanoparticles can provide a target specific and sustained release of these drugs, thus improving their bioavailabilty and associated side effects. In this direction, poly (isohexyl cyanate) nanoparticles of zidovudine have been synthesized for targeting the lymphoid tissue in the gastrointestinal tract. Use of this carrier system, when compared with aqueous drug solution resulted in higher of the drug levels in the Peyer's patches. In another study, polyhexylcyanoacrylate nanoparticles were employed for the delivery of zidovudine (Lobenberg et al., 1998), thus improving its bioavailability. In a distinct experiment, PLGA nanoparticles containing multiple antiretroviral drugs, i.e ritonavir, lopinavir, and efavirenz were formulated and results showed that drugs could be detected in peripheral blood mononuclear cells in vitro for 28 days (Destache et al., 2009). In a study with zidovudine-loaded poly(isohexyl cyanate) nanoparticles, zidovudine was accumulated in the cells of the reticuloendothelial system (Lobenberg et al., 1998). Poly(epsilon-caprolactone) nanoparticles loaded with saquinavir were also successfully used for targeting the phagocytic mononuclear system by modifying the surface of the nanoparticles (Shah & Amiji, 2006). Results showed that the intracellular drug concentrations were found to be higher with encapsulated saquinavir compared with free drug solution. In separate experiments, stavudine, zidovudine and lamivudine have been entrapped in polybutylcyanoacrylate (PBCA) and methylmethacrylate-sulfopropylmethacrylate (MMA-SPM) nanoparticles for brain targeting. The permeability of zidovudine and lamivudine was 8–20 fold higher and 10–18 fold higher, respectively, with PBCA nanoparticles and MMA-SPM nanoparticles led to a 2-fold increase in the BBB permeability of both drugs (Kuo, 2005). In a similar experiment, stavudine, delavirdine, and saquinavir were delivered as PBCA and MMA-SPM nanoparticles and their delivery to the brain was studied. The results showed that the permeability of all three drugs increased about 12–16 fold with PBCA nanoparticles and 3–7-fold with MMA-SPM nanoparticles (Kuo & Su, 2006). Dendrimers have also been used to deliver antiretroviral drugs. Tuftsin-conjugated poly(propyleneimine) dendrimers loadedwith efavirenz was evaluated for targeted delivery to macrophages. These dendrimer formulations showed reduced cytotoxicity compared with nonconjugated poly(propyleneimine) dendrimers in vitro and enhanced cellular uptake by mononuclear phagocytic cells, with greater anti-HIV activity in vitro (Dutta et al., 2008). SLNs have also been used for antiretroviral drugs with success. SLNs loaded with stavudine, delavirdine, and saquinavir have been evaluated for their ability to cross the BBB in vitro using human brain microvascular endothelial cells. The permeability of the drugs was improved 4–11 fold when incorporated into SLNs (Kuo & Su, 2007). Similarly, SLNs incorporating atazanavir with Pluronic F68 as an emulsifier were evaluated. In vitro studies using hCMEC/D3, a human brain microvessel endothelial cell line, showed a higher uptake of the drug when delivered in SLN form, as compared with free atazanavir (Chattopadhyay et al., 2008). Regarding liposomal formulations, stavudine loaded into mannosylated and galactosylated liposomes exhibited greater cellular uptake by cells of the mononuclear phagocytic system and greater accumulation in organs of the reticuloendothelial system as compared with free drug solution or even non-modified liposomes (Garg et al., 2006). PLGA nanoparticles containing ritonavir, lopinavir and efavirenz led to an increased uptake of the drugs by macrophages (Destache et al., 2009). Quite similarly, PHCA nanoparticles containing zidovudine showed a higher drug concentration in the organs of the reticuloendothelial system. An interesting finding was the higher levels of zidovudine in the brain when the nanoparticles were coated with polysorbate 80 (Bender et al., 1994). Further studies evaluated PBCA and MMSPM nanoparticles for brain targeting of zidovudine and lamivudine. The permeability of both the drugs to BBB was found to be significantly increased (Kuo & Chen, 2006). In a similar study, stavudine, delaviridine and saquinavir loaded PBCA and MMSPM nanoparticles coated with PS-80 and SLNs showed a higher drug permeability to brain (Kuo & Su, 2007). In an important finding, researchers observed a significant enhancement of brain localization of zidovudine when it was delivered by transferrin-anchored PEGylated albumin nanoparticles (Mishra et al., 2006). In another study, PLGA nanoparticles loaded ritonavir, lopinavir and efavirenz showed a sustained release for 28 days and anti-HIV inhibition was comparable to that of free drugs. Besides, PPI dendrimer-based nanocontainers have been used for targeting of efavirenz macrophages. The haemolytic activity and cytotoxicity of PPI dendrimer was found to be very high and there was a significant increase in cellular uptake of efavirenz by macrophages (Dutta et al., 2007).

7. Conclusion

Nanotechnology provides a wide range of techniques and strategies that can optimize the delivery of pharmaceutical agents. Nano-carrier mediated delivery offers sustained release of drugs in the body as well as protecting them from premature in-vivo degradation or clearance, subsequently increasing the bioavailability and therapeutic potential. By shielding the drug in nanoparticles, the otherwise toxic effects of the drug can be reduced. Most importantly, site-specific delivery of drugs allows increased local concentrations of the drugs and significantly lowers the undesirable systemic toxicity. Nano-carriers have another unprecedented potential that they can allow for new patent opportunities in the case of dugs with expired patents. Thus, nanotechnology can be applied at all stages of drug development, from formulations for optimal delivery to therapeutic applications in clinical trials.

8. References

Abraham, M.H.; Chadha, H.S. & Mitchell, R.C. (1994). Factors that influence the distribution of solutes between blood and brain, *Journal of Pharmaceutical Sciences,* Vol.83, No.9, pp. 1257–1268

Abu-Dahab, R.; Schäfer, U.F. & Lehr, C.M. (2001). Lectin-functionalized liposomes for pulmonary drug delivery: effect of nebulization on stability and bioadhesion, *European Journal of Pharmaceutical Sciences,* Vol.14, pp. 37–46

Ahmad, Z. & Khuller, G.K. (2008). Alginate-based sustained release drug delivery systems for tuberculosis, *Expert Opinion in Drug Delivery,* Vol.5, No.12, pp. 1323-1334

Ahmad, Z.; Pandey, R.; Sharma. S. & Khuller, G.K. (2006). Alginate nanoparticles as antituberculosis drug carriers: formulation development, pharmacokinetics and therapeutic potential, *Indian Journal of Chest Diseases and Allied Sciences*, Vol.48, No.3, pp. 171-176

Ahmad, Z.; Sharma, S. & Khuller, G.K. (2007). Chemotherapeutic evaluation of alginate nanoparticle-encapsulated azole antifungal and antitubercular drugs against murine tuberculosis, *Nanomedicine,* Vol.3, No.3, pp. 239-243

Allemann, E.; Gurny, R. & Doelker E. (1993). Drug loaded nanoparticles preparation methods and drug targeting issues, *European Journal of Pharmaceutics and Biopharmaceutics*, Vol.39, pp. 173-191

Allen, D.D. & Smith, Q.R. (2001). Characterization of the blood–brain barrier choline transporter using the in situ rat brain perfusion technique, *Journal of Neurochemistry,* Vol.76, No.4, pp. 1032–1041

Alyautdin, R.N.; Tezikov, B.E.; Ramge, P.; Kharkevich, D.A.; Begley, D.J. & Kreuter, J. (1998). Significant entry of tubocurarine into the brain of rats by adsorption to polysorbate-80 coated polybutylcyanoacrylate nanoparticles: an in situ brain perfusion study, *Journal of Microencapsulation,* Vol.15, No.1, pp. 67–74

Alyautidin, R.N.; Gother, D. & Petrov, V. (1995). Analgesic activity of the hexapeptide dalagrin adsorbed on the surface of polysorbate-80 coated polybutylcyano-acrylate nanoparticles, *European Journal of Pharmaceutics and Biopharmaceutics,* Vol.41, pp. 44–48

Anand, P.; Nair, H.B.; Sung, B.; Kunnumakkara, A.B.; Yadav, V.R.; Tekmal, R.R. & Aggarwal, B.B. (2010). Design of curcumin-loaded PLGA nanoparticles formulation with enhanced cellular uptake, and increased bioactivity in vitro and superior bioavailability *in vivo, Biochemical Pharmacology,* Vol.79, pp. 330-338

Antohe, F.; Dobrila, L.; Heltianu, C.; Simionescu, N. & Simionescu, M. (1993). Albumin-binding proteins function in the receptor-mediated binding and transcytosis of albumin across cultured endothelial cells, *European Journal of Cell Biology,* Vol.60, pp. 268–275

Antohe, F.; Heltianu, C. & Simionescu, M. (1991). Albumin-binding proteins of endothelial cells: Immunocytochemical detection of the 18 kDa peptide, *European Journal of Cell Biology,* Vol.56, pp. 34–42

Azarmi, S.; Tao, X.; Chen, H.; Wang, Z.; Finlay, W.H.; Löbenberg, R.; Roa, W.H. (2006). Formulation and cytotoxicity of doxorubicin nanoparticles carried by dry powder aerosol particles, *International Journal of Pharmacology,* Vol.319, pp. 155–161

Bai, S. & Ahsan, F. (2009). Synthesis and evaluation of pegylated dendrimeric nanocarrier for pulmonary delivery of low molecular weight heparin, *Pharmaceutical Research,* Vol.26, pp. 539–548

Bai, S.; Thomas, C. & Ahsan, F. (2007). Dendrimers as a carrier for pulmonary delivery of enoxaparin, a low-molecular weight heparin, *Journal of Pharmaceutical Sciences,* Vol.96, pp. 2090–2106

Bailey MM, Berkland CJ. (2009). Nanoparticle formulations in pulmonary drug delivery, *Medicine Research Reviews,* Vol.29, pp. 196–212

Bangham, A.D. & Horne, R.W. (1964). Negative Staining of Phospholipids + Their Structural Modification by-Surface Active Agents as Observed in Electron Microscope, *Journal of Molecular Biology,* Vol.8, pp. 660-668

Basu, S.; Harfouche, R.; Soni, S.; Chimote, G.; Mashelkar, R.A. & Sengupta, S. (2009). Nanoparticle-mediated targeting of MAPK signaling predisposes tumor to chemotherapy, *Proceedings of the National Academy of Sciences USA*, Vol.106, pp. 7957-7961

Batist, G.; Gelmon, K.A.; Chi, K.N.; Miller, W.H. Jr.; Chia, S.K.; Mayer, L.D.; Swenson, C.E.; Janoff, A.S. & Louie, A.C. (2009). Safety, pharmacokinetics, and efficacy of CPX-1 liposome injection in patients with advanced solid tumors, *Clinical Cancer Research*, Vol.15, pp. 692-700

Benameur, H.; Latour, N.; Schandene, L.; Van Vooren, J.P.; Flamion, B.; Legros, F.J. (1995). Liposome-incorporated dexamethasone palmitate inhibits in-vitro lymphocyte response to mitogen, *Journal of Pharmaceutics and Pharmacology*, Vol.47, pp. 812–817

Bender, A.; Schfer, V.; Steffan, A.M.; Royer, C.; Kreuter, J.; Rübsamen-Waigmann, H. & von Briesen, H. (1994). Inhibition of HIV in vitro by antiviral drug-targeting using nanoparticles, *Research Virology*, Vol.145, pp. 215-220

Boado, R.J.; Black, K.L. & Pardridge, W.M. (1994). Gene expression of GLUT3 and GLUT1 glucose transporters in human brain tumors, *Molecular Brain Research*, Vol.27, No.1, pp. 51–57

Bosman, A.W.; Janssen, H.M. & Meijer, E.W. (1999). About dendrimers: Structure, physical properties, and applications, *Chemical Reviews*, Vol.99, No.7, pp. 1665–1688

Burch, W.M.; Sullivan, P.J. & McLaren. C.J. (1986). Technegas - A new ventilation agent for lung scanning, *Nuclear Medicine Communications*, Vol.7, pp. 865-871

Butte, A.M.; Jones, H.C. &Abbot, N.J. (1990). Electrical resistance across the blood-brain barrier in anaesthetized rats: a developmental study, *Journal of Physiology*, Vol.429, pp. 47–62

Chang, J.; Jallouli, Y.; Kroubi, M.; Yuan, X.; Feng, W.; Kang, C.; Pu, P. & Betbeder, D. (2009). Characterization of endocytosis of transferrin-coated PLGA nanoparticles by the blood-brain barrier, *International Journal of Pharmaceutics*, Vol.379, No.2, pp. 285-292

Chattopadhyay, N.; Zastre, J.; Wong, H.L.; Wu, X.Y. & Bendayan, R. (2008). Solid lipid nanoparticles enhance the delivery of the HIV protease inhibitor, atazanavir, by a human brain endothelial cell line, *Pharmaceutical Research*, Vol.25, No.10, pp.2262–2271

Chaudhuri, P.; Harfouche, R.; Soni, S.; Hentschel, D.M. & Sengupta, S. (2010). Shape effect of carbon nanovectors on angiogenesis, *ACS Nano*, Vol.4, pp. 574-582

Choy, H. (1999). Taxanes in combined-modality therapy for solid tumors, *Oncology (Williston Park)*, Vol.13, pp. 23–38

Chun, T.W.; Justement, J.S.; Moir, S.; Hallahan, C.W.; Maenza, J.; Mullins, J.I.; Collier, A.C.; Corey, L. & Fauci, A.S. (2007). Decay of the HIV reservoir in patients receiving antiretroviral therapy for extended periods: implications for eradication of virus, *Journal of Infectious Diseases*, Vol.195, pp. 1762-1764

Cihlar, T. & Ray, A.S. (2010). Nucleoside and nucleotide HIV reverse transcriptase inhibitors: 25 years after zidovudine, *Antiviral Research*, Vol.85, pp. 39-58

Cornford, E.M.; Braun, L.D. & Oldendorf, W.H. (1978). Carrier mediated blood–brain barrier transport of choline and certain choline analogs, *Journal of Neurochemistry*, Vol.30, No.2, pp. 299–308

Crown, J. & O'Leary, M. (2000). The taxanes: An update, *Lancet*, Vol.355, pp. 1176–1178

Cryan, S.A.; Devocelle, M.; Moran, P.J.; Hickey, A.J. & Kelly JG. (2006). Increased intracellular targeting to airway cells using octaarginine-coated liposomes: In vitro assessment of their suitability for inhalation, *Molecular Pharmacology*, Vol.3, pp. 104–112

Cullis, P.R.; Mayer, L.D. & Bally, M.B. (1989). Generating and loading of liposomal systems for drug delivery systems, *Advanced Drug Delivery Reviews*, Vol.3, pp. 267–282

Daniels, T.R.; Delgado, T.; Helguera, G. & Penichet, M.L. (2006). The transferrin receptor part II: targeted delivery of therapeutic agents into cancer cells, *Clinical Immunology*, Vol.121, No.2, pp. 159–176

Dellamary, L.A.; Tarara, T.E.; Smith, D.J.; Woelk, C.H.; Adractas, A.; Costello, M.L.; Gill, H. & Weers, J.G. (2000). Hollow porous particles in metered dose inhalers, *Pharmaceutical Research*, Vol.17, pp. 168–174

Densmore, C.L. (2006). Advances in noninvasive pulmonary gene therapy, *Current Drug Delivery*, Vol.3, pp. 55–63

Desai, N.; Trieu, V.; Yao, Z.; Louie, L.; Ci, S.; Yang, A.; Tao, C.; De, T.; Beals, B.; Dykes, D.; Noker, P.; Yao, R.; Labao, E.; Hawkins, M. & Soon-Shiong, P. (2006). Increased antitumor activity, intratumor paclitaxel concentrations, and endothelial cell transport of Cremophor-free, albumin-bound paclitaxel, ABI-007, compared with Cremophor-based paclitaxel, *Clinical Cancer Research*, Vol.12, pp. 1317–1324

Desgrosellier, J.S. & Cheresh, D.A. (2010). Integrins in cancer: biological implications and therapeutic opportunities, *Nature Review Cancer*, Vol.10, pp. 9-22

Destache, C.J.; Belgum, T.; Christensen, K.; Shibata, A.; Sharma, A. & Dash, A. (2009). Combination antiretroviral drugs in PLGA nanoparticle for HIV-1, *BMC Infectetious Diseases*, Vol.9, pp.198

Dickinson, P.A.; Howells, S.W. & Kellaway, I.W. (2001). Novel Nanoparticles for Pulmonary Drug Administration, *Journal of Drug Targeting*, Vol.9, No.4, pp. 295-302

du Toit, L.C.; Pillay, V. & Choonara, Y.E. (2010). Nano-microbicides: Challenges in drug delivery, patient ethics and intellectual property in the war against HIV/AIDS, *Advanced Drug Delivery Reviews*, Vol.62, No.4–5, pp. 532–546

Dutta, T.; Agashe, H.B.; Garg, M.; Balakrishnan, P.; Kabra, M. & Jain, N.K. (2007). Poly (propyleneimine) dendrimer based nanocontainers for targeting of efavirenz to human monocytes/macrophages *in vitro*, *Journal of Drug Targeting*, Vol.15, No.1, pp. 89-98

Dutta, T.; Garg, M. & Jain, N.K. (2008). Targeting of efavirenz loaded tuftsin conjugated poly(propyleneimine) dendrimers to HIV infected macrophages *in vitro*, *European Journal of Pharmaceutical Sciences*, Vol.34, No.2–3, pp.181–189

Dvorak, H.F.; Senger, D.R.; Dvorak, A.M.; Harvey, V.S. & McDonagh, J. (1985). Regulation of extravascular coagulation by microvascular permeability, *Science*, Vol.227, pp. 1059–1061

Eavarone, D.A.; Yu, X. & Bellamkonda, R.V. (2000). Targeted drug delivery to C6 glioma by transferrin-coupled liposomes, *Journal of Biomedical Materials Research*, Vol.51, No.1, pp. 10–14

Emerich, D.F. & Thanos, C.G. (2007). Targeted nanoparticle-based drug delivery and diagnosis. *Journal of Drug Targeting*, Vol.15, pp. 163-183

Farokhzad, O.C.; Cheng, J.;Teply, B.A.; Sherifi, I.; Jon, S.; Kantoff, P.W.; Richie, J.P. & Langer, R. (2006). Targeted nanoparticle-aptamer bioconjugates for cancer chemotherapy *in vivo, Proceedings of the National Academy of Sciences USA,* Vol.103, pp. 315- 6320

Farr, C.P.; Taylor, S.G.; Smith, G. & Wyatt, D. (1992). The pharmacokinetics of pulmonary-delivered insulin: A comparison of intratracheal and aerosol administration to the rabbit, *Pharmaceutical Research,* Vol.9, pp. 764-768

Fenart, L.; Casanova, A.; Dehouck, B.; Duhem, C.; Slupek, S.; Cecchelli, R. & Betbeder, D. (1999). Evaluation of effect of charge and lipid coating on ability of 60 nm nanoparticles to cross an in vitro model of the blood-brain barrier, *Journal of Pharmacology and Experimental Therapeutics,* Vol.291, No.3, pp. 1017-1022

Fogal, V.; Zhang, L. & Ruoslahti, E. (2008). Mitochondrial/ Cell surface protein p32/gC1qR as a molecular target in tumor cells and tumor stroma, *Cancer Research,* In press

Folkman, J. (1995). Angiogenesis in cancer, vascular, rheumatoid and other disease, *Nature Medicine,* Vol.1, No.1, pp. 27-31

Folkman, J. (2003). Fundamental concepts of the angiogenic process, *Current Molecular Medicine,* Vol.3, pp. 643-651

Fortin, D.; McCormick, C.I.; Remsen, L.G.; Nixon, R. & Neuwelt, E.A. (2000). Unexpected neurotoxicity of etoposide phosphate administered in combination with other chemotherapeutic agents after blood-brain barrier modification to enhance delivery, using propofol for general anesthesia, in a rat model, *Neurosurgery,* Vol.47, pp. 199-207

Garg, M.; Asthana, A.; Agashe, H.B.; Agrawal, G.P. & Jain, N.K. (2006). Stavudine-loaded mannosylated liposomes: In-vitro anti-HIV-I activity, tissue distribution and pharmacokinetics, *Journal of Pharmaceutics and Pharmacology,* Vol.58, pp. 605-616

Gelderblom, H.; Verweij, J.; Nooter, K. & Sparreboom, A. (2001). Cremophor EL: The drawbacks and advantages of vehicle selection for drug formulation, *European Journal of Cancer,* Vol.37, pp. 1590-1598

Gelperina, S.E.; Khalansky, A.S.; Skidan, I.N.; Smirnova, Z.S.; Bobruskin, A.I.; Severin, S.E.; Turowski, B.; Zanella, F.E. & Kreuter, J. (2002). Toxicological studies of doxorubicin bound to polysorbate 80-coated poly(butyl cyanoacrylate) nanoparticles in healthy rats and rats with intracranial glioblastoma, *Toxicological Letters,* Vol.126, No.2, pp. 131-141

Ghebrehiwet, B.; Lim, B.L.; Peerschke, E.I.; Willis, A.C & Reid, K.B. (1994). Isolation, cDNA cloning, and overexpression of a 33-kD cell surface glycoprotein that binds to the globular "heads" of C1q, *Journal of Experimental Medicine,* Vol.179, pp. 1809-1821

Golden, P.L. & Pollack, G.M. (2003). Blood-brain barrier efflux transport, *Journal of Pharmaceutical Sciences,* Vol.92, No.9, pp. 1739-1753

Gonzalez-Rothi, R.J. & Schreier, H. (1995). Pulmonary delivery of liposome-encapsulated drugs in asthma therapy, *Clinical Immunotherapy,* Vol.4, pp. 331-337

Goppert, T.M. & Muller, R.H. (2005). Polysorbate-stabilized solid lipid nanoparticles as colloidal carriers for intravenous targeting of drugs to the brain: comparison of plasma protein adsorption patterns, *Journal of Drug Targeting,* Vol.13, No.3, pp. 179-187

Goren, D.; Horwitz, A.T.; Tzemach, D.; Tarshish, M.; Zalipsky, S. & Gabizon, A. (2000). Nuclear delivery of doxorubicin via folate-targeted liposomes with bypass of multidrug-resistance efflux pump, *Clinical Cancer Research,* Vol.6, pp. 1949-1957

Gradishar, W.J.; Tjulandin, S.; Davidson, N.; Shaw, H.; Desai, N.; Bhar, P.; Hawkins, M. & O'Shaughnessy, J. (2005). Superior efficacy of albumin-bound paclitaxel, ABI-007, compared with polyethylated castor oil-based paclitaxel in women with metastatic breast cancer: results of a phase III trial, *Journal of Clinical Oncology*, Vol.23, pp. 7794-7803

Greig, N.H. (1989). Drug delivery to the brain by blood–brain barrier circumvention and drug modification. In: Implications of the Blood–Brain Barrier and its Manipulation; Neuwelt, E.A., Ed.; Plenum Press: New York, pp. 311–367

Guarneri, V. & Conte, P.F. (2004). The curability of breast cancer and the treatment of advanced disease, *European Journal of Nuclear Medicine and Molecular Imaging*, Vol.31, pp. S149–S161

Gulyaev, A.E.; Gelperina, S.E.; Skidan, I.N.; Antropov, A.S.; Kivman, G.Y. & Kreuter, J. (1999). Significant transport of doxorubicin into the brain with polysorbate-80 coated nanoparticles, *Pharmaceutical Research*, Vol.16, pp. 1564–1569

Gururangan, S. & Friedman, H.S. (2002). Innovations in design and delivery of chemotherapy for brain tumors, *Neuroimaging Clinics of North America*, Vol.12, No.4, pp. 583–597

Hall, W.A. (1991). Transferrin receptor on glioblastoma multiforme, *Journal of Neurosurgery*, Vol.74, No.2, pp. 313–314

Hamaguchi, T.; Matusmura, Y.; Suzuki, M.; Shimizu, K.; Goda, R.; Nakamura, I.; Nakatomi, I.; Yokoyama, M.; Kataoka, K. & Kakizoe, T.(2005). NK105, a paclitaxel-incorporating micellar nanoparticle formulation, can extend in vivo antitumor activity and reduce the neurotoxicity of paclitaxel, *British Journal of Cancer*, Vol.92, pp. 1240–1246

Hänninen, M.M.; Haapasalo, J.; Haapasalo, H.; Fleming, RE.; Britton, R.S.; Bacon, B.R. & Parkkila, S. (2009). Expression of iron-related genes in human brain and brain tumors, *BMC Neuroscience*, Vol.10, pp. 36

Hardebo, J.E. & Kahrstrom, J. (1985). Endothelial negative surface charge areas and blood–brain barrier function, *Acta Physiologica Scandinavica*, Vol.125, pp. 495–499

Harfouche, R.; Basu, S.; Soni, S.; Hentschel, D.M.; Mashelkar, R.A. & Sengupta, S. (2009). Nanoparticle-mediated targeting of phosphatidylinositol-3-kinase signaling inhibits angiogenesis, *Angiogenesis*, Vol.12, No.4, pp. 325-38

Hatakeyama, H.; Akita, H.; Maruyama, K.; Suhara, T. & Harashima, H. (2004). Factors governing the in vivo tissue uptake of transferrin-coupled polyethylene glycol liposomes *in vivo*, *International Journal of Pharmacology*, Vol.281, No.1-2, pp. 25–33

Hawkins, M.J.; Soon-Shiong, P. & Desai, N. (2008). Protein nanoparticles as drug carriers in clinical medicine, *Advanced Drug Delivery Reviews*, Vol.60, pp. 876–885

Hochman, J.H.; Chiba, M.; Nishime, J.; Yamazaki, M. & Lin, A.H. (2000). Influence of P-glycoprotein on the transport and metabolism of indinavir in Caco-2 cells expressing cytochrome P-450 3A4, *Journal of Pharmacological and Experimental Therapeutics*, Vol.292, pp. 310-318

Hu, S. & Zhang, Y. (2010). Endostar-loaded Peg-PLgA nanoparticles: in vitro and in vivo evaluation, *International Journal of Nanomedicine*, Vol.5, pp. 1039–1048

Ibrahim, N.K.; Desai, N.; Legha, S.; Soon-Shiong, P.; Theriault, R.L.; Rivera, E.; Esmaeli, B.; Ring, S.E.; Bedikian, A.; Hortobagyi, G.N. & Ellerhorst, J.A. (2002). Phase I and pharmacokinetic study of ABI-007, a Cremophor-free, protein-stabilized, nanoparticle formulation of paclitaxel, *Clinical Cancer Research*, Vol.8, pp. 1038-1044

Ibrahim, N.K.; Samuels, B.; Page, R.; Doval, D.; Patel, K.M.; Rao, S.C.; Nair, M.K.; Bhar, P.; Desai, N. & Hortobagyi, G.N. (2005). Multicenter phase II trial of ABI-007, an albumin- bound paclitaxel, in women with metastatic breast cancer, *Journal of Clinical Oncology*, Vol.23, No.25, pp. 6019-6026

Jain, K.K. (2010). Advances in the field of nanooncology, *BMC Medicine*, Vol.8, pp. 83

Jefferies, W.A.; Brandon, M.R.; Hunt, S.V.; Williams, A.F.; Gatter, K.C. & Mason, D.Y. (1984). Transferrin receptor on endothelium of brain capillaries, *Nature*, Vol.312, No.5990, pp. 162-163

Jemal, A.; Siegel, R. & Ward E. (2008) Cancer statistics. *CA: A Cancer Journal for Clinicians*, Vol.58, No.2, pp. 71-96

Jenning, V.; Lippacher, A. & Gohla, SH. (2002) Medium scale production of solid lipid nanoparticles (SLN) by high pressure homogenization, *Journal of Microencapsulation*, Vol.19, pp. 1-10

John, T.A.; Vogel, S.M.; Tiruppathi, C.; Malik, A.B. & Minshall, R.D. (2003). Quantitative analysis of albumin uptake and transport in the rat microvessel endothelial monolayer, *Lung Cellular and Molecular Physiology*, Vol.284, pp. L187-L196

Justo, O.R. & Moraes, A.M. (2003). Incorporation of antibiotics in liposomes designed for tuberculosis therapy by inhalation, *Drug Delivery*, Vol.10, pp. 201-207

Kabanov, A.V.; Batrakova, E.V. & Alakhov, V.Y. (2002). Pluronic block copolymers as novel polymer therapeutics for drug and gene delivery, *Journal of Control Release*, Vol.82, pp. 189-212

Kang, K.W.; Chun, M.K.; Kim, O.K.; Subedi, R.K.; Ahn, S.G.; Yoon, J.H. & Choi, H.K. (2010). Doxorubicin-loaded solid lipid nanoparticles to overcome multidrug resistance in cancer therapy, *Nanomedicine Nanotechnology Biology and Medicine*, Vol.6, No.2, pp. 210-213

Kang, Y.S.; Terasaki, T.; Ohnishi, T. & Tsuji, A. (1990). In vivo and in vitro evidence for a common carrier mediated transport of choline and basic drugs through the blood-brain barrier, *Journal of Pharmacobiodyn*, Vol.13, No.6, pp. 353-360

Kimura, S.; Egashira, K.; Chen, L.; Nakano, K.; Iwata, E.; Miyagawa, M.; Tsujimoto, H.; Hara, K.; Morishita, R.; Sueishi, K.; Tominaga, R. & Sunagawa, K. (2009). Nanoparticle-mediated delivery of nuclear factor {kappa}B decoy into lungs ameliorates monocrotaline-induced pulmonary arterial hypertension, *Hypertension, 2009 May;53(5):877-83*

Knight, V.; Koshkina, N.; Waldrep, C.; Giovanella, B.C.; Kleinerman, E. & Gilbert, B. (2000). Anti-cancer activity of 9-nitrocamptothecin liposome aerosol in mice. *Transactions of the American Clinical and Climatological Association*, Vol.11, pp. 135-145

Koziara, J.M.; Lockman, P.R.; Allen, D.D. & Mumper, R.J. (2004). Paclitaxel nanoparticles for the potential treatment of brain tumors, *Journal of Controlled Release*, Vol.99, pp. 259-269

Kreuter, J. (2001). Nanoparticulate systems for brain delivery of drugs, *Advanced Drug Delivery Reviews*, Vol.47, pp. 65-81

Kreuter, J.; Alyautdin, R.N.; Kharkevich, D.A. & Ivanov, A.A. (1995). Passage of peptides through the blood-brain barrier with colloidal polymer particles (nanoparticles), *Brain Research*, Vol.674, No.1, pp. 171-174

Kreuter, J.; Petrov, V.E.; Kharkevich, D.A. & Alyautdin, R.N. (1997). Influence of the type of surfactant on the analgesic effects induced by the peptide dalargin after its delivery across the blood–brain barrier using surfactant-coated nanoparticles, *Journal of Controlled Release*, Vol.49, No.1, pp. 81–87

Kumagai, A.K.; Eisenberg, J.B. & Pardridge, W.M. (1987). Absorptive-mediated endocytosis of cationized albumin and a b-endorphin-cationized albumin chimeric peptide by isolated brain capillaries. Model system of blood–brain barrier transport, *Journal of Biological Chemistry*, Vol.262, No.31, pp. 15214–15219

Kuo, Y.C. & Chen, H.H. (2006). Effect of nanoparticulate polybutylcyanoacrylate and methylmethacrylate-sulfopropylmethacrylate on the permeability of zidovudine and lamivudine across the in vitro blood-brain barrier, *International Journal of Pharmaceutics*, Vol.327, pp. 160-169

Kuo, Y.C. & Su, F.L. (2007). Transport of stavudine, delavirdine, and saquinavir across the blood-brain barrier by polybutylcyanoacrylate, methylmethacrylate-sulfopropylmethacrylate, and solid lipid nanoparticles, *Journal of Pharmaceutics*, Vol.340, No.1–2, pp. 143–152

Kuo, Y.C. (2005). Loading efficiency of stavudine on polybutylcyanoacrylate and methylmethacrylate-sulfopropylmethacrylate copolymer nanoparticles, *International Journal of Pharmaceutics*, Vol.290, No.1–2, pp.161–172

Kurihara, A. & Pardridge, W.M. (1999). Imaging brain tumors by targeting peptide radiopharmaceuticals through the blood–brain barrier, *Cancer Research*, Vol.59, No.24, pp. 6159–6163

Laakkonen, P.; Porkka, K.; Hoffman, J.A. & Ruoslahti, E. (2002). A tumor-homing peptide with a targeting specificity related to lymphatic vessels, *Nature Medicine*, Vol.8, pp. 751–755

Lai, S.K.; Fu, J.; Man, S.T. & Hanes, J. (2005). Doxorubicin-loaded transferrin-targeted polymeric micelles rapidly enter cancer cells and accumulate near the cell nucleus. AIChE Annual Meeting, Conference Proceedings, pp. 14370

Lam, W.; Leung, C.H.; Chan, H.L. & Fong, W.F. (2000). Toxicity and DNA binding of dextran-doxorubicin conjugates in multidrug-resistant KB-V1 cells: optimization of dextran size, *Anticancer Drugs*, Vol.11, pp. 377-384

Laske, D.W.; Youle, R.J. & Oldfield, E.H. (1997). Tumor regression with regional distribution of the targeted toxin TF-CRM107 in patients with malignant brain tumors, *Nature Medicine*, Vol.3, No.12, pp. 1362–1368

Lee, R.J.; Wang, S. & Low, P.S. (1996). Measurement of endosome pH following folate receptor-mediated endocytosis, *Biochimca Biophysca Acta*, Vol.1312, No.3, pp. 237–242

Li, F.Q.; Hu, J.H.; Lu, B.; Yao, H. & Zhang, W.G. (2001). Ciprofloxacin-loaded bovine serum albumin microspheres: preparation and drug-release *in vitro*, *Journal of Microencapsulation*, Vol.18, pp. 825–829

Li, S.; Wang, A.; Jiang, W. & Guan, Z. (2008). Pharmacokinetic characteristics and anticancer effects of 5-Fluorouracil loaded nanoparticles, *BMC Cancer*, Vol.8, pp. 103

Li, X. & Chan, K.W. (1999). Transport, metabolism and elimination mechanisms of anti-HIV agents, *Advanced Drug Delivery Reviews*, Vol.39, pp. 81-103

Liu, J.; Gong, T.; Fu, H.; Wang, C.; Wang, X.; Chen, Q.; Zhang, Q.; He, Q. & Zhang, Z. (2008). Solid lipid nanoparticles for pulmonary delivery of insulin, *International Journal of Pharmaceutics*, Vol.356, pp. 333-344

Liu, Y.; Huang, L. & Liu, F. (2010). Paclitaxel Nanocrystals for Overcoming Multidrug Resistance in Cancer. *Molecular Pharmaceutics*, Vol.7, No.3, pp. 863-869

Lobenberg, R.; Maas, J. & Kreuter, J. (1998). Improved body distribution of 14C-labelled AZT bound to nanoparticles in rats determined by radioluminography, *Journal of Drug Targeting*, Vol.5, No.3, pp. 171-179

Lockman, P.R., Mumper, R.J., Khan, M.A. & Allen, D.D. (2002). Nanoparticle technology for drug delivery across the blood-brain barrier, *Drug Development and Industrial Pharmacy*, Vol.28, pp. 1-13

Lockman, P.R.; Koziara, J.M.; Mumper, R.J. & Allen, D.D. (2004). Nanoparticle surface charges alter blood-brain barrier integrity and permeability, *Journal of Drug Targeting*, Vol.12, No.9-10, pp. 635-641

Mallipeddi, R.; & Rohan, L.C. (2010). Progress in antiretroviral drug delivery using nanotechnology, *International Journal of Nanomedicine*, Vol.5, pp. 533-547

Marsh, D.; Bartucci, R. & Sportelli, L. (2003). Lipid membranes with grafted polymers: physicochemical aspects, *Biochimica Biophysica Acta - Biomembranes*, Vol.1615, pp. 33-59

Martin, F.J. (1998). Clinical pharmacology and antitumor efficacy of DOXIL (pegylated liposomal doxorubicin). In: Lasic DD, Papahadjopoulos D, editors. Medical Applications of Liposomes, New York: Elsevier Science BV, pp. 635-688

Matsumura, Y.; Gotoh, M.; Muro, K.; Yamada, Y.; Shirao, K.; Shimada, Y.; Okuwa, M.; Matsumoto. S.; Miyata, Y.; Ohkura, H.; Chin, K.; Baba, S.; Yamao, T.; Kannami, A.; Takamatsu, Y.; Ito, K. & Takahashi, K. (2004). Phase I and pharmacokinetic study of MCC-465, a doxorubicin (DXR) encapsulated in PEG immunoliposome, in patients with metastatic stomach cancer, *Annals of Oncology*, Vol.15, pp. 517-525

Miele, E.; Spinelli, G.P.; Miele, E.; Tomao, F. & Tomao, S. (2009). Albumin-bound formulation of paclitaxel (Abraxane® ABI-007) in the treatment of breast cancer, *International Journal of Nanomedicine*, Vol.4, pp. 99-105

Minko, T.; Batrakova, E.V.; Li, S.; Li, Y.; Pakunlu, R.I.; Alakhov, V.Y. & Kabanov, A.V. (2005). Pluronic block copolymers alter apoptotic signal transduction of doxorubicin in drug-resistant cancer cells, *Journal of Control Release*, Vol.105, pp. 269-278

Minshall, R.D.; Sessa, W.C. & Stan, R.V. (2003). Caveolin regulation of endothelial function, *Lung Cellular and Molecular Physiology*, Vol.285, pp. L1179-L1183

Mishra. V.; Mahor, S.; Rawat, A.; Gupta, P.N.; Dubey, P.; Khatri, K. & Vyas, S.P. (2006). Targeted brain delivery of AZT via transferrin anchored pegylated albumin nanoparticles, *Journal of Drug Targeting*, Vol.14, pp. 45-53

Moghimi, S.M.; Hunter, A.C. & Murray, J.C. (2001). Long-circulating and target-specific nanoparticles: theory to practice, *Pharmacological Reviews*, Vol.53, No.2, pp. 283-318

Moorthi, C.; Manavalan, R. & Kathiresan, K. (2011). Nanotherapeutics to Overcome Conventional Cancer Chemotherapy Limitations, *Journal of Pharmacy and Pharmaceutical Sciences*, Vol.14, No.1, pp. 67 - 77

Muckerheide, A.; Apple, R.J.; Pesce, A.J. & Michael, J.G. (1987). Cationization of protein antigens. I. Alteration of immunogenic properties, *Journal of Immunology*, Vol.138, No.3, pp. 833–837

Muller, R.H.; Mader, K. & Gohla, S. (2000). Solid lipid nanoparticles (SLN) for controlled drug delivery - a review of the state of the art, *European Journal of Pharmaceutics Biopharmaceutics*, Vol.50, pp. 161–177

Murakami, M.; Ushio, Y.; Morino, Y.; Ohta T. & Matsukado Y. (1988). Immunohistochemical localization of apolipoprotein E in human glial neoplasms, *Journal of Clinical Investigation*, Vol.82, No.1, pp. 177–188

Nagy, Z., Peters, H. & Huttner, I. (1983). Charge-related alterations of the cerebral endothelium, *Laboratory Investigation*, Vol.49, pp. 662–671

National Comprehensive Cancer Network, Clinical Practice Guidelines in Oncology: Breast Cancer v2, (2008). Available at http://www.nccn.org/professionals/physician_gls/default.asp

Naumov, G.N.; Akslen, L.A. & Folkman J. (2006). Role of angiogenesis in human tumor dormancy: animal models of the angiogenic switch, *Cell Cycle*, Vol.5, pp. 1779-1787

Newman, L.A. & Singletary, S.E. (2007). Overview of adjuvant systemic therapy in early stage breast cancer, *Surgical Clinics of North America*, Vol.87, No.2, pp. 499–509

Ng, K.; Stringer, K.A. & Cohen, Z. (1998). Alveolar macrophage cell line is not activated by exposure to polymeric microspheres, International Journal of Pharmaceutics, Vol.170, pp. 41–49

Nimesh, S.; Kumar, R. & Chandra, R. (2006). Novel polyallylamine- dextran sulfate-DNA nanoplexes: Highly efficient non-viral vector for gene delivery, *International Journal of Pharmaceutics*, Vol.320, No.12, pp. 143-149

Nishiyama, N. & Kataoka, K. (2006). Current state, achievements, and future prospects of polymeric micelles as nanocarriers for drug and gene delivery, *Pharmacological Therapeutics*, Vol.112, No.3, pp. 630–648

Olbrich, C.; Gessner, A.; Schroder, W.; Kayser, O. & Muller, R.H. (2004). Lipid-drug conjugate nanoparticles of the hydrophilic drug diminazene-cytotoxicity testing and mouse serum adsorption, *Journal of Controlled Release*, Vol.96, pp. 425–435

Pandey, R. & Khuller, G.K. (2005). Solid lipid particle-based inhalable sustained drug delivery system against experimental tuberculosis, *Tuberculosis (Edinb)*, Vol.85, pp. 227-234

Pandey, R. & Khuller, G.K. (2006). Nanotechnology based drug delivery system(s) for the management of tuberculosis, *Indian Journal of Experimental Biology*, Vol.44, No.5, pp. 357-366

Pandey, R.; Sharma, A.; Zahoor, A.; Sharma, S.; Khuller, G.K. & Prasad, B. (2003). Poly(DL-lactide-co-glycolide) nanoparticle-based inhalable sustained drug delivery system for experimental tuberculosis, *Journal of Antimicrobial Chemotherapy*, Vol.52, pp. 981–986

Pappas, G.D. & Tennyson, V.M. (1962). An electron microscopic study of the passage of colloidal particles from the blood vessels of the ciliary processes and choroid plexus of the rabbit, *Journal of Cell Biology*, Vol.15, pp. 227–239

Pardridge, W.M. (1995). Transport of small molecules through the blood-brain barrier: biology and methodology, *Advanced Drug Delivery Reviews*, Vol.15, No.1–3, pp. 5–36

Pardridge, W.M. (1997). Drug delivery to the brain, *Journal of Cerebral Blood Flow & Metabolism,* Vol.17, No.7, pp. 713-731

Pardridge, W.M. (1999). Non-invasive drug delivery to the human brain using endogenous blood-brain barrier transport systems, *Pharmaceutical Science & Technology Today,* Vol.2, No.2, pp. 49-59

Pardridge, W.M. (2001). BBB-genomics: creating new openings for brain-drug targeting, *Drug Discovery Today,* Vol.6, No.8, pp. 381-383

Pardridge, W.M. (2002). Drug and gene targeting to the brain with molecular Trojan horses, *Nature Reviews Drug Discovery,* Vol.1, No.2, pp. 131-139

Pardridge, W.M.; Buciak, J.L. & Friden, P.M. (1991). Selective transport of an anti-transferrin receptor antibody through the blood-brain barrier *in vivo, Journal of Pharmacology and Experimental Therapeutics,* Vol.259, No.1, pp. 66-70

Pardridge, W.M.; Eisenberg, J. & Yang, J. (1987). Human blood-brain barrier transferrin receptor, *Metabolism,* Vol.36, No.9, pp. 892-895

Pardridge, W.M.; Triguero, D. 7 Buciak, J.L. (1990). Beta-endorphin chimeric peptides: transport through the blood-brain barrier in vivo and cleavage of disulfide linkage by brain, *Endocrinology,* Vol.126, No.2, pp. 977-984

Park, E.K.; Kim, S.Y.; Lee, S.B. & Lee, Y.M. (2005). Folate-conjugated methoxy poly(ethylene glycol)/poly(E-caprolactone) amphiphilic block copolymeric micelles for tumor-targeted drug delivery, *Journal of Controlled Release,* Vol.109, No.1-3, pp. 158-168

Park, J.H.; Kwon, S.; Nam, J.O.; Park, R.W.; Chung, H.; Seo, S.B.; Kim, I.S.; Kwon, I.C. & Jeong, S.Y. (2004). Self-assembled nanoparticles based on glycol chitosan bearing 5beta-cholanic acid for RGD peptide delivery, *Journal of Control Release,* Vol.95, pp. 579-588

Patton, J.S. & Byron, P.R. (2007). Inhaling medicines: delivering drugs to the body through the lungs, *Nature Reviews Drug Discovery,* Vol.6, pp. 67-74

Perez, C.; Sanchez, A.; Putnam, D.; Ting, D.; Langer, R. & Alonso, M.J. (2001). Poly(lactic acid)-poly(ethylene glycol) nanoparticles as new carriers for the delivery of plasmid DNA, *Journal of Controlled Release,* Vol.75, No.1-2, pp. 211-224

Poduslo, J.F. & Curran, G.L. (1996). Polyamine modification increases the permeability of proteins at the blood-nerve and blood-brain barriers, *Journal of Neurochemistry,* Vol.66, pp. 1599-1609

Ramge, P.; Unger, R.E. & Oltrogge, J.B. (2000). Polysorbate-80 coating enhances uptake of polybutylcyanoacrylate (PBCA)-nanoparticles by human, bovine, and murine primary brain capillary endothelial cells, *European Journal of Neurology,* Vol.12, pp. 1935-1940

Reese, T.S. & Karnovsky, M.J. (1967). Fine structural localization of a blood-brain barrier to exogenous peroxidase, *Journal of Cell Biology,* Vol.34, No.1, pp. 207-217

Remsen, L.G.; Trail, P.A.; Hellstrom, I.; Hellstrom, K.E. & Neuwelt, E.A. (2000). Enhanced delivery improves the efficacy of a tumor-specific doxorubicin immunoconjugate in a human brain tumor xenograft model, *Neurosurgery,* Vol.46, pp. 704-709

Richman, D.D.; Margolis, D.M.; Delaney, M.; Greene, W.C.; Hazuda, D. & Pomerantz, R.J. (2009). The challenge of finding a cure for HIV infection, *Science,* Vol.323, pp. 1304-1307

Ross, J.F.; Chaudhuri, P.K. & Ratnam, M. (1994). Differential regulation of folate receptor isoforms in normal and malignant tissues in vivo and in established cell lines. Physiologic and clinical implications, *Cancer*, Vol.73, No.9, pp. 2432–2443

Rowinsky, E.K.; Cazenave, L.A. & Donehower, R.C. (1990). Taxol: a novel investigational antimicrotubule agent, *Journal of the National Cancer Institute*, Vol.82, pp. 1247–1259

Saari, S.M.; Vidgren, M.T.; Koskinen, M.O.; Turjanmaa, V.M.; Waldrep, J.C. & Nieminen, M.M. (1998). Regional lung deposition and clearance of 99mTc-labeled beclomethasone-DLPC liposomes in mild and severe asthma, *Chest*, Vol.113, No.6, pp. 1573-1579

Saito, Y. & Wright, E.M. (1983). Bicarbonate transport across the frog choroid plexus and its control by cyclic nucleotides, *Journal of Physiology*, Vol.336, pp. 635–648

Sarkar, K. & Yang, H. (2008). Encapsulation and Extended Release of Anti-CancerAnastrozole by Stealth Nanoparticles, *Drug Delivery*, Vol.15, pp. 343–346

Satchi-Fainaro, R.; Mamluk, R.; Wang, L.; Short, S.M.; Nagy, J.A.; Feng, D.; Dvorak, A.M.; Dvorak, H.F.; Puder, M.; Mukhopadhyay, D.; Folkman, J. (2005). Inhibition of vessel permeability by TNP-470 and its polymer conjugate, caplostatin, *Cancer Cell*, Vol.7, pp. 251-261

Sauer, I.; Nikolenko, H.; Keller, S.; Abu Ajaj, K.; Bienert, M. & Dathe, M. (2006). Dipalmitoylation of a cellular uptake-mediating apolipoprotein E-derived peptide as a promising modification for stable anchorage in liposomal drug carriers, *Biochimca Biophysica Acta-Biomembranes*, Vol.1758, No.4, pp. 552–561

Saul, J.M.; Annapragada, A.; Natarajan, J.V. & Bellamkonda, R.V. (2003). Controlled targeting of liposomal doxorubicin via the folate receptor *in vitro*, *Journal of Controlled Release*, Vol.92, No.1–2, pp. 49–67

Schöler, N.; Krause, K.; Kayser, O.; Müller, R.H.; Borner, K.; Hahn, H. & Liesenfeld, O. (2001). Atovaquone nanosuspensions show excellent therapeutic effect in a new murine model of reactivated toxoplasmosis, *Antimicrobial Agents and Chemotherapy*, Vol.45, No.6, pp. 1771–1779

Schroder, U.; Sommerfeld, P.; Ulrich, S. & Sabel, B.A. (1998). Nanoparticle technology for delivery of drugs across the blood-brain barrier, *Journal of Pharmaceutical Sciences*, Vol.87, pp. 1305–1307

Seymour, L.W.; Ferry, D.R.; Kerr, D.J.; Rea, D.; Whitlock, M.; Poyner, R.; Boivin, C.; Hesslewood, S.; Twelves, C.; Blackie, R.; Schatzlein, A.; Jodrell, D.; Bissett, D.; Calvert, H.; Lind, M.; Robbins, A.; Burtles, S.; Duncan, R. & Cassidy, J. (2009). Phase II studies of polymer-doxorubicin (PK1, FCE28068) in the treatment of breast, lung and colorectal cancer, *International Journal of Oncology*, Vol.34, pp. 1629-1636

Shah, L. & Amiji, M. (2006). Intracellular delivery of saquinavir in biodegradable polymeric nanoparticles for HIV/AIDS, *Pharmaceutical Research*, Vol.23, No.11, pp. 2638–2645

Shahiwala, A. & Misra, A. (2004). Pulmonary absorption of liposomal levonorgestrel, *AAPS PharmSciTech*, Vol.5, No.1, E13

Sharma, A.; Pandey, R.; Sharma, S. & Khuller, G.K. (2004). Chemotherapeutic efficacy of pol(DL-lactide-co-glycolide) nanoparticle encapsulated antitubercular drugs at sub-therapeutic dose against experimental tuberculosis, *International Journal of Antimicrobial Agents*, Vol.24, No.6, pp. 599-604

Shmeeda, H.; Mak, L.; Tzemach, D.; Astrahan, P.; Tarshish, M. & Gabizon, A. (2006). Intracellular uptake and intracavitary targeting of folate-conjugated liposomes in a mouse lymphoma model with up-regulated folate receptors, *Molecular Cancer Therapeutics*, Vol.5, No.4, pp. 818-824

Singla, A.K.; Garg, A. & Aggarwal, D. (2002). Paclitaxel ant its formulations, *International Journal of Pharmaceutics*, Vol.235, pp. 179-192

Smith, Q.R. (2003). A review of blood-brain barrier transport techniques, *Methods in Molecular Medicine*, Vol.89, pp. 193-208

Smola, M.; Vandamme, T. & Sokolowski, A. (2008). Nanocarriers as pulmonary drug delivery systems to treat and to diagnose respiratory and non respiratory diseases, *International Journal of Nanomedicine*, Vol.3, No.1, pp. 1-19

Soni, V.; Kohli, D.V. & Jain, S.K. (2005). Transferrin coupled liposomes as drug delivery carriers for brain targeting of 5-florouracil, *Journal of Drug Targeting*, Vol.13, No.4, pp. 245-250

Sosnik, A.; Chiappetta, D.A. & Carcaboso, A.M. (2009). Drug delivery systems in HIV pharmacotherapy: what has been done and the challenges standing ahead, *Journal of Controlled Release*, Vol.138, pp. 2-15

Stark, B.; Debbage, P.; Andreae, F.; Mosgoeller, W. & Prassl, R. (2007). Association of vasoactive intestinal peptide with polymer-grafted liposomes: structural aspects for pulmonary delivery, *Biochim Biophys Acta*, Vol.1768, pp. 705-714

Steiniger, S.C.; Kreuter, J.; Khalansky, A.S.; Skidan, I.N.; Bobruskin, A.I.; Smirnova, Z.S.; Severin, S.E.; Uhl, R.; Kock, M.; Geiger, K.D. & Gelperina, S.E. (2004). Chemotherapy of glioblastoma in rats using doxorubicin-loaded nanoparticles, *International Journal of Cancer*, Vol.109, No.5, pp.759-767

Stella, B.; Arpicco, S.; Peracchia, M.T.; Desmaële, D.; Hoebeke, J.; Renoir, M.; D'Angelo, J.; Cattel, L. & Couvreur, P. (2000). Design of folic acid-conjugated nanoparticles for drug targeting, *Journal of Pharmaceutical Science*, Vol.89, No.11, pp. 1452-1464

Sudimack, J. & Lee, R.J. (2000). Targeted drug delivery via the folate receptor, *Advanced Drug Delivery Reviews*, Vol.41, pp. 147-162

Sun, W.; Xie, C.; Wang, H. & Hu, Y. (2004). Specific role of polysorbate 80 coating on the targeting of nanoparticles to the brain, *Biomaterials*, Vol.25, No.15, pp. 3065-3071

Suntres, Z.E. & Shek, P.N. (1998). Liposomes promote pulmonary glucocorticoid delivery, *Journal of Drug Targeting*, Vol.6, pp. 175-182

Svenson, S. & Tomalia, D.A. (2005). Dendrimers in biomedical applications-reflections on the field, *Advanced Drug Delivery Reviews*, Vol.57, No.15, pp. 2106-2129

Takeuchi, H.; Yamamoto, H. & Kawashima, Y. (2001). Mucoadhesive nanoparticulate systems for peptide drug delivery, *Advanced Drug Delivery Reviews*, Vol.47, pp. 39-54

Taylor, K.M.G. & Farr, S.J. (1993). Liposomes for drug delivery to the respiratory tract, *Drug Development and Industrial Pharmacy*, Vol.19, pp. 123-142

Tedeschi, G.; Lundbom, N.; Raman, R.; Bonavita, S.; Duyn, J.H.; Alger, J.R. & Di Chiro, G. (1997). Increased choline signal coinciding with malignant degeneration of cerebral gliomas: a serial proton magnetic resonance spectroscopy imaging study, *Journal of Neurosurgery*, Vol.87, No.4, pp. 516-524

Terzano, C.; Allegra, L.; Alhaique, F.; Marianecci, C. & Carafa, M. (2005). Non phospholipids vesicles for pulmonary glucocorticoid delivery, *European Journal of Pharmaceutics and Biopharmaceutics*, Vol.59, pp. 57-62

Thole, M.; Nobmanna, S.; Huwyler, J.; Bartmann, A. & Fricker G. (2002). Uptake of cationzied albumin coupled liposomes by cultured porcine brain microvessel endothelial cells and intact brain capillaries, *Journal of Drug Targeting*, Vol.10, No.4, pp. 337-344

Tomalia, D.A; Reyna, L.A. & Svenson, S. (2007). Dendrimers as multi-purpose nanodevices for oncology drug delivery and diagnostic imaging, *Biochemical Society Transactions*, Vol.35, (Pt 1), pp. 61-67

Torchilin, V.P. (2005). Recent advances with liposomes as pharmaceutical carriers, *Nature Reviews Drug Discovery*, Vol.4, pp. 145-159

Triguero, D.; Buciak, J. & Pardridge, W.M. (1990). Capillary depletion method for quantification of blood-brain barrier transport of circulating peptides and plasma proteins, *Journal of Neurochemistry*, Vol.54, No.6, pp. 1882-1888

Tsukamoto, H.; Boado, R.J. & Pardridge, W.M. (1996).Differential expression in glioblastoma multiforme and cerebral hemangioblastoma of cytoplasmic proteins that bind two different domains within the 30-untranslated region of the human glucose transporter 1 (GLUT1) messenger RNA, *Journal of Clinical Investigation*, Vol.97, No.12, pp. 2823-2832

Umezawa, F. & Eto, Y. (1988). Liposome targeting to mouse brain: mannose as a recognition marker, *Biochemical and Biophysical Research Communications*, Vol.153, No.3, pp. 1038-1044

Uner, M. & Yener, G. (2007). Importance of solid lipid nanoparticles (SLN) in various administration routes and future perspectives. *International Journal of Nanomedicine*, Vol.2, No.3, pp. 289-300

Vaishampayan, U.; van Zuylen, L.; Verweij, J. & Sparreboom, A. (2001). Role of formulation vehicles in taxane pharmacology, *Investigational New Drugs*, Vol.19, pp. 125-141

Valle, J.W.; Armstrong, A.; Newman, C.; Alakhov, V.; Pietrzynski, G.; Brewer, J.; Campbell, S.; Corrie, P.; Rowinsky, E.K. & Ranson, M.: (2010). A phase 2 study of SP1049C, doxorubicin in P-glycoprotein-targeting pluronics, in patients with advanced adenocarcinoma of the esophagus and gastroesophageal junction, *Investigational New Drugs*, 2010. [Epub ahead of print]

Veronese, F.M. & Pasut, G. (2005). PEGylation, successful approach to drug delivery, *Drug Discovery Today*, Vol.10, pp. 1451-1458

Videira, M.A.; Gano, L.; Santos, C.; Neves, M. & Almeida, A.J. (2006). Lymphatic uptake of lipid nanoparticles following endotracheal administration, *Journal of Microencapsulation*, Vol.23, pp. 855-862

Vinogradov, S.V.; Bronich, T.K. & Kabanov, A.V. (2002). Nanosized cationic hydrogels for drug delivery: preparation properties and interactions with cells, *Advanced Drug Delivery Reviews*, Vol.54, pp. 135-147

Vorbrodt, A.W., Lossinsky, A.S., Dobrogowska, D.H. & Wisniewski, H.M. (1990). Sequential appearance of anionic domains in the developing blood-brain barrier, *Brain Research. Developmental Brain Research*, Vol.52, pp. 31-37

Vyas, S.P. & Sihorkar, V. (2000). Endogenous carriers and ligands in non-immunogenic site-specific drug delivery, *Advanced Drug Delivery Reviews*, Vol.43, No.2-3, pp. 101-164

Wahl, M.; Schilling, L.; Unterberg A. & Baethmann A. (1993). Mediators of vascular and parenchymal mechanisms in secondary brain damage, *Acta Neurochir Suppl*, Vol.57, pp. 64-72

Waldrep, J.C.; Gilbert, B.E.; Knight, C.M.; Black, M.B.; Scherer, P.W.; Knight, V. & Eschenbacher, W. (1997). Pulmonary delivery of beclomethasone liposome aerosol in volunteers, *Chest*, Vol.111, pp. 316-323

Wall, D.A. (1995). Pulmonary absorption of peptides and proteins, *Drug Delivery*, Vol.2, pp. 1-20

Wang, A.Z.; Gu, F.; Zhang, L.; Chan, J.M.; Radovic-Moreno ,A.; Shaikh, M.R. & Farokhzad, O.C. (2008). Biofunctionalized targeted nanoparticles for therapeutic applications, *Expert Opinion on Biological Therapy*, Vol.8, No.8, pp. 1063-1070

Wang, Y.; Yu, L.; Han, L.; Sha, X. & Fang, X. (2007). Difunctional Pluronic copolymer micelles for paclitaxel delivery: Synergistic effect of folate-mediated targeting and Pluronic-mediated overcoming multidrug resistance in tumor cell lines, *International Journal of Pharmaceutics*, Vol.337, pp. 63-73

Weidner, N.; Folkman, J.; Pozza, F.; Bevilacqua, P.; Allred, E.N.; Moore, D.H.; Meli, S. & Gasparini, G. (1992). Tumor angiogenesis: a new significant and independentprognostic indicator in early-stage breast carcinoma, *Journal of the National Cancer Institute*, Vol.84, pp. 1875-1887

Weidner, N.; Semple, J.P.; Welch, W.R. & Folkman J. (1991). Tumor angiogenesis and metastasis- correlation in invasive breast carcinoma, *The New England Journal of Medicine*, Vol.324, pp. 1-8

Weitman, S.D.; Lark, R.H.; Coney, L.R.; Fort, D.W.; Frasca, V.; Zurawski, V.R. Jr & Kamen, B.A. (1992). Distribution of the folate receptor GP38 in normal and malignant cell lines and tissues, *Cancer Research*, Vol.52, No.12, pp. 3396-3401

Wiedenmann, N.; Valdecanas, D.; Hunter, N.; Hyde, S.; Buchholz, T.A.; Milas, L. & Mason, K.A. (2007). 130-nm albumin-bound paclitaxel enhances tumor radiocurability and therapeutic gain, *Clinical Cancer Research*, Vol.13, No.6, pp. 1868-1874

Wolburg, H.; Wolburg-Buchholz, K.; Liebner, S. & Engelhardt B. (2001). Claudin-1, claudin-2 and claudin-11 are present in tight junctions of choroid plexus epithelium of the mouse, *Neuroscience Letters*, Vol.307, No.2, pp. 77-80

World Health Organization. Cancer. (2009). http://www.who.int/mediacentre/factsheets/fs297/en/index.html.

Wu, D. & Pardridge, W.M. (1999). Blood-brain barrier transport of reduced folic acid, *Pharmaceutical Research*, Vol.16, No.3, pp. 415-419

Xiang, G.; Wu, J.; Lu, Y.; Liu, Z. & Lee, R.J. (2008). Synthesis and Evaluation of a Novel Ligand for Folate-mediated Targeting liposomes, *International Journal of Pharmacology*, Vol.356, No.1-2, pp. 29-36

Xu, Y.; Wen, Z. & Xu, Z. (2009). Chitosan nanoparticles inhibit the growth of human hepatocellular carcinoma xenografts through an antiangiogenic mechanism, *Anticancer Research*, Vol.29, pp. 5103-5109

Yang, C.S.; Lu, F.L. & Cai, Y. (1999). Body distribution in mice of intravenously injected camphotothericin solid lipid nanoparticles and targeting eect on the brain, *Journal of Controlled Release*, Vol.59, pp. 299-307

Yang, W.; Peters, J.I. & Williams, R.O. (2008). Inhaled nanoparticles-a current review, *International Journal of Pharmacology*, Vol.356, pp. 239-247

Yoo, H.S. & Park, T.G. (2004). Folate receptor targeted biodegradable polymeric doxorubicin micelles, *Journal of Controlled Release,* Vol.96, No.2, pp. 273–283

Zahoor, A.; Sharma, S. & Khuller, G.K. (2005). Inhalable alginate nanoparticles as antitubercular drug carriers against experimental tuberculosis, *International Journal of Antimicrobial Agents,* Vol.26, pp. 298–303

Zeng, X.M.; Martin, G.P. & Marriott, C. (1995). Preparation and in vitro evaluation of tetrandrine-entrapped albumin microspheres as an inhaled drag delivery system, *European Journal of Pharmaceutical Sciences,* Vol.3, pp. 87–93

Zhang, C.; Zhao, L.; Dong, Y.; Zhang, X.; Lin, J. & Chen, Z. (2010). Folate-mediated poly (3-hydroxybutyrate-co-3-hydroxyoctanoate) nanoparticles for targeting drug delivery. *European Journal of Pharmaceutics and Biopharmaceutics,* Vol.76, No.1, pp. 10-16

Zhang, J.A.; Anyarambhatla, G.; Ma, L.; Ugwu, S.; Xuan, T.; Sardone, T. & Ahmad, I. (2005). Development and characterization of a novel Cremophor® EL free liposome-based paclitaxel (LEP-ETU) formulation, *European Journal of Pharmaceutics and Biopharmaceutics,* Vol.59, No.1, pp. 177-187

Zhang, L. & Granick, S. (2006). How to stabilize phospholipid liposome (using nanoparticles), *Nano Letters,* Vol.6, pp. 694-698

Zhao, R.; Seither, R.; Brigle, K.E.; Sharina, I.G.; Wang, P.J. & Goldman, I.D. (1997). Impact of overexpression of the reduced folate carrier (RFC1), an anion exchanger, on concentrative transport in murine L1210 leukemia cells, *Journal of Biological Chemistry,* Vol.272, No.34, pp. 21207–21212

Zhuo, W.; Luo, C.; Wang, X.; Song, X.; Fu, Y. & Luo, Y. (2010). Endostatin inhibits tumour lymphangiogenesis and lymphatic metastasis via cell surface nucleolin on lymphangiogenic endothelial cells, *Journal of Pathology,* Vol.222, No.3, pp. 249–260

20

Silver Nanoparticles – Universal Multifunctional Nanoparticles for Bio Sensing, Imaging for Diagnostics and Targeted Drug Delivery for Therapeutic Applications

Anitha Sironmani[1] and Kiruba Daniel[2]
[1]*School of Biotechnology, Madurai Kamaraj University, Madurai*
[2]*Dept.Nanocience and Nanotechnology, AnnaUniversiy of Technology, Trichy, India*

1. Introduction

Nanotechnology is a multidisciplinary scientific field undergoing explosive development. Nanometer-sized particles offer novel structural, optical and electronic properties that are not attainable with individual molecules or bulk solids. Advances in nanomedicine can be made by engineering nanoparticles that are capable of targeted delivery of drugs. This leads toward the concept and possibility of personalized medicine for the potential of early detection of diseases and most importantly, molecular targeted therapy. Promoting nanotechnology for diagnosis, prevention and treatment is the focus of the recently developing multifunctional nanotechnology. Engineered nanoparticles have the potential to revolutionize the diagnosis and treatment of many diseases; for example, by allowing the targeted delivery of a drug to particular subsets of cells. However, so far, such nanoparticles have not proved capable of surmounting all of the biological barriers required to achieve this goal. Nevertheless, advances in nanoparticle engineering, as well as advances in understanding the importance of nanoparticle characteristics such as size, shape and surface properties for biological interactions, are creating new opportunities for the development of nanoparticles for therapeutic applications.

Silver nanoparticles as an arch product from the field of nanotechnology, has gained interest because of distinctive properties, such as good conductivity, chemical stability, catalytic , antibacterial activity, antifungal, anti-viral, anti-inflammatory (Mukherjee et al., 2001; Sondi and Branka, 2004; Chen and Schluesener, 2008). Silver-based medical products, ranging from topical ointments and bandages for wound healing to coated stents, have been proven to be effective in retarding and preventing bacterial infections (Chen, 2007). Improvements in the development of novel silver nanoparticles-containing products are continuously sought. In particular, there is an increasing interest towards the exploitation of silver nanoparticles technology in the development of bioactive biomaterials, aiming at combining the relevant antibacterial properties of the metal with the peculiar performance of the biomaterial.

Compared with larger particles of the bulk material nanoparticles exhibit completely new or improved properties based on specific characteristics such as size, distribution and morphology. Nanoparticles present a higher surface-to-volume ratio is relevant for catalytic reactivity and other related properties such as antimicrobial activity in silver nanoparticles.

Nanoenabled drug delivery has already been successful in delivering drugs to specific tissues within the body, and promises capabilities that will enhance drug penetration into cells, as well as other means to improve drug activity. A very promising prospect of nanoparticles is its use in targeted drug delivery and also "multi-targeting", which is essential in the case of several diseases (Woodleand and Lu, 2005).

Recently, synthesis of silver nanoparticles has attracted considerable attention owing to their diverse properties like catalysis (Shiraishi and Toshima, 2000), magnetic and optical polarizability (Shiraishi and Toshima, 2000), electrical conductivity (Chang and Yen, 1995), antimicrobial activity (Sharverdi et al., 2007) and Surface Enhanced Raman Scattering (Matejka et al., 1992).

Recently it was shown that highly concentrated and nonhazardous nanosized silver particles can easily be prepared in a cost-effective manner and tested as a new type of bactericidal nanomaterial.

2. Synthesis of silver nanoparticles

The synthesis of metal nanoparticles is an expanding research area due to the potential applications for the development of novel technologies.

Silver nanoparticles have increasingly attracted more attentions because of their promising applications in the fields of catalysis (Musi et al.,2009; Shin et al., 2009; Tian et al.,2009) electronics, (Xia et al.,2003) sensing, (Guo et al.,2009; Zhao et al., 2009) and surface-enhanced Raman scattering, (Sun et al., 2009).For most applications, the properties of metal nanoparticles are determined by their size, shape, composition, and structure (Skrabalak and Xia, 2009; Xia et al., 2009). It is of great importance to prepare high quality silver nanoparticles with controllable chemical-physical properties.

Generally, nanoparticles are prepared by a variety of chemical and physical methods such as chemical reduction (Yu, 2007; Tan et al., 2002; Petit et al., 1993; Vorobvova et al., 1999), photochemical reduction (Vorobvova et al., 1999; Mallick et al., 2005; Keki et al., 2000; Pileni, 2000; Sun et al., 2001), electrochemical reduction (Liu and Lin, 2004; Sandmann et al., 2000), heat vaporation (Bae et al., 2002; Smetana et al., 2005) etc. These reagents could be inorganic such as sodium/potassium borohydrate, hydrazine and salts of tartarate, or organic ones like sodium citrate, ascorbic acid and amino acids capable of being oxidized. Various reagents have been reported to serve as stabilizing agent.

A number of reports adjusted the shape and size of silver nanoparticles using capping agents such as dendrimer, (Esumi et al., 2004) chitosan, (Murugadoss and Chattopadhyay, 2008) ionic liquid, (Zhang et al., 2009) and poly(vinylpyrrolidone) (PVP) (Sun and Xia, 2002), based on controlling the growth of silver nanoparticles through reaction confinement within the matrix or through preferential adsorption on specific crystal facets.

Most of these methods are extremely expensive and they also involve the use of toxic, hazardous chemicals which are not environmental friendly.

The biomedical applications of silver nanoparticle can be effective by the use of synthesized nanoparticles which minimize the factors such as toxicity and cost and are found to be exceptionally stable like other nanomaterials. Hence the development of better experimental procedures for the synthesis of nanoparticles of different chemical compositions, sizes, shapes and controlled polydispersity is vital for its advancement (Bhattacharya and Mukherjee, 2008).

Recently, a number of inorganic nanomaterials have been synthesized by bioreduction processes employing different microorganisms. Nanocrystals of gold, silver and their alloys have been synthesized within cells of lactic acid bacteria (Nair and Pradeep, 2002), *Pseudomonas stutzeri* AG259, (Joerger et al., 2000; Klaus et al., 2001). In addition, eukaryotic organisms such as fungi have also been used to grow nanoparticles of different chemical composition and sizes like *Verticillum sp.* (Mukherjee et al., 2001); *Fusarium oxysporum* (Ahmad et al., 2003) and *Aspergillus flavus* (Vigneshwaran et al., 2003) and also with enzymes (Willner et al., 2006). On the other hand, to mimic natural biomineralization, even live plants have been studied as templates for silver nanoparticles synthesis (Sanghi and Verma, 2009).

Synthesis of nanomaterial such as silver, gold, platinum and palladium using plants or plant extracts (Shankar et al., 2004) have been suggested as possible ecofriendly alternatives to chemical and physical methods. Nanoparticles synthesis using plants can be advantageous over other biological processes because it eliminates the elaborate process of maintaining cell cultures and can also be suitably scaled up for large-scale synthesis of nanoparticles (Shankar et al., 2004). Bioreduction of gold and silver ions to yield metal nanoparticles using living plants, (Gardea-Torresdey et al., 2003; Gardea-Torresdey et al., 2005), Geranium leaf broth (Shivshankar et al., 2003), Neem leaf broth, (Shivshankar et al., 2004) Lemongrass extract (Shivshankar et al., 2005), Tamarind leaf extract (Ankamwar et al., 2005) and Aloe Vera plant extracts (Prathap et al., 2006), have been reported.

Kasthuri et al., (2009) adopted a bioreductive approach of anisotropic gold and quasi-spherical silver nanoparticles by using apiin compound. Kasthuri et al., (2009) synthesized the anisotropic gold and spherical- quasi-spherical silver nanoparticles using extract of phyllanthin at room temperature. Spent mushroom substrate (Vigneshwaran et al., 2007), *Gliricidia sepium* extract (Jae Yong Song and Beom Soo Kim, 2008; Raut Rajesh et al., 2009) and *C. zeylanicum* bark powder (Sathishkumar et al., 2009) were used to synthesize nanoparticles. Krishna raj et al., (2010) studied the rapid synthesis of silver nanoparticles using aqueous leaves extract of *A. indica* and evaluated its antibacterial activity against water borne pathogens such as *Escherichia coli* and *Vibrio cholerae*. Daizy Philip (2009) studied mushroom mediated green chemistry approach towards the synthesis of gold, silver and gold-silver nanoparticles. Synthesis of metallic nanoparticles using green resources like Jatropha (*J. curcas* latex) (Harekrishna Bar et al.,2009), Hibiscus, (Daizy Philip,2010), *Ocimum tenuiflorum* (Kiruba Daniel et al.,2011b) and *Achyranthus aspera* (Kiruba Daniel et al., 2011c).

Silver nanoparticles can be synthesized and stabilized by peptides, proteins, DNA and chemical/biological polymers (Sengupta et al., 2009; Shemer et al., 2006). Several synthesis methods exist thus displaying different characteristics of the nanoparticles (Kiruba Daniel et al., 2010, 2011a 2011d;Nimroth Ananth et al., 2011)[Figure-1]

3. Characterization

Basically nanoparticles can be spectroscopically characterized on the basis of their sizes and the method can reveal the concentration of the synthesized nanoparticles too.

Nanoparticles are characterized by a variety of techniques such as dynamic light scattering (DLS), electron microscopy (TEM or SEM), atomic force microscopy (AFM), fourier transform infrared spectroscopy (FTIR), X-ray photoelectron spectroscopy (XPS), powder X-ray diffraction (XRD), matrix-assisted laser desorption/ionization time-of-flight mass spectrometry (MALDI-TOF), and magnetic resonance (NMR).

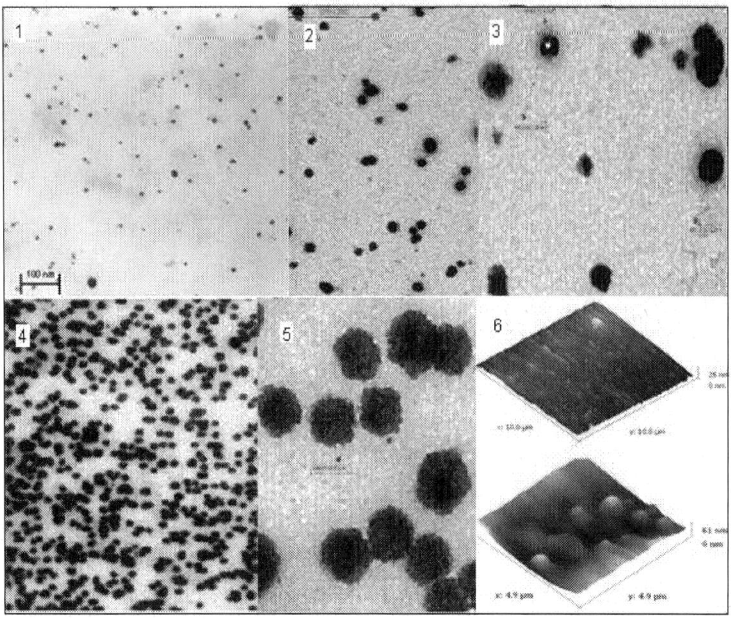

Fig. 1. Transmission electron microscopic pictures of Silver nanoparticles prepared using starch (1) , Plant extracts (2),(4) lower magnification , 3 & 5 higher magnification and atomic force microscopic picture of silver nanoparticles prepared using polyvinyl alcohol (top) and Bovine serum albumin (bottom)(6)

4. Structure and functional properties of nanoparticles

Most inorganic nanoparticles share the same basic structure. This consists of a central core that defines the fluorescence, optical, magnetic, and electronic properties of the particle, with a protective organic coating on the surface. This outside layer protects the core from degradation in a physiologically aggressive environment and can form electrostatic or covalent bonds, or both, with positively charged agents and biomolecules that have basic functional groups such as amines and thiols. Several research groups have successfully linked fluorescent nanoparticles to peptides, proteins, and oligonucleotides.
Of the three metals (silver, gold, copper) that display plasmon resonances in the visible spectrum, silver exhibits the highest efficiency of plasmon excitation (Kneipp et al., 2002). Moreover, optical excitation of plasmon resonances in nanosized silver particles is the most efficient mechanism by which light interacts with matter. A single silver nanoparticle

interacts with light more efficiently than a particle of the same dimension composed of any known organic or inorganic chromophore. The light-interaction cross-section for Ag can be about ten times that of the geometric cross-section, which indicates that the particles capture much more light than is physically incident on them (Esumi et al., 1997). Silver is also the only material whose plasmon resonance can be tuned to any wavelength in the visible spectrum.

The UV-Visible absorption spectrum of this preparation is given in Figure 2. The typical peak at 420 nm corresponds to the characteristic surface plasmon resonance of silver nanoparticles. Also, the plasmon band is symmetric which indicates that the solution does not contain many aggregated particles, a conclusion that agrees with the electron micrograph observation (below). It is well known that colloidal silver nanoparticles exhibit absorption at the wavelength from 390 to 420 nm due to Mie scattering (Kleemann, 1993). Hence, the band at 420 nm can be attributed to the property of Mie scattering.This may not include the protecting agent, because the Mie scattering responds only to the silver metal (Aoki, 2003). The plasmon bands are broad with an absorption tail in the longer wavelengths, which could be in principle due to the size distribution of the particles (Chalmers, 2002). Since the varying intensity of the plasmon resonance depends on the cluster size, the number of particles cannot be related linearly to the absorbance intensities (Klabunde, 2001).

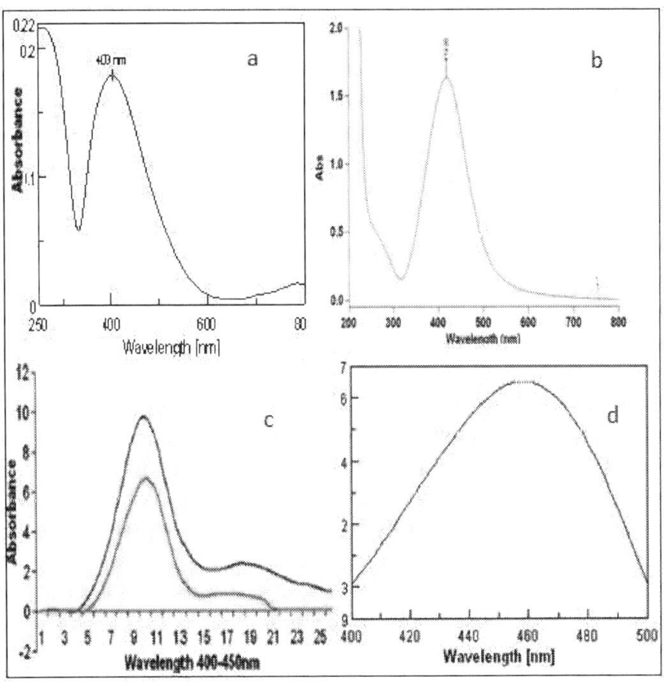

Fig. 2. UV-Visible spectral pattern of Clay stabilized(a), Starch stabilized (b), polyvinyl alcohol (Ag-PVA) and Bovine serum albumin (Ag-BSA) stabilized(c) and Plant extract stabilized (d) silver nanoparticles.

According to Mie's theory, only a single SPR band is expected in the absorption spectra of spherical nanoparticles, whereas anisotropic particles could give rise to two or more SPR bands depending on the shape of the particles. The number of SPR peaks increases as the symmetry of the nanoparticle decreases (Esumi et al., 2004; Murugadoss and Chattopadhyay, 2008; Zhang et al., 2009) [Figure-2].

5. Advantages of nanoparticles

a. Longer shelf-stability
b. High carrier capacity
c. Ability to incorporate hydrophilic and hydrophobic drug molecules
d. Can be administered via different routes
e. Longer clearance time
f. Ability to sustain the release of drug
g. Can be utilized for imaging studies
h. Increase the bioavailability of drugs
i. Targeted delivery of drugs at cellular and nuclear level
j. Development of new medicines which are safer
k. Prevent the multi-drug resistance mediated efflux of chemotherapeutic agents
l. Product life extension
m. Does not involve higher manufacturing costs and decrease in the cost of formulation
n. Does not involve use of harsh toxic solvents in the preparation process
o. Does not trigger immune response and allergic reactions
p. Tissues take only optimum concentrations nanoparticles and hence drug over dose does not occur

First-generation nanoparticles have been clinically translated as pharmaceutical drug delivery carriers for their ability to improve on drug tolerability, circulation half-life, and efficacy. Toward the development of the next-generation nanoparticles, researchers have designed novel multifunctional platforms for sustained release, molecular targeting, and environmental responsiveness.

6. Toxicity, immunological activity and pharmacodynamics *in vivo* and *in vitro* system

The lack of information regarding the toxicity of manufactured nanoparticles poses serious problems. Understanding the unique characteristics of engineered nanomaterials and their interactions with biological systems is key to the safe implementation of these materials in biomedical diagnostics and therapeutics and hence, the potential toxicity, the biological distribution and cellular uptake of silver nanoparticles were studied. For nanoparticles, like conventional chemical compounds, there are three main routes of exposure: inhalation, skin absorption and ingestion. It should be noted that nanoparticles have certain intrinsic properties (such as pinocytosis) that make it easy for them to enter cells. At the cellular level, nanoparticles can be found in various compartments, and even in the cell nucleus, which contains all the genetic information (Lovric et al., 2005; Asharani et al., 2009).

The animal study in swiss mice demonstrated that the silver nanoparticles were

1. non toxic, 2. showed no immune response. The silver nanoparticles were distributed in all organs (Figure 3 and 4) including liver and spleen that contained phagocytes similar to that

observed by Raynal et al., (2004); Bourrinet et al., (2006); Briley-Saebo et al., (2006); Chang et al., (2006) and Cai et al., (2007) in the case of iron oxide nanoparticles and AUNP-PEG nanoparticles because of the absence of renal excretion by glomerular filtration, as the size of the nanoparticles was larger (20 nm). In general, the spacing of cell membranes is in the range of 6 to 10 nm and the macromolecular contrast agents with a molecular size of less than 8 nm in diameter are cleared from blood by glomerular filtration and by tubular excretion of the kidney (Kobayashi et al., 2004) although the electrostatic charge properties of those particles also have a significant role in their ability to penetrate the glomerular basement membrane. Garnacho et al., (2008) have demonstrated enhanced accumulation of anti-ICAM/I125 ASM nanocarriers in the kidney, heart, liver, spleen and primarily the lungs both in wild type and ASM Knockout mice.

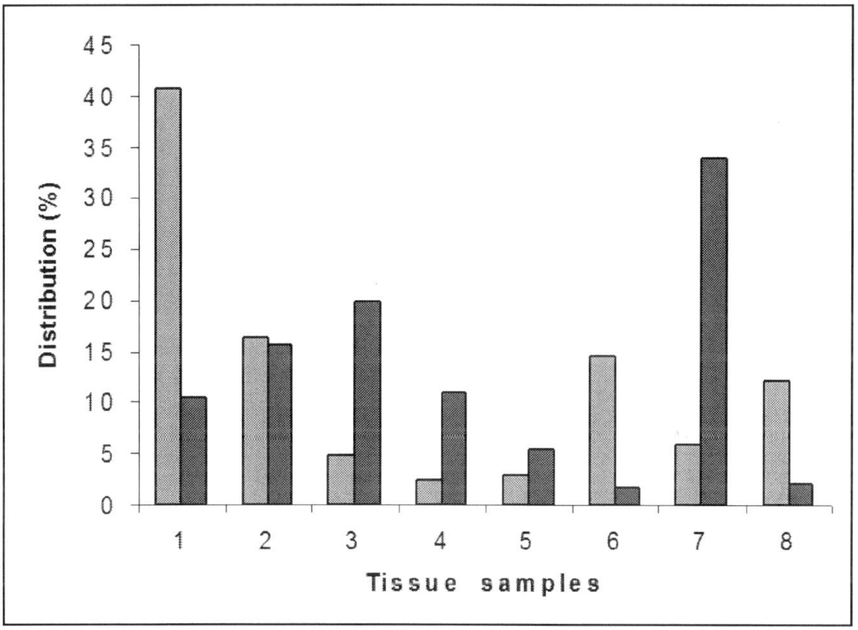

Fig. 3. Distribution pattern of Slver - polyvinyl alcohol / Silver - Bovine serum albumin nanoparticles in 1.Liver 2.Kidney 3.Spleen 4.Lungs 5.Heart 6.Intestine 7.Brain 8.Blood (420nm)

The presence of nanoparticles in the brain (Figure 5) indicated the penetration of nanosilver materials across the blood brain barrier (BBB) without producing apparent toxicity but upregulating the brain function by increasing the glutamine synthase activity of the brain that is important for neurotransmission and other activities. The nanoparticles were detected in the brain in UV-Visible analysis. To evaluate the potential effects of silver nanoparticles on brain neurophysiology, the level of glutamine synthase was tested. Approximately a two fold increase in the glutamine synthase activity was found. Glutamine synthase is the key enzyme responsible for the conversion of glutamate to glutamine and for the detoxification of ammonia in the brain (Caroline et al., 1999). Reactive oxygen radicals are known to cause the reduction in specific activity of glutamine synthase (Friedman and McDonald, 1997). The higher glutamine synthase activity indirectly showed the low level of free radicals.

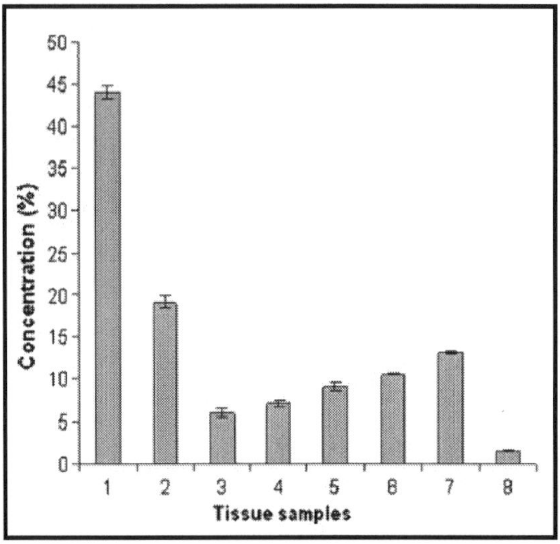

Fig. 4. Concentration of immuno-precipitated Silver - Bovine serum albumin(Ag-BSA) nanoparticles with rabbit antiBSA antibody in 1. Liver 2.Kidney 3.Spleen 4.Lungs 5.Heart 6.Intestine 7.Brain 8.Blood of mice as per the UV-visible spectrum pattern.

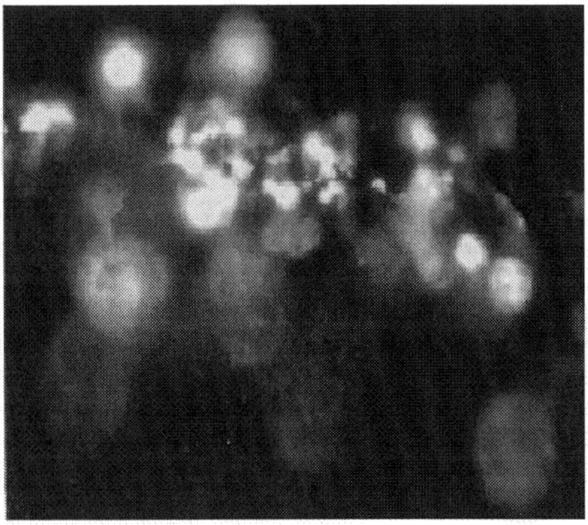

Fig. 5. Fluorescent microscopic images of Silver-Starch treated rat brain cells in suspension.

The silver nanoparticles were observed in other tissues especially in lungs at saturation with 5mg dose and no increase in uptake was observed in lungs when 20mg of silver nanoparticles were given revealing that the lung attained saturation at exposure to 5mg or less than that of silver nanoparticles. Increased half-life of silver nanoparticles in blood observed in this study was also reported earlier by Kobayashi et al., (2004) for AUNPs-PEG. Hainfeld et al., (2006) showed that the blood half-life of ultra small particles was increased by the redirection of the elimination pathways from reticulo-endothelial system to the mononuclear phagocyte systems with reference to gold nanoparticles. The lower concentration of silver nanoparticles particles in the spleen may be the reason for the less immune response.

7. Applications

Nanomaterials are at the leading edge of the rapidly developing field of nanotechnology. Their unique size-dependent properties make these materials superior and indispensable in many areas of human activity.

Living organisms are built of cells that are typically 10 µm across. The proteins are a typical size of just 5 nm, which is comparable with the dimensions of smallest man made nanoparticles. This gives an idea of using nanoparticles as very small probes that would allow unraveling and studying all physiological mechanism at the cellular machinery without introducing too much interference. Understanding of biological processes on the nanoscale level is a strong driving force behind development of nanotechnology.

A list of some of the applications of nanomaterials to biology or medicine is given below:

- Fluorescent biological labels - Drug and gene delivery - Bio detection of pathogens - Detection of proteins - Probing of DNA structure - Tissue engineering,- Tumor destruction via heating (hyperthermia) - Separation and purification of biological molecules and cells - MRI contrast enhancement - Phagokinetic studies and to use nanoparticles as biological tags.

8. Antimicrobial activity

Silver has long been known to exhibit a strong toxicity to a wide range of micro-organisms [5]; for this reason silver-based compounds have been used extensively in many bactericidal applications [6]. Silver compounds have also been used in the medical field to treat burns and a variety of infections. Several salts of silver and their derivatives are commercially employed as antimicrobial agents [7].

Silver nanoparticles exhibit a broad size distribution and morphologies with highly reactive facets. The major mechanism through which silver nanoparticles manifested antibacterial properties is by anchoring to and penetrating the bacterial cell wall, and modulating cellular signaling by dephosphorylating putative key peptide substrates on tyrosine residues. The antibacterial effect of nanoparticles is independent of acquisition of resistance by the bacteria against antibiotics.

Recently it was shown that highly concentrated and non hazardous nanosized silver particles can easily be prepared in a cost-effective manner and tested as a new type of bactericidal nanomaterial.

It was hypothesized that the exposed sulfur-bearing residues of the glycoprotein knobs would be attractive sites for nanoparticles interaction but the mechanism underlying the

HIV-inhibitory activity of silver nanoparticles are fully elucidated recently by Elechiguerra et al., (2005). They have done several assays like antiviral activity of silver nanoparticles against various HIV-1 strains, virus adsorption assays, cell-based fusion assays, a gp120/CD4 capture ELISA, time-of-addition experiments, virucidal activity assays with cell-free and cell-associated HIV-1 virus. From these assays, authors come into conclusion that the silver nanoparticles possess anti-HIV activity at an early stage of viral replication, most likely as a virucidal agent or viral entry inhibitor.

Drugs with the ability to dissolve have much stronger efficacy, however many drugs are insoluble. In order to compensate, drugs often need to be administered in higher doses. This increases the possibility of bacteria and other organisms mutating as the high doses make it easier for them to build resistance to the drugs. This leads to treatments becoming obsolete and the need for new medicines to be developed.

Recent data has shown that in some cases, low concentrations of insoluble drugs in a nanoparticle form can be more active than previously thought, offering the potential to administer drugs in low dosages without reducing the effectiveness of the treatment. The new technology is allowing the scientists to develop new medicines by converting currently available drugs into a nanoparticle form.

9. Imaging

One of the greatest values of nanotechnology will be in the development of new and effective medical diagnostics and treatments (i.e. nanomedicine). The ability to image cellular migration *in vivo* could be very useful for studying inflammation, tumors, immune response, and effects of stem cell therapy. Imaging to deliver fluorescent imaging agents to cells--the tiny spheres could help explain how some biological materials such as peptides are able to enter cells.

However, various imaging contrast agents were conjugated to these nanoparticles and results showed the feasibility of tumor imaging using these nanoparticles. Importantly, therapeutic agents can be conjugated or encapsulated to nanoparticles through surface modification and bioconjugation of the nanoparticles. Nanoparticles have been used in experimental paradigms to label and track transplanted human mesenchymal stem cells, neural stem cells, hematopoietic cells, Schwann cells, olfactory ensheathing cells, and oligodendrocyte precursors among others. Several promising cellular transplantation therapies for central nervous system diseases and injury are currently entering human clinical trials. There are many promising research directions that require concerted effort for success. Foremost is the design and development of nanoparticles with mono-, dual- or multiple functions, allowing detection, diagnosis, imaging, transport and controlled release of cargo, and cell destruction. Greater efficacy of lower doses of drugs and destruction of solely the cancer cells could be achieved by selective targeting of unique surface signatures of tumor cells.

Silver was chosen here instead of the traditional gold for several reasons. Silver exhibits slightly stronger and sharper plasmon resonance peaks than gold. This differential implies that silver would provide slightly better absorption of light and thus, stronger photoacoustic signal. Silver is also used in a host of biomedical applications as an antibacterial agent. Some of the most recent advances include silver coated catheters or other orthopedic implant devices. Silver has been shown *in vitro* to be more cytotoxic than gold, especially where the concentration of the silver ion exceeds 5 mg/ml, but silver toxicity is highly debated and it is shown as low concentration as 16-20 ng is sufficient for its antibacterial activity without any toxicity (Kiruba Daniel et al., 2010, 2011 a, b, c, d, and Nimroth Ananth, 2011) [Figure-6].

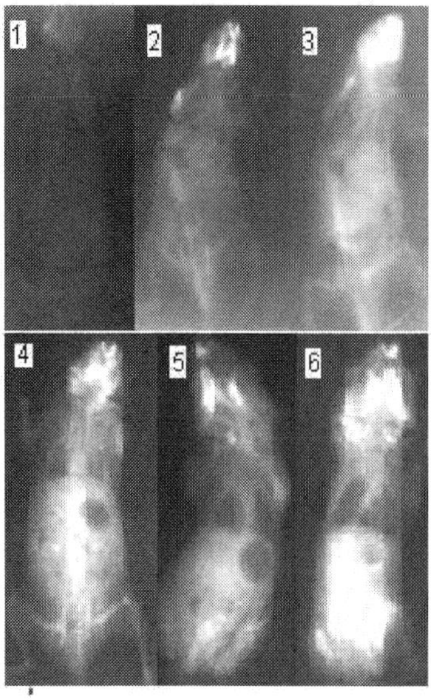

Fig. 6. The whole body X-ray of control mice (1), Silver - polyvinyl alcohol nanoparticle (2) and Silver - Bovine serum albumin nanoparticle injected (3) mice and Drug treated mice (4-6).

10. Multifunctional nanoparticles

Nanoparticles are emerging as promising candidates for various biomedical applications such as enhanced resolution magnetic resonance imaging, drug delivery, tissue repair, cell and tissue targeting and transfection, etc especially for *in vivo* applications, such as drug delivery.

Nanoparticles have a further advantage over larger microparticles, because they are better suited for intravenous delivery. The smallest capillaries in the body are 5-6 mm in diameter. The size of particles being distributed into the bloodstream must be significantly smaller than 5 mm, without forming aggregates, to ensure that the particles do not form an embolism. Nanoparticles can be used to deliver hydrophilic drugs, hydrophobic drugs, proteins, vaccines, biological macromolecules, etc. They can be formulated for targeted delivery to the lymphatic system, brain, arterial walls, lungs, liver, spleen, or made for long-term systemic circulation. Four of the most important characteristics of nanoparticles are their size, encapsulation efficiency, zeta potential (surface charge), and release characteristics.

In practice, silver and gold nanoparticles are the most commonly used nanoparticles for diagnostics and drug delivery. The unique chemical properties of colloidal silver make it a promising targeted delivery approach for drugs or gene specific cells.

11. Biosensor

In order to interact with biological target, a biological or molecular coating or layer acting as a bioinorganic interface should be attached to the nanoparticle. Examples of biological coatings may include antibodies, biopolymers like collagen, or monolayers of small molecules that make the nanoparticles biocompatible. In addition, as optical detection techniques are wide spread in biological research, nanoparticles should either fluoresce or change their optical properties.

A tight control of the average particle size and a narrow distribution of sizes allow creating very efficient fluorescent probes that emit narrow light in a very wide range of wavelengths. This helps with creating biomarkers with many and well distinguished colors. The core itself might have several layers and be multifunctional. For example, combining magnetic and luminescent layers one can both detect and manipulate the particles. Organic molecules that are adsorbed or chemisorbed on the surface of the particle are also used for this purpose. One group is aimed at attaching the linker to the nanoparticle surface and the other is used to bind various moieties like biocompatibles (dextran), antibodies, fluorophores etc., depending on the function required by the application.

12. Protein biosensor

Proteins are the important part of the cell machinery and structure, and understanding their functionalities is extremely important. Surface-enhanced Raman scattering spectroscopy is a well-established technique for detection and identification of single dye molecules. Antibodies are attached to the metal nanoparticles, and the antigen recognition is monitored via the change of light absorption when this binding event occurs.

Silver nanoparticles functionalized with bioreceptors (BSA) for biosensing applications were attempted. Upon binding of proteins to the silver particles, changes in both the intensity and the wavelength of the particle were observed. It can be used for biosensing using silver nanoparticle coated with any protein or any antibody, based on a resonance enhancement. Furthermore, this novel approach is promising as an alternative for conventional biosensing techniques [Figure 2] Nimroth Ananth et al.2011)[Figure-7 and 8].

13. Genosensors/diagnostic agent

The nanoparticles are coated with hydrophilic oligonucleotides containing a Raman dye at one end and terminally capped with a small molecule recognition element (e.g. biotin). Moreover, this molecule is catalytically active and will be coated with silver in the solution of silver (I) and hydroquinone. After the probe is attached to a small molecule or an antigen it is designed to detect, the substrate is exposed to silver and hydroquinone solution. A silver-plating is happening close to the Raman dye, which allows for dye signature detection with a standard Raman microscope. Apart from being able to recognize small molecules this probe can be modified to contain antibodies on the surface to recognize proteins. When tested in the protein array format against both small molecules and proteins, the probe has shown no cross-reactivity. Not only is the absorbance originating from plasmon resonances of the particles influenced by the dielectric properties of molecules attached to the nanospheres but also the inter band absorption of the particles changes [Figure-9]. This change in absorption can be very large when adhered molecules are at resonance (inter band transitions). In addition, the presented type of biosensing can be a cost-effective and easy to use alternative to conventional biosensing techniques.

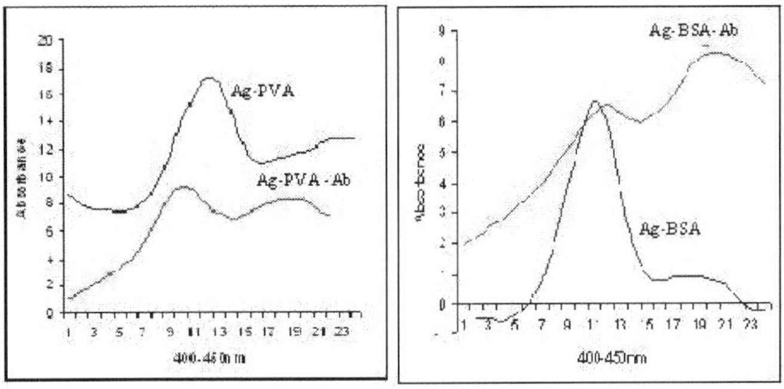

Fig. 7. Fluorescence Spectrum of Silver - polyvinyl alcohol and Silver - Bovine serum albumin nanoparticles with mice(3) and without antibody binding .

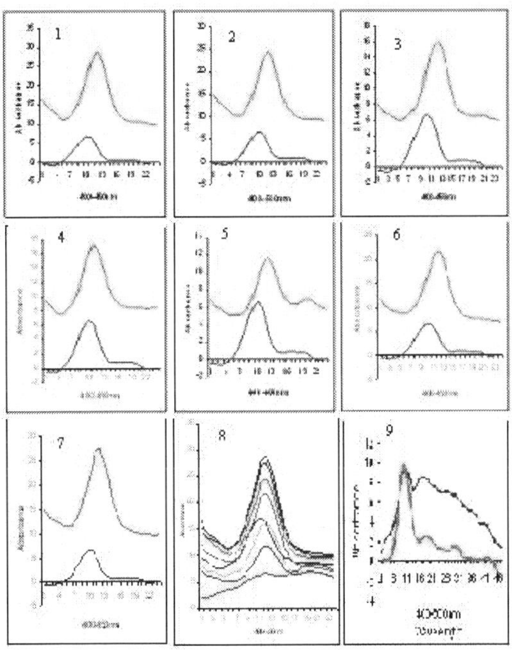

Fig. 8. UV-visible absorption pattern of Silver - Bovine serum albumin with (pink) and without (blue line) antiBSA in the visible region (400-450 nm) in different tissue samples 1. Liver 2.Kidney 3.Spleen 4.Lungs 5.Heart 6.Intestine 7.Brain 8.Comparitive pattern of all tissues 9. Positive control.

Applications of DNA-conjugated nanostructures have shown improvement in not only size, but also performance. For example, noncomputational tiling arrays have been used as molecular scale circuit components (He et al., 2009) either by the chemistry between DNA and molecular electrodes (He et al., 2009), or by the use of gold beads (Martin et al., 1999). Nano mechanical devices have also been created that undergo conformational change due to environmental change, (Mao et al., 1999; Chen et al., 2004; Liu et al., 2007) strand displacement, (Yan et al., 2002) such as the nano walker, (Sherman & Seeman, 2004; Shin & Pierce, 2004) or enzymatic activity, (Yin et al., 2004; Park et al., 2002). Lastly, the optical properties brought about by aggregation and network formation can be used as a tool in DNA-detection. Some examples include the diagnosis of genetic diseases, RNA profiling, biodefense, (Kushon et al., 2003; Lockhart and Winzeler, 2000; Hill et al. 2000; gene chips, (Lipshutz et al. 1999) detection of UV damage, (Jiang et al. 2007) and single-molecule sequencing, (Austin et al. 1997) including the use of nanopores,(Branton et al. 2008; Storm et al. 2003; Gerland et al. 2004). Our study is only one type of many novel biosensors developed using SPR technology [Figure-8].

14. Cancer treatment

Nanotechnology has become an enabling technology for personalized medicine in which cancer detection, diagnosis, and therapy. The promises of nanotechnology in cancer research lie in the potential to overcome the drawbacks such as side effects and toxicity to healthy cells that come across in the current cancer treatment (surgery, radiation, and chemotherapy).

Rational design of nanoparticles requires the knowledge of tumor-specific receptors that would allow endocytosis of nanoparticles, tumor-specific biomarkers that facilitate identification of cancers, and tumor-specific homing proteins and enzymes that can permit selective uptake into cells or accumulation in tumor micro environments.

Several nanobiotechnologies mostly based on nanoparticles, have been used to facilitate drug delivery in cancer. As tumor architecture causes nanoparticles to preferentially accumulate at the tumor site, their use as drug delivery vectors results in the localization of a greater amount of the drug load at the tumor site; thus improving cancer therapy.

Nanotechnology has tremendous potential to make an important contribution in cancer prevention, detection, diagnosis, imaging and treatment. It can target a tumor, carry imaging capability to document the presence of tumor, sense pathophysiological defects in tumor cells, deliver therapeutic genes or drugs based on tumor characteristics, respond to external triggers Gene delivery offers the potentials to (a) replace missing or defective genes; (b) deliver genes that catalyze the destruction of cancer cells; (c) cause cancer cells to revert back to normal tissue,(O'Connor et al., 2006).

Nanoshells are layered colloids with a nonconducting nanoparticle core covered by a thin metal shell, whose thickness can be changed to precisely tune the plasmon resonance. Proteins that bind only with tumor cells can be attached to the surface, creating tumor-seeking nanoparticles. By tuning the shells to strongly absorb 820 nm NIR light, where optical transmission through body tissue is optimal and harmless, low-power extracorporeally applied laser light shone at the patient induces a response signal from injected nanoshells clustered around a tumor. Increasing the laser power to a still moderately low exposure heats the nanoshells just enough to destroy the tumor without harming healthy tissue. On exposure to 35 W/cm^2 NIR light, human breast carcinoma cells incubated with nanoshells *in vitro* undergo photothermally induced morbidity. Cells without nanoshells display no loss in viability. Likewise, *in vivo* studies under magnetic resonance guidance reveal that exposure to low-dose (4 W/cm^2) NIR light in solid tumors treated with nanoshells incur a temperature increase of 37.4±6.6°C within 4-6 minutes. The tissue displays coagulation, cell shrinkage, and loss of nuclear staining, indicating irreversible thermal damage. Controls treated without nanoshells demonstrated significantly lower temperatures and appeared undamaged. Miniscule beads coated with gold are also Nanoshells. By manipulating the thickness of the layers making up the nanoshells, scientists can design these beads to absorb specific wavelengths of light. The most useful nanoshells are those that absorb near-infrared light, which can easily penetrate several centimeters of human tissue. The absorption of light by the nanoshells creates an intense heat that is lethal to cells.

Researchers can already link nanoshells to antibodies that recognize cancer cells. Scientists envision letting these nanoshells seek out their cancerous targets, then applying near-infrared light. In laboratory cultures, the heat generated by the light-absorbing nanoshells has successfully killed tumor cells while leaving neighboring cells intact. To achieve tumor-targeted drug delivery, nanoparticle systems must address technical and biological concerns that influence their distribution.

15. Gene/Drug delivery

Gene delivery systems are used in the field of gene therapy to introduce foreign DNA encoding therapeutic protein sequences into cells. Several gene delivery systems have been developed to promote gene expression either *in vitro* or *in vivo*. Among them, viral methods are well known and can be extremely efficient (viral vectors were used in the first human gene therapy test), but the safety (including the immunogenicity and the risk associated with replication-competent viruses) and production issues of viral vectors have stimulated efforts toward the development of nonviral gene delivery systems such as cationic lipids, polymers and other mechanical and electrical methods. Among the nonviral gene delivery systems, novel biocompatible polymers have gained increasing attention and been examined for their properties as gene carriers. Although the use of polymeric gene carriers may overcome the current problems associated with viral vectors in safety, immunogenicity and mutagenesis, they are usually inefficient and toxic. Inefficient endosomal release, cytoplasmic transport and nuclear entry of plasmids are currently the limiting factors in the use of polymers for effective plasmid-based gene therapy.

Gene expression detection can provide powerful insights into the chemistry and physiology of biological systems. Better understanding of the molecular mechanisms underlying biological processes can be achieved by comparing gene expression between cells in different states or between cells from different tissues. Furthermore,an abnormally expressed gene can be used as a new drug target or as a genetic marker for diagnosis.

A major requirement for gene therapy is the efficient transport of DNA through the cell membrane by processes that are not well defined.Because potentially a large number of different genes need to be transported, and different types of organs and tissues whose cells need to be targeted for genetic therapy of different diseases, a broad range of gene delivery technologies is necessary for effective treatments.

Development of efficient gene therapeutics would depend largely on the availability of vectors that allow an efficient and selective delivery of therapeutic genes to target cells with minimal toxicity (Wagner et al.,2004; Wang and Yuan,2006; Niidome and Huang,2002). Because potentially a large variety of very different genes need to be delivered and many types of organs and tissues that cells need to be targeted for the therapy of different diseases, an immensely broad range of gene delivery technologies is foreseen to be necessary to cater for all the conceivable applications and treatments, (Lawson, 2006; Glover et al.,2005; Larin et al.2004).

Silver nanoparticles have increasingly attracted more attentions because of their promising applications in the fields of catalysis, (Musi et al. 2009; Shin et al. 2009; Tian et al. 2009) electronics, (Xia et al. 2003) sensing, (Guo et al., 2009; Zhao et al., 2009; Nimroth Ananth et al., 2011) and surface-enhanced Raman scattering (Sun et al., 2009) etc.

DNA has particular advantages to produce silver nanomaterials, (Shemer et al., 2006; Sengupta et al., 2009) because of its unique self-assembly and mechanical properties, as well as the high affinity with silver cations. As silver cations prefer to associate with heterocyclic bases rather than balance negative charges of the phosphate backbone, (Eichhorn, 1973) it is intriguing to investigate the influence of particular DNA structures on the formation and the properties of silver nanoparticles.

The nanoparticles are usually coated with hydrophilic and biocompatible polymers/molecules. Clays are naturally occurring aluminosilicate materials composed primarily of alumina, silica and water with small amounts of metal cations such as Ca^{2+}, Fe^{3+}, K^{+}, Mg^{2+} and Na^{+} also present,(Izatt et al., 1971). Clays have interesting chemical and physical characteristics, e.g., montmorillonite has a high modulus, high cation exchange capacity, a large surface area to mass ratio, and the ability to form stable dispersions in aqueous solutions (Marzilli, 1977).

The unique features of clays have led to their widespread use in materials developed for the automotive, medical, food and cosmetics industries (Marzilli, 1977). In addition, clays have been used successfully as vectors for delivery of DNA into cells in recent experiments (Shamsi and Geckeler, 2008). The concept of green nanoparticles preparation using b-D-glucose as the reducing agent was first reported by Raveendran et al., (2003) where starch played the role of stabilizer. Soluble starch, the amylose component of starch, is a linear polymer formed by the alpha-(1-4) linkages between D-glucose units and adopts a left-handed helical conformation in aqueous solution. In this report, the aldehyde terminal of soluble starch is used to reduce silver nitrate while the starch itself stabilized the silver nanoparticles. Temperature accelerates the reduction process by aldehydes. The extensive number of hydroxyl groups present in soluble starch facilitates the complexation of silver ions to the molecular matrix while the aldehyde terminals helped in reduction of the same (Pinnavaia and Beall, 2000).

Synthesis of silver nanoparticles using citrate and poly lysine was also reported earlier. Organics like sodium citrate, ascorbic acid and amino acids capable of being oxidized also used as alternate methods,(Rivas et al., 2001;Zhu Shiguo et al., 2002). All the silver nanoparticles preparations showed partical size of 20-25nm.

Plasmid pCDNA-GFP was studied in terms of their degree of adsorption on montmorillonite, silver nanoparticles stabilized with montmorillonite clay, starch, citrate, polylysine and multiwalled carbon nanotubes [Figure 7].

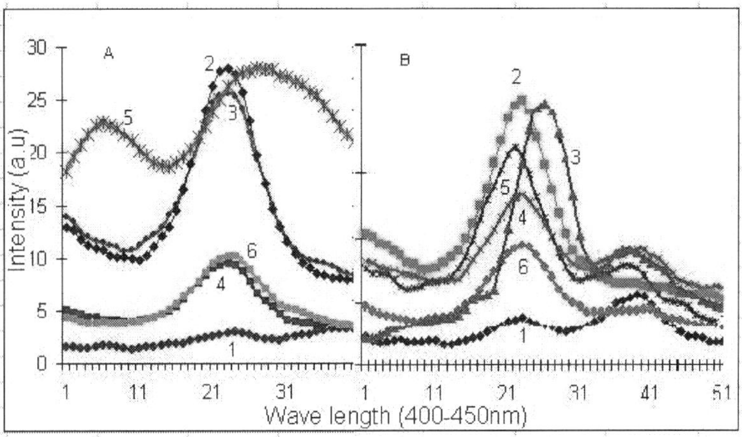

Fig. 9. The fluorescence spectrum (400-500nm) of control and plasmid DNA functionalized nanopreparations. 1.clay 2.silver- clay 3.silver-starch 4.silver-citrate 5.silver-poly lysine nanoparticles 6.Multiwalled carbon nanotubes.

DNA molecules are net negatively-charged, and they can adsorb to net positively-charged surfaces, such as the edges of clay minerals (Nath et al., 2007) as well as to net negatively-charged surfaces, such as the surfaces of clays, by electrostatic bridges with the water of hydration of charge-compensating cations (Paul et al., 2010). Under acidic conditions (generally below pH 5), DNA becomes positively charged by protonation of adenine and cytosine, followed by guanine, and by protonation of the negative charges of phosphate groups. This protonation produces cationic groups in the DNA molecule that can bind to negatively-charged sites on clays. The location and strength of the acidic groups of DNA determine the interaction between clay and DNA. Super coiled plasmid DNA interacts by a low number of strongly acidic groups, presumably located at the maximum of bending of the double strand where a high charge density exists. Linear chromosomal molecules appear to attach on the clay surface and edges, as demonstrated by previous observations, through acidic groups distributed along the DNA molecules.

Citric acid forms only two bonds with silver (1 0 0) because of the geometry mismatch. Migration of a hydrogen atom within citric acid activates the electrons of the carboxyl oxygen and provides additional binding affinity towards silver (1 1 1). The preferential binding energy of citric acid to silver (1 1 1) promotes crystal growth along the silver (1 0 0) surface (Rivas et al., 2001). Cationic Poly-L-lysine interacts with DNA cooperatively at high sodium chloride concentrations and in excess of DNA, and produces DNA particles with various structures, depending upon the concentration of monovalent ions in the medium (Zhu Shiguo et al., 2002).

Cationic carbon nanotubes are able to condense DNA to varying degrees, indicating that both nanotube surface area and charge density are critical parameters that determine the interaction and electrostatic complex formation between functionalized carbon nanotubes with DNA. Upon the addition of divalent metal ions super coiled plasmid DNA forms relatively stable complexes with carbon nanotubes due to chelation. The degree of binding

and tight association between DNA and nanotubes is a desirable trait to increase gene expression efficiency *in vitro* or *in vivo* (Khanna et al., 1998).
Transfection efficiency of these nanoparticles was then assessed on liver cells *in vitro*, using a plasmid containing a fusion of an enhanced green fluorescent protein (pCDNA-GFP) reporter gene [Figure-10]. The intensity was measured and transfection efficiencies were compared [Figure-11]. These results implied that this gene vector based on silver nanoparticles prepared with starch and clay as stabilizing agents could be a promising gene delivery system. Differences in the levels of gene expression were correlated with the structural and biophysical data obtained for the various products including multiwalled carbon nanotube -DNA complexes to suggest that large surface area leading to very efficient DNA condensation is not necessary for effective gene transfer.

Fig. 10. Transfection of Liver cells with Silver -starch funtionalized with pCDNA-GFP.
1. Cells under phase contrast microscope 2. Cells under Fluorescence microscope.

16. Therapeutics

Nanoparticles based diagnostics and therapeutics hold great promise because multiple functions can be built into the particles. Among noble-metal nanoparticles, silver nanoparticles have received considerable attention due to their attractive physicochemical properties and the strong toxicity that to a wide range of microorganisms.
Therapeutics and protection of ornamental gold fishes against red spot and white spot diseases was attempted. The results demonstrated the uptake of nano particles by fish via the gills and body surface, and a cure within 7days with a weight gain and without showing any toxicity. The starch stabilized silver nanoparticles could penetrate all tissues including the brain through BBB. The fishes showed resistance to re infection and hence life time protection can be given to diseased fishes at very low concentration (0.016ng/ml) by simple bathing method. This is the first report on silver nanoparticle therapy against protozoan and fungal infections in fishes [Figure-12] (paper communicated).
Surface modification of metal nanostructures can create multifunctional materials potentially very useful in many application fields and consequently, Silver has been used as therapeutic molecule.

Silver nanoparticles offer a wide range of surface functional groups allowing conjugation to multiple diagnostic and therapeutic agents. Multifunctional nanostructures could be used for simultaneous targeting, imaging and treatment, a major goal in nanomedicine.

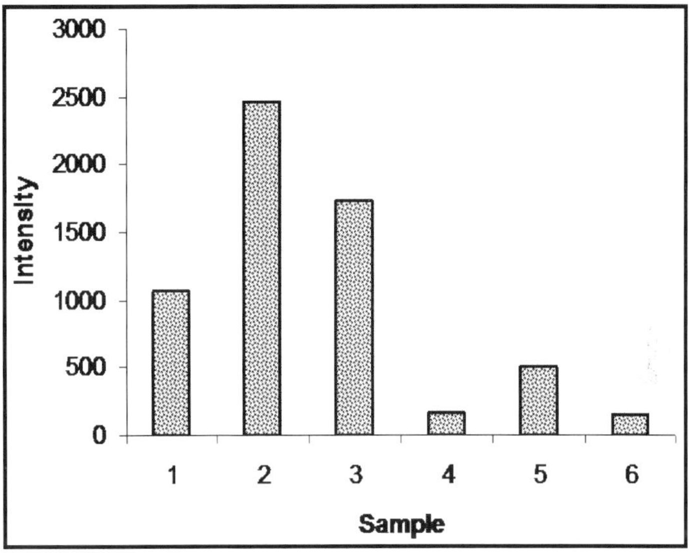

Fig. 11. Gene expression pattern of (GFP intensity) plasmid DNA functionalized nanopreparations. 1. clay, 2. silver- clay, 3. silver-starch, 4. silver-citrate, 5. silver-poly lysine nanoparticles, 6. Multiwalled carbon nanotubes.

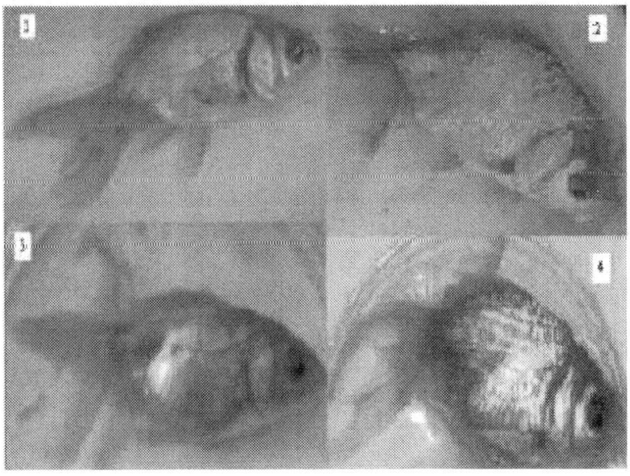

Fig. 12. Red Spot diseased fish before(1) & after treatment (3) White Spot diseased fish before (2) and after treatment (4) Silver nanoparticle treatment.

17. Development and commercialization of nanomaterials

Drug delivery techniques were established to deliver or control the amount, rate and, sometimes location of a drug in the body to optimize its therapeutic effect, convenience and dose. Combining a well established drug formulation with a new delivery system is a relatively low risk activity and can be used to enhance a company's product portfolio by extending the drug's commercial life-cycle. Although not exhausting, this is a representative selection reflecting current industrial trends. Many companies are involved in the development and commercialisation of nanomaterials in biological and medical applications.

Most companies are developing pharmaceutical applications, mainly for drug delivery. Most major and established pharmaceutical companies have internal research programs on drug delivery that are on formulations or dispersions containing components down to nano sizes.

Most of the companies are developing pharmaceutical applications, mainly for drug delivery. Several companies exploit quantum size effects in semiconductor nanocrystals for tagging biomolecules, or use bio-conjugated gold nanoparticles for labelling various cellular parts. A number of companies are applying nano-ceramic materials to tissue engineering and orthopaedics

Colloidal silver is widely used in anti-microbial formulations and dressings. The high reactivity of titania nanoparticles, either on their own or then illuminated with UV light, is also used for bactericidal purposes in filters. Enhanced catalytic properties of surfaces of nano-ceramics or those of noble metals like platinum are used to destruct dangerous toxins and other hazardous organic materials.

Nanotechnology is the application of nanoscience. Nanotechnology is being seen as a science having potential to create many new materials with specific properties and devices with wide ranging applications in medicine, electronics and energy production. A lot of research is being carried out in all the branches of science which is expected to result in revolutionary progress in the field of nanoscience and nanotechnology. Already many nanotechnology based industries have come up with products like flat plate display unit using the concept of electron field emission by carbon nano tubes; devices using antimicrobial activity of nano-silver, water purification, crease free textile material, nano sensors and nano probes etc are in the market. The near future nanotechnology based products being envisaged are fuel cell, hydrogen storage, solar cell, super capacitors, lithium battery, microwave absorption, bullet proof jackets, drug delivery, diagnostic devices etc. The desire to be part of the global market, nanotechnology is diversifying into many innovative new fields which have generated lots of hope and hype. Research & Development with an eye on commercialization efforts of this young technology are continuing unabatedly across the globe.

Sustained world class R&D through funding multidisciplinary research and development is the prerequisite. Infrastructure availability is crucial to assist businesses, especially small companies that cannot afford the cost of nanotechnology instrumentation, equipment and facilities. There should be cooperation between university and industry. This will suffice the need of basic science innovations, expensive laboratories, and for highly trained workers.

18. Future opportunities and challenges

Nanotechnology has received much attention from scientists and journalists in the last few years raising hopes of revolutionary developments in a wide range of technologies on an increasingly small scale, dramatic improvements to standards of living, and solutions to a variety of environmental, medical and communications problems.

Silver nanoparticles have already been applied as drug delivery systems with great success. Nanoparticles provides massive advantages regarding drug targeting, delivery and release and with their potential for combine diagnosis and therapy and one of the major tools in nanomedicine. These are many technical challenges in developing the following techniques:- virus- like systems for intracellular systems, architecting of biomimetic polymers, control of sensitive drugs, functions of active drug targeting, bioresponsive triggered systems, systems interacting with the person (body smart delivery), nanochips for nanoparticle release, carriers for advanced polymers for the delivery of therapeutic peptide / proteins.

As it stands now, the majority of commercial nanoparticle applications in medicine are geared towards drug delivery. In biosciences, nanoparticles are replacing organic dyes in the applications that require high photo-stability as well as high multiplexing capabilities. There are some developments in directing and remotely controlling the functions of nano-probes, for example driving magnetic nanoparticles to the tumour and then making them either to release the drug load or just heating them in order to destroy the surrounding tissue. The major trend in further development of nanomaterials is to make them multifunctional and controllable by external signals or by local environment thus essentially turning them into nano-devices.

19. Biosafety

Silver nanoparticles have been shown to damage brain cells (Hussain et al., 2006), liver cells (Hussain et al., 2005) and stem cells (Braydich-Stolle et al., 2005). Even with prolonged exposure to colloidal silver salt deposits of metallic silver under the skin cause skin diseases like argyria or argyrosis (Chen et al.,2007). Silver nanoparticles at 10 ug/ml and above concentration showed dramatic changes like necrosis and apoptosis of cells. Silver at 5-10 ug/ml,drastically reduced mitochondrial function and cell viability.

Silver metal and silver dressings, when used in reasonable has no negative effects on the human body and it has a natural antimicrobial (Margaret et al.,2006; Sarkar et al., 2007) towards many pathogens such as bacteria (Hill and Pillsbury,1939;Zhang and Sun,2007), viruses, fungi, yeast etc. New silver coated catheters are used because they stop the infections that were common place with the old ones. To protect us from food poisoning, silver particles are now being put in cutting boards, table tops, surface disinfectants and refrigerators. Silver is woven and impregnated into fabrics to kill bacteria that cause body odor.

In vivo tests have been completed, both injected and ingested at silver levels as high as 5000 milligrams per kilogram of a 32 part per million product.LD-50 tests have also been completed at a level of up to 200 times the normal adult dosage.Cellular or cyto-toxicity tests have also been completed on both the 10 ppm and also the 22 ppm products on both human epithelial cells and also on African green monkey cells. The products were found to be completely safe; they did not hurt the human or monkey cells in any way, shape or form.

20. Environmental safety

Silver nanoparticles will grow to biologically far less active clumps even if one dumps 27 liters of 20 ppm colloidal silver on each ton of soil. Because of the low concentrations in which silver nanoparticles based products are sold, the total amount which could be released in any part of the environment would still be expected to be very low. Silver nanoparticles are not water soluble, and therefore, silver colloids will not release silver ions into the environment. Silver nanoparticles do not last as nanoparticles in nature for very long, but grow to harmless clumps of silver metal which has existed in nature from the beginning of our planet.

Silver nanoparticles based diagnostics and therapeutics hold great promise because multiple functions can be built onto the particles. The potential applicability of these silver nanoparticles in the present approach is simple, sensitive and selective for the versatile applications related to diagnostics and therapeutics. The usage of silver nanoparticles is safe to consumer health and environment.

21. References

[1] Mukherjee P, Ahmad A, Mandal D, Senapati S, Sainkar Sudhakar R, Khan MI, et al. (2001) Nano Lett.1:515.

[2] Sondi I, Branka SS (2004) J.Colloid Interface Sci.275:177.

[3] Chen X, Schluesener HJ (2008) Toxicol Lett.176:1.

[4] Chen JP (2007) J. InVasiVe Cardiol. 19 (9): 395.

[5] Woodleand MC, Lu PY (2000) Nanotoday 8:34.

[6] Shiraishi Y, Toshima N (2000) Colloids Surf A Physicochem. Eng. Asp.169:59. doi:10.1016/S0927-7757(00)00417-9

[7] Chang LT, Yen CC (1995) J. Appl.Polym.Sci.55(2):371. doi:10. 1002/ app. 1995. 070550219)

[8] Sharverdi AR, Mianaeian S, Shahverdi HR, Jamalifar H, Nohi AA (2007) Process Biochem.42:919 doi:10.1016/j.procbio.2007.02.005.

[9] Matejka P, Vlckova B, Vohlidal J, Pancoska P, Baumruk V (1992) J.Phys. Chem. 96(3):1361 doi:10.1021/j100182a063.

[10] Musi A, Massiani P, Brouri D, Trichard JM, Da Costa P (2009) Catal Lett. 128:25.

[11] Shin KS, Choi JY, Park CS, Jang HJ, Kim K (2009) Catal Lett.133:1.

[12] Tian D, Yong GP, Dai Y, Yan XY, Liu SM (2009) Catal Lett.130:211.

[13] Xia YN, Yang PD, Sun YG, Wu YY, Mayers B, Gates B, Yin YD,Kim F, Yan YQ (2003) Adv Mater 15:353.

[14] Guo WW, Yuan JP, Wang EK (2009) Chem. Commun. (23):3395.

[15] Zhao K, Chang QF, Chen X, Zhang BC, Liu JH (2009) Mater Sci.Eng. C 29:1191.

[16] Sun L, Sun Y, Xu F, Zhang Y, Yang T, Guo C, Liu Z, Li Z (2009) Nanotechnology 20:125502.

[17] Skrabalak SE, Xia YA (2009) ACS Nano 3:10.

[18] Xia Y, Xiong YJ, Lim B, Skrabalak SE (2009) Angew Chem Int.Ed 48:60.

[19] Yu DG (2007) Colloid Surf. B 59: 171.

[20] Tan Y, Wang Y, Jiang L, et al. (2002) J. Colloid Interf. Sci. 249:336.

[21] Petit C, Lixon P, Pileni MP (1993) J. Phys. Chem. 97:12974.

[22] Vorobyova SA, Lesnikovich AI, Sobal NS (1999)Colloid Surf. A 152:375.

[23] Mallick K, Witcombb MJ, Scurrella MS (2005) Mater. Chem. Phys. 90:221.

[24] Keki S, Torok J, Deak G, et al. (2000) J. Colloid Interf. Sci. 229:550.

[25] Pileni, MP(2000) Pure Appl.Chem.72:53. doi:10.1351/pac200072010053

[26] Sun YP, Atorngitjawat P, Meziani MJ (2001) Langmuir 17(19):5707. doi:10.1021/la0103057.

[27] Liu YC, Lin LH (2004) Electrochem. Commun. 6:1163.
[28] Sandmann G, Dietz H, Plieth W (2000) J. Electroanal. Chem. 491:78.
[29] Bae CH, Nam SH, Park SM (2002) Appl. Surf. Sci. 197:628.
[30] Smetana AB, Klabunde KJ, Sorensen CM (2005)J. Colloid Interf.Sci.284:521.
[31] Esumi K, Isono R, Yoshimura T (2004) Langmuir 20:237.
[32] Murugadoss A, Chattopadhyay A (2008) Nanotechnology 19:1.
[33] Zhang HJ, Li XY, Chen GH (2009) J Mater Chem./8223.
[34] Sun YG, Xia YN (2002) Science 298:2176.
[35] Bhattacharya R, Mukherjee P.(2008) AdvDrug Deliv Rev.60:1289.
[36] Nair B, Pradeep T (2002) Cryst Growth Des.2(4):293. doi:10.1021/cg0255164
[37] Joerger R, Klaus T, Granqvist CG (2000) Adv Mater 12(6):407. doi:10.1002/(SICI)1521-4095(200003)12:6\407::AID-ADMA407[3.0.CO;2-O
[38] Klaus T, Joergere R, Olsson E, Granqvist CG (2001) Trends Biotechnol.19:15. doi:10.1016/S0167-7799(00)01514-6
[39] Ahmad A, Mukherjee P, Senapati S, Mandal D, Khan MI,Kumar R, Sastry M (2003) Colloids Surf B Biointerfaces 28:313.
[40] Vigneshwaran N, Ashtaputre NM, Varadarajan PV, N9achane RP, Paralikar KM, Balasubramanya RH (2007) Mater Lett.61:1413. doi:10.1016/j.matlet.2006.07.042
[41] Willner I, Baron R, Willner B, (2006) Adv. Mater., 18:1109.
[42] Shankar SS, Rai A, Ahmad A, Sastry M, (2004)J. Colloid Interf.Sci. 275: 496.
[43] Sanghi R, Verma P (2009) Bioresour Technol. 100:501.
[44] Gardea-Torresdey JL, Gomez E, Peralta-Videa JR, Parsons JG, Troiani H, Jose-Yacaman M (2003) Langmuir 19:1357.
[45] Gardea-Torresdey JL, Rodriguez E, Parsons-Jason G, Peralta-Videa JR, Meitzner EG, Cruz-Jimenez G (2005) Anal. Bioanal. Chem. 382: 347.
[46] Shivshankar S, Ahmad A, Sastry M (2003) Biotechnol. Prog.19:1627.
[47] Shivshankar S, Rai A, Ahmad A, Sastry M (2004) Colloid Interface Sci.275: 496.
[48] Shivshankar S, Rai A, Ahmad A, Sastry M (2005) Chem. Mater.17:566.
[49] Ankamwar B, Chaudhary M, Sastry M (2005) Synth. React. Inorg. Metal-Org. Nanometal. Chem.35: 19.
[50] Prathap SC, Chaudhary M, Pasricha R, Ahmad A, Sastry M (2006) Biotechnol. Prog. 22: 577.
[51] Kasthuri J, Veerapandian S, Rajendiran N (2009) Colloids and Surfaces B: Biointerfaces 68:55.
[52] Kasthuri J, Kathiravan K, Rajendiran N (2009) J Nanopart Res.11:1075.
[53] Jae Yong Song, Beom Soo Kim (2008) Korean J. Chem. Eng. 25(4): 808.
[54] Raut Rajesh W1, Lakkakula Jaya R1, Kolekar Niranjan S1, Mendhulkar Vijay D1, Kashid Sahebrao B (2009) Current Nanoscience, 5: 117.
[55] Sathishkumar M, Sneha K, Won SW, Cho CW, Kim S, Yun YS (2009) Colloids and Surfaces B: Biointerfaces 73:332.
[56] Krishnaraj C, Jagan EG, Rajasekar S, Selvakumar P, Kalaichelvan PT, Mohan N (2010) Colloids and Surfaces B: Biointerfaces 76: 50.
[57] Daizy Philip (2009) Spectrochimica Acta Part A 73: 374.
[58] Daizy Philip (2010) Physica E 42: 1417.
[59] Harekrishna Bar, Dipak Kr. Bhui, Gobinda P. Sahoo, Priyanka Sarkar, Santanu Pyne, Ajay Misra (2009) Colloids and Surfaces A: Physicochem. Eng. Aspects 348: 212.

[60] Kiruba Daniel SCG, Ayyappan S, John Paul Philiphan N, Sivakumar M, Menaga G, Anitha Sironmani T (2011) Int.J.Nanoscience and Nanotechnology (in press)
[61] Kiruba Daniel SCG, Kumar R, Sathish V, Sivakumar M, Sunitha S, Anitha Sironmani T (2011) Int.J.Nanoscience and Nanotechnology 2(2)103.
[62] Sengupta B, Springer K, Buckman JG, Story SP, Abe OH, Hasan ZW, Prudowsky ZD, Rudisill SE, Degtyareva NN, Petty JT (2009) J.Phys.Chem.C 113:19518.
[63] Shemer G, Krichevski O, Markovich G, Molotsky T, Lubitz I, Kotlyar AB(2006) J.Am.Chem.Soc.128:11006.
[64] Nimrodh Ananth A, Kiruba Daniel SCG, Anitha Sironmani T, Umapathi(2011) Colloids and surfaces B 85: 138.
[65] Kneipp K, Kneipp H, Itzkan I, Dasari RR, Feld MS (2002) J. Phys. 14:R597.
[66] Kneipp K, Wang Y, Kneipp H, Perelman LT, Itzkan I, Dasari RR, Feld MS (1997) Phys. Rev. Lett. 78: 1667.
[67] Kleemann W (1993) Int. J. Mod. Phys. B 7: 2469.
[68] Aoki K, Chen J, Yang N, Nagasawa H (2003) Langmuir 19: 9904.
[69] Chalmers JM, Griffiths PR (2002) Handbook of Vibrational Spectroscopy; Wiley: New York.
[70] Klabunde KJ (2001) Nanoscale Materials in Chemistry; Wiley:New York.
[71] Lovric J, Bazzi HS, Cuie Y, Fortin GR, Winnik FM, Maysinger D (2005) J Mol Med.83: 377.
[72] Asharani PV, Low GKM, Hande MP, Valiyaveettil S (2009). ACS Nano 3: 279.
[73] Raynal I, Prigent P, Peyramaure S, Najid A, Rebuzzi C, Corot C (2004) Invest. Radiol. 39: 56.
[74] Bourrinet P, Bengele HH, Bonnemain B, DenCausse A, Idee JM, Jacobs PM, Lewis JM (2006) Invest.Radiol. 41: 313.
[75] Briley-Saebo KC, Johansson LO, Hustvedt SO, Haldorsen AG (2006) Invest. Radiol. 41: 560.
[76] Chang JM, Lee JM, Lee MW, Han JK, Kim SH, Lee JY, Choi SH, Choi BI (2006) Invest. Radiol. 41: 168.
[77] Cai, Quan-Yu, Kim, Sun Hee, Choi, Kyu Sil, Kim, Soo Yeon, Byun, Seung Jae, Kim, Kyoung Woo, Park, Seong Hoon, Juhng, Seon Kwan, Yoon, Kwon-Ha (2007) Invest. Radiol. 42: 797.
[78] Kobayashi H, Jo SK, Kawamoto S, Yasuda H, Hu X, Knopp MV, Brechbiel MW, Choyke PL, Star RA (2004) J. Magn. Reson. Imaging 20(3): 512.
[79] Garnacho, Carmen, Dhami, Rajwinder, Simone, Eric, Dziubla, Thomas, Leferovich, John,Schuman, Edward H, Muzvkantov, Vladimir, Muro, Silvia (2008) J. Pharmacol. Exp. Ther. 107: 133298.
[80] Caroline MF, Graeme JS, George GFGT, Martin JB (1999) Br. J. Pharmacol. 126 (7):1634.
[81] Friedman M, McDonald GM (1997) Crit. Rev. Plant Sci. 16: 55.
[82] Hainfeld JF, Slatkin DN, Focella TM, Smilowitz HM (2006) Br. J. Radiol. 79: 248.
[83] Morones JR, Elechiguerra JL, Camacho A, Holt K, Kouri JB, Ramirez JT, Yacaman MJ (2005) J.Nanotechnology 16:2346.
[84] He J, Lin L, Liu H, Zhang P, Lee M, Sankey OF, Lindsay SM (2009) Nanotechnology 20:075102-1-8
[85] Martin BR, Dermody DJ, Reiss BD, Fang M, Lyon LA, Natan MJ, Mallouk TE (1999) Adv.Mater. 11:1021.

[86] Mao C, Sun W, Shen Z, Seeman NC (1999) Nature 397:144.
[87] Chen Y, Lee SH, Mao C (2004) Angew Chem.Int.Ed.43: 5335.
[88] Liu H, Xu Y, Li F, Yang Y, Wang W, Song Y, Liu D (2007) Angew Chem.Int.Ed. 46: 2515.
[89] Yan H, Zhang X, Shen Z, Seeman NC (2002) Nature 415:62.
[90] Sherman WB, Seeman NC (2004) Nano Lett. 4:1203.
[91] Shin JS, Pierce NA (2004) J.Am. Chem.Soc.126:10834.
[92] Yin P, Yan H, Daniell XG, Turberfield AJ, Reif JH (2004) Angew Chem.Int. Ed.43, 4906.
[93] Park SJ, Taton TA, Mirkin CA (2002) Science 295:1503.
[94] Kushon SA, Bradford K, Marin V, Suhrada C, Armitage BA, McBranch D, Whitten D (2003) Langmuir 19: 6456.
[95] Lockhart DJ, Winzeler EA (2000) Nature 405: 827.
[96] Hill AA, Hunter CP, Tsung BT, Tucker-Kellogg G, Brown EL (2000) Science 290: 809.
[97] Lipshutz RJ, Fodor SP, Gingeras TR, Lockhart DJ (1999) Nat.Genet. 21: 20.
[98] Jiang YC, Mieczkowski PA, Marszalek PE (2007) Biophys.Journal 93: 1758.
[99] Austin RH, Brody JP, Cox EC, Duke T, Volkmuth W (1997) Phys .Today 50:32.
[100] Branton et al.(2008) Nature- Biotechnology 26:1146.
[101] Storm AJ, Chen JH, Ling XS, Zandbergen HW, Dekker C (2003) Natural Materials 2: 537.
[102] Gerland U, Bundschuh R, Hwa T (2004) Phys. Biol.1:19.
[103] O'Connor TP, Crystal RG (2006) Nat Rev Genet 7: 261.
[104] Wagner E, Kircheis R, Walker GF (2004) Biomed Pharmacother. 58: 152.
[105] Wang Y, Yuan F (2006) Ann.Biomed Eng. 34: 114.
[106] Niidome T, Huang L.(2002) Gene Ther. 9: 1647.
[107] Lawson C (2006) Methods Mol Biol.333: 175.
[108] Glover DJ, Lipps HJ, Jans DA (2005) Nat Rev Genet. 6: 299.
[109] Larin SS, Georgiev GP, Kiselev SL (2004) Gene Ther. 11(1): S18.
[110] Eichhorn GL (1973) In: Eichhorn GL (ed) Inorganic biochemistry, chapter33, vol 2. Elsevier, New York
[111] Izatt RM, Christensen JJ, Rytting JH (1971) Chem.Rev.71:439.
[112] Marzilli LG (1977) In: Lippard SJ (ed) Progress in inorganic chemistry,vol 23. John Wiley and Sons, New York.
[113] Shamsi MH, Geckeler KE (2008) Nanotechnology 19:1.
[114] Raveendran P, Fu J, Wallen SL (2003) J.Am.Chem.Soc.125:13940.
[115] Pinnavaia TJ, Beall GW (2000) editors. Polymer-clay nanocomposites. Wiley Press; Chichester, UK.
[116] Rivas L, Sanchez-Cortes S, Garcia-Ramos JV, Morcillo G (2001) Langmuir 17:574.
[117] Zhu Shiguo, Lu Hongbin, Xiang Juanjuan, Tang Ke, Zhang Bicheng, Zhou Ming, Tan Chen, Li Guiyuan (2002) Chinese Science Bulletin 47(8): 654.
[118] Nath SS, Chakdar D, Gope G (2007) Nanotrends: J. Nanotechnol. Appl. 2
[119] Paul P, Hossain M, Yadav RC, Kumar GS (2010) Biophysical Chemistry148(1-3): 93. 0301-4622.
[120] Khanna MM, Yoder L, Calamai, Stotzky G (1998) Sci.Soils 3:1.
[121] Hussain SM, Javorina MK, Schrand AM, Duhart HM, Ali SF, Schlager JJ (2006) Toxicol.Sci.92:456.
[122] Hussain SM, Hess KL, Gearhart JM, Geiss KT, Schlager JJ (2005) Toxicol.in Vitro. 19:975.

[123] Margaret IP, Lui SL, Poon VKM, Lung I, Burd A (2006) J.Med.Microbiol.55: 59.
[124] Sarkar R, Pal SK (2006) Biopolymers 83: 675.
[125] Hill WR, Pillsbury DM. Argyria: The Pharmocology of Silver.MD:Williams & Wilkins Company,Baltimore 4.

21

Mesenchymal Stem Cells as Vehicles for Targeted Therapies

Gabriele Putz Todd, Michelle A LeRoux and Alla Danilkovitch-Miagkova
Osiris Therapeutics, Inc.
USA

1. Introduction

1.1 Challenges of conventional drug delivery

Traditional drug delivery systems include oral drug administration, injection, infusion, and topical administration, where the drug is applied to body surfaces such as the skin or mucous membranes. Many of the conventional drug delivery systems distribute the pharmaceutical compound proportionally to the regional blood flow through the systemic blood circulation. Consequently, the drug is delivered indiscriminately throughout the whole body to diseased and healthy tissues. As a result, patients suffer from side effects due to the non-specific delivery of the drug. Systemic delivery of a drug with body-wide distribution also results in a limited availability of the therapeutic agent at the site of interest, lowering the ability of the drug to produce a beneficial effect. To compensate for the low availability of the drug at the affected site, the drug has to be administered in large quantities, resulting in increased drug toxicity as well as high therapy costs. Another drawback of systemic drug delivery is the short circulation half-life of many drugs, which leads to the administration of high drug concentrations or high dosing frequencies (Branco & Schneider, 2009).

Pain and discomfort caused by frequent drug applications are another challenge of conventional drug delivery, especially for children and the elderly. First steps have been made in the development of micro needle injection and needle-free injection to reduce the pain and inconvenience of injections (Brunner, 2004; Stoeber & Liepmann, 2002). As beneficial as mechanical improvements in drug delivery will be for the patient's comfort and compliance, they will not reduce the number of administrations or the amount of required therapeutic. They also will not affect drug toxicity or effectiveness. To maximize the therapeutic effect of a drug, the appropriate concentration of the drug has to be available at the right location and time, while sparing healthy tissues. Therefore, new tools are needed that enable the delivery of drugs directly to the diseased area, and/or release the therapeutic agent in a controlled way.

In this chapter, vehicles for the targeted delivery of drugs will be discussed, with special focus on the potential use of human mesenchymal stem cells (hMSCs) for targeted therapies. Besides the development of targeted drug delivery tools, efforts in the medical field attempt to increase the efficiency of conventional applications. An example is topical drug delivery, which has profited from the introduction of new topical applications including transdermal patches (Brunner, 2004), use of microneedles (Henry et al., 1998), electroporation techniques

(Escobar-Chavez et al., 2009), and the development of pulmonary delivery methods (Brunner, 2004). Additional methods to improve conventional drugs include sustained and controlled release technologies and enhanced absorption technology to provide more efficient drug absorption and increased bioavailability, as well as reduce pain from administration and improve ease of use (Brunner, 2004). These topics will not be further addressed in this chapter.

1.2 Advantages of targeted drug delivery

The ultimate goal of drug delivery is the efficient and timely transport of a drug to a diseased tissue, within the therapeutic and outside the toxic range, while sparing any healthy tissue. To progress towards this end, controlled drug delivery systems are being developed that can 1) control the rate of drug release, 2) control the location of drug release (spatial/targeted delivery), 3) or achieve both, temporal and spatial control of drug delivery (Hilt, 2010). Controlled delivery systems require the ability to localize and target drug action, extend drug action at a predetermined rate, and provide a physiologically/therapeutically based drug release system, which controls the rate of drug release based on the physiological/therapeutic needs of the body (Ding et al., 2006).

Targeted drug delivery seeks to concentrate the medication in the tissues of interest while reducing the relative concentration of the medication in the remaining tissues. As a result, a high local drug concentration and low systemic exposure is achieved which helps to improve the drug's effectiveness while lowering its damaging effects on healthy tissue. Especially in cancer therapy requiring highly toxic drugs, there is a great need for vehicles that transport drugs in a safe manner, very specifically to the diseased sites.

Targeted drug delivery can rely on passive or active mechanisms. Passive targeting is mediated by the enhanced permeability and retention (EPR) effect, which is based on the longevity of the pharmaceutical carrier in the blood and its accumulation in pathological sites with compromised vasculature (Haley & Frenkel, 2008; Ruoslahti et al., 2010). Delivery tools relying on passive targeting mechanisms have limited target specificity, as passive targeting depends on the EPR effect, and thus on the degree of vascularization and angiogenesis of the targeted site. In cancer therapy, passive targeting makes extravasation of nanocarriers dependent on tumor type and tumor location. Active targeting, in contrast, is based on the attachment of specific ligands to the surface of pharmaceutical carriers to recognize and bind pathological target cells. The targeting ligands can be monoclonal antibodies, antibody fragments or non-antibody ligands, some of which will be discussed in the review. Despite the discrimination of active and passive mechanisms, it is important to keep in mind that active targeting cannot be separated from the passive because it occurs only after passive accumulation in the targeted site (Bae, 2009; Danhier et al., 2010).

In summary, targeted drug delivery systems have several advantages over common systemic drug delivery methods (see Figure 1). The ability to convey the therapeutically active molecule only to the site of action, without affecting other organs and tissues, increases the therapeutic index, and allows for a lower required drug dose or dose frequency. This in turn increases the safety profile of the drug, and reduces side effects and risks, as less healthy tissue is targeted (Ruggiero et al., 2010). Equally important is the impact on the patient's comfort, which will improve as a result of lower drug dose and side effects. Finally, the economic benefits of decreased drug use should be appreciated. The next section provides an overview of recent progress in the development of active and passive systems for the targeted delivery of drugs, with a brief description of intracellular targeting strategies.

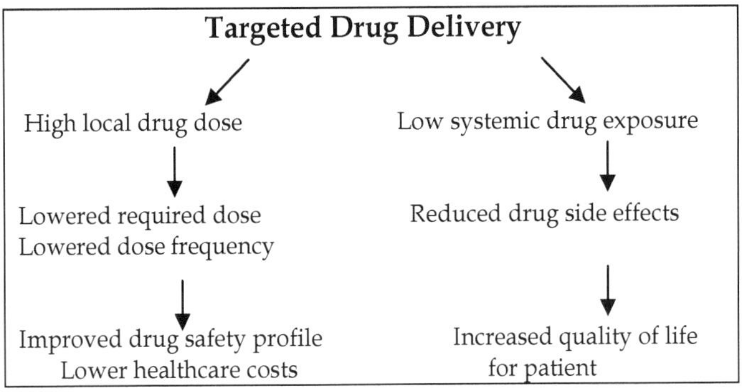

Fig. 1. Advantages of targeted delivery tools over conventional drug delivery methods

2. Recent progress in the development of targeted drug delivery tools

2.1 Nanoparticles

Among other targeted drug delivery systems, nanoparticles have recently drawn strong interest in the medical community because of their utility as carriers. Nanoparticles come in a variety of sizes and shapes, like spheres, tubes, shells, and branched structures, and include among others, liposomes, quantum dots, nanospheres, nanocapsules, nanotubes, dentrimers, micelles, and fullerenes. One important aspect of nanoparticles is their limited size of up to 100nm (although the upper limit can vary in the literature), which enables them to pass through fenestrations of compromised leaky endothelium. As leaky epithelium is characteristic for tumors and their environment, nanoparticles can accumulate at tumor sites mediated by the EPR effect, and therefore can be used as a carrier for cancer therapeutics to the tumor (Danhier et al., 2010; Haley & Frenkel, 2008; Lowery et al., 2011). Besides being used in a passive drug delivery process, nanoparticles can be coupled to ligands which interact with their receptors at the target cell site and used in an active targeting process (Haley & Frenkel, 2008). Therapeutics can be encapsulated, entrapped, or attached to the nanoparticle surface and delivered to the tumor by the nanoparticles.

The small size of nanoparticles also has a drawback. It results in the fast clearance of nanoparticles by the mononuclear phagocyte system (MPS), also called reticulo-endothelial system (RES), which is predominantly distributed in liver, lung, spleen, and bone marrow. Unless there is desired drug delivery to those organs, nanoparticles have to be surface modified with molecules like polyethylene glycol (PEG) to escape the MPS (Haley & Frenkel, 2008). PEG creates a steric barrier and prevents the interaction of nanoparticles with opsonins and phagocytic cells (Ishihara et al., 2009). Yang et al. (Yang et al., 2007) showed that the PEGylated liposomal formulation of paclitaxel significantly reduced the uptake by the MPS, while accumulation of liposomes at the tumor site, as well as biological half-life, were increased. Several drugs using nanoparticle carriers are already in preclinical and clinical use (Adiseshaiah et al., 2009; Bawa, 2008; Haley & Frenkel, 2008; Kim et al., 2010; Lowery et al., 2011; Ochekpe et al., 2009; Tuscano et al., 2010; Zhang et al., 2008), like

PEGylated doxorubicin (Doxil), and PEGylated daunorubicine (DaunoXome). Table 1 lists examples of approved nanoparticle-based therapeutics in clinical use.

Brand Name	Description	Nanostructure	Approved Indications
Abelcet	Amphotericin B lipid complex injection	Liposomes	• Invasive fungal infections in patients refractory or intolerant to amphotericin B
Abraxane	Albumin-bound nanoparticle formulation of Paclitaxel (Taxol)	Protein nanoparticles	• Breast cancer after failure of combination chemotherapy for metastatic disease or relapse within 6 months of adjuvant chemotherapy
Adagen	Pegademase bovine	Polymeric nanoparticles	• Adenosine deaminase deficiency in patients with severe combined immunodeficiency disease who failed or are not suitable candidates for bone marrow transplantation
AmBisome	Liposomal amphotericin B	Liposomes	• Systemic or disseminated infections due to Candida, Aspergillus, or Cryptococcus in patients who are refractory to or intolerant of conventional amphotericin B therapy, or have renal impairment • Visceral leishmaniasis
Amphotec	Amphotericin B lipid complex	Lipid colloidal dispersion	• Invasive aspergillosis in patients refractory, or intolerant to amphotericin B
Copaxone	Glatiramer acetate injection	Polymeric nanoparticles	• Relapsing-remitting multiple sclerosis, including patients who have experienced a first clinical episode and have MRI features consistent with multiple sclerosis
DaunoXome	Daunorubicin citrate liposome injection	Liposomes	• Advanced AIDS-related Kaposi's sarcoma
Depocyt	Cytarabine liposome injection	Liposomes	• Intrathecal treatment of lymphomatous meningitis
Diprivan	Propofol liposomes	Liposomes	• Induction and maintenance of anesthesia
Doxil / Caelyx	Doxorubicin HCl liposome injection	Liposomes	• Progressed or refractory ovarian cancer • AIDS-related Kaposi's sarcoma in patients with intolerance to, or failure of prior systemic chemotherapy • Myeloma in combination with bortezomib in patients who have not previously received bortezomib and have received at least one prior therapy
Elestrin	Estradiol gel incorporating calcium phosphate nanoparticles	Calcium phosphate nanoparticles	• Moderate-to-severe vasomotor symptoms (hot flashes) associated with menopause

Brand Name	Description	Nanostructure	Approved Indications
Epaxal* (Switzerland, Canada)	Hepatitis A vaccine adjuvanted with immunopotentiating reconstituted influenza virosomes	Liposomes	• Active immunization against hepatitis A
Estrasorb	Estradiol micellar nanoparticles	Liposomes	• Vasomotor symptoms in menopausal women
Feridex	Ferumoxides injectable solution	Iron oxide Nanoparticles	• Contrast agent for magnetic resonance imaging of liver lesions
Macugen	Pegylated anti-VEGF aptamer	Polymeric nanoparticles	• Neovascular age-related macular degeneration
Myocet* (Europe, Canada)	Nonpegylated liposomal doxorubicin	Liposomes	• Metastatic breast cancer in combination with cyclophosphamide
Oncaspar	Pegaspargase	Polymeric nanoparticles	• First-line treatment of patients with acute lymphoblastic leukemia as a component of a multiagent chemotherapy regimen
Neulasta	Pegfilgrastim (PEG-rmetHuG-CSF)	Polymeric nanoparticles	• Decrease incidence of infection manifested by febrile neutropenia in patients with non-myeloid malignancies receiving myelosuppressive anti-cancer drugs associated with a clinically significant incidence of febrile neutropenia
Pegasys	Peginterferon alfa-2a	Polymeric nanoparticles	• Chronic hepatitis C in patients coinfected with hepatitis C and HIV
PEGIntron	Peginterferon alfa-2b	Polymeric nanoparticles	• Chronic hepatitis C infection with compensated liver disease
Resovist	Carboxydextran superparamagnetic iron oxide formulation	Iron oxide nanoparticles	• Contrast agent for magnetic resonance imaging of liver lesions
Somavert	Pegvisomant	Polymeric nanoparticles	• Acromegaly in patients with inadequate response to surgery and/or radiation therapy and/or other medical therapies, or for whom these therapies are not appropriate
Triglide	Nanocrystalline fenofibrate	Nanocrystals	• Primary hypercholesterolemia, mixed dyslipidemia, and hypertriglyceridemia, for use in conjuction with diet
Verigene	Gold nanoparticles	Gold nanoparticles	• *In vitro* diagnostics: genetic test for warfarin sensitivity

* Not U.S. Food and Drug Administration (FDA) approved

Table 1. Examples of approved nanoparticle-based therapeutics in clinical use

2.2 Ligand-targeted therapeutics

Ligand-targeted therapeutics are based on the selective delivery of drugs to target cells by associating drugs with molecules that bind to antigens or receptors uniquely expressed or over-expressed on the target cell relative to normal cells (Allen, 2002). Such targeting ligands can be monoclonal antibodies, antibody fragments, and non-antibody ligands (Danhier et al., 2010). The drug of interest is directly conjugated to these targeting ligands, or loaded onto high capacity drug carriers, which are directly conjugated to targeting proteins or derivatized for interactions with specific adapters that are conjugated to the targeting protein (Backer et al., 2002). Ligand-targeted delivery systems rely on active targeting mechanisms, which help to improve target specificity, as the target ligands can act as "homing devices", improving the selective delivery of drug to specific tissue and cells (Danhier et al., 2010).

Non-antibody targeting ligands include small molecules (folic acid, galactose), peptides (Arginine-Glycine-Aspartic acid (RGD), Vascular Endothelial Growth Factor (VEGF) peptide), aptamers (pegaptanib), and proteins, like transferrin and luteinizing hormone releasing hormone (Allen, 2002; Yu et al., 2010). Despite the advantage that non-antibody ligands are often readily available and inexpensive to manufacture, many of them bind relatively non-selectively to target and non-target tissue (Allen, 2002). For this reason, antibody ligands with higher cell selectivity, e.g. Anti-Human Epidermal Growth Factor Receptor 2 (HER2/neu/ERBB2), Anti-Vascular Endothelial Growth Factor Receptor (VEGFR), Anti-CD20, and Anti-CD33, have gained research attention (Allen, 2002; Park et al., 1997, 2002). However, the fact that antibody-targeted therapies rely on the expression of specific antigens is at the same time a drawback, as antigen expression is likely to change between patients, type of disease and time (Loebinger & Janes, 2010).

To enable the delivery of highly potent cytotoxic agents to antigen-expressing cells, antibody-drug conjugates (ADCs) were designed, which take advantage of the site specificity of antibodies. The key components of an ADC are 1) the cytotoxic agent, 2) a monoclonal antibody targeting a tumor-enriched or tumor specific antigen, and 3) a linker that covalently binds these components together (Alley et al., 2010; Chari, 2008; Krop et al., 2010). Unfortunately, the clinical success of ADCs so far has been very limited. Only gemtuzumab ozogamicin (Pfizer), an anti-CD33 monoclonal antibody linked to calicheamicin, had been approved by the FDA in the year 2000 for the treatment of patients with acute myeloid leukemia, but the product was voluntarily withdrawn from the US market in 2010 after results from a clinical trial raised concerns about the product's safety and clinical benefit (Beck et al., 2010, 2011). Several ADC therapies are in clinical testing, including trastuzumab-DM1 (T-DM1) for breast cancer, brentuximab vedotin (SGN-35) for Hodgkin lymphoma (HL) and anaplastic large cell lymphoma (ALCL), and inotuzumab ozogamicin (CMC-544) for non-Hodgkin lymphoma (NHL) (Alley et al., 2010). T-DM1 is an antibody-drug conjugate which uses the HER2-binding antibody trastuzumab to deliver the potent antimicrotubule agent DM1 to HER2-expressing cells (Krop et al., 2010). A first clinical study with HER2-directed ADC in patients with HER2-positive metastatic breast cancer showed a clinical benefit rate (objective response plus stable disease at 6 months) of 73% among 15 patients treated at the maximum tolerated-dose. The confirmed response rate among patients with measurable disease in this group was 44%. Based on those results, Burries et al. (Burris et al., 2011) evaluated T-DM1 treatment in patients with HER2-positive metastatic breast cancer who experienced progression on HER2-directed therapy in a single-arm phase II study (study ID: TDM4258g). Among 112 treated patients, an objective response rate (ORR) of 26% was observed by independent assessment, which is comparable to the ORR of other HER2 therapies (Burris et al., 2011). The fact that response rates were higher among patients with confirmed HER2-positive tumors and among patients whose tumor HER2 expression levels were above the median, emphasizes the need for patient prescreening for HER2 target expression levels to obtain optimal results.

Another ADC in advanced clinical development is SGN-35 (Seattle Genetics and Millennium Pharmaceuticals), comprised of an anti-CD30 monoclonal antibody linked to monomethyl auristatin E. CD30, is a defining marker of HL, but also expressed on other cancers, including ALCL. HL and ALCL patients were treated intravenously with SGN-35 every 3 weeks for up to 16 cycles. With an objective response rate of 75% in HL and 86% in ALCL, SGN-35 represents the most active ADC reported. In February 2011, a biologics license application was submitted to the FDA (Beck et al., 2011; Deutsch et al., 2011). Many other ADCs are in early clinical trials and future results will reveal their benefit for clinical use.

2.3 Cell penetrating peptides

The transport of a therapeutic from the site of administration to the site of interest is not the only phase in drug delivery that can be controlled. After arrival of the drug at the site of a diseased tissue, it might also be necessary to control the transport of the drug across the plasma membrane of the targeted cells. Vehicles that facilitate and control intracellular transport are being developed and include physical delivery strategies, like electroporation, and biochemical delivery strategies, like cell-penetrating peptides (CPPs). CPPs are also named protein transduction domains and comprise short and usually basic amino acids-rich peptides originating from proteins able to cross biological barriers (Chou et al., 2011; Hassan & Elshafeey, 2010; Vives et al., 2008). They are able to act as vectors for the delivery of chemically conjugated biomolecules like peptides or oligonucleotides, and allow for viral-free transduction which eliminates the risk of virus vector induced complications. Besides the protein transduction domains (penetratin and TAT (48-60)), there are chimeric CPPs (MPG, transportan), synthetic CPPs (oligoarginine), and peptidic vectors designed from structure-activity studies on already known CPPs (Pip2b, stearylated-Tp10). The mechanisms of internalization of CPPs are still controversial, and might be diverse, depending on CPP, cell type and cell cargo (Hassan & Elshafeey, 2010; Sawant & Torchilin, 2011).

The most frequently used CPP is the TAT peptide (TATp), derived from the transcription activator protein encoded by human immunodeficiency virus type 1 (Torchilin, 2008). TATp can be covalently linked to many drug classes, including large protein molecules, and was used to transduce attached cargoes into cells of all organ types (Sawant & Torchilin, 2011). Responsible for the transduction ability of the TAT protein is the positive charge in the transduction domain which extends from residue 47 to 57. As for other CPPs, different mechanisms have also been proposed for the endocytic uptake of TATp, including classical clathrin-mediated endocytosis and clathrin-independent lipid raft-mediated caveolae endocytosis (Torchilin, 2008).

Still, there are some challenges that must be overcome, like sequestration and entrapment of internalized material within endocytic vesicles, before CPPs can become a valuable clinical tool. Tools to enhance endosomal escape of CPP-attached cargos are developed and include the use of pH sensitive proteins, fusogenic lipids, membrane disruptive peptides, polymers, and lysomotropic agents. Another drawback is the lack of selectivity of certain CPPs, which raises concerns about drug-induced toxicity in normal tissues (Chou et al., 2011; Sawant & Torchilin, 2011). The problem might be solved by combining target specific drug carriers with CPPs, to assure both delivery of the drug to the target cell and delivery of the drug from the outside of the cell into the cytoplasm of the target cell.

2.4 Cells as delivery vehicles

The ability of hematopoietic and non-hematopoietic cells to migrate to sites of injury, inflammation, and infection makes them attractive for investigation as a potential drug delivery vehicle. Cells can be loaded with drugs or modified to produce them, and then be used to carry the drug to the site of interest. The cell modifications can be done in many ways, including genetic cell engineering, and culture-induced modifications.

Genetically-modified cells used in clinical trials are mainly autologous hematopoietic cells which are isolated from the patient, modified and reintroduced into the patient. Among hematopoietic cells, lymphocytes are the most commonly genetically modified cell population used in clinical trials, with lymphocytes expressing T-cell receptor (TCR) or Interleukin-12 (IL-12) for the treatment of advanced melanoma, and lymphocytes expressing Anti-P53 TCR, Anti-carcinoembryonic antigen (CEA), Anti-melanoma antigen family (MAGE)-A3/12 TCR, Anti-HER2, and Anti-NY ESO-1 (a cancer/testis antigen) TCR for the treatment of other metastatic cancers (see clinicaltrials.gov). The disadvantage of hematopoietic cells as delivery vehicle, and in transfusion medicine in general, is their immunogenicity. To avoid immune reactions of the patient's immune system against the introduced cells, and attacks of the transplanted material against the recipient's body, autologous cells or AB0- and human leukocyte antigen (HLA)-matched cells must be used.

An alternative to the use of hematopoietic cells are non-hematopoietic mesenchymal stem cells (MSCs), which are known for their low immunogenicity. The ability to use MSCs in an allogeneic setting eliminates the time consuming step of collecting stem cells from the patient and allows for the use of frozen, off-the-shelf cell products. The delay between diagnosis and availability of cells would be eliminated. In the following sections, MSCs in general and their use as potential drug delivery vehicles are discussed.

3. Mesenchymal Stem Cell biology

The therapeutic potential of MSCs is linked to a broad spectrum of MSC biological activities such as anti-inflammatory, immunomodulative and tissue reparative activities via paracrine mechanisms. Besides those activities, MSCs have the unique ability to home to sites of inflammation/injury and tumors, which makes them useful for the delivery of therapeutics to these sites. Cells are an ideal vehicle for targeted drug delivery, since they can be loaded with therapeutic agents and have the ability to migrate to sites of disease. This section describes current understanding of MSCs, their characteristics and biological activities, and current experience with MSCs in clinical trials that supports their use for targeted drug delivery.

3.1 Background on MSCs

The ability to generate an embryo from a single fertilized oocyte or to regenerate tissues upon injury or natural physiological turnover is a direct result of stem cells. As the embryo first develops, an undifferentiated mass of totipotent embryonic stem cells (ESCs) will form a multicellular organism. As development proceeds, totipotent ESCs disappear as more restricted somatic stem cells (SSCs) give rise to the tissues and organs. Although cell diversification is mostly completed at or shortly after birth, organs must have a mechanism to replenish cells as they die as a result of natural homeostasis or injury. Therefore, after birth life-long reservoirs of SSCs are present in the body. Major characteristics of stem cells that distinguish them from all other cells include (1) self-renewal, or the ability to generate at least one daughter cell with characteristics similar to the initiating cell; (2) multi-lineage differentiation potential of a single cell; and (3) *in vivo* functional reconstruction of a given tissue. Adult SSCs fulfill these criteria, however the degree of self-renewal and differentiation potential are restricted in comparison to ESCs. There are several types of SSCs in the body including MSCs.

MSCs were described as precursors of fibroblasts, which were isolated from bone marrow by Friedenstein in 1970 (Friedenstein et al., 1970). Upon culture at low density either as whole bone marrow or after cell separation over a density gradient, the cultured cells form characteristic colonies derived from a single precursor, referred to as colony forming unit fibroblasts or CFU-F. After ectopic transplantation under the kidney capsule, these cells gave rise to a broad spectrum of differentiated connective tissues including bone, cartilage, adipose and myelosupportive stroma (Owen, 1988; Prockop, 1997). Based on these observations it was proposed that these mesenchymal origin tissues are derived from a common precursor cell residing in bone marrow, termed the mesenchymal stem cell. These observations also led to the development and wide use of the colony forming unit-fibroblasts (CFU-F) assay used to estimate MSC frequency among bone marrow nucleated cells. Using this technique, MSCs have been identified as a rare population of cells in bone marrow, representing ~0.001-0.01% of the nucleated cells (Pittenger & Martin, 2004). Estimation of MSC frequency in bone marrow using CFU-F shows that MSC number declines with age (Caplan, 2007), which correlates with poor mesenchymal tissue healing. This poor capacity for healing is evident, for example, in broken bones in elderly individuals.

Adult, tissue specific stem cells are found in specialized niches in their corresponding tissues of origin. For example, hematopoietic stem cells (HSCs) can be found in bone marrow and epidermal stem cells are located in mammalian hair follicles. In contrast, cell types originated from MSCs are present through the entire body, and it has been shown that MSCs can be isolated from virtually all organs. There are three hypotheses regarding the location of MSCs in the body. In the first, MSCs are located in only one specific organ or tissue, from which they can migrate to other sites via the blood circulation to replenish the cell population. However, the number of MSCs circulating in blood is extremely low or undetectable. The difficulty establishing MSC culture from peripheral blood votes against this possibility. The second possibility is that MSCs are present in different tissues: MSCs have been successfully isolated from various tissues in addition to bone marrow. These tissues include adipose, periosteum, tendon, muscle, synovial membrane, skin and many others. When cultured *in vitro*, MSCs derived from different tissues show very similar characteristics and functionality, suggesting that different tissue-intrinsic stem cells might behave as MSCs when characterized *in vitro*. And the third possibility is that the MSC niche *in vivo* is the perivascular zone of blood vessels, and pericytes have all characteristics of MSCs. In this scenario, MSCs can actively participate in tissue repair after the release from blood vessels upon the damage in any tissue. Several experimental data support this hypothesis (da Silva Meirelles et al., 2008).

3.2 MSC immune privilege

One of the most significant advantages of MSCs is that they can be used allogeneically. *In vivo* studies have demonstrated that tissues of mesodermal origin including bone, cartilage, and connective tissues, derived from MSCs, can be successfully transplanted without matching with a low incidence of acute rejection (Bacsich & Wyburn, 1947; Girdler, 1997). Thus, the mesodermal origin of MSCs suggests they are not recognized as foreign by the recipient immune system. Data accumulated *in vitro* and *in vivo* support the concept of MSCs as universally tolerated stem cells, rationalizing the transplantation of allogeneic MSCs without donor-recipient HLA matching. The universality is based on the low immunogenicity profile of MSCs. *In vitro* characterization has shown that MSCs constitutively express low levels of HLA class I molecules and do not express HLA class II molecules on the cell surface and co-stimulatory molecules like CD40, 80 and 86, which are essential for initiation of the immune response (Klyushnenkova et al., 2005; Tse et al., 2003). The absence of co-stimulatory molecules may lead to tolerance induction instead of rejection of allogeneic MSCs. The absence of host immune response against allogeneic MSCs has been demonstrated *in vitro* (Bartholomew et al., 2002; Di Nicola et al., 2002; Tse et al., 2003) and *in vivo* in animals (Atoui et al., 2008; Chen et al., 2009) and humans (Kebriaei et al., 2009; Le Blanc et al., 2004; Prasad et al., 2011; Sundin et al., 2007).

3.3 MSC biological activities

3.3.1 Regulation of hematopoiesis (stromal support)

The critical role of bone marrow stroma for homing and long-term maintenance of hematopoiesis in mammalian bone was demonstrated early on by Friedenstein (Friedenstein et al., 1974). MSCs secrete a variety of cytokines, chemokines, and growth factors supporting hematopoietic cell expansion and maturation (Caplan, 2007; Deans & Moseley, 2000). Stromal Derived Factor-1 (SDF-1), which is produced by bone marrow stromal cells and mediates HSC homing and engraftment to the bone marrow, is one example of such chemokines. MSCs also play a critical role in megakaryocyte development: MSCs express thrombopoetin (TPO), IL-6, IL-11, Leukemia inhibitory factor (LIF) and Stem Cell Factor (SCF), which are critical regulators of megakaryopoiesis (Cheng et al., 2000). In addition to the regulation of megakaryopoiesis, MSCs also support cells of myeloid and lymphoid lineages. The ability of MSCs to support hematopoiesis was used in patients with hematopoietic cell graft failures. Co-administration of MSCs together with hematopoietic stem cells enhanced engraftment and accelerated neutrophil, platelet, and lymphoid cell recovery (Ball et al., 2007; Fouillard et al., 2003, 2007; Koc et al., 2000; Lazarus et al., 2005; Le Blanc et al., 2007). However, administration of MSCs together with hematopoietic cells resulted in high chimerism for hematopoietic cells in both blood and bone marrow, and microchimerism for MSCs - the majority of MSCs remained of host origin (Bacher et al., 2010; Bartsch et al., 2009). The low number of engrafted donor MSCs in bone marrow suggests that the support of hematopoietic cell engraftment and recovery is unlikely to be due to a stromal support function of donor MSCs. This MSC effect can be mediated rather by the MSC's ability to modulate immune response, and thus, to prevent the hematopoietic graft rejection.

3.3.2 Tissue protection and repair

Accumulated data in animal models indicate that MSCs have the potential to protect and repair tissues in the body by several different mechanisms. First, mesenchymal tissue repair can occur via MSC differentiation into cells of mesenchymal tissues. Since MSCs can be differentiated into distinctive mesenchymal phenotypes, they have been used for mesenchymal tissue regeneration by implanting MSCs *in vivo* into different tissue sites in tissue specific scaffolds. For example, MSCs can be delivered to bone or cartilage repair sites in calcium phosphate porous ceramics or hyaluronan and polymeric scaffolds for bone and cartilage repair, respectively (Bruder et al., 1998; Kon et al., 2000; Murphy et al., 2003; Solchaga et al., 2005). This approach resulted in well integrated, newly differentiated tissues (Kadiyala et al., 1997; Kon et al., 2000; Murphy et al., 2003), and showed that MSC-based tissue engineering is feasible for clinical use. MSCs have also been shown potential to trans-differentiate into mature cells of non-mesenchymal origin. Reported data indicate that MSCs can be transdifferentiated into hepatocytes (Ong et al., 2006; Sato et al.; 2005), islet beta cells (Moriscot et al., 2005; Sun et al., 2007), endothelial cells (Oswald et al., 2004) and neural (Phinney & Isakova, 2005) or kidney tissues (Yokoo et al., 2005). These data show plasticity of MSCs and point to the possible use of MSCs for regenerative medicine of non-mesenchymal tissues. In addition to the differentiation mechanism, the paracrine mechanism plays an important role in MSC-mediated tissue protection and repair. A set of MSC-derived factors with proangiogenic/proarteriogenic activities is shown by Kinnaird et al. (Kinnaird et al., 2004). Under hypoxic conditions MSCs promote proliferation and migration of endothelial and smooth muscle cells via secretion of VEGF and basic Fibroblast Growth Factor (bFGF), augmenting collateral remodeling that is critical for recovery from tissue ischemia. The effects of MSC-secreted biological active molecules can be direct, indirect, or both: direct by triggering intracellular signaling, or indirect by triggering another cell in the vicinity to secrete other biologically active factors. This indirect effect has been termed a "trophic" effect (Caplan & Dennis, 2006). In a variety of animal models, including myocardial infarction and stroke, MSC-mediated trophic effects are the primary mechanism involved in tissue repair (Caplan & Dennis, 2006).

3.3.3 MSC-mediated immunomodulation

An important function of MSCs is their role as potent immunomodulators. It was first observed by Osiris scientists, as well as others, that MSCs can inhibit T-cell proliferation both *in vitro* and *in vivo* (Bartholomew et al., 2002; Di Nicola et al., 2002). Subsequently, further studies have demonstrated that MSCs are able to regulate the immune system through cells of both the innate (macrophages, dendritic and natural killer cells) and adaptive (T- and B-cells) immune systems (Newman et al., 2009). A simplified schematic representation of MSC effects on different subsets of immune cells reflecting our current knowledge is captured in Figure 2. The ability of MSCs to inhibit immune response and down regulate secretion of inflammatory cytokines suggests that MSCs have the potential to treat inflammatory immune-mediated diseases such as graft versus host disease (GvHD), organ rejection, and autoimmune diseases. However, MSCs are not constitutively immunosuppressive. In a non-inflammatory environment, MSCs express low levels of COX-2 (cyclooxygenase 2), Prostaglandin E2 (PGE2), Transforming growth factor β (TGF-β), Indoleamine 2,3-dioxygenase (IDO), and other factors that can inhibit immune response, however, pro-inflammatory cytokines such as Interferon γ (IFN-γ) and Tumor Necrosis Factor-α (TNF-α) dramatically up-regulate the secretion of anti-inflammatory factors by MSCs (Aggarwal & Pittenger, 2005; English et al., 2007; Krampera et al., 2006; Meisel et al.,

2004; Ryan et al., 2007). These *in vitro* data support a hypothesis of dynamic MSC response to inflammatory stimuli released from activated immune cells. *In vivo* animal data further demonstrate that MSCs require an ongoing immune response to exert their immunosuppressive functions (Renner et al., 2009). The dynamic response to cells and factors present in the microenvironment is an important feature and benefit of MSCs. Such regulated immunosuppressive activity of MSCs will help to avoid treatment-related complications that are common for traditional immunosuppressive drugs, particularly high rate of infections and multiple organ toxicities.

The MSCs' ability to regulate hematopoiesis, protect and repair tissues, and regulate immune reactions equips the cells with a great therapeutic potential. The therapeutic effects are well documented in animal models and are investigated in ongoing clinical trials (Parekkadan & Milwid, 2010). Whether those biological activities still play a role after MSCs modification for the transport of therapeutic drugs has to be determined. Especially for the treatment of inflammatory diseases it could be beneficial to combine the immunomodulatory effect of the MSCs with the therapeutic effect of MSC-delivered drug. Also, tissue repair activities would be beneficial in combination with therapeutic drugs, when injured tissue is targeted.

3.4 MSC biodistribution and migration ability

3.4.1 MSC biodistribution

Understanding the biodistribution of MSCs in the body in its healthy, or baseline state is important for the development of MSCs as targeted drugs. For this reason, MSC biodistribution after infusion was studied in healthy animals (Allers et al., 2004). Allers et al. infused human bone marrow-derived technetium-99m (^{99m}Tc)-labeled MSCs intravenously into unconditioned mice. Fifteen minutes after infusion, radioactivity was detected in lungs and heart, suggesting blood vessel circulation of the infused labeled cells. Three hours later, MSCs were scattered in the body, but still accumulated in the lungs and also in the liver. The MSCs became temporarily entrapped in the lungs, probably as a consequence of significant differences in the diameter of MSC and inner lung capillary lumen. Whole-body scanning 24 hours after infusion revealed no or scarce radioactivity in the body, except for lungs, liver, and spleen. A similar pattern of short-term distribution of MSCs was observed in rats after syngeneic transplantation of indium-111-oxine–labeled rat MSCs (Gao et al., 2001). After intraarterial (IA) and intravenous (IV) infusion, radioactivity associated with MSCs was first detected in the lungs and secondarily in the liver and other organs. Forty-eight hours later, the radioactivity was observed primarily in the liver with considerable amounts detected in the lungs and kidneys (Gao et al., 2001). The long-term fate of systemically infused autologous and allogeneic MSCs was studied in non-human primates (Devine et al., 2003). Following lethal total body irradiation, which causes major damage to the bone marrow, baboons received green fluorescent protein (GFP)-labeled baboon MSCs by IV infusion. Tissue collection after 9 to 21 months after infusions showed that allogeneic and autologous MSCs appeared to distribute in a similar manner. The highest concentrations of engrafted cells per microgram of deoxyribonucleic acid (DNA) were found in gastrointestinal tissues including colon, duodenum, jejunum, and ileum. Kidney, lung, liver, thymus, and skin also harbored high amounts of DNA equivalents. Estimated levels of engraftment ranged from 0.1% to 2.7%. The data show that MSCs not only migrate to certain tissues, but can also engraft in low numbers at those sites.

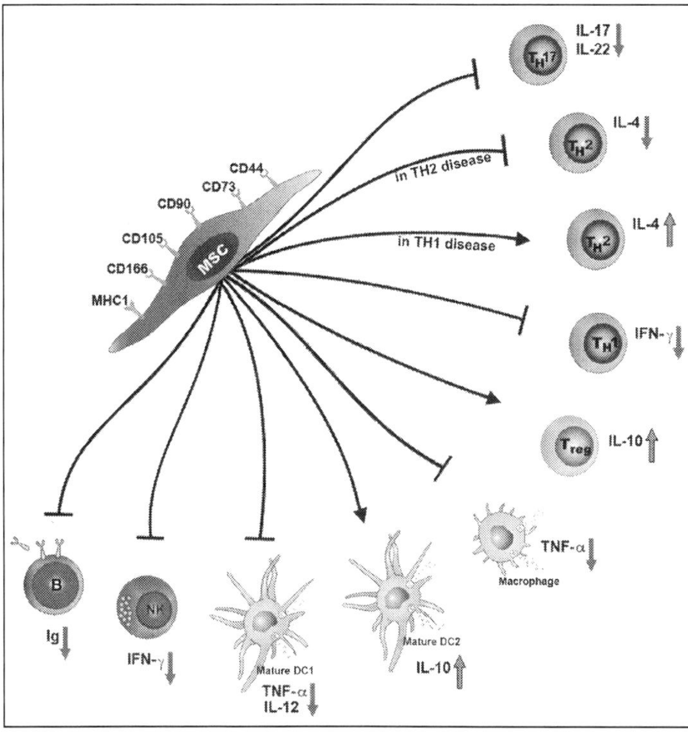

Fig. 2. MSC effects on different types of immune cells. MSCs have both immunostimulative and suppressive activity, which is driven by type of immune cells and presence of cellular and molecular signals in local tissue microenvironment. Abbreviations: B = B-cells; CD = cluster of differentiation, molecules expressed on cell surface; DC1 and DC2 = dendritic cells types 1 and 2; IFN-γ = interferon gamma; Ig = immunoglobulin; IL-4, 10, 12, 17 and 22 = interleukin 4, 10, 12, 17, and 22; MHC1 = major histocompatibility complex class I; MSC = mesenchymal stem cell; NK = natural killer cells; Th1, 2, and 17 = T helper cells 1, 2, and 17; TNF-α = tumor necrosis factor alpha; Treg = regulatory T-cells. Red arrows - decrease/inhibition. Green arrows - increase/stimulation. Black stealth arrows - stimulation of immune cells; black lines with blunt ends- suppression of immune cells

3.4.2 Migration of MSCs towards injured tissue

MSCs reside in various tissues including bone marrow, adipose tissues, amniotic membrane, and the umbilical cord (Motaln et al., 2010). In case of tissue damage, MSCs can be mobilized by signals such as cytokines and chemokines released from the damaged tissue and migrate to the sites of injury to participate in wound repair and tissue regeneration (Ramirez et al., 2006). Animal studies demonstrated that MSCs migrate to injured sites in the body, including the heart (Assis et al., 2010; Detante et al., 2009; Kraitchman et al., 2005; Wu et al., 2003), kidney (Herrera et al., 2007; Morigi et al., 2004), skin (Li et al., 2006), and bone (Horwitz et al., 1999; Mackenzie & Flake, 2001; Mosca et al., 2000). In rats bearing Lewis cardiac allografts, Wu et al. (Wu et al., 2003) found that IV injected β-galactosidase (lacZ) labeled MSCs can migrate into lesions of chronic rejection in the cardiac grafts and home to the bone marrow. In a myocardial infarction model in rats, Assis et al. (Assis et al., 2010) showed that systemically delivered ^{99m}Tc -labeled hexamethylpropyleneamine oxime (^{99m}Tc-HMPAO) and 4',6-diamidino-2-phenylindole (DAPI)-labeled MSCs migrate to the infarcted area. One hour after MSC injection, the radioactivity in infarcted hearts was 23-fold higher than in control hearts, and a week later DAPI-labeled MSCs were still detected in the infarcted areas of the heart (Assis et al., 2010). In a similar study, ^{99m}Tc-hMSCs were injected into the saphenous vein of rats one week after cerebral ischemia (Detante et al., 2009). After initial entrapment of the cells in the lungs, they were able to migrate towards the ischemic brain lesion. Finally, the MSCs were sequestered in the spleen and eliminated predominantly by the kidneys. MSC migration was also studied in mice with induced renal injury. After IV injection of MSCs into syngeneic female mice one day after induction of kidney injuries, MSCs were detected in the context of the well-differentiated tubular epithelial lining. MSCs strongly protected renal function as reflected by significantly lower blood urea nitrogen values (Morigi et al., 2004). In a canine model, MSCs were also shown to migrate to the bone marrow after myeloablation of dogs via total body irradiation (Mosca et al., 2000). After MSC transfusion, 58% of the bone marrow samples analyzed were transgene positive. Engrafted MSCs were viable at least 6 months after infusion. The animal studies clearly show the MSCs' ability to migrate to sites of injury to participate in tissue repair processes and demonstrate their potential as vehicles for gene delivery.

The migration ability of MSCs was also studied in human patients with osteogenesis imperfecta (Horwitz et al., 2002). Osteogenesis imperfecta is a genetic disorder of mesenchymal cells in which generalized osteopenia leads to bony deformities, excessive fragility with fracturing, and short stature mostly due to a mutation in one of the two genes encoding type I collagen. Intravenous infusions of allogeneic, gene-marked, marrow-derived MSCs in patients with osteogenesis imperfecta resulted in the migration of the cells to the bone, skin, and marrow stroma, and their engraftment in one or more of these sites (Horwitz et al., 2002).

3.4.3 MSC migration to cancer tissue

MSCs do not only show tropism to sites of injury, but also to sites of tumorigenesis. In both cases, inflammatory mediators are involved in recruitment of MSCs. Factors involved include cytokines and growth factors like Epidermal Growth factor (EGF), Hepatocyte Growth Factor (HGF), Insulin like Growth Factor 1(IGF-1), IL-1-β, IL-8, Platelet Derived Growth Factor (PDGF), SDF-1, TGF-β, TNF-α, and VEGF (Birnbaum et al., 2007; Forte et al., 2006; Ji et al., 2004; Klopp et al., 2007; Motaln et al., 2010; Nakamizo et al., 2005; Ponte et al., 2007; Ries et al., 2007; Xu et al., 2010). Many of the same inflammatory mediators secreted by wounds are also found in tumor microenvironment and thought to be involved in attracting MSCs to these sites (Spaeth et al., 2008). Dvorak actually described the tumor as an unhealed wound that produces a continuous source of inflammatory mediators (Dvorak, 1986). Inflammation is a component present during all steps of tumor development and in all types of tumors (Sansone & Bromberg, 2011; Spaeth et al., 2008; von Hertzen et al., 2011; Wallace et al., 2010).

The migration of MSCs to tumors is well documented (Loebinger et al., 2009a, 2009b; Nakamizo et al., 2005; Studeny et al., 2002, 2004; Xin et al., 2007). Loebinger et al. studied MSC migration in metastatic xenograft cancer models (Loebinger et al., 2009a, 2009b). Metastatic lung tumors were produced by the delivery of MDA-MB-231 cells into the lateral tail vein of mice, and visualized as focal regions of increased signal with magnetic resonance imaging (MRI). Thirty-five days after setup of the animal model, human MSCs double-labeled with DiI and iron nanoparticles were injected into the lateral tail vein of the animals. MRI one hour after injection showed a decrease in signal intensity caused by the iron oxide in MSCs in areas of metastatic deposits detected in pre-MSC delivery images (Loebinger et al., 2009b). The *in vivo* experiments confirmed results from *in vitro* transwell migration studies, which had demonstrated tumor homing of iron nanoparticle-labeled and unlabeled MSCs. The migration potential of MSCs towards tumors could also be shown for murine osteosarcoma (Xu et al., 2009), murine fibrosarcoma (Xiang et al., 2009), and murine glioma models (Nakamizo et al., 2005).

The number of MSCs that reaches a site of injury or tumorigenesis after systemic administration may not always be sufficient to have a therapeutic effect. In those cases, ways have to be found to enhance MSC migration. As radiation increases the expression of inflammatory mediators, it was argued that it might also enhance the recruitment of MSCs. Klopp et al. addressed the question by irradiation of murine breast carcinomas and showed that migration of MSCs to the tumor environment can indeed be enhanced by irradiation. Twenty-four hours after unilateral irradiation of 4T1 breast carcinomas, MSCs expressing firefly luciferase were injected intravenously into the animals. Forty-eight hours post irradiation, levels of MSC engraftment were 34% higher in tumors receiving 2 Gy ($p = 0.004$) than in the contralateral unirradiated limb. Immuohistochemistry also revealed higher levels of MSCs in the parenchyma of radiated tumors. Irradiated 4T1 cells resulted in increased expression of the cytokines, TGF-β1, VEGF, and PDGF-BB, known to be involved in MSC migration (Klopp et al., 2007). Similar results were obtained in murine colon cancer xenograft models (Zielske et al., 2009). Thus, low dose irradiation might be a potential clinical tool to increase the tropism for and engraftment of MSCs in the tumor microenvironment. Another option to increase the *in vivo* migratory and adhesion capacity of MSCs is the activation of MSCs with proinflammatory cytokines like TNF-α prior to treatment (Dwyer et al., 2007; Spaeth et al., 2008).

3.5 Safety of human MSCs in clinical trials

The clinical use of MSCs started in the 1990's (Horwitz et al., 1999; Koc et al., 2000; Lazarus et al., 1995). There were no adverse events linked to MSCs, and some clinical benefits were observed after MSC infusions. Today more than 100 clinical trials are registered at clinicaltrials.gov. These clinical trials are using bone marrow, adipose or placenta-derived MSCs and are covering a wide spectrum of diseases (see Table 2). More than half of the registered trials utilize autologous MSCs. The routes of delivery include both systemic and local administration.

Osiris Therapeutics has experience with numerous clinical trials utilizing expanded human allogeneic MSCs (Prochymal® (remestemcel-L)), which allow for immediate treatment of patients with no delay due to cell processing that occurs with the use of autologous MSCs. Human MSCs have been used by Osiris for the treatment of immunologic, gastrointestinal, cardiac, and orthopedic indications. Prochymal® is being evaluated in Phase III clinical trials for several indications, such as acute GvHD and Crohn's disease. Chondrogen™, an injectable formulation of MSCs, is under investigation for the treatment of arthritis in the knee. Altogether, more than 1,300 patients have been treated in Osiris clinical trials. With much of the data from double-blinded, placebo-controlled studies, the results provide strong support for the positive safety profile of MSCs.

MSC Type	MSC Source	Therapeutic Areas
• Autologous • Allogeneic	• Bone Marrow • Adipose • Placental-derived	• Inflammatory and immune-mediated • Cardiovascular • Orthopedic • Gastrointestinal/Liver/Pancreatic • Neurological • Pulmonary • Nephrological • Dermatological • Hematological • Metabolic • Genetic

Table 2. MSCs in clinical trials

Valuable safety information has been obtained from these studies because of the diverse patient population, including adult and pediatric patients, and the wide range of dosing regimens studied in Osiris clinical trials. No infusional toxicities were observed in both adult and pediatric populations. Overall review of safety data, including adverse events, has detected no trends or signals in the events experienced by patients attributed to administration of MSCs (Hare et al., 2009; Kebriaei et al., 2009; Lazarus et al., 2005; Prasad et al., 2011). Consistent with Osiris' data, the safe use of MSCs has also been reported by other investigators (e.g. Chen et al., 2004; Ciccocioppo et al., 2011; Duijvestein et al., 2010; Le Blanc et al., 2008; Lucchini et al., 2010; Williams et al., 2011). The safety of MSCs, together with the ability to use unmatched allogeneic MSCs and the potential of MSCs to home to the sites of inflammation or injury, makes these cells a promising candidate for drug delivery vehicles.

4. MSCs - A drug delivery tool

The unique ability of MSCs to migrate to sites of inflammation, modulate immune and inhibit inflammatory responses, and prevent and repair tissue damage, make MSCs an attractive cell therapy for the treatment of diseases with inflammatory components (Newman et al., 2009). It is those features, as well as MSCs' low immunogenicity profile allowing for allogeneic, off-the-shelf use, that makes MSCs promising as a cell therapy. Table 3 summarizes the important features of MSCs for use in drug delivery.

Characteristics supporting the use of MSCs as a vehicle for drug delivery
• Selective MSCs homing to sites of inflammation and cancer • Low immunogenicity profile of MSCs which allows for allogeneic use of MSCs • Allogeneic use of MSCs enables development of "off-the-shelf" drugs • Established biodistribution and toxicology profile • Positive safety profile of MSCs in clinical trials to date • Easy availability of MSCs from adult bone marrow donors and other sources • Potential for GMP-compliant, large-scale manufacturing processes • Cryopreservation for long-term storage of MSC products

Table 3. Features of MSCs for use as a drug delivery system

4.1 MSCs as vehicle for therapeutic drugs

4.1.1 MSCs as vehicle for cancer therapeutics

Recent data providing evidence that MSCs migrate to sites of tumorigenesis in some instances suggest another therapeutic area for MSCs: the use of MSCs as a vehicle for the targeted delivery of cytotoxic agents to tumor tissue (Hall et al., 2007; Hu et al., 2010). Cells, like MSCs, which are able to target cancer cells, and are, at the same time, non-immunogenic and non-toxic to the host are the ideal vehicle for tumor-selective drug delivery. Several preclinical studies support the rationale for genetically modified MSC to deliver therapeutics to tumor sites. Successful animal models include sarcoma, melanoma, carcinoma, and several cancer metastasis models. Table 4 gives an overview of preclinical studies focusing on the delivery of genetically modified MSCs for cancer therapy.

Genes Delivered By MSCs	Treated Tumor	Reference
Cytosine deaminase in combination with 5-FC	Colon cancer Melanoma	(Kucerova et al., 2007) (Kucerova et al., 2008)
CD : UPRT	Human prostate tumor	(Cavarretta et al., 2010)
CRAd	Ovarian carcinoma Intracranial glioma Tumor metastasis	(Komarova et al., 2006) (Sonabend et al., 2008) (Stoff-Khalili et al., 2007)
CX3CL1 (Fractalkine)	Tumor metastasis	(Xin et al., 2007)
EGFRvIII	Glioma	(Balyasnikova et al., 2010)
Interferon-α	Tumor metastasis	(Ren et al., 2008a)
Interferon-β	Glioma Tumor metastasis Tumor metastasis	(Nakamizo et al., 2005) (Ren et al., 2008b) (Studeny et al., 2004)
Interleukin-2	Glioma Melanoma	(Nakamura et al., 2004) (Stagg et al., 2004)
Interleukin-12	Tumor metastasis Ewing sarcoma tumors Melanoma	(Chen et al., 2008) (Duan et al., 2009) (Elzaouk et al., 2006)
iNOS	Fibrosarcoma	(Xiang et al., 2009)
NK4 (adenovirus)	Tumor metastasis	(Kanehira et al., 2007)
(Delta)24-RGD (adenovirus)	Glioma	(Yong et al., 2009)
TRAIL	Tumor metastasis Glioma Carcinoma	(Loebinger et al., 2009a) (Sasportas et al., 2009) (Mohr et al., 2008)

Abbreviations: CD: UPRT = cytosine deaminase: uracil phosphoribosyltransferase; CRADs = conditionally replicating adenoviruses; EGFRvIII = mutant epidermal growth factor receptor; 5FC = 5-fluorocytosine; iNOS = inducible nitric oxide synthase; TRAIL = tumor necrosis factor related apoptosis-inducing ligand

Table 4. Preclinical studies of genetically engineered MSCs for the delivery of anti-cancer agents to tumors.

Among others, recent efforts focused on the delivery of anti-proliferative and pro-apoptotic therapeutics, like Interferon-β (IFN-β) (Chawla-Sarkar et al., 2001; Johns et al., 1992). The therapeutic efficacy of IFN-β had been limited by its toxicity associated with systemic administration (Menon et al., 2009). To be able to minimize toxicity and increase the local concentration of IFN-β, MSCs were selected as delivery vehicle. Murine MSCs were engineered to release IFN-β and injected via tail vein into immunocompetent mice with prostate cancer lung metastasis (Ren et al., 2008b). Following IFN-β-expressing MSC therapy, the mice showed a reduction of tumor volume in the lung, increased tumor cell apoptosis, decreased tumor cell proliferation and blood vessel counts, and an increase in the natural killer cell activity. The systemic level of IFN-β was not significantly elevated by the targeted cell therapy (Ren et al., 2008b).

MSCs expressing IFN-β were also used for targeted delivery of interferon to metastatic breast carcinoma and melanoma models (Studeny et al., 2004). To establish pulmonary metastases, mice were injected MDA-MB-231 tumor cells in the lateral tail vein. Eight days after tumor cell injection, mice started treatment with recombinant IFN-β, IFN-β-MSCs, or MSC-Gal by intravenous injection (Studeny et al., 2004). Whole lung weight was used as a surrogate endpoint of MDA-MB-231 tumor burden in the lung. Tumor mice treated intravenously with MSC-IFN-β cells had significantly smaller lungs then untreated control mice injected with tumor cells only (mean lung weight 0.408 g versus 0.977 g; $p = 0.021$). By contrast, there was no statistically significant difference in the mean lung weight of mice treated with recombinant IFN-β or MSC-Gal cells and control mice injected with tumor cells only. Intravenous administration of human IFN-β-MSCs also prolonged the survival of animals with established metastases of MDA-MB-231 breast carcinoma (median survival 60 days versus 37 days in control mice, $p < 0.001$) and A375SM melanoma tumor in the lung (median survival 73.5 days versus 30 days in control mice, $p < 0.001$) (Studeny et al., 2004).

Another therapeutic with encouraging preclinical results in MSC-targeted cancer therapy is the tumor necrosis factor-related apoptosis-inducing ligand (TRAIL), a transmembrane protein, which induces apoptosis in various tumor cell types (Hao et al., 2001; Kagawa et al., 2001). Loebinger and coauthors (Loebinger et al., 2009a) showed that directly delivered TRAIL-expressing MSCs were able to significantly reduce tumor growth ($p < 0.001$) in subcutaneous xenograft experiments. In a pulmonary metastasis model, systemically delivered TRAIL-expressing MSCs localized to lung metastasis, and the controlled local delivery of TRAIL completely cleared lung metastases in 38% of mice compared to none of the controls ($p < 0.05$) (Loebinger et al., 2009a). Anti-tumorigenic effects of MSC-delivered recombinant TRAIL were also reported from human glioma models (Sasportas et al., 2009). The ability of MSCs to target primary tumors and their metastases suggests an important therapeutic role for MSCs as drug delivery vehicles in the future.

4.1.2 MSCs as vehicle for prodrug gene therapy

A very promising approach to reduce cancer drug toxicity is prodrug gene therapy, based on the delivery of genes encoding enzymes that convert nontoxic prodrugs into toxic antimetabolites (Menon et al., 2009). One of the chemotherapeutic agents of interest for prodrug gene therapy is the prodrug 5-Fluorocytosine. This prodrug is converted to the potent chemotherapeutic substrate 5-fluorouracil by the bacterial and/or yeast cytosine deaminase enzyme. 5-Fluorouracil has been used successfully for colorectal and pancreatic cancer therapy for about 40 years. Despite the fact that it is a potent chemotherapeutic agent, its high toxicity results in severe side effects in treated patients. The development of a prodrug, which is only converted into the toxic chemotherapeutic agent at the site of tumorigenesis, is an important step to achieve lower toxicity of 5-fluorouracil. Kucerova et al. combined MSC-driven targeted delivery of the prodrug converting enzyme cytosine deaminase: uracil phosphoribosyltransferase with the systemic administration of the prodrug 5-fluorocytosine (Kucerova et al., 2007, 2008). The administration of MSCs expressing the prodrug converting enzyme (CDy-AT-MSCs) in combination with systemic delivery of 5-Fluorocytosine, inhibited subcutaneous human colon cancer growth in immunocompromised mice. By day 18, significant inhibition of tumor growth of up to 69% was observed in all animals injected with CDy-AT-MSC. The animals did not show any signs of toxic side effects of the therapeutic regimen.

Also in a murine melanoma model, systemic administration of CDy-AT-MSC resulted in cell homing into subcutaneous melanoma and mediated tumor growth inhibition (Kucerova et al., 2008). A similar study on pancreatic cancer was recently conducted by Cararetta et al. (Cavarretta et al., 2010). After induction of PC3 tumors in mice, the animals received systemic administration of CDy-AT-MSCs and were daily treated with 5-Fluorocytosine. On day 24, average tumor volume had decreased in all treated animals compared to control animals. In a second group with repeated CDy-AT-MSC injections, complete regression of the tumor was observed at day 36 in three out of six mice. The studies confirm that MSC have the potential to travel to site of tumorigenesis and to effectively deliver prodrug converting enzymes. Targeted delivery of prodrug-converting enzymes in combination with the systemic delivery of the according prodrug might substantially reduce side effects of otherwise highly toxic therapeutics.

4.1.3 MSCs as vehicle for biological pacemaker genes

In addition to the development of MSCs as delivery vehicles for cancer therapeutics, much research in MSC delivery tools focuses on the delivery of biological pacemakers for the treatment of heart diseases. Electronic pacemakers, the standard of care for heart block and other electrophysiological abnormalities, still have shortcomings, like limitations on exercise tolerance and cardiac rate-response to emotion; limited battery life, interference with neural stimulators, metal detectors, and MRI equipment; effects on electrophysiological or contractile function; and sizing challenges for growing pediatric patients (Rosen et al., 2004, 2008). Biological pacemakers that would create a stable physiological rhythm, not require electronic equipment and adapt to changes in activity and emotion, would be an attractive alternative. MSCs might serve as a platform for the delivery of pacemaker genes. First proof of concept was collected in a canine study by Potapova et al. (Potapova et al., 2004). Human MSCs were engineered to express the biological pacemaker gene mHCN2 and administered into the left ventricular wall of adult dogs. The animals were subjected to a pericardiectomy and within ten days, vagal stimulation was performed to induce atrioventricular block and to analyze whether escape pacemaker function occurred. Five of six animals receiving hMSCs expressing the biological pacemaker and the enhanced green fluorescent protein (EGFP) reporter gene developed rhythms originating from the left ventricle and pace-mapped to the injection site. Only two out of four control animals, which had received MSCs expressing EGFP alone, developed right ventricular escape rhythms. Dogs who had received the biological pacemaker gene developed idioventricular rhythms with rates approximating on average 61 beats per minute (bpm), while the rates of control animals only reached 45 bpm ($p < 0.05$; (Potapova et al., 2004)). Nests of adult human MSCs were found at the site of injection, as well as evidence for gap junctional coupling between adult MSCs and myocytes.

In another study from the same group (Plotnikov et al., 2007), mHCN2 expressing MSCs were administered into the left ventricular wall of adult dogs in complete heart block and with backup electronic pacemakers to operate in "tandem" mode. After stabilization around day 10 to 12, the biological pacemaker functioned stably and with little time-dependent variation in dogs that had received at least 700,000 hMSCs. The pacemaker function was stable until the end of the study at day 42. Following Plotnikov et al., no cellular or humoral rejection, loss of function, or apoptosis was observed during this time (Plotnikov et al., 2007). A later analysis by Rosen et al. (Rosen et al., 2008) assessed the observation of loss of function and histological evidence of rejection in some of the xenotransplants. The studies show that, despite great progress in the development of MSCs as vehicles for biological pacemakers, some questions remain unanswered. Further studies are needed to investigate how reliable and durable pacemaker function can be obtained without rejection and how the cells can be maintained in the target area.

4.1.4 Clinical progress with MSCs delivering therapeutics

While many preclinical studies have shown proof of concept for the use of MSCs as targeted delivery vehicle, clinical studies are focused on unmodified human MSCs. Additional modification of the cells may help to increase levels of therapeutics generated by the cells, or induce the production of therapeutics which are not present in naïve cells. MSCs can be modified using genetic and non-genetic techniques, including the pre-differentiation of MSCs in growth factor containing media. In a first clinical study, adipose-derived insulin-producing MSCs (h-AD-MSC) were used for the treatment of type 1 diabetes mellitus (DM), an autoimmune disorder with disturbed glucose/insulin metabolism, which has no medical treatment other than life-long insulin therapy (Trivedi et al., 2008). To obtain MSCs that produce insulin, the adipose-tissue derived MSCs were cultured in differentiation medium. The DM patients received intraportal administration of h-AD-MSC together with xenogeneic-free, cultured bone marrow-derived hematopoietic stem cell transplantation. Five insulinopenic DM patients at the age of 14 to 28 years received a mean dose of 3 million h-AD-MSC. The patients showed 30% to 50% decreased insulin requirements with 4- to 26-fold increased serum c-peptide levels, at a mean follow-up of 2.9 months. No adverse side effects related to the stem cell infusion or the administration of induction therapy were reported. The study provided initial evidence of potential treatment of insulinopenic diabetics using insulin-producing h-AD-MSC in conjunction with hematopoietic stem cell transplants. It is a first step in the use of modified MSCs in clinical settings, and additional larger studies will be important to assess the durability of the response.

Another clinical study with autologous cultured mesenchymal bone marrow stromal cells secreting neurotrophic factors (MSC-NTF, NurOwn™) is planned by the Hadassah Medical Organization in Jerusalem, Israel, in collaboration with Brainstorm Cell Therapeutics Ltd. The study will evaluate the safety and therapeutic effects of MSC-NTFs injections as a treatment for patients with amyotrophic lateral sclerosis (ALS). ALS, also called Lou Gehrig's disease, is a progressive neurodegenerative disease that affects nerve cells in the brain and the spinal cord, characterized by progressive degeneration of motor neurons. Animal studies have shown that glial-derived neurotrophic factor (GDNF) can protect motor neurons from degeneration *in vitro* (Henderson et al., 1994; Suzuki et al., 2007). For this clinical study, adult bone marrow cells capable of releasing neurotrophic factors, including GDNF, will be generated and transplanted into ALS patients. In early ALS subjects, MSC-NTF cells will be transplanted intramuscularly, while cells will be administered intrathecally in progressive ALS patients. The hypothesis is that the administration of MSCs expressing GDNF might protect motor neurons from further neurodegeneration. Results are not available yet, as the study is in its early stages.

4.2 MSCs as vehicle for nanoparticles

Nanoparticles can be used not only as a carrier for drugs, but also as a diagnostic and therapeutic tool. As nanoparticles reach their target site by passive targeting via the EPR effect, their target specificity is limited. Target specificity, however, could be improved by using MSCs as a vehicle to deliver nanoparticles specifically to sites of inflammation and tumorigenesis. At the site of interest, the nanoparticles could serve different purposes, dependent on the nanoparticle material and therapeutic aim.

An essential requirement for the development of nanoparticle-carrying MSCs as a diagnostic or therapeutic tool is the successful uptake of nanoparticles by the cells and low toxicity of the nanoparticles within the cell. Studies have shown that, among other factors, nanoparticle size, shape and surface charge play an important role in the uptake of nanoparticles in cells (Chithrani & Chan, 2007; Chithrani et al., 2006; Jo et al., 2010; Patra et al., 2010). Chithrani et al. investigated the intracellular uptake of different sized and shaped colloidal gold nanoparticles in HeLa cells and other mammalian cell lines (Chithrani & Chan, 2007; Chithrani et al., 2006). Gold nanoparticles were used as a model nanoparticle system, as their size and shape can be easily controlled during synthesis, and quantification of the nanoparticles is possible in biological samples. Among spherical nanoparticles with diameters between 14 nm and 100 nm, the maximum uptake by a cell occurred at a nanoparticle size of 50 nm. Similar findings were made by other research groups (Malugin & Ghandehari, 2010). The uptake of rod-shaped gold nanoparticles was lower, and the fraction of exocytosed rod-shaped nanoparticles higher, than that of their spherical counterpart. In general, exocytosis occurred at a higher rate and higher percentage in smaller compared to larger nanoparticles. Thus, both, uptake and removal of nanoparticles were highly dependent upon the size of the nanoparticles, but the trends were different (Chithrani & Chan, 2007). Besides nanoparticle size and form, the type of ligand coating the cells also influenced the cellular uptake. The number of transferrin-coated gold nanoparticles that entered the cells was about three times less than that of the citrate-stabilized gold nanoparticles (Chithrani et al., 2006). The uptake of gold nanoparticles was also investigated in MSCs (Koshevoy et al., 2010; Yamada et al., 2009). In-depth knowledge of nanoparticle properties crucial for cellular uptake will help to accelerate the development of nanoparticle candidates for targeted cell therapies.

4.2.1 Nanoparticle labeled cells as diagnostic tool

The development of nanoparticle-loaded MSCs in the recent past has concentrated on diagnostic applications. The nanoparticles of choice for such cell labeling studies in MSCs were superparamagnetic iron oxide (SPIO) particles which can be used to track the biodistribution and migration of transplanted cells by MRI and other imaging methods (Arbab et al., 2004; Bulte et al., 2005; Chen et al., 2010a; Jo et al., 2010; Kostura et al., 2004; Loebinger et al., 2009b; Reddy et al., 2010; Walczak et al., 2005). Tracking labeled MSCs after transplantation will enable a better understanding of the dynamics of cell-tissue interactions and help improve the design of stem cell therapies by optimizing cell manufacturing and cell delivery protocols (Bulte et al., 2005; Srinivas et al., 2010). The impact of nanoparticle uptake on cell viability and cell functionality was analyzed in *in vitro* studies. Bulte et al. injected poly-L-lysine coated ferumoxide (PLL-Feridex) labeled canine MSCs via MR fluoroscopy in a canine myocardial infarction model, and followed their biodistribution (Bulte et al., 2005). The cells could be serially tracked by MRI for at least eight weeks following implantation. Feridex-labeling did not affect cell proliferation, adipogenesis, or osteogenesis, but markedly diminished the cells' ability to undergo chondrogenesis (Bulte et al., 2005; Kostura et al., 2004). This could also be shown for human MSCs labeled with SPIO nanoparticles coated with carboxydextran (Resovist) by Reddy et al. (Reddy et al., 2010), while Schäfer et al. (Schäfer et al., 2010) did not observe such effect. In contrast, human MSCs labeled with chitosan-coated superparamagnetic iron oxide did not exhibit any significant alterations in the surface marker expression or adipo /osteo /chondrogenic differentiation potential when compared to unlabeled control cells (Reddy et al., 2010).

These studies show that careful selection of the MR contrast agent and modification protocol are required to retain full functionality of the cells after modification. Extensive *in vitro* and *in vivo* analyses of nanoparticle-loaded cells have to be conducted to ensure safety and effectiveness of the cell based diagnostic tool. As mammalian cells are well adapted to regulation of iron homeostasis, the use of ferumoxides appears clinically safe. So far, the iron oxide-based contrast agents Feridex and Resovist have been approved by the FDA. Despite technical challenges that still have to be addressed, the studies show that MSCs can be successfully loaded with the MR contrast agents and tracked via MRI. Besides MRI, other non-optical cell tracking methods are available, like positron emission tomography (PET) and single photon emission computed tomography (SPECT). An overview of stem cell tracking methods addressing their pros and cons can be found in reviews by Reagan and Kaplan (Reagan & Kaplan, 2011) and Srinivas et al. (Srinivas et al., 2010).

Clinical studies tracking radiolabeled or SPIO labeled cells have been conducted with different cell types, including dendritic cells, neural stem cells, hematopoietic stem cells, and cadaveric islet cells (Bulte, 2009; Srinivas et al., 2010). With increasing clinical use of MSCs, the *in vivo* tracking of MSCs has become useful because it can help to evaluate and optimize MSC therapies. One phase I/II clinical study conducted in Jerusalem, Israel involved the administration of autologous Feridex-labeled MSCs in patients with multiple sclerosis and amyotrophic lateral sclerosis in an effort to prevent further neurodegeneration (Karussis et al., 2010). The Feridex-tag was added to allow cell tracking via MRI and evaluate migration of the transplanted cells. Intrathecal and intravenous administration were combined to maximize the potential therapeutic benefit by accessing the central nervous system through the cerebrospinal fluid and the systemic circulation. Of the 34 patients enrolled, nine patients received SMIO labeled (Feridex) MSCs. MRIs of the brain and whole spine performed at different time points after MSC injection indicated possible dissemination of the MSCs from the lumbar site of inoculation to the occipital horns, meninges, spinal roots, and spinal cord parenchyma. The results, however, need to be interpreted with caution, as the number of patients in the study is small and it is not ruled out that macrophages phagocytized the iron oxide magnetic resonance contrast agent and migrated to the inflammatory lesions.

The ability of MSCs to migrate to sites of tumorigenesis might also allow for the development of labeled MSCs as a clinical tool for cancer detection. In support of this idea, Loebinger et al. showed that intravenously injected iron-labeled MSCs could be tracked *in vivo* to multiple lung metastases using MRI (Loebinger et al., 2009b). Human MSCs were labeled with starch-coated FluidMAG iron nanoparticles and injected via the lateral tail vein into mice with metastatic lung tumors. MRI and immunohistological staining confirmed the localization of SPIO-loaded MSCs to lung metastases one hour after injection. Preceding experiments with mice carrying subcutaneous MDA-MB-231 tumors showed that as few as 1,000 Feridex-labeled MSCs could be visualized in tumors using MRI (Loebinger et al., 2009b). The ability to track MSCs homing to primary tumors and metastases using a noninvasive scanning method could be of great benefit for future diagnostic applications.

4.2.2 Nanoparticle-loaded cells as therapeutic tool

Besides diagnostic applications, nanoparticle-carrying cells are also interesting for therapeutic use. High Z-elements like gold can be utilized for radiotherapy enhancement (Butterworth et al., 2010; Chang et al., 2008; Chithrani et al., 2010; Hainfeld et al., 2004, 2008; Herold et al., 2000; Kong et al., 2008; Liu et al., 2010; Rahman et al., 2009; Rose et al., 1999), photothermal ablation of cancer cells by heating with near-infrared lasers (Atkinson et al., 2010; Chen et al., 2010b; Cherukuri et al., 2010; Diagaradjane et al., 2008; Gobin et al., 2010; Kennedy et al., 2011), and thermal destruction of cancer cells by radiofrequency field-induced heating (Gannon et al., 2008). Radiotherapy is one of the most commonly used methods in cancer therapy. Gold nanoparticles were shown to increase radiotherapy efficiency when accumulated in tumors due to their high absorption of X-rays (Hainfeld et al., 2008). However, injections of gold did not result in the delivery of gold nanoparticles to the tumor sites only. Although some nanoparticles were transported to the tumor via the EPR effect, others were detected in the blood, liver, spleen, and muscle, before renal clearance (Hainfeld et al., 2006). MSCs have been shown to home to sites of tumorigenesis and represent a potential vehicle for the targeted delivery of radiotherapy enhancers to tumor sites. Delivering a curative dose of radiation to tumor tissues, while sparing normal tissues, would help to reduce side effects of radiotherapy treatment and increase radiotherapy efficiency.

First steps towards the development of cells carrying nanoparticles for radiotherapy enhancement have been made. Radiation enhancement was quantified in HELA cells by irradiating the cells with 220 kVp X-rays in the absence and presence of different sized internalized gold nanoparticles. Radiosensitization was dependent on the number of gold nanoparticles internalized in the cells, with gold nanoparticles of 50 nm diameter showing the highest radiosensitization enhancement factor (1.43 at 220 kVp) among gold nanoparticles ranging from 14 to 74 nm diameter. Radiation sensitization in HELA cells carrying 50 nm gold nanoparticles also depended on the energy of the radiation source (Chithrani et al., 2010).

The enhancement of radiation effects by gold nanoparticles was also studied in bovine aortic endothelial (BAEC) cells (Rahman et al., 2009). Tumor growth and survival are critically linked to the proliferation of endothelial cells comprising the tumor blood vessel network (Sieman, 2006). Targeting the blood vessel network of a tumor with radiation aims to impair the nutritional support system of the tumor. Rahman et al. exposed BAEC cells carrying 1.9 nm gold nanoparticles to kilovoltage X-ray radiation therapy and megavoltage electron radiation therapy. Dose enhancement in cells irradiated with superficial X-ray reached a dose enhancement factor of 24.6 with X-ray beams of 80 kVp and correlated with the concentration of internalized gold nanoparticles. Dose enhancement in cells irradiated with electron beams reached a factor of 4.1. The study showed that gold nanoparticles can be used to enhance the effect of radiation doses from kilovoltage X-ray radiation therapy and megavoltage electron radiation therapy beams. As lower radiation doses destroy the same fraction of cells when gold nanoparticles are present as do larger radiation doses without radiosensitizers, the use of gold nanoparticles in radiotherapy might help to reduce radiation doses in the future (Rahman et al., 2009).

4.3 Outlook on MSCs as targeted delivery tools

Safety and ready availability of MSCs, together with their ability to home to sites of injury and tumorigenesis, and their low immunogenicity profile, makes them an attractive delivery vehicle for diagnostic and therapeutic purposes. Still, there are hurdles to be overcome before drug-loaded MSCs will be ready for clinical use. One of the challenges to be mastered is the effective loading of the vehicle cell with the therapeutic. MSCs must be loaded with drugs or modified to produce high enough concentrations of agent to reach therapeutic effectiveness without compromising cell viability and properties necessary for effective drug delivery (e.g. homing or migration potential). Several animal models have shown that therapeutically effective, modified MSCs can be generated (as discussed in section 4.1), and clinical trials will show whether those results can be translated into human use. Another necessity is the development of effective drug release mechanisms. Such mechanisms to initiate the release of the therapeutic from the MSCs to gain access to or enter the target cell remain to be found.

Furthermore, for access to target sites, biological barriers, like the blood-brain barrier (Gabathuler, 2010; Patel et al., 2009), have to be crossed for the cells to be able to reach their target, which makes the route of administration another important factor to consider. In one study following intravenous injection of MSCs into rats after resuscitation from cardiac arrest, MSCs were detected in the brain. The number of detected cells was low, however neurologic recovery of the animals appeared to improve (Wang et al., 2008). Future studies have to demonstrate whether the number of MSCs crossing the blood-brain barrier is sufficient for therapeutically effective drug delivery. Alternatively, other routes of drug delivery could be chosen. Intranasally administered MSCs were shown to bypass the blood-brain barrier by migrating from the nasal mucosa through the cribriform plate along the olfactory neural pathway into the brain and cerebrospinal fluid (Danielyan et al., 2009). Also local injections of drug-loaded MSCs might be considered to gain access to diseased tissue that is difficult to target. In this case, MSCs would be responsible for the "micro-targeting" of the drug very specifically within the target area.

In addition to biological complications, there will also be technical hurdles in the development of drug-carrying MSCs. The successful transfer of MSC modification processes at the research scale to manufacturing levels could be challenging. Large-scale production of drug-loaded MSCs, whether it involves genetic modifications, culture-induced modification of cells, or loading of cells with nanoparticles, can be very expensive and time-consuming. Results from small-scale experiments cannot always easily be translated into large-scale production without significant additional efforts. Overall, MSCs are a very promising drug delivery tool. However, this new technology will only support widespread clinical use if effective drug loading and successful drug release at the site of interest can be ensured, and robust manufacturing processes are developed.

5. References

Adiseshaiah, P. P., Hall, J. B. & McNeil, S. E. (2009). Nanomaterial standards for efficacy and toxicity assessment. *Wiley Interdiscip Rev Nanomed Nanobiotechnol,* 2, 99-112

Aggarwal, S. & Pittenger, M. F. (2005). Human mesenchymal stem cells modulate allogeneic immune cell responses. *Blood,* 105, 1815-22

Allen, T. M. (2002). Ligand-targeted therapeutics in anticancer therapy. *Nat Rev Cancer,* 2, 750-63

Allers, C., Sierralta, W. D., Neubauer, S., Rivera, F., Minguell, J. J. & Conget, P. A. (2004). Dynamic of distribution of human bone marrow-derived mesenchymal stem cells after transplantation into adult unconditioned mice. *Transplantation,* 78, 503-8

Alley, S. C., Okeley, N. M. & Senter, P. D. (2010). Antibody-drug conjugates: targeted drug delivery for cancer. *Curr Opin Chem Biol,* 14, 529-37

Arbab, A. S., Yocum, G. T., Kalish, H., Jordan, E. K., Anderson, S. A., Khakoo, A. Y., Read, E. J. & Frank, J. A. (2004). Efficient magnetic cell labeling with protamine sulfate complexed to ferumoxides for cellular MRI. *Blood,* 104, 1217-23

Assis, A. C., Carvalho, J. L., Jacoby, B. A., Ferreira, R. L., Castanheira, P., Diniz, S. O., Cardoso, V. N., Goes, A. M. & Ferreira, A. J. (2010). Time-dependent migration of systemically delivered bone marrow mesenchymal stem cells to the infarcted heart. *Cell Transplant,* 19, 219-30

Atkinson, R. L., Zhang, M., Diagaradjane, P., Peddibhotla, S., Contreras, A., Hilsenbeck, S. G., Woodward, W. A., Krishnan, S., Chang, J. C. & Rosen, J. M. (2010). Thermal enhancement with optically activated gold nanoshells sensitizes breast cancer stem cells to radiation therapy. *Sci Transl Med,* 2, 55ra79

Atoui, R., Asenjo, J. F., Duong, M., Chen, G., Chiu, R. C. & Shum-Tim, D. (2008). Marrow stromal cells as universal donor cells for myocardial regenerative therapy: their unique immune tolerance. *Ann Thorac Surg,* 85, 571-9

Bacher, U., Asenova, S., Badbaran, A., Zander, A. R., Alchalby, H., Fehse, B., Kroger, N., Lange, C. & Ayuk, F. (2010). Bone marrow mesenchymal stromal cells remain of recipient origin after allogeneic SCT and do not harbor the JAK2V617F mutation in patients with myelofibrosis. *Clin Exp Med,* 10, 205-8

Backer, M. V., Aloise, R., Przekop, K., Stoletov, K. & Backer, J. M. (2002). Molecular vehicles for targeted drug delivery. *Bioconjug Chem,* 13, 462-7

Bacsich, P. & Wyburn, G. M. (1947). The significance of the mucoprotein content on the survival of homografts of cartilage and cornea. *Proc R Soc Edinb Biol,* 62, 321-7

Bae, Y. H. (2009). Drug targeting and tumor heterogeneity. *J Control Release,* 133, 2-3

Ball, L. M., Bernardo, M. E., Roelofs, H., Lankester, A., Cometa, A., Egeler, R. M., Locatelli, F. & Fibbe, W. E. (2007). Cotransplantation of ex vivo expanded mesenchymal stem cells accelerates lymphocyte recovery and may reduce the risk of graft failure in haploidentical hematopoietic stem-cell transplantation. *Blood,* 110, 2764-7

Balyasnikova, I. V., Ferguson, S. D., Sengupta, S., Han, Y. & Lesniak, M. S. (2010). Mesenchymal stem cells modified with a single-chain antibody against EGFRvIII successfully inhibit the growth of human xenograft malignant glioma. *PLoS One,* 5, e9750

Bartholomew, A., Sturgeon, C., Siatskas, M., Ferrer, K., McIntosh, K., Patil, S., Hardy, W., Devine, S., Ucker, D., Deans, R., Moseley, A. & Hoffman, R. (2002). Mesenchymal stem cells suppress lymphocyte proliferation in vitro and prolong skin graft survival in vivo. *Exp Hematol,* 30, 42-8

Bartsch, K., Al-Ali, H., Reinhardt, A., Franke, C., Hudecek, M., Kamprad, M., Tschiedel, S., Cross, M., Niederwieser, D. & Gentilini, C. (2009). Mesenchymal stem cells remain host-derived independent of the source of the stem-cell graft and conditioning regimen used. *Transplantation,* 87, 217-21

Bawa, R. (2008). Nanoparticle-based therapeutics in humans: a survey. *Nanotechnology Law and Business,* 135-55

Beck, A., Haeuw, J. F., Wurch, T., Goetsch, L., Bailly, C. & Corvaia, N. (2010). The next generation of antibody-drug conjugates comes of age. *Discov Med,* 10, 329-39

Beck, A., Senter, P. D. & Chari, R. J. (2011). World Antibody Drug Conjugate Summit Europe: February 21-23, 2011; Frankfurt, Germany. *MAbs,* 3:4, 1-7

Birnbaum, T., Roider, J., Schankin, C. J., Padovan, C. S., Schichor, C., Goldbrunner, R. & Straube, A. (2007). Malignant gliomas actively recruit bone marrow stromal cells by secreting angiogenic cytokines. *J Neurooncol,* 83, 241-7

Branco, M. C. & Schneider, J. P. (2009). Self-assembling materials for therapeutic delivery. *Acta Biomater,* 5, 817-31

Bruder, S. P., Kraus, K. H., Goldberg, V. M. & Kadiyala, S. (1998). The effect of implants loaded with autologous mesenchymal stem cells on the healing of canine segmental bone defects. *J Bone Joint Surg Am,* 80, 985-96

Brunner, C. S. (2004). Challenges and Opportunities in Emerging Drug Delivery Technologies. Product Genesis, Cambridge. PG Report Emerging Drug Delivery Technologies 0403

Bulte, J. W., Kostura, L., Mackay, A., Karmarkar, P. V., Izbudak, I., Atalar, E., Fritzges, D., Rodriguez, E. R., Young, R. G., Marcelino, M., Pittenger, M. F. & Kraitchman, D. L. (2005). Feridex-labeled mesenchymal stem cells: cellular differentiation and MR assessment in a canine myocardial infarction model. *Acad Radiol,* 12 Suppl 1, S2-6

Bulte, J. W. (2009). In vivo MRI cell tracking: clinical studies. *AJR Am J Roentgenol,* 193, 314-25

Burris, H. A., 3rd, Rugo, H. S., Vukelja, S. J., Vogel, C. L., Borson, R. A., Limentani, S., Tan-Chiu, E., Krop, I. E., Michaelson, R. A., Girish, S., Amler, L., Zheng, M., Chu, Y. W., Klencke, B. & O'Shaughnessy, J. A. (2011). Phase II study of the antibody drug conjugate trastuzumab-DM1 for the treatment of human epidermal growth factor receptor 2 (HER2)-positive breast cancer after prior HER2-directed therapy. *J Clin Oncol,* 29, 398-405

Butterworth, K. T., Coulter, J. A., Jain, S., Forker, J., McMahon, S. J., Schettino, G., Prise, K. M., Currell, F. J. & Hirst, D. G. (2010). Evaluation of cytotoxicity and radiation enhancement using 1.9 nm gold particles: potential application for cancer therapy. *Nanotechnology,* 21, 295101

Caplan, A. I. & Dennis, J. E. (2006). Mesenchymal stem cells as trophic mediators. *J Cell Biochem,* 98, 1076-84

Caplan, A. I. (2007). Adult mesenchymal stem cells for tissue engineering versus regenerative medicine. *J Cell Physiol,* 213, 341-7

Cavarretta, I. T., Altanerova, V., Matuskova, M., Kucerova, L., Culig, Z. & Altaner, C. (2010). Adipose tissue-derived mesenchymal stem cells expressing prodrug-converting enzyme inhibit human prostate tumor growth. *Mol Ther,* 18, 223-31

Chang, M. Y., Shiau, A. L., Chen, Y. H., Chang, C. J., Chen, H. H. & Wu, C. L. (2008). Increased apoptotic potential and dose-enhancing effect of gold nanoparticles in combination with single-dose clinical electron beams on tumor-bearing mice. *Cancer Sci,* 99, 1479-84

Chari, R. V. (2008). Targeted cancer therapy: conferring specificity to cytotoxic drugs. *Acc Chem Res,* 41, 98-107

Chawla-Sarkar, M., Leaman, D. W. & Borden, E. C. (2001). Preferential induction of apoptosis by interferon (IFN)-beta compared with IFN-alpha2: correlation with TRAIL/Apo2L induction in melanoma cell lines. *Clin Cancer Res,* 7, 1821-31

Chen, C. L., Zhang, H., Ye, Q., Hsieh, W. Y., Hitchens, T. K., Shen, H. H., Liu, L., Wu, Y. J., Foley, L. M., Wang, S. J. & Ho, C. (2010a). A New Nano-sized Iron Oxide Particle with High Sensitivity for Cellular Magnetic Resonance Imaging. *Mol Imaging Biol,* Epub ahead of print

Chen, J., Glaus, C., Laforest, R., Zhang, Q., Yang, M., Gidding, M., Welch, M. J. & Xia, Y. (2010b). Gold nanocages as photothermal transducers for cancer treatment. *Small,* 6, 811-7

Chen, L., Tredget, E. E., Liu, C. & Wu, Y. (2009). Analysis of allogenicity of mesenchymal stem cells in engraftment and wound healing in mice. *PLoS One,* 4, e7119

Chen, S. L., Fang, W. W., Ye, F., Liu, Y. H., Qian, J., Shan, S. J., Zhang, J. J., Chunhua, R. Z., Liao, L. M., Lin, S. & Sun, J. P. (2004). Effect on left ventricular function of intracoronary transplantation of autologous bone marrow mesenchymal stem cell in patients with acute myocardial infarction. *Am J Cardiol,* 94, 92-5

Chen, X., Lin, X., Zhao, J., Shi, W., Zhang, H., Wang, Y., Kan, B., Du, L., Wang, B., Wei, Y., Liu, Y. & Zhao, X. (2008). A tumor-selective biotherapy with prolonged impact on established metastases based on cytokine gene-engineered MSCs. *Mol Ther,* 16, 749-56

Cheng, L., Qasba, P., Vanguri, P. & Thiede, M. A. (2000). Human mesenchymal stem cells support megakaryocyte and pro-platelet formation from CD34(+) hematopoietic progenitor cells. *J Cell Physiol,* 184, 58-69

Cherukuri, P., Glazer, E. S. & Curley, S. A. (2010). Targeted hyperthermia using metal nanoparticles. *Adv Drug Deliv Rev,* 62, 339-45

Chithrani, B. D., Ghazani, A. A. & Chan, W. C. (2006). Determining the size and shape dependence of gold nanoparticle uptake into mammalian cells. *Nano Lett,* 6, 662-8

Chithrani, B. D. & Chan, W. C. (2007). Elucidating the mechanism of cellular uptake and removal of protein-coated gold nanoparticles of different sizes and shapes. *Nano Lett,* 7, 1542-50

Chithrani, D. B., Jelveh, S., Jalali, F., van Prooijen, M., Allen, C., Bristow, R. G., Hill, R. P. & Jaffray, D. A. (2010). Gold nanoparticles as radiation sensitizers in cancer therapy. *Radiat Res,* 173, 719-28

Chou, L. Y., Ming, K. & Chan, W. C. (2011). Strategies for the intracellular delivery of nanoparticles. *Chem Soc Rev,* 40, 233-45

Ciccocioppo, R., Bernardo, M. E., Sgarella, A., Maccario, R., Avanzini, M. A., Ubezio, C., Minelli, A., Alvisi, C., Vanoli, A., Calliada, F., Dionigi, P., Perotti, C., Locatelli, F. & Corazza, G. R. (2011). Autologous bone marrow-derived mesenchymal stromal cells in the treatment of fistulising Crohn's disease. *Gut,* 60, 788-98

da Silva Meirelles, L., Caplan, A. I. & Nardi, N. B. (2008). In search of the in vivo identity of mesenchymal stem cells. *Stem Cells,* 26, 2287-99

Danhier, F., Feron, O. & Preat, V. (2010). To exploit the tumor microenvironment: Passive and active tumor targeting of nanocarriers for anti-cancer drug delivery. *J Control Release,* 148, 135-46

Danielyan, L., Schäfer, R., von Ameln-Mayerhofer, A., Buadze, M., Geisler, J., Klopfer, T., Burkhardt, U., Proksch, B., Verleysdonk, S., Ayturan, M., Buniatian, G. H., Gleiter, C. H. & Frey, W. H., 2nd. (2009). Intranasal delivery of cells to the brain. *Eur J Cell Biol,* 88, 315-24

Deans, R. J. & Moseley, A. B. (2000). Mesenchymal stem cells: biology and potential clinical uses. *Exp Hematol,* 28, 875-84

Detante, O., Moisan, A., Dimastromatteo, J., Richard, M. J., Riou, L., Grillon, E., Barbier, E., Desruet, M. D., De Fraipont, F., Segebarth, C., Jaillard, A., Hommel, M., Ghezzi, C. & Remy, C. (2009). Intravenous administration of ^{99m}Tc-HMPAO-labeled human mesenchymal stem cells after stroke: in vivo imaging and biodistribution. *Cell Transplant,* 18, 1369-79

Deutsch, Y. E., Tadmor, T., Podack, E. R. & Rosenblatt, J. D. (2011). CD30: an important new target in hematologic malignancies. *Leuk Lymphoma,* 52, 1641-54

Devine, S. M., Cobbs, C., Jennings, M., Bartholomew, A. & Hoffman, R. (2003). Mesenchymal stem cells distribute to a wide range of tissues following systemic infusion into nonhuman primates. *Blood,* 101, 2999-3001

Di Nicola, M., Carlo-Stella, C., Magni, M., Milanesi, M., Longoni, P. D., Matteucci, P., Grisanti, S. & Gianni, A. M. (2002). Human bone marrow stromal cells suppress T-lymphocyte proliferation induced by cellular or nonspecific mitogenic stimuli. *Blood,* 99, 3838-43

Diagaradjane, P., Shetty, A., Wang, J. C., Elliott, A. M., Schwartz, J., Shentu, S., Park, H. C., Deorukhkar, A., Stafford, R. J., Cho, S. H., Tunnell, J. W., Hazle, J. D. & Krishnan, S. (2008). Modulation of in vivo tumor radiation response via gold nanoshell-mediated vascular-focused hyperthermia: characterizing an integrated antihypoxic and localized vascular disrupting targeting strategy. *Nano Lett,* 8, 1492-500

Ding, X., Alani, A. & Robinson, J. M. (2006). Extended-release and targeted drug delivery systems. In: *Remington, The Science and Practice of Pharmacy, 21st edition,* ed Troy, D. B., 939-64, Lippincot Williams and Wilkins, Philadelphia

Duan, X., Guan, H., Cao, Y. & Kleinerman, E. S. (2009). Murine bone marrow-derived mesenchymal stem cells as vehicles for interleukin-12 gene delivery into Ewing sarcoma tumors. *Cancer,* 115, 13-22

Duijvestein, M., Vos, A. C., Roelofs, H., Wildenberg, M. E., Wendrich, B. B., Verspaget, H. W., Kooy-Winkelaar, E. M., Koning, F., Zwaginga, J. J., Fidder, H. H., Verhaar, A. P., Fibbe, W. E., van den Brink, G. R. & Hommes, D. W. (2010). Autologous bone marrow-derived mesenchymal stromal cell treatment for refractory luminal Crohn's disease: results of a phase I study. *Gut,* 59, 1662-9

Dvorak, H. F. (1986). Tumors: wounds that do not heal. Similarities between tumor stroma generation and wound healing. *N Engl J Med,* 315, 1650-9

Dwyer, R. M., Potter-Beirne, S. M., Harrington, K. A., Lowery, A. J., Hennessy, E., Murphy, J. M., Barry, F. P., O'Brien, T. & Kerin, M. J. (2007). Monocyte chemotactic protein-1 secreted by primary breast tumors stimulates migration of mesenchymal stem cells. *Clin Cancer Res,* 13, 5020-7

Elzaouk, L., Moelling, K. & Pavlovic, J. (2006). Anti-tumor activity of mesenchymal stem cells producing IL-12 in a mouse melanoma model. *Exp Dermatol,* 15, 865-74

English, K., Barry, F. P., Field-Corbett, C. P. & Mahon, B. P. (2007). IFN-gamma and TNF-alpha differentially regulate immunomodulation by murine mesenchymal stem cells. *Immunol Lett,* 110, 91-100

Escobar-Chavez, J. J., Bonilla-Martinez, D., Villegas-Gonzalez, M. A. & Revilla-Vazquez, A. L. (2009). Electroporation as an efficient physical enhancer for skin drug delivery. *J Clin Pharmacol,* 49, 1262-83

Forte, G., Minieri, M., Cossa, P., Antenucci, D., Sala, M., Gnocchi, V., Fiaccavento, R., Carotenuto, F., De Vito, P., Baldini, P. M., Prat, M. & Di Nardo, P. (2006). Hepatocyte growth factor effects on mesenchymal stem cells: proliferation, migration, and differentiation. *Stem Cells,* 24, 23-33

Fouillard, L., Bensidhoum, M., Bories, D., Bonte, H., Lopez, M., Moseley, A. M., Smith, A., Lesage, S., Beaujean, F., Thierry, D., Gourmelon, P., Najman, A. & Gorin, N. C. (2003). Engraftment of allogeneic mesenchymal stem cells in the bone marrow of a patient with severe idiopathic aplastic anemia improves stroma. *Leukemia,* 17, 474-6

Fouillard, L., Chapel, A., Bories, D., Bouchet, S., Costa, J. M., Rouard, H., Herve, P., Gourmelon, P., Thierry, D., Lopez, M. & Gorin, N. C. (2007). Infusion of allogeneic-related HLA mismatched mesenchymal stem cells for the treatment of incomplete engraftment following autologous haematopoietic stem cell transplantation. *Leukemia,* 21, 568-70

Friedenstein, A. J., Chailakhjan, R. K. & Lalykina, K. S. (1970). The development of fibroblast colonies in monolayer cultures of guinea-pig bone marrow and spleen cells. *Cell Tissue Kinet,* 3, 393-403

Friedenstein, A. J., Deriglasova, U. F., Kulagina, N. N., Panasuk, A. F., Rudakowa, S. F., Luria, E. A. & Ruadkow, I. A. (1974). Precursors for fibroblasts in different populations of hematopoietic cells as detected by the in vitro colony assay method. *Exp Hematol,* 2, 83-92

Gabathuler, R. (2010). Approaches to transport therapeutic drugs across the blood-brain barrier to treat brain diseases. *Neurobiol Dis,* 37, 48-57

Gannon, C. J., Patra, C. R., Bhattacharya, R., Mukherjee, P. & Curley, S. A. (2008). Intracellular gold nanoparticles enhance non-invasive radiofrequency thermal destruction of human gastrointestinal cancer cells. *J Nanobiotechnology,* 6, 2

Gao, J., Dennis, J. E., Muzic, R. F., Lundberg, M. & Caplan, A. I. (2001). The dynamic in vivo distribution of bone marrow-derived mesenchymal stem cells after infusion. *Cells Tissues Organs,* 169, 12-20

Girdler, N. M. (1997). The role of mandibular condylar cartilage in articular cartilage repair. *Ann R Coll Surg Engl*, 79, 28-37

Gobin, A. M., Watkins, E. M., Quevedo, E., Colvin, V. L. & West, J. L. (2010). Near-infrared-resonant gold/gold sulfide nanoparticles as a photothermal cancer therapeutic agent. *Small*, 6, 745-52

Hainfeld, J. F., Slatkin, D. N. & Smilowitz, H. M. (2004). The use of gold nanoparticles to enhance radiotherapy in mice. *Phys Med Biol*, 49, N309-15

Hainfeld, J. F., Slatkin, D. N., Focella, T. M. & Smilowitz, H. M. (2006). Gold nanoparticles: a new X-ray contrast agent. *Br J Radiol*, 79, 248-53

Hainfeld, J. F., Dilmanian, F. A., Slatkin, D. N. & Smilowitz, H. M. (2008). Radiotherapy enhancement with gold nanoparticles. *J Pharm Pharmacol*, 60, 977-85

Haley, B. & Frenkel, E. (2008). Nanoparticles for drug delivery in cancer treatment. *Urol Oncol*, 26, 57-64

Hall, B., Dembinski, J., Sasser, A. K., Studeny, M., Andreeff, M. & Marini, F. (2007). Mesenchymal stem cells in cancer: tumor-associated fibroblasts and cell-based delivery vehicles. *Int J Hematol*, 86, 8-16

Hao, C., Beguinot, F., Condorelli, G., Trencia, A., Van Meir, E. G., Yong, V. W., Parney, I. F., Roa, W. H. & Petruk, K. C. (2001). Induction and intracellular regulation of tumor necrosis factor-related apoptosis-inducing ligand (TRAIL) mediated apoptosis in human malignant glioma cells. *Cancer Res*, 61, 1162-70

Hare, J. M., Traverse, J. H., Henry, T. D., Dib, N., Strumpf, R. K., Schulman, S. P., Gerstenblith, G., DeMaria, A. N., Denktas, A. E., Gammon, R. S., Hermiller, J. B., Jr., Reisman, M. A., Schaer, G. L. & Sherman, W. (2009). A randomized, double-blind, placebo-controlled, dose-escalation study of intravenous adult human mesenchymal stem cells (prochymal) after acute myocardial infarction. *J Am Coll Cardiol*, 54, 2277-86

Hassan, A. O. & Elshafeey, A. H. (2010). Nanosized particulate systems for dermal and transdermal delivery. *J Biomed Nanotechnol*, 6, 621-33

Henderson, C. E., Phillips, H. S., Pollock, R. A., Davies, A. M., Lemeulle, C., Armanini, M., Simmons, L., Moffet, B., Vandlen, R. A., Simpson, L. C. & et al. (1994). GDNF: a potent survival factor for motoneurons present in peripheral nerve and muscle. *Science*, 266, 1062-4

Henry, S., McAllister, D. V., Allen, M. G. & Prausnitz, M. R. (1998). Microfabricated microneedles: a novel approach to transdermal drug delivery. *J Pharm Sci*, 87, 922-5

Herold, D. M., Das, I. J., Stobbe, C. C., Iyer, R. V. & Chapman, J. D. (2000). Gold microspheres: a selective technique for producing biologically effective dose enhancement. *Int J Radiat Biol*, 76, 1357-64

Herrera, M. B., Bussolati, B., Bruno, S., Morando, L., Mauriello-Romanazzi, G., Sanavio, F., Stamenkovic, I., Biancone, L. & Camussi, G. (2007). Exogenous mesenchymal stem cells localize to the kidney by means of CD44 following acute tubular injury. *Kidney Int*, 72, 430-41

Hilt, Z. (2010). Nanotechnology for Responsive and Feedback-Controlled systems for Protein and Drug Delivery.

http://mediaserver.aaps.org/meetings/2010PSWC/Slides/Short_Courses/Short_Course_4/Hilt_(Peppas).pdf

Horwitz, E. M., Prockop, D. J., Fitzpatrick, L. A., Koo, W. W., Gordon, P. L., Neel, M., Sussman, M., Orchard, P., Marx, J. C., Pyeritz, R. E. & Brenner, M. K. (1999). Transplantability and therapeutic effects of bone marrow-derived mesenchymal cells in children with osteogenesis imperfecta. *Nat Med,* 5, 309-13

Horwitz, E. M., Gordon, P. L., Koo, W. K., Marx, J. C., Neel, M. D., McNall, R. Y., Muul, L. & Hofmann, T. (2002). Isolated allogeneic bone marrow-derived mesenchymal cells engraft and stimulate growth in children with osteogenesis imperfecta: Implications for cell therapy of bone. *Proc Natl Acad Sci U S A,* 99, 8932-7

Hu, Y. L., Fu, Y. H., Tabata, Y. & Gao, J. Q. (2010). Mesenchymal stem cells: a promising targeted-delivery vehicle in cancer gene therapy. *J Control Release,* 147, 154-62

Ishihara, T., Takeda, M., Sakamoto, H., Kimoto, A., Kobayashi, C., Takasaki, N., Yuki, K., Tanaka, K., Takenaga, M., Igarashi, R., Maeda, T., Yamakawa, N., Okamoto, Y., Otsuka, M., Ishida, T., Kiwada, H., Mizushima, Y. & Mizushima, T. (2009). Accelerated blood clearance phenomenon upon repeated injection of PEG-modified PLA-nanoparticles. *Pharm Res,* 26, 2270-9

Ji, J. F., He, B. P., Dheen, S. T. & Tay, S. S. (2004). Interactions of chemokines and chemokine receptors mediate the migration of mesenchymal stem cells to the impaired site in the brain after hypoglossal nerve injury. *Stem Cells,* 22, 415-27

Jo, J., Aoki, I. & Tabata, Y. (2010). Design of iron oxide nanoparticles with different sizes and surface charges for simple and efficient labeling of mesenchymal stem cells. *J Control Release,* 142, 465-73

Johns, T. G., Mackay, I. R., Callister, K. A., Hertzog, P. J., Devenish, R. J. & Linnane, A. W. (1992). Antiproliferative potencies of interferons on melanoma cell lines and xenografts: higher efficacy of interferon beta. *J Natl Cancer Inst,* 84, 1185-90

Kadiyala, S., Jaiswal, N. & Buder, S. P. (1997). Culture-expanded, bone marrowderived mesenchymal stem cells regenerate a critical-sized segmental bone defect. *Tissue Eng.,* 3, 173-85

Kagawa, S., He, C., Gu, J., Koch, P., Rha, S. J., Roth, J. A., Curley, S. A., Stephens, L. C. & Fang, B. (2001). Antitumor activity and bystander effects of the tumor necrosis factor related apoptosis inducing ligand (TRAIL) gene. *Cancer Res,* 61, 3330-8

Kanehira, M., Xin, H., Hoshino, K., Maemondo, M., Mizuguchi, H., Hayakawa, T., Matsumoto, K., Nakamura, T., Nukiwa, T. & Saijo, Y. (2007). Targeted delivery of NK4 to multiple lung tumors by bone marrow-derived mesenchymal stem cells. *Cancer Gene Ther,* 14, 894-903

Karussis, D., Karageorgiou, C., Vaknin-Dembinsky, A., Gowda-Kurkalli, B., Gomori, J. M., Kassis, I., Bulte, J. W., Petrou, P., Ben-Hur, T., Abramsky, O. & Slavin, S. (2010). Safety and immunological effects of mesenchymal stem cell transplantation in patients with multiple sclerosis and amyotrophic lateral sclerosis. *Arch Neurol,* 67, 1187-94

Kebriaei, P., Isola, L., Bahceci, E., Holland, K., Rowley, S., McGuirk, J., Devetten, M., Jansen, J., Herzig, R., Schuster, M., Monroy, R. & Uberti, J. (2009). Adult human mesenchymal stem cells added to corticosteroid therapy for the treatment of acute graft-versus-host disease. *Biol Blood Marrow Transplant,* 15, 804-11

Kennedy, L. C., Bickford, L. R., Lewinski, N. A., Coughlin, A. J., Hu, Y., Day, E. S., West, J. L. & Drezek, R. A. (2011). A new era for cancer treatment: gold-nanoparticle-mediated thermal therapies. *Small*, 7, 169-83

Kim, B. Y., Rutka, J. T. & Chan, W. C. (2010). Nanomedicine. *N Engl J Med*, 363, 2434-43

Kinnaird, T., Stabile, E., Burnett, M. S., Lee, C. W., Barr, S., Fuchs, S. & Epstein, S. E. (2004). Marrow-derived stromal cells express genes encoding a broad spectrum of arteriogenic cytokines and promote in vitro and in vivo arteriogenesis through paracrine mechanisms. *Circ Res*, 94, 678-85

Klopp, A. H., Spaeth, E. L., Dembinski, J. L., Woodward, W. A., Munshi, A., Meyn, R. E., Cox, J. D., Andreeff, M. & Marini, F. C. (2007). Tumor irradiation increases the recruitment of circulating mesenchymal stem cells into the tumor microenvironment. *Cancer Res*, 67, 11687-95

Klyushnenkova, E., Mosca, J. D., Zernetkina, V., Majumdar, M. K., Beggs, K. J., Simonetti, D. W., Deans, R. J. & McIntosh, K. R. (2005). T cell responses to allogeneic human mesenchymal stem cells: immunogenicity, tolerance, and suppression. *J Biomed Sci*, 12, 47-57

Koc, O. N., Gerson, S. L., Cooper, B. W., Dyhouse, S. M., Haynesworth, S. E., Caplan, A. I. & Lazarus, H. M. (2000). Rapid hematopoietic recovery after coinfusion of autologous-blood stem cells and culture-expanded marrow mesenchymal stem cells in advanced breast cancer patients receiving high-dose chemotherapy. *J Clin Oncol*, 18, 307-16

Komarova, S., Kawakami, Y., Stoff-Khalili, M. A., Curiel, D. T. & Pereboeva, L. (2006). Mesenchymal progenitor cells as cellular vehicles for delivery of oncolytic adenoviruses. *Mol Cancer Ther*, 5, 755-66

Kon, E., Muraglia, A., Corsi, A., Bianco, P., Marcacci, M., Martin, I., Boyde, A., Ruspantini, I., Chistolini, P., Rocca, M., Giardino, R., Cancedda, R. & Quarto, R. (2000). Autologous bone marrow stromal cells loaded onto porous hydroxyapatite ceramic accelerate bone repair in critical-size defects of sheep long bones. *J Biomed Mater Res*, 49, 328-37

Kong, T., Zeng, J., Wang, X., Yang, X., Yang, J., McQuarrie, S., McEwan, A., Roa, W., Chen, J. & Xing, J. Z. (2008). Enhancement of radiation cytotoxicity in breast-cancer cells by localized attachment of gold nanoparticles. *Small*, 4, 1537-43

Koshevoy, I. O., Lin, Y. C., Chen, Y. C., Karttunen, A. J., Haukka, M., Chou, P. T., Tunik, S. P. & Pakkanen, T. A. (2010). Rational reductive fusion of two heterometallic clusters: formation of a highly stable, intensely phosphorescent Au-Ag aggregate and application in two-photon imaging in human mesenchymal stem cells. *Chem Commun (Camb)*, 46, 1440-2

Kostura, L., Kraitchman, D. L., Mackay, A. M., Pittenger, M. F. & Bulte, J. W. (2004). Feridex labeling of mesenchymal stem cells inhibits chondrogenesis but not adipogenesis or osteogenesis. *NMR Biomed*, 17, 513-7

Kraitchman, D. L., Tatsumi, M., Gilson, W. D., Ishimori, T., Kedziorek, D., Walczak, P., Segars, W. P., Chen, H. H., Fritzges, D., Izbudak, I., Young, R. G., Marcelino, M., Pittenger, M. F., Solaiyappan, M., Boston, R. C., Tsui, B. M., Wahl, R. L. & Bulte, J. W. (2005). Dynamic imaging of allogeneic mesenchymal stem cells trafficking to myocardial infarction. *Circulation*, 112, 1451-61

Krampera, M., Cosmi, L., Angeli, R., Pasini, A., Liotta, F., Andreini, A., Santarlasci, V., Mazzinghi, B., Pizzolo, G., Vinante, F., Romagnani, P., Maggi, E., Romagnani, S. & Annunziato, F. (2006). Role for interferon-gamma in the immunomodulatory activity of human bone marrow mesenchymal stem cells. *Stem Cells,* 24, 386-98

Krop, I. E., Beeram, M., Modi, S., Jones, S. F., Holden, S. N., Yu, W., Girish, S., Tibbitts, J., Yi, J. H., Sliwkowski, M. X., Jacobson, F., Lutzker, S. G. & Burris, H. A. (2010). Phase I study of trastuzumab-DM1, an HER2 antibody-drug conjugate, given every 3 weeks to patients with HER2-positive metastatic breast cancer. *J Clin Oncol,* 28, 2698-704

Kucerova, L., Altanerova, V., Matuskova, M., Tyciakova, S. & Altaner, C. (2007). Adipose tissue-derived human mesenchymal stem cells mediated prodrug cancer gene therapy. *Cancer Res,* 67, 6304-13

Kucerova, L., Matuskova, M., Pastorakova, A., Tyciakova, S., Jakubikova, J., Bohovic, R., Altanerova, V. & Altaner, C. (2008). Cytosine deaminase expressing human mesenchymal stem cells mediated tumour regression in melanoma bearing mice. *J Gene Med,* 10, 1071-82

Lazarus, H. M., Haynesworth, S. E., Gerson, S. L., Rosenthal, N. S. & Caplan, A. I. (1995). Ex vivo expansion and subsequent infusion of human bone marrow-derived stromal progenitor cells (mesenchymal progenitor cells): implications for therapeutic use. *Bone Marrow Transplant,* 16, 557-64

Lazarus, H. M., Koc, O. N., Devine, S. M., Curtin, P., Maziarz, R. T., Holland, H. K., Shpall, E. J., McCarthy, P., Atkinson, K., Cooper, B. W., Gerson, S. L., Laughlin, M. J., Loberiza, F. R., Jr., Moseley, A. B. & Bacigalupo, A. (2005). Cotransplantation of HLA-identical sibling culture-expanded mesenchymal stem cells and hematopoietic stem cells in hematologic malignancy patients. *Biol Blood Marrow Transplant,* 11, 389-98

Le Blanc, K., Rasmusson, I., Sundberg, B., Gotherstrom, C., Hassan, M., Uzunel, M. & Ringden, O. (2004). Treatment of severe acute graft-versus-host disease with third party haploidentical mesenchymal stem cells. *Lancet,* 363, 1439-41

Le Blanc, K., Samuelsson, H., Gustafsson, B., Remberger, M., Sundberg, B., Arvidson, J., Ljungman, P., Lonnies, H., Nava, S. & Ringden, O. (2007). Transplantation of mesenchymal stem cells to enhance engraftment of hematopoietic stem cells. *Leukemia,* 21, 1733-8

Le Blanc, K., Frassoni, F., Ball, L., Locatelli, F., Roelofs, H., Lewis, I., Lanino, E., Sundberg, B., Bernardo, M. E., Remberger, M., Dini, G., Egeler, R. M., Bacigalupo, A., Fibbe, W. & Ringden, O. (2008). Mesenchymal stem cells for treatment of steroid-resistant, severe, acute graft-versus-host disease: a phase II study. *Lancet,* 371, 1579-86

Li, H., Fu, X., Ouyang, Y., Cai, C., Wang, J. & Sun, T. (2006). Adult bone-marrow-derived mesenchymal stem cells contribute to wound healing of skin appendages. *Cell Tissue Res,* 326, 725-36

Liu, C. J., Wang, C. H., Chen, S. T., Chen, H. H., Leng, W. H., Chien, C. C., Wang, C. L., Kempson, I. M., Hwu, Y., Lai, T. C., Hsiao, M., Yang, C. S., Chen, Y. J. & Margaritondo, G. (2010). Enhancement of cell radiation sensitivity by pegylated gold nanoparticles. *Phys Med Biol,* 55, 931-45

Loebinger, M. R., Eddaoudi, A., Davies, D. & Janes, S. M. (2009a). Mesenchymal stem cell delivery of TRAIL can eliminate metastatic cancer. *Cancer Res,* 69, 4134-42

Loebinger, M. R., Kyrtatos, P. G., Turmaine, M., Price, A. N., Pankhurst, Q., Lythgoe, M. F. & Janes, S. M. (2009b). Magnetic resonance imaging of mesenchymal stem cells homing to pulmonary metastases using biocompatible magnetic nanoparticles. *Cancer Res,* 69, 8862-7

Loebinger, M. R. & Janes, S. M. (2010). Stem cells as vectors for antitumour therapy. *Thorax,* 65, 362-9

Lowery, A., Onishko, H., Hallahan, D. E. & Han, Z. (2011). Tumor-targeted delivery of liposome-encapsulated doxorubicin by use of a peptide that selectively binds to irradiated tumors. *J Control Release,* 150, 117-24

Lucchini, G., Introna, M., Dander, E., Rovelli, A., Balduzzi, A., Bonanomi, S., Salvade, A., Capelli, C., Belotti, D., Gaipa, G., Perseghin, P., Vinci, P., Lanino, E., Chiusolo, P., Orofino, M. G., Marktel, S., Golay, J., Rambaldi, A., Biondi, A., D'Amico, G. & Biagi, E. (2010). Platelet-lysate-expanded mesenchymal stromal cells as a salvage therapy for severe resistant graft-versus-host disease in a pediatric population. *Biol Blood Marrow Transplant,* 16, 1293-301

Mackenzie, T. C. & Flake, A. W. (2001). Human mesenchymal stem cells persist, demonstrate site-specific multipotential differentiation, and are present in sites of wound healing and tissue regeneration after transplantation into fetal sheep. *Blood Cells Mol Dis,* 27, 601-4

Malugin, A. & Ghandehari, H. (2010). Cellular uptake and toxicity of gold nanoparticles in prostate cancer cells: a comparative study of rods and spheres. *J Appl Toxicol,* 30, 212-7

Meisel, R., Zibert, A., Laryea, M., Gobel, U., Daubener, W. & Dilloo, D. (2004). Human bone marrow stromal cells inhibit allogeneic T-cell responses by indoleamine 2,3-dioxygenase-mediated tryptophan degradation. *Blood,* 103, 4619-21

Menon, L. G., Shi, V. S. & Carroll, R. S. (2009). Mesenchymal stromal cells as drug delivery system. *StemBook,* ed Girard, L., Harvard Stem Cell Institute, http://www.stembook.org/node/534

Mohr, A., Lyons, M., Deedigan, L., Harte, T., Shaw, G., Howard, L., Barry, F., O'Brien, T. & Zwacka, R. (2008). Mesenchymal stem cells expressing TRAIL lead to tumour growth inhibition in an experimental lung cancer model. *J Cell Mol Med,* 12, 2628-43

Morigi, M., Imberti, B., Zoja, C., Corna, D., Tomasoni, S., Abbate, M., Rottoli, D., Angioletti, S., Benigni, A., Perico, N., Alison, M. & Remuzzi, G. (2004). Mesenchymal stem cells are renotropic, helping to repair the kidney and improve function in acute renal failure. *J Am Soc Nephrol,* 15, 1794-804

Moriscot, C., de Fraipont, F., Richard, M. J., Marchand, M., Savatier, P., Bosco, D., Favrot, M. & Benhamou, P. Y. (2005). Human bone marrow mesenchymal stem cells can express insulin and key transcription factors of the endocrine pancreas developmental pathway upon genetic and/or microenvironmental manipulation in vitro. *Stem Cells,* 23, 594-603

Mosca, J. D., Hendricks, J. K., Buyaner, D., Davis-Sproul, J., Chuang, L. C., Majumdar, M. K., Chopra, R., Barry, F., Murphy, M., Thiede, M. A., Junker, U., Rigg, R. J., Forestell, S.

P., Bohnlein, E., Storb, R. & Sandmaier, B. M. (2000). Mesenchymal stem cells as vehicles for gene delivery. *Clin Orthop Relat Res*, S71-90

Motaln, H., Schichor, C. & Lah, T. T. (2010). Human mesenchymal stem cells and their use in cell-based therapies. *Cancer*, 116, 2519-30

Murphy, J. M., Fink, D. J., Hunziker, E. B. & Barry, F. P. (2003). Stem cell therapy in a caprine model of osteoarthritis. *Arthritis Rheum*, 48, 3464-74

Nakamizo, A., Marini, F., Amano, T., Khan, A., Studeny, M., Gumin, J., Chen, J., Hentschel, S., Vecil, G., Dembinski, J., Andreeff, M. & Lang, F. F. (2005). Human bone marrow-derived mesenchymal stem cells in the treatment of gliomas. *Cancer Res*, 65, 3307-18

Nakamura, K., Ito, Y., Kawano, Y., Kurozumi, K., Kobune, M., Tsuda, H., Bizen, A., Honmou, O., Niitsu, Y. & Hamada, H. (2004). Antitumor effect of genetically engineered mesenchymal stem cells in a rat glioma model. *Gene Ther*, 11, 1155-64

Newman, R. E., Yoo, D., LeRoux, M. A. & Danilkovitch-Miagkova, A. (2009). Treatment of inflammatory diseases with mesenchymal stem cells. *Inflamm Allergy Drug Targets*, 8, 110-23

Ochekpe, N. A., Olorunfemi, P. O. & Ngwuluka, N. C. (2009). Nanotechnology and Drug Delivery Part 2: Nanostructures for Drug Delivery. *Tropical Journal of Pharmaceutical Research*, 8, 275-87

Ong, S. Y., Dai, H. & Leong, K. W. (2006). Inducing hepatic differentiation of human mesenchymal stem cells in pellet culture. *Biomaterials*, 27, 4087-97

Oswald, J., Boxberger, S., Jorgensen, B., Feldmann, S., Ehninger, G., Bornhauser, M. & Werner, C. (2004). Mesenchymal stem cells can be differentiated into endothelial cells in vitro. *Stem Cells*, 22, 377-84

Owen, M. (1988). Marrow stromal stem cells. *J Cell Sci Suppl*, 10, 63-76

Parekkadan, B. & Milwid, J. M. (2010). Mesenchymal stem cells as therapeutics. *Annu Rev Biomed Eng*, 12, 87-117

Park, J. W., Hong, K., Kirpotin, D. B., Meyer, O., Papahadjopoulos, D. & Benz, C. C. (1997). Anti-HER2 immunoliposomes for targeted therapy of human tumors. *Cancer Lett*, 118, 153-60

Park, J. W., Hong, K., Kirpotin, D. B., Colbern, G., Shalaby, R., Baselga, J., Shao, Y., Nielsen, U. B., Marks, J. D., Moore, D., Papahadjopoulos, D. & Benz, C. C. (2002). Anti-HER2 immunoliposomes: enhanced efficacy attributable to targeted delivery. *Clin Cancer Res*, 8, 1172-81

Patel, M. M., Goyal, B. R., Bhadada, S. V., Bhatt, J. S. & Amin, A. F. (2009). Getting into the brain: approaches to enhance brain drug delivery. *CNS Drugs*, 23, 35-58

Patra, C. R., Bhattacharya, R., Mukhopadhyay, D. & Mukherjee, P. (2010). Fabrication of gold nanoparticles for targeted therapy in pancreatic cancer. *Adv Drug Deliv Rev*, 62, 346-61

Phinney, D. G. & Isakova, I. (2005). Plasticity and therapeutic potential of mesenchymal stem cells in the nervous system. *Curr Pharm Des*, 11, 1255-65

Pittenger, M. F. & Martin, B. J. (2004). Mesenchymal stem cells and their potential as cardiac therapeutics. *Circ Res*, 95, 9-20

Plotnikov, A. N., Shlapakova, I., Szabolcs, M. J., Danilo, P., Jr., Lorell, B. H., Potapova, I. A., Lu, Z., Rosen, A. B., Mathias, R. T., Brink, P. R., Robinson, R. B., Cohen, I. S. & Rosen, M. R. (2007). Xenografted adult human mesenchymal stem cells provide a platform for sustained biological pacemaker function in canine heart. *Circulation,* 116, 706-13

Ponte, A. L., Marais, E., Gallay, N., Langonne, A., Delorme, B., Herault, O., Charbord, P. & Domenech, J. (2007). The in vitro migration capacity of human bone marrow mesenchymal stem cells: comparison of chemokine and growth factor chemotactic activities. *Stem Cells,* 25, 1737-45

Potapova, I., Plotnikov, A., Lu, Z., Danilo, P., Jr., Valiunas, V., Qu, J., Doronin, S., Zuckerman, J., Shlapakova, I. N., Gao, J., Pan, Z., Herron, A. J., Robinson, R. B., Brink, P. R., Rosen, M. R. & Cohen, I. S. (2004). Human mesenchymal stem cells as a gene delivery system to create cardiac pacemakers. *Circ Res,* 94, 952-9

Prasad, V. K., Lucas, K. G., Kleiner, G. I., Talano, J. A., Jacobsohn, D., Broadwater, G., Monroy, R. & Kurtzberg, J. (2011). Efficacy and safety of ex vivo cultured adult human mesenchymal stem cells (Prochymal) in pediatric patients with severe refractory acute graft-versus-host disease in a compassionate use study. *Biol Blood Marrow Transplant,* 17, 534-41

Prockop, D. J. (1997). Marrow stromal cells as stem cells for nonhematopoietic tissues. *Science,* 276, 71-4

Rahman, W. N., Bishara, N., Ackerly, T., He, C. F., Jackson, P., Wong, C., Davidson, R. & Geso, M. (2009). Enhancement of radiation effects by gold nanoparticles for superficial radiation therapy. *Nanomedicine,* 5, 136-42

Ramirez, M., Lucia, A., Gomez-Gallego, F., Esteve-Lanao, J., Perez-Martinez, A., Foster, C., Andreu, A. L., Martin, M. A., Madero, L., Arenas, J. & Garcia-Castro, J. (2006). Mobilisation of mesenchymal cells into blood in response to skeletal muscle injury. *Br J Sports Med,* 40, 719-22

Reagan, M. R. & Kaplan, D. L. (2011). Concise review: mesenchymal stem cell tumor-homing: detection methods in disease model systems. *Stem Cells,* 29, 920-7

Reddy, A. M., Kwak, B. K., Shim, H. J., Ahn, C., Lee, H. S., Suh, Y. J. & Park, E. S. (2010). In vivo tracking of mesenchymal stem cells labeled with a novel chitosan-coated superparamagnetic iron oxide nanoparticles using 3.0T MRI. *J Korean Med Sci,* 25, 211-9

Ren, C., Kumar, S., Chanda, D., Chen, J., Mountz, J. D. & Ponnazhagan, S. (2008a). Therapeutic potential of mesenchymal stem cells producing interferon-alpha in a mouse melanoma lung metastasis model. *Stem Cells,* 26, 2332-8

Ren, C., Kumar, S., Chanda, D., Kallman, L., Chen, J., Mountz, J. D. & Ponnazhagan, S. (2008b). Cancer gene therapy using mesenchymal stem cells expressing interferon-beta in a mouse prostate cancer lung metastasis model. *Gene Ther,* 15, 1446-53

Renner, P., Eggenhofer, E., Rosenauer, A., Popp, F. C., Steinmann, J. F., Slowik, P., Geissler, E. K., Piso, P., Schlitt, H. J. & Dahlke, M. H. (2009). Mesenchymal stem cells require a sufficient, ongoing immune response to exert their immunosuppressive function. *Transplant Proc,* 41, 2607-11

Ries, C., Egea, V., Karow, M., Kolb, H., Jochum, M. & Neth, P. (2007). MMP-2, MT1-MMP, and TIMP-2 are essential for the invasive capacity of human mesenchymal stem cells: differential regulation by inflammatory cytokines. *Blood,* 109, 4055-63

Rose, J. H., Norman, A., Ingram, M., Aoki, C., Solberg, T. & Mesa, A. (1999). First radiotherapy of human metastatic brain tumors delivered by a computerized tomography scanner (CTRx). *Int J Radiat Oncol Biol Phys,* 45, 1127-32

Rosen, M. R., Brink, P. R., Cohen, I. S. & Robinson, R. B. (2004). Genes, stem cells and biological pacemakers. *Cardiovasc Res,* 64, 12-23

Rosen, M. R., Brink, P. R., Cohen, I. S. & Robinson, R. B. (2008). The utility of mesenchymal stem cells as biological pacemakers. *Congest Heart Fail,* 14, 153-6

Ruggiero, C., Pastorino, L. & Herrera, O. L. (2010). Nanotechnology based targeted drug delivery. *Conf Proc IEEE Eng Med Biol Soc,* 2010, 3731-2

Ruoslahti, E., Bhatia, S. N. & Sailor, M. J. (2010). Targeting of drugs and nanoparticles to tumors. *J Cell Biol,* 188, 759-68

Ryan, J. M., Barry, F., Murphy, J. M. & Mahon, B. P. (2007). Interferon-gamma does not break, but promotes the immunosuppressive capacity of adult human mesenchymal stem cells. *Clin Exp Immunol,* 149, 353-63

Sansone, P. & Bromberg, J. (2011). Environment, inflammation, and cancer. *Curr Opin Genet Dev,* 21, 80-5

Sasportas, L. S., Kasmieh, R., Wakimoto, H., Hingtgen, S., van de Water, J. A., Mohapatra, G., Figueiredo, J. L., Martuza, R. L., Weissleder, R. & Shah, K. (2009). Assessment of therapeutic efficacy and fate of engineered human mesenchymal stem cells for cancer therapy. *Proc Natl Acad Sci U S A,* 106, 4822-7

Sato, Y., Araki, H., Kato, J., Nakamura, K., Kawano, Y., Kobune, M., Sato, T., Miyanishi, K., Takayama, T., Takahashi, M., Takimoto, R., Iyama, S., Matsunaga, T., Ohtani, S., Matsuura, A., Hamada, H. & Niitsu, Y. (2005). Human mesenchymal stem cells xenografted directly to rat liver are differentiated into human hepatocytes without fusion. *Blood,* 106, 756-63

Sawant, R. & Torchilin, V. (2011). Intracellular delivery of nanoparticles with CPPs. *Methods Mol Biol,* 683, 431-51

Schäfer, R., Bantleon, R., Kehlbach, R., Siegel, G., Wiskirchen, J., Wolburg, H., Kluba, T., Eibofner, F., Northoff, H., Claussen, C. D. & Schlemmer, H. P. (2010). Functional investigations on human mesenchymal stem cells exposed to magnetic fields and labeled with clinically approved iron nanoparticles. *BMC Cell Biol,* 11:22

Sieman, D. W. (2006). Tumor vasculature: a target for anticancer therapies. In: *Vascular-targeted Therapies in Oncology,* ed Sieman, D. W., 1-8, John Wiley & Sons, Chichester, UK

Solchaga, L. A., Temenoff, J. S., Gao, J., Mikos, A. G., Caplan, A. I. & Goldberg, V. M. (2005). Repair of osteochondral defects with hyaluronan- and polyester-based scaffolds. *Osteoarthritis Cartilage,* 13, 297-309

Sonabend, A. M., Ulasov, I. V., Tyler, M. A., Rivera, A. A., Mathis, J. M. & Lesniak, M. S. (2008). Mesenchymal stem cells effectively deliver an oncolytic adenovirus to intracranial glioma. *Stem Cells,* 26, 831-41

Spaeth, E., Klopp, A., Dembinski, J., Andreeff, M. & Marini, F. (2008). Inflammation and tumor microenvironments: defining the migratory itinerary of mesenchymal stem cells. *Gene Ther,* 15, 730-8

Srinivas, M., Aarntzen, E. H., Bulte, J. W., Oyen, W. J., Heerschap, A., de Vries, I. J. & Figdor, C. G. (2010). Imaging of cellular therapies. *Adv Drug Deliv Rev,* 62, 1080-93

Stagg, J., Lejeune, L., Paquin, A. & Galipeau, J. (2004). Marrow stromal cells for interleukin-2 delivery in cancer immunotherapy. *Hum Gene Ther,* 15, 597-608

Stoeber, B. & Liepmann, D. (2002). Design, fabrication and testing of a MEMS syringe. *Proceedings of Solid-State Sensor and Actuator Workshop,* Transducers Research Foundation, Hilton Head Island, SC, USA, 2002

Stoff-Khalili, M. A., Rivera, A. A., Mathis, J. M., Banerjee, N. S., Moon, A. S., Hess, A., Rocconi, R. P., Numnum, T. M., Everts, M., Chow, L. T., Douglas, J. T., Siegal, G. P., Zhu, Z. B., Bender, H. G., Dall, P., Stoff, A., Pereboeva, L. & Curiel, D. T. (2007). Mesenchymal stem cells as a vehicle for targeted delivery of CRAds to lung metastases of breast carcinoma. *Breast Cancer Res Treat,* 105, 157-67

Studeny, M., Marini, F. C., Champlin, R. E., Zompetta, C., Fidler, I. J. & Andreeff, M. (2002). Bone marrow-derived mesenchymal stem cells as vehicles for interferon-beta delivery into tumors. *Cancer Res,* 62, 3603-8

Studeny, M., Marini, F. C., Dembinski, J. L., Zompetta, C., Cabreira-Hansen, M., Bekele, B. N., Champlin, R. E. & Andreeff, M. (2004). Mesenchymal stem cells: potential precursors for tumor stroma and targeted-delivery vehicles for anticancer agents. *J Natl Cancer Inst,* 96, 1593-603

Sun, Y., Chen, L., Hou, X. G., Hou, W. K., Dong, J. J., Sun, L., Tang, K. X., Wang, B., Song, J., Li, H. & Wang, K. X. (2007). Differentiation of bone marrow-derived mesenchymal stem cells from diabetic patients into insulin-producing cells in vitro. *Chin Med J (Engl),* 120, 771-6

Sundin, M., Ringden, O., Sundberg, B., Nava, S., Gotherstrom, C. & Le Blanc, K. (2007). No alloantibodies against mesenchymal stromal cells, but presence of anti-fetal calf serum antibodies, after transplantation in allogeneic hematopoietic stem cell recipients. *Haematologica,* 92, 1208-15

Suzuki, M., McHugh, J., Tork, C., Shelley, B., Klein, S. M., Aebischer, P. & Svendsen, C. N. (2007). GDNF secreting human neural progenitor cells protect dying motor neurons, but not their projection to muscle, in a rat model of familial ALS. *PLoS One,* 2, e689

Torchilin, V. P. (2008). Tat peptide-mediated intracellular delivery of pharmaceutical nanocarriers. *Adv Drug Deliv Rev,* 60, 548-58

Trivedi, H. L., Vanikar, A. V., Thakker, U., Firoze, A., Dave, S. D., Patel, C. N., Patel, J. V., Bhargava, A. B. & Shankar, V. (2008). Human adipose tissue-derived mesenchymal stem cells combined with hematopoietic stem cell transplantation synthesize insulin. *Transplant Proc,* 40, 1135-9

Tse, W. T., Pendleton, J. D., Beyer, W. M., Egalka, M. C. & Guinan, E. C. (2003). Suppression of allogeneic T-cell proliferation by human marrow stromal cells: implications in transplantation. *Transplantation,* 75, 389-97

Tuscano, J. M., Martin, S. M., Ma, Y., Zamboni, W. & O'Donnell, R. T. (2010). Efficacy, biodistribution, and pharmacokinetics of CD22-targeted pegylated liposomal doxorubicin in a B-cell non-Hodgkin's lymphoma xenograft mouse model. *Clin Cancer Res,* 16, 2760-8

Vives, E., Schmidt, J. & Pelegrin, A. (2008). Cell-penetrating and cell-targeting peptides in drug delivery. *Biochim Biophys Acta,* 1786, 126-38 von Hertzen, L. C., Joensuu, H. & Haahtela, T. (2011). Microbial deprivation, inflammation and cancer. *Cancer Metastasis Rev*, 30, 211-23

Walczak, P., Kedziorek, D. A., Gilad, A. A., Lin, S. & Bulte, J. W. (2005). Instant MR labeling of stem cells using magnetoelectroporation. *Magn Reson Med*, 54, 769-74

Wallace, A. E., Gibson, D. A., Saunders, P. T. & Jabbour, H. N. (2010). Inflammatory events in endometrial adenocarcinoma. *J Endocrinol*, 206, 141-57

Wang, T., Tang, W., Sun, S., Xu, T., Wang, H., Guan, J., Huang, Z. & Weil, M. H. (2008). Intravenous infusion of bone marrow mesenchymal stem cells improves brain function after resuscitation from cardiac arrest. *Crit Care Med*, 36, S486-91

Williams, A. R., Trachtenberg, B., Velazquez, D. L., McNiece, I., Altman, P., Rouy, D., Mendizabal, A. M., Pattany, P. M., Lopera, G. A., Fishman, J., Zambrano, J. P., Heldman, A. W. & Hare, J. M. (2011). Intramyocardial stem cell injection in patients with ischemic cardiomyopathy: functional recovery and reverse remodeling. *Circ Res*, 108, 792-6

Wu, G. D., Nolta, J. A., Jin, Y. S., Barr, M. L., Yu, H., Starnes, V. A. & Cramer, D. V. (2003). Migration of mesenchymal stem cells to heart allografts during chronic rejection. *Transplantation*, 75, 679-85

Xiang, J., Tang, J., Song, C., Yang, Z., Hirst, D. G., Zheng, Q. J. & Li, G. (2009). Mesenchymal stem cells as a gene therapy carrier for treatment of fibrosarcoma. *Cytotherapy*, 11, 516-26

Xin, H., Kanehira, M., Mizuguchi, H., Hayakawa, T., Kikuchi, T., Nukiwa, T. & Saijo, Y. (2007). Targeted delivery of CX3CL1 to multiple lung tumors by mesenchymal stem cells. *Stem Cells*, 25, 1618-26

Xu, F., Shi, J., Yu, B., Ni, W., Wu, X. & Gu, Z. (2010). Chemokines mediate mesenchymal stem cell migration toward gliomas in vitro. *Oncol Rep*, 23, 1561-7

Xu, W. T., Bian, Z. Y., Fan, Q. M., Li, G. & Tang, T. T. (2009). Human mesenchymal stem cells (hMSCs) target osteosarcoma and promote its growth and pulmonary metastasis. *Cancer Lett*, 281, 32-41

Yamada, S., Fujita, S., Uchimura, E., Miyake, M. & Miyake, J. (2009). Reverse transfection using gold nanoparticles. *Methods Mol Biol*, 544, 609-16

Yang, T., Cui, F. D., Choi, M. K., Cho, J. W., Chung, S. J., Shim, C. K. & Kim, D. D. (2007). Enhanced solubility and stability of PEGylated liposomal paclitaxel: in vitro and in vivo evaluation. *Int J Pharm*, 338, 317-26

Yokoo, T., Ohashi, T., Shen, J. S., Sakurai, K., Miyazaki, Y., Utsunomiya, Y., Takahashi, M., Terada, Y., Eto, Y., Kawamura, T., Osumi, N. & Hosoya, T. (2005). Human mesenchymal stem cells in rodent whole-embryo culture are reprogrammed to contribute to kidney tissues. *Proc Natl Acad Sci U S A*, 102, 3296-300

Yong, R. L., Shinojima, N., Fueyo, J., Gumin, J., Vecil, G. G., Marini, F. C., Bogler, O., Andreeff, M. & Lang, F. F. (2009). Human bone marrow-derived mesenchymal stem cells for intravascular delivery of oncolytic adenovirus Delta24-RGD to human gliomas. *Cancer Res*, 69, 8932-40

Yu, B., Tai, H. C., Xue, W., Lee, L. J. & Lee, R. J. (2010). Receptor-targeted nanocarriers for therapeutic delivery to cancer. *Mol Membr Biol*, 27, 286-98

Zhang, L., Gu, F. X., Chan, J. M., Wang, A. Z., Langer, R. S. & Farokhzad, O. C. (2008). Nanoparticles in medicine: therapeutic applications and developments. *Clin Pharmacol Ther*, 83, 761-9

Zielske, S. P., Livant, D. L. & Lawrence, T. S. (2009). Radiation increases invasion of gene-modified mesenchymal stem cells into tumors. *Int J Radiat Oncol Biol Phys*, 75, 843-53